IMPLANT AND REGENERATIVE THERAPY IN DENTISTRY

A GUIDE TO DECISION MAKING

IMPLANT AND REGENERATIVE THERAPY IN DENTISTRY

A GUIDE TO DECISION MAKING

Paul A. Fugazzotto, DDS

WILEY-BLACKWELL
A John Wiley & Sons, Ltd., Publication

Edition first published 2009

Blackwell Publishing was acquired by John Wiley & Sons in February 2007. Blackwell's publishing program has been merged with Wiley's global Scientific, Technical, and Medical business to form Wiley-Blackwell.

Editorial Office
2121 State Avenue, Ames, Iowa 50014-8300, USA

For details of our global editorial offices, for customer services, and for information about how to apply for permission to reuse the copyright material in this book, please see our website at www.wiley.com/wiley-blackwell.

Library of Congress Cataloging-in-Publication Data

Fugazzotto, Paul A.
Implant and regenerative therapy: a guide to decision making / Paul A. Fugazzotto.
p. ; cm.
Includes bibliographical references and index.
ISBN 978-0-8138-2962-3 (hardback : alk. paper)
1. Dental implants. 2. Guided bone regeneration. I. Title.
[DNLM: 1. Dental Implantation—methods. 2. Dental Implants.
3. Guided Tissue Regeneration, Periodontal—methods.
4. Periodontal Diseases—therapy. 5. Tooth Loss—therapy.
WU 640 F957i 2009]
RK667.I45F84 2009
617.6′92–dc22
2008053892

A catalog record for this book is available from the U.S. Library of Congress.

Set in 10.5/12 pt ITC Slimbach by Aptara® Inc., New Delhi, India
Printed in Singapore

2 2012

To Salvatore and Gloria Fugazzotto, without whom nothing was possible, and to Emily, without whom nothing is worthwhile.

Contents

Contributors

Editor/Author

Paul A. Fugazzotto, DDS
Private Practice
Milton, Massachusetts

Contributors

Jamil Alayan, BS, BDS, MDSc, FRACDS (Periodontics)
Brisbane, Queensland, Australia
Griffith University, School of Dentistry and Oral health
Southport, Queensland, Australia

Isabel Andía, PhD
Scientific researcher of BTI Biotechnology Institute
San Antonio
Vitoria, Spain

Eduardo Anitua, DDS, MD
Scientific director of BTI Biotechnology Institute
Private Practice in Vitoria (Spain)
San Antonio
Vitoria, Spain

Paulo M. Camargo, DDS, MS, MBA, FACD
UCLA School of Dentistry
Section of Periodontics
Los Angeles, California

Sergio De Paoli, MD, DDS
University of Ancona
Private Practice
Ancona, Italy

Anthony J. Dickinson, BDSc, MSD
Registered Specialist, Prosthodontist
Glen Iris
Victoria, Australia

Robert Jaffin, DMD
Private Practice
Director, Periodontal Services
Hackensack University Medical Center
Hackensack, New Jersey

Will Martin, DMD, MS, FACP
Clinical Associate Professor
University of Florida – College of Dentistry
Center for Implant Dentistry
Gainesville, Florida

Philip R. Melnick, DMD, FACD
UCLA School of Dentistry
Section of Periodontics
Los Angeles, California

Dean Morton, BDS, MS, FACP
Professor and Assistant Dean
Department of Diagnostic Sciences,
Prosthodontics and Restorative Dentistry
University of Louisville School of Dentistry
Louisville, Kentucky

Gorka Orive, PhD
Scientific researcher of BTI Biotechnology Institute
San Antonio
Vitoria, Spain

Acknowledgment

I would be remiss to not send the appropriate gratitude and thanks to Sophia Joyce of Wiley-Blackwell for first proposing this project to me and helping me to formulate its conceptual framework, and to Shelby Allen for her perseverance and patience in putting up with me. Finally, I need to thank Samantha for risking her dexterity in compiling and working on the manuscript.

IMPLANT AND REGENERATIVE THERAPY IN DENTISTRY

A GUIDE TO DECISION MAKING

Chapter 1

Tooth Retention and Implant Placement: Developing Treatment Algorithms

Paul A. Fugazzotto, DDS and Sergio De Paoli, MD, DDS

Outline

There is no doubt that the introduction and evolution of regenerative and implant therapies affords clinicians the opportunity to provide patients with previously undreamt-of treatment outcomes. However, such therapeutic approaches must not be visualized as an end to themselves.

The goals of conscientious and comprehensive therapy remain the maximization of patient comfort, function, and esthetics in both the short and long terms. While it has become popular to speak of paradigm shifts in clinical dentistry, these shifts represent nothing more than alterations in the treatment approaches utilized to attain the aforementioned therapeutic goals. In addition, efforts must be made to utilize the least involved and least expensive therapies possible for ensuring these treatment outcomes.

Maximization of oral health and amelioration of patient concerns remain the sine qua non of ethical practice. When considering the utilization of various regenerative or implant reconstructive approaches, it is important to listen to patient desires, determine patient needs, and ensure that the therapy to be employed is truly in the best interests of the patient. These interests may not always be optimally served through use of tooth extraction, complex regenerative therapies, and placement of multiple implants. Such treatment options should never be viewed as a means by which to supplant all other therapeutic approaches. Rather, a thorough understanding of the predictability of appropriately performed therapies around natural teeth is crucial to the formulation of an ideal treatment plan for a given patient. This treatment plan is based on a precise diagnosis of the patient's condition, and recognition of all contributing etiologies. Such a diagnosis takes into consideration the entire dentition, treating each site as both an individual entity, and a component in the masticatory unit.

Nowhere is this fact more evident than when considering management of the periodontally diseased dentition.

When faced with active periodontal disease, one of seven therapies may be employed.

- **No treatment:** Such a decision may be due to the patient's refusal of active therapy; or the patient's physical, financial, or psychological inability to undergo the necessary treatments. In such a scenario, it is imperative that the patient be made aware of the short- and long-term risks to both his or her oral and overall health represented by such a decision. It is important to realize that periodontal disease is a self-propagating disease. If no active therapy is carried out to halt disease progress, extension of the disease will result in tooth loss. When a patient chooses to pursue no active therapy, it is imperative that this concern be explained to the patient, and that every effort be made to both motivate the patient to seek treatment, and to adapt the treatment to the individual patient and the specific characteristics of his or her problems.

Regardless of which active therapeutic course is chosen, patients are always instructed in appropriate plaque control measures, so as to obtain an acceptable level of home debridement and bacterial control. A reevaluation is then carried out to determine which sites have healed through only the patient's plaque control efforts, and which areas still demonstrate signs of inflammation. Such a reevaluation is carried out in concert with a patient's specific risk assessment.

- **Subgingival debridement and institution of a regular professional prophylaxis schedule:** While this option seems attractive to many clinicians and patients, it is important to realize that, in many cases, such an approach does not halt the ongoing periodontal disease processes when significant pocketing is present. At best, the rate of attachment loss is slowed. This treatment option is indicated for patients who are physically, financially, or psychologically unable to undergo more comprehensive therapy, but who would at least agree to periodic debridement and prophylaxis in an attempt to delay tooth loss. This option is most appropriate for patients of an advanced age, who have demonstrated moderate attachment loss. Younger patients, or older patients with more aggressive periodontal disease problems, are less suited to actuarial therapeutic regimens. In addition, the potential dangers to adjacent teeth must be recognized and planned for.
- **Surgical therapies aimed at defect debridement and/or pocket reduction:** As explained above, these treatment approaches represent a significant compromise in therapy. A patient who has undergone surgical intervention is left with a milieu which is highly susceptible to further periodontal breakdown. It is important to consider the need for retreatment and the potential damage to the attachment apparati of adjacent teeth. This treatment option offers minimal advantages over the aforementioned treatment approach, and no advantages compared to the subsequent treatment approach.
- **Resective periodontal surgical therapy, including elimination of furcation involvements, in an effort to ensure a posttherapeutic attachment apparatus characterized by a short connective tissue attachment to the root surface, a short junctional epithelial adhesion, and elimination of probing depths greater than 3 mm:** This treatment approach offers the greatest chance of preventing reinitiation of periodontal disease processes. However, such a treatment regimen must be utilized appropriately. Osseous resective therapy that results in irreversible compromise of a given tooth, the initiation of secondary occlusal trauma due to reduced periodontal support and a poor crown to root ratio, or an esthetically unacceptable treatment result should not be considered ideal therapy. The advent of regenerative and implant therapies affords additional treatment options in previously untenable scenarios.
- **Periodontal regenerative therapy aimed at rebuilding lost attachment apparatus and surrounding alveolar bone:** Long viewed as an ideal to be strived for, periodontal regenerative therapy has a history of misunderstanding, misuse, and abuse. There is no doubt that predictable regenerative techniques are available for utilization in appropriate defects. There is also no doubt that the indications for the employment of these therapies are poorly understood. The net result is inconsistent treatment outcomes and condemnation of otherwise useful therapies by a large number of clinicians. When utilized in the appropriate manner in stringently selected defects, guided tissue regeneration yields highly predictable treatment outcomes. The advent of new materials offers the potential for even more impressive regenerative results. Unfortunately, the field of periodontal therapy continues to be handicapped by an incomplete understanding of diagnostic and technical criteria for success

with regenerative therapy. Many of these criteria have been elucidated in a previous publication (1). Advances in tissue engineering also offer preliminary regenerative results which are highly impressive. However, while the use of available growth factors is promising, the precise parameters of utilization, questions of cost, and reasonable treatment results are yet to be defined.

- **Tooth removal with either simultaneous regenerative therapy and implant insertion or guided bone regeneration with subsequent implant placement and restoration:** While highly predictable in almost every situation, regenerative and implant therapies must not be viewed as a panacea. To remove teeth, which may be predictably maintained through more conservative therapies and which will yield acceptable treatment outcomes, is unconscionable. However, to maintain compromised teeth which will eventually be lost, or to subject a patient to an inordinate amount of therapy or expense to keep teeth which may be more simply and predictably replaced by implants, is unacceptable.
- **A combination of the above therapies:** An uncomfortable and irresponsible dichotomy is developing in which the patient is viewed as either a "periodontal patient" or an "implant patient." A patient is neither.

Prior to the initiation of active therapy, a thorough examination and diagnosis must be carried out, and a comprehensive interdisciplinary treatment plan must be formulated. A high-quality full series of radiographs must be taken. When necessary, three-dimensional images are utilized as well. Panorex films are not utilized, as their accuracy is insufficient for providing useful information for comprehensive therapy. The components of a thorough clinical examination, including periodontal probing depths, hard and soft tissue examination, models and facebow records, are well established and will be discussed in subsequent chapters. However, it is important to realize that a thorough examination begins with an open discussion with the individual patient. It is crucial that the clinician determines the patient's needs and desires. In this way, treatment plans may be formulated which are in the best interest of the patient and which represent a greater value for the patient.

Prior to formulating a comprehensive treatment plan, all potential etiologies must be identified and assessed. In addition to systemic factors, these etiologies include periodontal disease, parafunction, caries, endodontic lesions, and trauma.

The treating clinician should always formulate an "ideal" treatment plan and present it to every patient. Appropriate and predictable treatment alternatives must be offered to the patient, thus allowing the patient to choose the treatment option to which he or she is best suited physically, financially, and psychologically.

Clinicians who fail to incorporate regenerative and implant therapies into their treatment armamentaria are depriving their patients of predictable therapeutic possibilities which afford unique treatment outcomes in a variety of situations.

Regenerative and implant therapies impact the partially edentous patient in a number of ways, including:

- replacement of less predictable therapies
- replacement of more costly therapies
- augmentation of existing therapies
- introduction of newer therapies

Conversely, teeth which can be predictably restored to health through reasonable means should be maintained if their retention is advantageous to the final treatment plan. Clinicians who claim to be implantologists, performing only implant therapy while ignoring periodontal and other pathologies, do patients a disservice. Such clinicians include practitioners who either perform inadequate periodontal therapy to predictably halt the disease process, or remove teeth which could be treated through straightforward periodontal techniques.

It is inconceivable that any clinician would see only patients who require implant therapy, and demonstrate periodontal, endodontic, restorative, and occlusal health around all remaining teeth which are not to be extracted. This trend toward metallurgy at the expense of ethical, comprehensive care must be avoided at all times.

Resective Therapy: Applicable Today?

Pocket elimination has long been advanced as one of the primary end points of periodontal therapy. An excellent review of the evolution of the treatment modalities employed in pursuit of this goal has been published in the *Proceedings of the World Workshop in Clinical Periodontics* (2). A frequently utilized procedure when seeking pocket elimination is osseous resective surgery. Unfortunately, the ultimate objectives of this approach are rarely elucidated correctly and comprehensively.

The World Workshop states the objectives of osseous resective surgery as follows:

1. pocket elimination or reduction
2. a physiologic gingival contour that tightly adapted to the alveolar bone and apical to the presurgical position
3. a clinically maintainable condition

This formulation is incomplete. The primary goal of pocket elimination therapy is to deliver to the patient an environment which is conducive to predictable, long-term periodontal health, both clinically and histologically. With this fact in mind, the aforementioned objectives should be expanded to read:

1. Pocket elimination or reduction to such a level where thorough subgingival plaque control is predictable for both the patient and the practitioner.
2. A physiologic gingival contour is conducive to plaque control measures. This would include the elimination of soft tissue concavities, in the area of the interproximal col and elsewhere, soft tissue clefts, and marked gingival margin discrepancies.
3. The establishment of the most plaque-resistant attachment apparatus possible. This includes the elimination of long epithelial relationships to the tooth surface, where possible, and the minimization of areas of nonkeratinized marginal epithelium.
4. The elimination of all other physical relationships which compromise patient and professional plaque control measures. These include furcation involvements and subgingival restorative margins.
5. A clinically maintainable condition will evolve as a result of the previous four criteria having been met.

In short, pocket elimination is seen as a means of maintaining the plaque–host equilibrium in the host's favor by closing the window of host vulnerability as much as possible. While not always a realistic end point, this goal is most predictably maximized through pocket elimination procedures.

Two important questions present themselves:

Are the principles behind pocket elimination conceptually sound?

Does the clinical literature support the continued use of pocket elimination therapy?

The Rationale for Pocket Elimination Procedures through the Use of Osseous Resective Techniques

Periodontal pockets have long been recognized as complicating factors in thorough patient and professional plaque control. Waerhaug has shown that flossing and brushing are only effective to a depth of about 2.5 mm subgingivally (3). Beyond this depth, significant amounts of plaque remain attached to the root surface following a patient's oral hygiene procedures. Professional prophylaxis results are also compromised in the presence of deeper pockets. The failure of root planing to completely remove subgingival plaque and calculus in deeper pockets is well documented in the literature (4–8). Through the examination of extracted teeth which had been root planed until they were judged plaque-free by all available clinical parameters, Waerhaug demonstrated the correlation between pocket depth and failure to completely remove subgingival plaque (3). Instrumentation of pockets measuring 3 mm or less was successful with regard to total plaque removal in 83% of the cases. In pockets of 3–5 mm in depth, 61% of the teeth exhibited retained plaque after thorough root planing. When pocket depths were 5 mm or more, failure to completely remove adherent plaque was the finding 89% of the time. Tabita (9) noted that no tooth demonstrated a plaque-free surface 14 days after thorough root planing, if the pretreatment pocket depths were 4–6 mm. This was true even though patients exhibited excellent supragingival plaque control.

Reinfection of the treated site is a result of three different pathways (3, 9):

(a) Plaque that remains in root lacunae, grooves, etc. will begin to multiply and repopulate the root surface following therapy.

(b) Plaque which is adherent to the epithelial lining of the pocket will repopulate the root surface after healing. It has been demonstrated that, even if curettage is intentionally performed in conjunction with root planing, complete removal of the epithelial lining of the pocket is not a common finding (10–12).
(c) Supragingival plaque will extend subgingivally, beyond the reach of the patient, and adhere to the root surface.

The magnitude of the limitations imposed upon proper plaque removal and control by pocket depths led Waerhaug to state: "If the pocket depth is more than 5 mm, the chances of failure are so great that there is an obvious indication for surgical pocket elimination" (3).

In the absence of deep probings, poor soft tissue morphology may contribute to increased plaque accumulation. Deep, sharp clefts, and marked soft tissue marginal discrepancies in adjacent areas have been implicated as factors contributing to inadequate patient plaque control (13). Interproximally, the morphology of the soft tissue col must be considered. If the buccal and/or lingual peaks of tissue are coronal to the contact point, the gingiva must "dip" under the contact point to reach the other side, resulting in a concave col form (14–16). When the col tissue touches the contact point, whether it is composed of natural tooth or restorative material, the epithelium does not keratinize (17 [Ruben MP, Personal communication, Boston, 1980], 18) (Figures 1.1 and 1.2). Such lack of keratinization is not an inherent property of either col or sulcular epithelium, as the ability of this tissue to keratinize when it is no longer in contact with the tooth, either as a result of periodontal therapy or eversion, is well documented (18–20). Nonkeratinized epithelium is less resistant to disruption and penetration by bacterial plaque than its keratinized counterpart (21, 22). When a concave, nonkeratinized col form is present, the patient must try to control an area which is conducive to plaque accumulation, and more easily breached by the aforementioned plaque and its byproducts (Figures 1.3 and 1.4).

Management of the soft tissue col form is predictably achieved through the proper use of osseous resective techniques. In addition to eliminating interproximal osseous craters, the buccolingual dimension of the alveolar process must be taken into consideration. If buccal osseous ledging is not

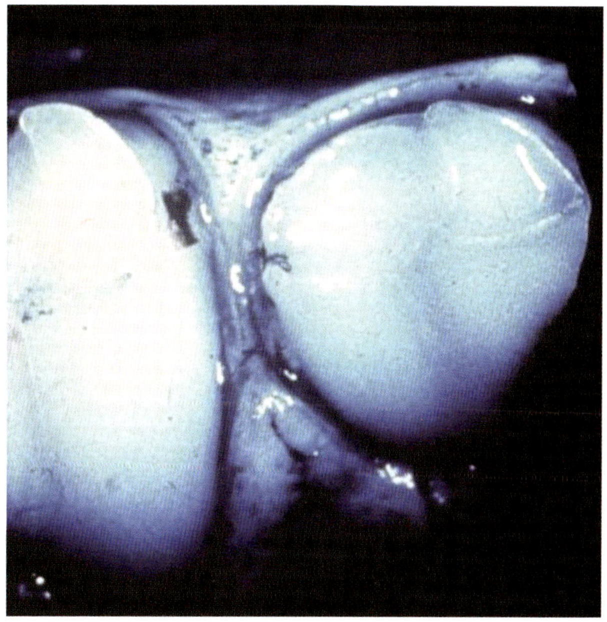

Figure 1.1 A decalcified section demonstrating the concave nature of the interproximal soft tissue col.

reduced adequately to allow for the smooth flow of soft tissues interproximally, without their first having to pass coronal to the contact point and "dip" underneath it, a concave col form will result (15, 23) (Figures 1.5 and 1.6). In addition, should the radicular bone be coronal to or at a height equal to the interproximal osseous septum, the soft tissues will not heal in tight adaptation to the underlying bone (16). Soft tissues will not heal in sharp angles, and will strive to regain a papillary form interproximally. All dimensions

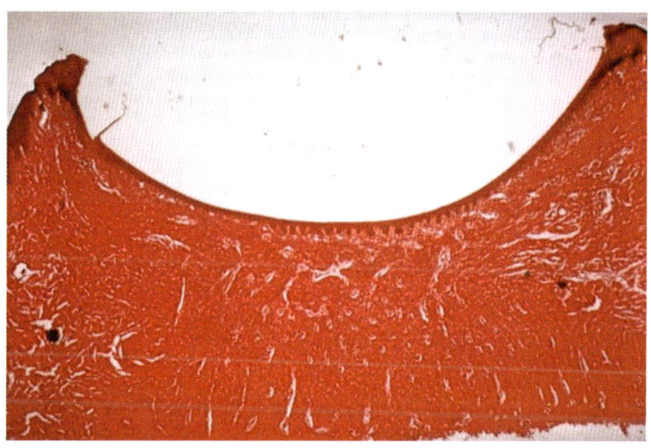

Figure 1.2 A histologic slide underscores the nonkeratinized nature of the col epithelium where it touches the contact point between the teeth.

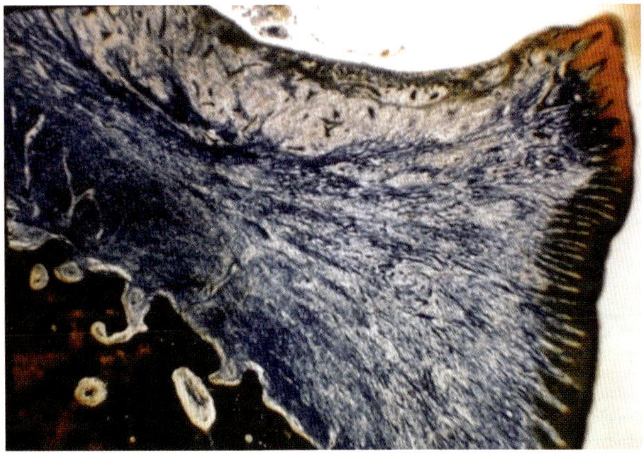

Figure 1.3 The nonkeratinized concave col epithelium is especially susceptible to bacterial penetration and inflammatory breakdown.

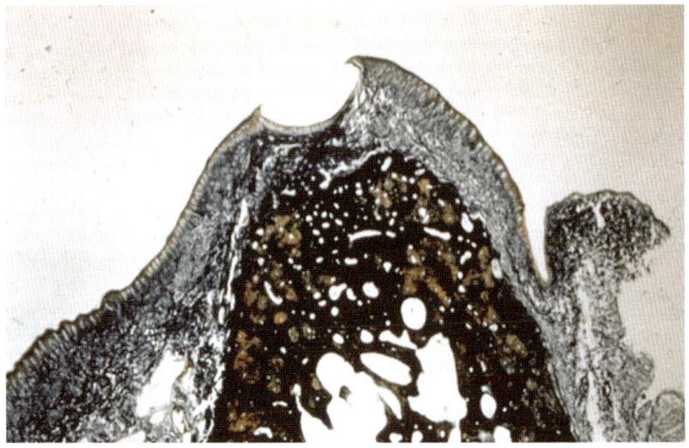

Figure 1.5 Despite the convex nature of the interproximal alveolar bone, the soft tissue col is concave due to its contacting the contact point between the teeth.

of the interproximal space (i.e., apico-occlusal, buccolingual, and mesiodistal) must be considered when evaluating the effects of existent osseous contours on the morphology of the overlying soft tissues. Matherson's work in monkeys demonstrated this fact clearly (24). The naturally occurring condition was one of a markedly concave soft tissue col. Replaced flap surgery without osseous therapy did not significantly alter the soft tissue col form. Interdental osteoplasty, resulting in the formation of an interproximal osseous peak, reduced the depth of the concavity in the col morphology. Osteoplasty which encompassed both the interproximal and radicular areas, thus reducing the buccolingual osseous ledging and eliminating reverse architecture, as well as forming an interproximal osseous peak, had the greatest effect on col

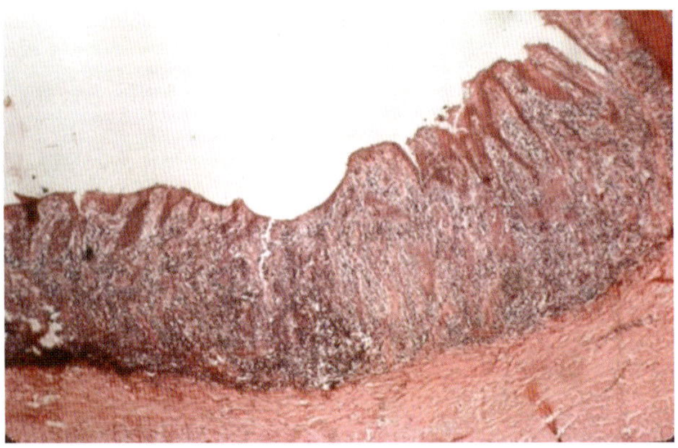

Figure 1.4 As the inflammatory lesion progresses through the nonkeratinized col epithelium and into the connective tissue, marked tissue destruction is noted.

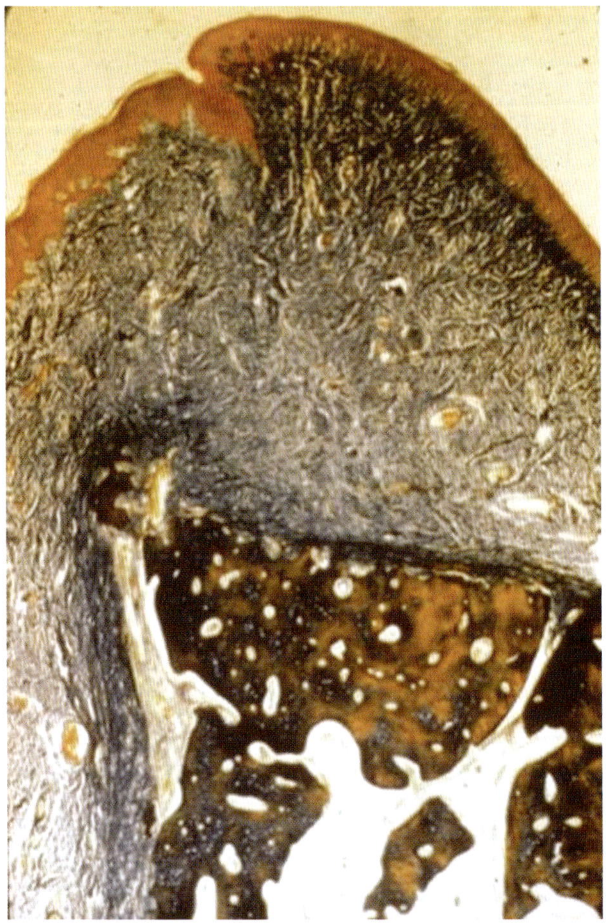

Figure 1.6 If the interproximal soft tissues are apical to the contact point, the convex interproximal bone contours are mimicked by covering keratinized soft tissues.

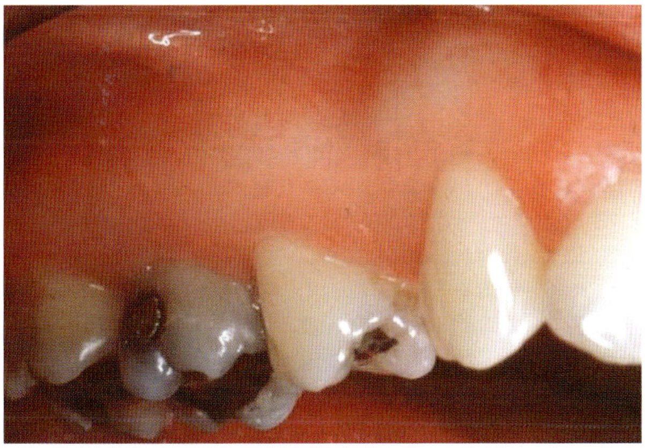

Figure 1.7 A patient presents with 6 mm pockets interproximally, which bleed upon gentle probing.

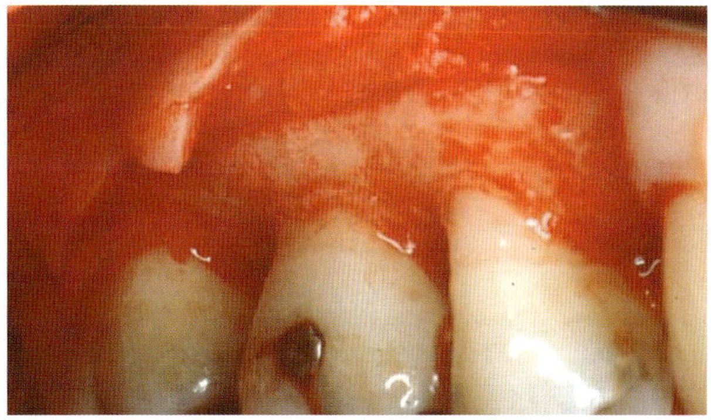

Figure 1.9 The appropriate osteoplasty has been performed. The soft tissues may now be replaced at osseous crest, and will heal in a concave, keratinized manner apical to the contact points between the teeth.

morphology. Formation of a covex col form postoperatively was limited by the contours of the monkeys' teeth. Their contact points are broader buccolingually and more apically placed than those found in man. Odontoplasty would have been necessary to allow for sufficient space for the regeneration of the interproximal soft tissues apical to the contact points of the natural teeth. There is no doubt, contrary to published interpretations (2), that osteoplasty affected the postsurgical col morphologies in the precise manner which would be expected by proponents of osseous resective surgery (Figures 1.7–1.9).

While keratinization of the col tissues and alteration of their morphology to one more conducive

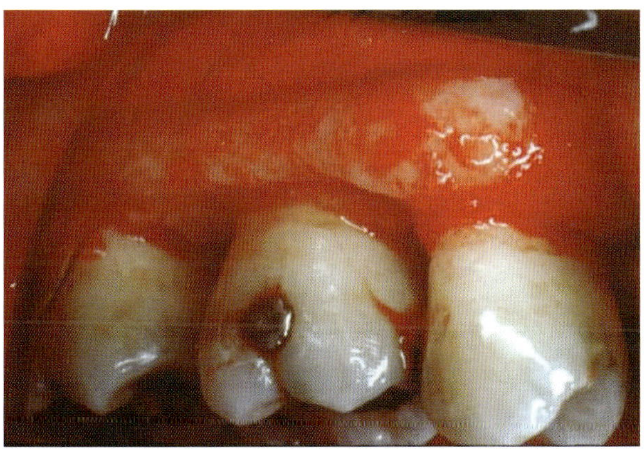

Figure 1.8 Flap reflection reveals extensive osseous ledging. Failure to eliminate this ledging will result in these soft tissues having to "dip under" the contact point, and the reestablishment of a nonkeratinized concave soft tissue col form.

to plaque control is achievable, this is not the case with the sulcular epithelium. Even if the sulcular epithelium could be predictably keratinized, it would serve no purpose, as the junctional epithelium is incapable of keratinization (25). The junctional epithelium is markedly different than other epithelia found in the oral cavity. In both keratinized and nonkeratinized oral epithelia, differentiation between the basal and superficial layers is a consistent finding (i.e., a decrease in Golgi vesicle and rough endoplasmic reticulum volumes, and an increase in tonofilament volume), as is a modification of the intercellular substance in the superficial layers, thus forming a permeability barrier (25). No evidence of differentiation is noted in the junctional epithelium. It has been suggested that this is due to the unique function of the junctional epithelium, which is to adhere to dissimilar tissues (26). If junctional epithelium was differentiated highly enough to keratinize, it would lose the ability to perform its primary function. Barnett (27) notes that, even in the presence of a keratinized sulcular epithelium, the junctional epithelium would still present a relatively easy mode of entry to the underlying structures for bacterial byproducts. Squiers (25) stated that "...it is reasonable to accept the junctional epithelium as a tissue which, by virtue of its adherent properties, is probably intrinsically permeable."

Saito et al. (28) examined clinically normal junctional epithelium in dogs via freeze-fracture and thin sectioning. Junctional epithelium was found to contain fewer desmosomes than other oral epithelium (5% in its most coronal aspect and only 3% apically). Very few cytoplasmic filaments were noted. Numerous gap junctions were noted, many of which were large in size. Tight junctions were only noted in freeze-fracture replicas, and these were underdeveloped or discontinuous in nature. These findings were in agreement with those of other researchers (29), and suggest that these areas leak, thus forming inadequate permeability barriers (30, 31). Saito et al. state that "...it is doubtful that the epithelium provides a complete barrier function because of the vast extent of the intercellular spaces and the sparseness of desmosomes" (28). Numerous studies have demonstrated the permeability of the junctional epithelium to a variety of substances (31–35). The relative impermeability of the sulcular epithelium, when compared to the junctional epithelium, has also been well documented. Substances were shown to penetrate the junctional epithelium, but not the sulcular epithelium (32, 33, 36).

The tenuous nature of the epithelial adherence to the tooth, and the ease with which it is separated, are well known (37). Listgarten (38) and others (39–43) have consistently shown that, in the presence of inflammation, the periodontal probe passes beyond the ulcerated junctional epithelium, stopping at the most coronal position of intact connective tissue fiber insertion into the root surface. This is not the case in noninflamed situations (44–46). The junctional epithelium therefore presents a dual-fold compromise. Not only is it more easily penetrated by bacterial enzymes, but it is also more easily detached in the presence of inflammation than inserted connective tissue fibers. In the stages of periodontal disease development, the "initial" lesion is seen as developing as follows:

1. bacterial accumulation in the gingival sulcus
2. an increase in the concentration of specific bacterial products
3. diffusion of these products through the more permeable junctional epithelium into the underlying connective tissue
4. dilation of the intercellular spaces of the junctional epithelium, and the presence of polymorphonuclear and mononuclear cells
5. perivascular collagen destruction
6. progression to the "early" lesion

Ideally, the expanse of the junctional epithelial adhesion to the tooth should be minimized in light of its relative biologic and mechanical inferiority when compared to connective tissue attachment to the root surface.

Following appropriate osseous resective surgery with apically positioned flaps, an attachment apparatus is formed which consists of approximately 1 mm of connective tissue fiber insertion into the root surface, followed by 1 mm of junctional epithelial adhesion coronally (47, 48). The connective tissue attachment is derived from a combination of outgrowth of the periodontal ligament and resorption of osseous crest (49). This is markedly different than the postsurgical attachment apparatus obtained with either curettage or replaced flap (modified Widman or open flap curettage) surgery. These procedures have all demonstrated healing to previously periodontally affected root surfaces by the formation of a long junctional epithelium (50–68). New connective tissue attachment supracrestally has not been a consistent finding, nor has cementogenesis (69). The components of the postoperative attachment apparatus of open flap curettage procedures without osseous resection are the same; connective tissue insertion for the first millimeter supracrestally, followed by a long junctional epithelium. The length of the junctional epithelium is dependent upon the distance between the osseous crest and the margin of the soft tissue. Only pocket elimination surgery will consistently result in a short junctional epithelium, and thus avoid the compromises inherent in a longer epithelial relationship.

Proper pocket elimination therapy is not only concerned with pocket depths, but also with plaque accumulation in a vertical direction. Horizontal destruction of periodontal support, resulting in furcation involvements, will lead to a major compromise in therapy if left untreated. The inaccessibility of even early furcation involvements to proper plaque control measures is well documented (3, 70–73). A review of the literature also underscores the inadequacy of many therapies in the treatment of the furcated tooth. "Maintenance" care, open and closed debridement, chemical treatment of the root surface, and placement of particulate materials without membrane use have failed to demonstrate predictable success in the treatment of the periodontally involved furcation. Removal of the vertical periodontal pocket, without eliminating the horizontal component of a furcation involvement, results in a compromised environment for the removal of plaque by the patient, leading to continued periodontal breakdown. This topic will be discussed in greater detail in Chapter 9.

Restorative margin position may also influence long-term periodontal health. Plaque accumulation at the restorative margin–tooth interface is a consistent finding in both research and clinical practice (74–81). If this margin is subgingival, the resultant increased plaque accumulation may lead to acceleration of periodontal breakdown and recurrent caries (81, 82) (Figure 1.10). This fact becomes more critical if the attachment apparatus attempting to maintain a healthy state includes a long junctional epithelium. The increased permeability and detachability of a long junctional epithelial adhesion in the face of inflammation lend the long junctional epithelium a greater vulnerability to the increased inflammatory insult inherent in subgingival margin placement.

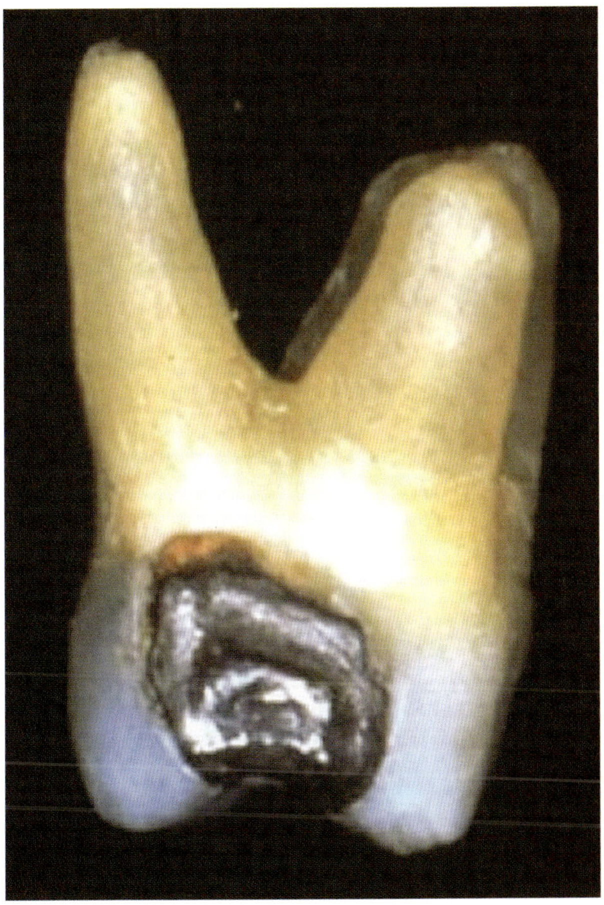

Figure 1.10 Recurrent caries is noted at the most apical extent of a deep subgingival interproximal restoration.

Results of Longitudinal Human Studies

Numerous clinical studies have attempted to compare short- and long-term results of various treatment modalities. The most widely read are probably those of Ramfjord and coworkers (83–91). As time progressed, these studies became more sophisticated in response to design shortcomings which were recognized by the authors. The first study, published in 1968 (83), compared the results of curettage versus pocket elimination in the treatment of periodontal pockets. The authors concluded that "subgingival curettage was followed by more favorable results than surgical elimination of periodontal pockets."

Being the first longitudinal study of this type, there were significant design flaws which the authors attempted to correct in subsequent studies. A split mouth design was not adopted until the third year of the study. For the first two years of data compilation, individual host response to therapy was an unaccounted for variable. Pockets were treated via gingivectomy procedures, if this could be accomplished within the bounds of the existing attached gingiva, if pocket depths were 5 mm or less and if extensive bone recontouring was not required to obtain acceptable gingival contours. This approach did not demonstrate a proper understanding of the rationale for pocket elimination therapy with osseous resection. Soft tissues will tend to reform interproximal papillae after periodontal surgery (92, 93). By eliminating interproximal osseous craters and reverse architecture, the clinician strives to achieve a closer adaptation of the reforming soft tissues to the underlying bone, helping to ensure the development of a postoperative attachment apparatus consisting of a connective tissue fiber insertion, followed by a short junctional epithelial adhesion. If interproximal osseous craters remained, which would have been the case where gingivectomy procedures were performed in the face of osseous defects, the long-term benefits of resective osseous therapy could not be properly assessed. In the 1968 study, no mention was made of the extent to which osteoplasty was carried out to eliminate buccal osseous ledging. If buccal ledging was allowed to remain, the resultant interproximal soft tissue morphology would be that of a concave col, due to the influence of the contact point. As previously discussed, this col would be more susceptible to inflammatory breakdown than the convex, keratinized interproximal soft tissues which would result from properly performed osseous resective therapy with apically positioned flaps.

Pocket measurements were taken at the "mesial side of the tooth," with no mention being made of probe angulation. Watts (94) has demonstrated that even small variations in probe angulation will result in significant probing errors. While 60% of the probing measurements were reproduced, the number dropped to 23% for reproducible site configurations. The most important source of probing error was variation of the probe position in a transverse plane, despite the use of a stent. If stents were not used, as is the case in the 1968 Ramfjord study, errors would be magnified. Measurements taken in the manner described do not accurately measure the differences between the attachment apparati obtained via pocket elimination surgery and curettage. One difference in these two attachment apparati is that of a short junctional epithelium following pocket elimination surgery, and a longer junctional epithelium following curettage. This difference is not as significant at the line angles of the teeth as it is interproximally between the base of an osseous crater and the most coronal extent of the junctional epithelial adhesion. If measurements are taken at the line angles of the teeth, the relative stabilities of the different attachment apparati over time are not taken into account.

Another significant weakness in the 1968 study is one of execution. The first postoperative measurements were recorded at one year. The mean pocket reduction following pocket elimination surgery was 1.6 mm, resulting in residual mean pocket depths greater than or equal to 2.4 mm. When the data were broken down, the range of residual pocket depths became evident. In initial pockets of greater than 6 mm, approximately a 0.4-mm change occurred, leaving residual pocket depths greater than or equal to 5.6 mm. One of the basic postulates of pocket elimination surgery is the inability of the patient to exhibit adequate subgingival plaque control in areas probing greater than 3 mm. By leaving pockets of greater than 5.6 mm after therapy, the efficacy of pocket elimination therapy was not tested. The 1973 study by Ramfjord and coworkers had an identical design to that of 1968, and thus suffered from the same problems (84).

In 1975, the study was expanded to include the modified Widman procedure (85) and patients were followed over time (86, 89). The modified Widman procedure employed, as described in 1974 (94), was essentially replaced flap curettage, with osseous therapy as needed to facilitate interproximal flap coaptation.

The authors concluded that pocket elimination surgery did not offer any long-term benefits with regard to pocket depth or progression of disease, and that "although all three methods result in gain of attachment in moderately deep pockets, the long-term gain is significant only after curettage and modified Widman flap" (89).

As already discussed, design and execution flaws masked the differences between pocket elimination therapy and curettage or modified Widman surgery.

Interproximal pocket depth measurements were recorded "at the mesio- and distobuccal surfaces close to the contacts and without tilting the probe" (89). Thus, the measurements were taken at the wrong positions to measure the differences between the attachment apparati of the various treatment modalities. Due to the limited buccal and/or lingual osseous resection performed with the modified Widman procedure, the attachment apparati at the line angles of the teeth were similar for both procedures. The only difference in underlying osseous morphologies existed in the interproximal craters. Measurements purporting to compare the two therapies must record these differences.

Appropriate osseous resection to eliminate defects and reverse architectures, followed by apically positioned flaps, routinely results in pocket depths of less than 3 mm. Such was not the case in these studies. In pockets which probed 4–6 mm initially, probing depths of 1.7–3.7 mm are noted one year postoperatively. Where pockets probed 7–12 mm before therapy, residual pocket depths were 2.6–7.6 mm. These readings are not indicative of pocket elimination having been achieved. What was tested was not pocket reduction (modified Widman) versus pocket elimination; but rather pocket reduction versus pocket reduction. It would be unusual if both situations did not behave identically over time.

Ramfjord and coworkers felt that "the fact that pockets and attachment levels on the four tooth surfaces behaved similarly when the initial severity was constant made it possible to collapse the data from the four surfaces and report the means" (89). This conclusion was based on the fact that all four tooth surfaces behaved the same with regard to pocket reduction and attachment gain one year postoperatively (95). However, one year is too short a time for proper evaluation of therapeutic results. Waerhaug has demonstrated the seemingly slow progression of untreated periodontal disease in data consisting of a large number of sites, and stated that a minimum of 3–5 years is necessary to evaluate treatment efficacy (3).

What was gained histologically following the various treatments was a short connective tissue insertion and a junctional epithelium of varying lengths. Where interproximal osseous craters are present, the junctional epithelium will be relatively longer; where there is a shorter distance from the osseous crest to the tissue margin (the buccal and lingual midradicular areas in most instances), the junctional epithelium will be relatively shorter. While areas of the same preoperative probing depth may appear to behave the same initially with regard to clinical response to therapy, they bear no resemblance to each other histologically. Collapsing the data in this manner masks the differences between the two clinical approaches.

One of the basic principles of pocket elimination therapy was ignored; that of the greater resistance of connective tissue fiber insertion than junctional epithelial adhesion to inflammatory breakdown. Buccal and lingual areas of long junctional epithelium are not subject to the same challenges as interproximal areas. Patient plaque control is easier and there are no concave col forms with retractable soft tissue peaks to trap plaque. Furthermore, restorative margins are more easily cleaned buccally than interproximally.

Ramfjord and coworkers also stated that "since the pockets and attachment levels from one year after treatment behaved essentially in a linear fashion, a grouping according to severity was adopted" (89). The progression of periodontal disease does not behave in a linear fashion, but rather is characterized by bursts of activity in specific sites, followed by periods of quiescence (96). The reporting of running medians is less effective in detecting site-specific changes in longitudinal periodontal studies than other statistical methods (97–99). By reworking statistics that reported no periodontal changes over time posttherapy, Lindhe was able to demonstrate the masking effect of reporting mean values (100).

The influence of furcations on the progression of periodontal breakdown was also ignored in the aforementioned studies. One facet of pocket elimination therapy is the elimination of furcation involvements through odontoplasty or root resection (101–104). Failure to eliminate the involved furcal areas renders complete plaque removal impossible due to local anatomy (105–108). Even with flap reflection, thorough debridement of an involved furcation is not a consistent finding (109, 110). An affected furcation will contribute to further periodontal breakdown both within the furcation itself and in adjacent structures. As the inflammatory lesion in the furcation spreads, it may also act in a "back door" manner, emerging from the internal aspect of the furcation to cause destruction of the attachment apparatus.

The effects of furcation involvements on the pathogenesis of periodontal disease were evident. Maxillary molars exhibited the greatest degree of periodontal breakdown following therapy, followed by mandibular molars and maxillary bicuspids.

The same limitations were evident in two studies carried out by Hill et al. and Ramfjord et al. (90, 91). Waerhaug's admonition with regard to leaving furcation involvements after therapy was borne out, as 16 of the 17 teeth lost in these studies were molars.

Pihlstrom et al. (111, 112), when comparing root planing alone and flap surgery with root planing, demonstrated greater pocket reduction initially with the flap procedure as a result of clinical attachment "gain." Repocketing of the areas treated with flap surgery, to the level of the root-planed sites, occurred within three years postoperatively. This is to be expected, as root planing and open flap curettage demonstrate the same compromised attachment apparati posttherapy.

Disturbing findings with all longitudinal studies evaluating treatment modalities which yield a long junctional epithelium as a posttherapeutic attachment apparatus (root planing, curettage, modified Widman, flap curettage without osseous therapy, etc.) were repocketing and continued attachment loss (90, 91, 113, 114).

Proponents of pocket elimination therapy contend that, when carried out and evaluated properly, pocket elimination is superior to pocket reduction with respect to patient maintainability and long-term periodontal health. Do longitudinal studies exist which support these contentions?

Ammon's group published two papers, one being a five-year follow-up of the initial patient data (115, 116), evaluating the relative efficacies of appropriately executed osseous resection with apically positioned flaps, and the other being apically positioned flaps with only root planing. Design modifications were made from the Ramfjord studies to help eliminate the problems already discussed. Data were first pooled by pocket depth, and then subdivided into tooth surfaces within a given pocket depth, to help elucidate the strengths and differences of the postsurgical attachment apparati. Mesial and distal probing depths were recorded with the probe placed as far interproximally as possible, angulated to follow the long axis of the tooth. Only lesions which were amenable to resective therapy, and could therefore properly evaluate its applicability, were treated in such a manner. Finally, surgical photographs were published which demonstrated the techniques employed.

Greater interproximal soft tissue cratering was noted upon initial healing following open flap curettage, as compared with osseous surgery. Six weeks postoperatively, the cratering had disappeared. This finding is in agreement with Lindhe and Nyman (117). Pocket reduction at six months was the same for sites treated by either modality; flap curettage reduction being a result of attachment "gain" while osseous surgery reduction was due to pocket elimination procedures. The attachment "gain" was a function of papillary regrowth and a subsequent long epithelial relationship to the root, as a connective tissue fiber attachment cannot be expected following flap curettage (51, 56, 69). Five years postoperatively, statistically significant interproximal pocket depth differences were noted between the sites treated with and without osseous therapy. Pocket depths in the flap curettage areas were approaching preoperative values while the pocket elimination attained with osseous therapy was maintained. On the buccal and lingual surfaces, pocket elimination was maintained with both treatment approaches. These results underscore both the fragility of the junctional epithelial adhesion and the danger of collapsing data. Radicularly, where patient plaque removal was easier and the junctional epithelium was shorter, pocket elimination was maintained following both therapies. In interproximal areas of more difficult plaque removal, coupled with a longer junctional epithelial relationship due to the presence of osseous craters, repocketing occurred in sites treated with open flap curettage. Flap curettage sites which initially probed 4 mm underwent repocketing at five years three times more often than sites treated via osseous resection. If initial probing depths were 5 mm, flap curettage sites repocketed 3.6 times as often as those treated with osseous resection. With initial probings of 6–8 mm, repocketing was 6 times as likely to occur with open flap curettage. When all sites with a preoperative probing depth greater than or equal to 4 mm were considered, bleeding upon probing was encountered 2.3 times more often in sites treated with open flap curettage than with osseous resection, five years postoperatively. There was a 91% correlation between the presence of subgingival plaque and bleeding upon probing.

Other authors have demonstrated the long-term efficacy of pocket elimination therapy. Lindhe and Nyman (100) reported the 14-year results of pocket elimination therapy in 61 patients with advanced periodontal disease preoperatively. All patients had remained on regular maintenance schedules. Only 0.49 teeth were lost per patient over 14 years. Disease progression was shown to be 20–30 times slower than in Swedes with untreated periodontal disease (118). Nabers et al. (119) reported the results of 1,435 patients treated via pocket elimination therapy. The patients lost an average of 0.29 teeth over a mean postoperative time of 12.9 years.

In contrast, McFall (120) demonstrated an average tooth loss of 2.6 teeth per patient 19 years posttherapy. Goldman et al. (121), 22.2 years postoperatively, documented a tooth mortality of 3.6 teeth per patient. Both of these studies employed treatment modalities which did not include pocket elimination therapy.

Kaldahl et al. (122, 123) compared treatment results in 82 periodontal patients treated in a split mouth design with either coronal scaling, root planing, modified Widman surgery, or flap surgery with osseous resection. All therapies produced mean pocket depth reductions, and there were no differences between the therapies with regard to residual pocket depths at the end of two years in sites which initially probed 4 mm or less. Subsequent breakdown of sites during supportive maintenance care of up to seven years was greater in areas treated with modified Widman surgery and scaling and root planing than in areas treated with osseous resective therapy. These differences in the number of sites breaking down increased as initial pocket depth increased, underscoring the superiority of osseous resective therapy as a clinical modality for eliminating pockets and rendering areas maintainable over time by patients. Shallower pocket depths, coupled with a biologically stronger attachment apparatus of a short connective tissue attachment and a short junctional epithelium attained after osseous resection, proved more resistant to subsequent breakdown during maintenance than an attachment apparatus of a short connective tissue attachment and a long junctional epithelial adhesion obtained following root planing or modified Widman surgery. As expected, these differences were greater in areas with deeper initial pocket depths, as the difference in posttherapeutic attachment apparatus would have been more marked in these areas than in their shallower counterparts.

The differences in tooth retention can be traced to the ability of the patient and the clinician to successfully and predictably effect thorough plaque removal. Properly performed pocket elimination therapy provides an environment of minimal probing depth which is conducive to plaque removal. Even in the face of excellent supragingival plaque removal, we know that the patient is only effective at removing plaque to a subgingival depth of 2.5 mm (3). Lindhe et al. have demonstrated that there is no relationship between supragingival plaque control and changes in probing depths or attachment levels (124), or between supragingival plaque control and bleeding upon probing. The clinician must not be misled by the supragingival scenario. Waerhaug spoke of the existence of subclinical inflammation (3), where the tissue appears healthy, but periodontal destruction is occurring subgingivally. Ammons and coworkers (116) found a direct correlation between pocket depth and bleeding upon probing. Greater postsurgical pocket depths resulted in a higher incidence of bleeding upon probing. Coupled with the previously discussed 91% correlation between bleeding upon probing and the presence of subgingival plaque, the problems inherent in deeper postoperative probing depths are obvious. Badersten et al. (125, 126) noted that bleeding upon probing was directly related to pocket depth, with deeper areas bleeding more often. Waite (127) found that areas with deeper probing depths exhibited a higher frequency of bleeding upon probing and a greater degree of inflammation. Additionally, the same limitations which apply to subgingival root planing in the face of pocket depths must be considered in the maintenance phase of therapy.

The deeper the residual probing depths, the more difficult debridement and maintenance become for both the patient and the dental professional (3, 128–137). Numerous longitudinal studies have demonstrated that sites with probing depths of greater than or equal to 6 mm are at significantly higher risk for future deterioration and development of additional attachment loss as a result of disease activity, if left untreated (138–143).

The scenario for continued loss of attachment in the face of posttherapeutic pocketing is as follows:

1. The patient presents with pocket depths in excess of 3 mm.
2. Patient plaque control removes plaque up to 2.5 mm subgingivally.
3. Subgingival scaling is increasingly less effective in areas probing greater than 3 mm.
4. Plaque left behind subgingivally following root planing begins to grow and repopulate the root surface within 14 days.
5. As the plaque front proceeds further subgingivally, its removal is less effective.
6. The attachment apparatus which results from curettage, modified Widman surgery, flap curettage, etc. has a long junctional epithelial component.
7. This epithelial adhesion exhibits greater permeability to plaque than a connective tissue fiber insertion.
8. Junctional epithelium is easily detached from the root in the presence of inflammation.
9. As the pocket deepens, the problems with plaque removal are exacerbated.
10. The presence of furcation involvements and/or subgingival restorations makes plaque removal even more difficult.
11. The result is continued periodontal breakdown.

Such continued periodontal breakdown following active therapy is avoidable. The technical aspects of osseous resective surgery have been clearly elucidated (16, 23). Employed in conjunction with selective extractions, root resective therapy, and prosthetic reconstruction, these techniques afford a high degree of predictability (23), albeit with significant temporal and financial costs.

Clinical Example One

In 1981, a 26-year-old female presented with a number of periodontal and restorative concerns. Postorthodontic blunting of the roots was noted (Figure 1.11). Class I furcation involvements were present on all maxillary and mandibular molars. Subgingival caries was present in many areas. Osseointegrated implants were not a viable treatment option at the time of patient examination.

The combination of the patient's young age, short root structures, and active periodontal and restorative pathologies mandated a comprehensive, coordinated effort in order to afford her with a predictable treatment outcome. The performance of periodontal surgical therapies which would not eliminate deeper pockets and furcation involvements, and render all caries and defective restorative margins supragingival for the restorative dentist's intervention, would be ill advised. When treating such a patient, the clinician has "one shot" at restoring the patient to health. The patient's limited attachment apparatus could not afford to withstand multiple surgical insults, nor be subject to continued periodontal breakdown following active care.

The patient was treated with an osseous resective approach. All furcation involvements were eliminated through odontoplasty. Tissues were positioned in such a manner as to allow placement of restorative margins supragingivally or intracrevicularly. A full series of radiographs taken 25 years after active therapy had been completed demonstrate the maintenance of periodontal support around the teeth, and the high degree of predictability afforded this patient through appropriate, coordinated care (Figure 1.12).

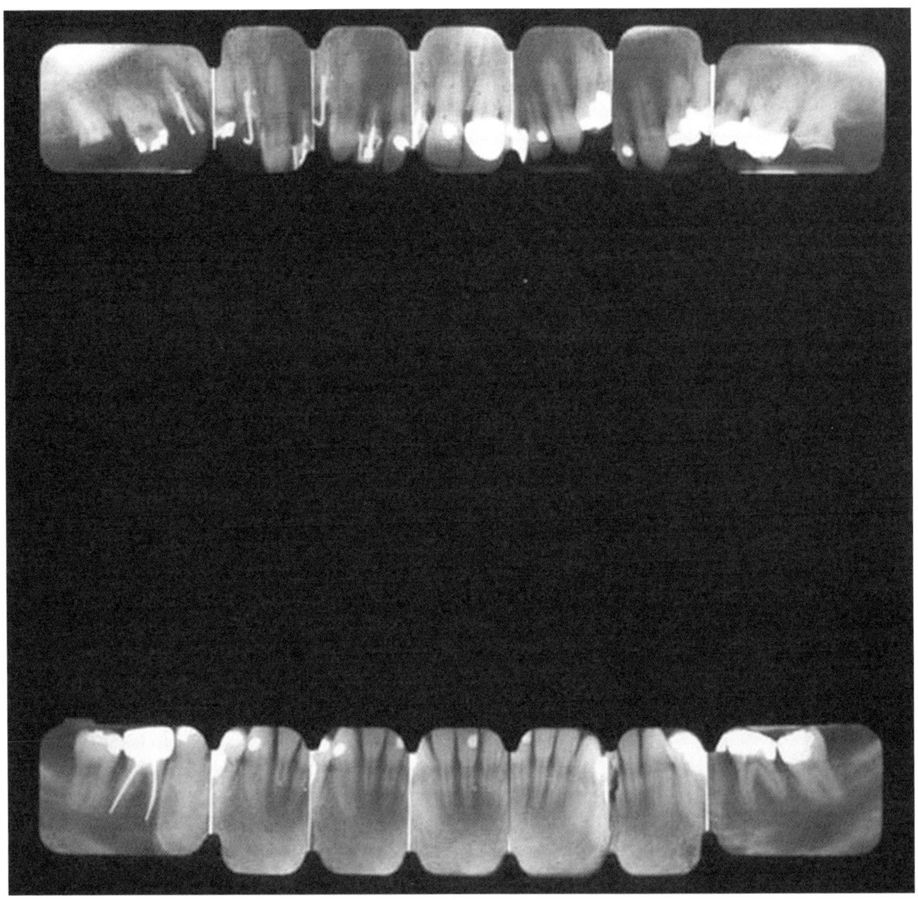

Figure 1.11 A patient presents with numerous oral health concerns including significant caries, blunted roots, and early-to-moderate periodontal destruction. Class I furcation involvements are noted on all molars.

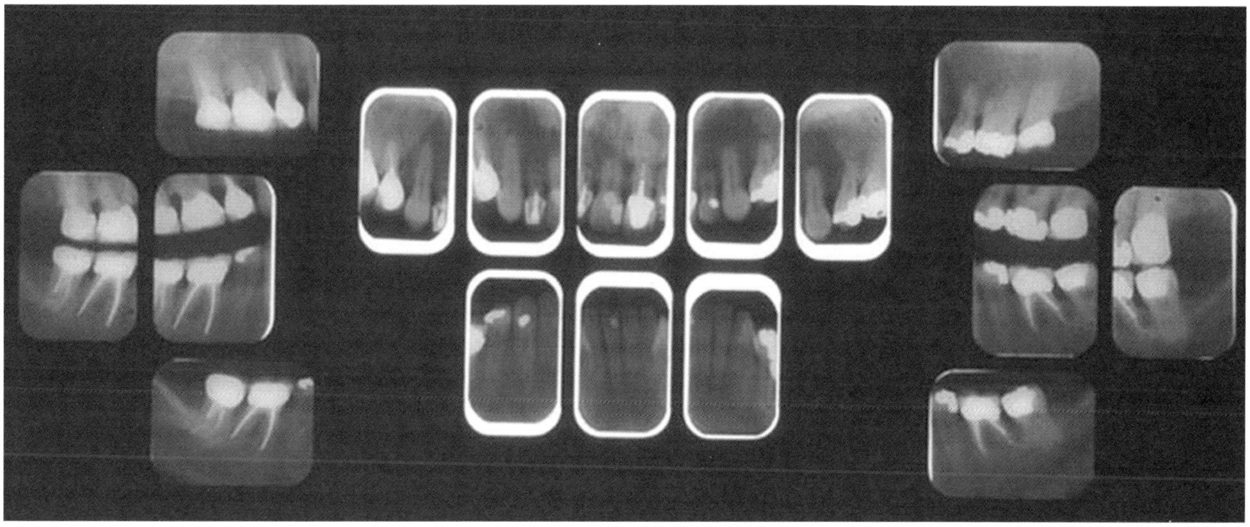

Figure 1.12 Twenty-five years after completion of active periodontal and restorative therapies, the patient demonstrates excellent periodontal and restorative stability.

While the therapy employed proved highly predictable, the question facing today's clinician is whether or not to perform such therapy on severely compromised teeth, or to remove selective teeth and utilize an implant reconstructive approach. This question is paramount when considering root resection therapy.

Root resective therapy is a highly predictable therapeutic modality in specific situations.

While various authors have reported a wide range of success and failure, this was often due to utilization of root resective therapies in less than ideal scenarios. It is imperative that the forces being placed upon a root-resected tooth be managed appropriately if a reasonable degree of predictability is to be attained. When this is accomplished, long-term treatment results rival those of osseointegrating implants. Seven hundred one root-resected molars were followed for a period of up to 15-plus years in function. The cumulative success rates of the root-resected teeth in function were 96.8% (144).

However, while such a treatment approach may yield a high degree of predictability, the technical acumen and financial commitment required for such care often prove daunting and unrealistic.

Clinical Example Two

A 41-year-old female presented with severe periodontal disease, characterized by moderate bone and attachment loss, Class II and III furcation involvements on all molars, and significant mobility patterns. The patient was temporized, underwent comprehensive periodontal therapy, including root resections and retention of a palatal root in the maxillary right second molar position; the mesiobuccal and distal buccal roots of the maxillary left first molar; and the distal root of the mandibular right first molar (Figure 1.13). The maxillary right cuspid was missing.

A maxillary full fixed reconstruction and a mandibular posterior reconstruction were carried out (Figures 1.14 a–f). The patient remained on a regular maintenance schedule. Radiographs taken 15 years after therapy had been performed, demonstrated stability of both the prosthesis and the supporting periodontium around the remaining teeth and or portions of teeth, despite the lack of a maxillary right cuspid (Figure 1.15).

After 15 years in function, the patient underwent significant life changes. The patient was not seen for one year, and had begun to clench and grind heavily. The net result was that the abutments in the maxillary right quadrant fractured. These abutments were most prone to parafunctional overload, as no cuspid was present. The loss of the established force equilibrium resulted in root fracture, tooth loss, and loss of the maxillary prosthesis.

While it is impossible to predict the future with regard to trauma and/or increased parafunction, the utilization of implants affords the

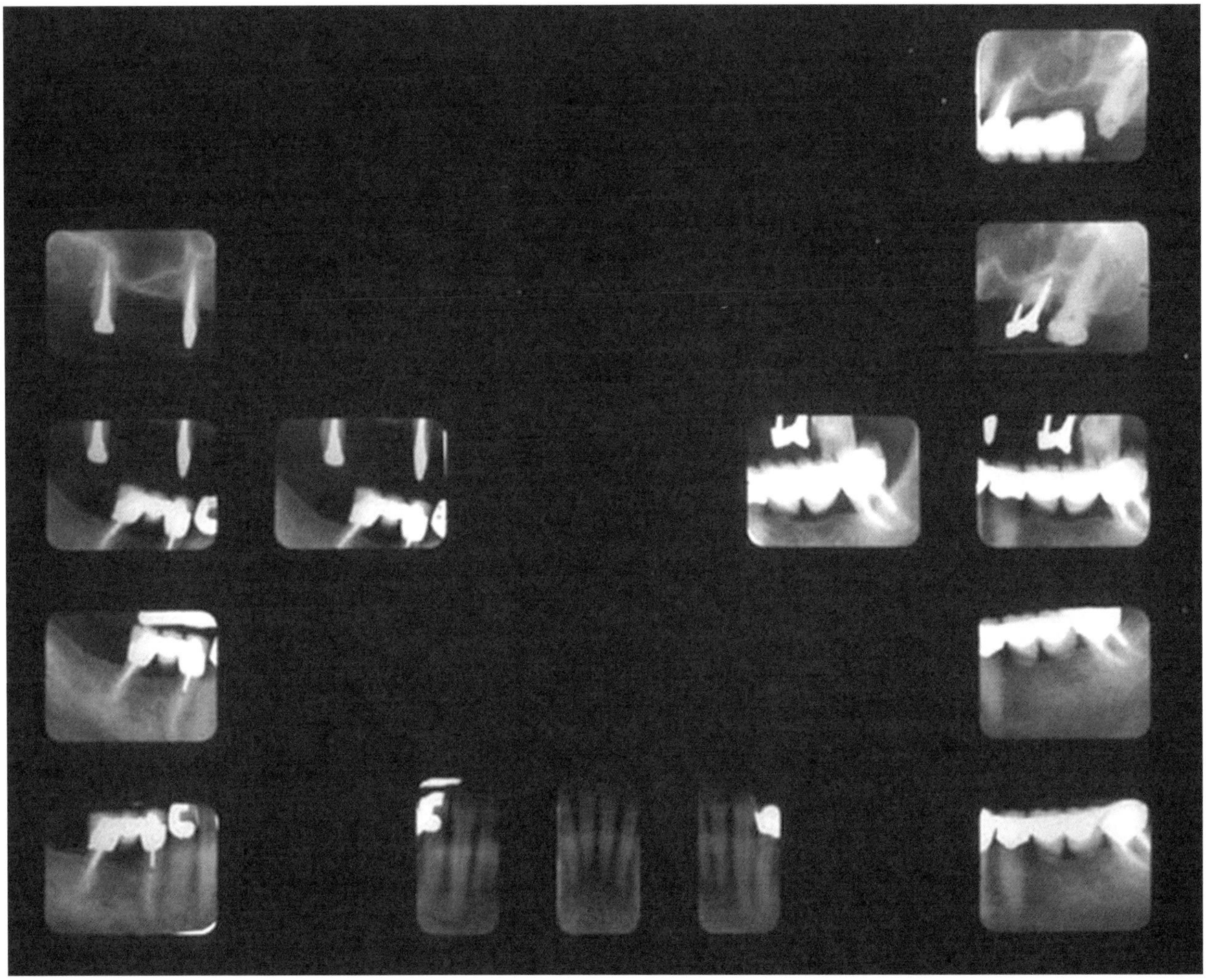

Figure 1.13 A patient who presented with severe periodontal disease has been temporized and treated with resective periodontal therapy, including root resections. The palatal root of the maxillary right second molar; the mesiobuccal and distal buccal roots of the maxillary left first molar; and a distal root of the mandibular right first molar have been maintained.

opportunity to build a greater margin of safety into reconstructive therapy.

FINANCIAL ALGORITHMS

Assessment of various treatment options in a given clinical scenario must also take into account the financial commitment entailed with each therapeutic approach. A recent survey polled over 100 periodontists and their referring dentists in 20 metropolitan areas regarding the costs for various therapies (145). The costs for periodontal surgical therapies, endodontic therapy on single- and multirooted teeth, posts and crowns on natural teeth, tooth extraction, implant placement, and implant abutments and crowns were assessed relative to a given value X (Table 1.1). Such information must be available to the clinician when formulating and presenting various treatment options to the patient.

SPECIFIC CLINICAL SCENARIOS

Scenario One: The Single-Rooted Decayed Tooth

When faced with a tooth which is decayed subgingivally at or near the osseous crest, the following treatment options present themselves:

(a) Crown-lengthening osseous surgery followed by endodontic therapy and post and

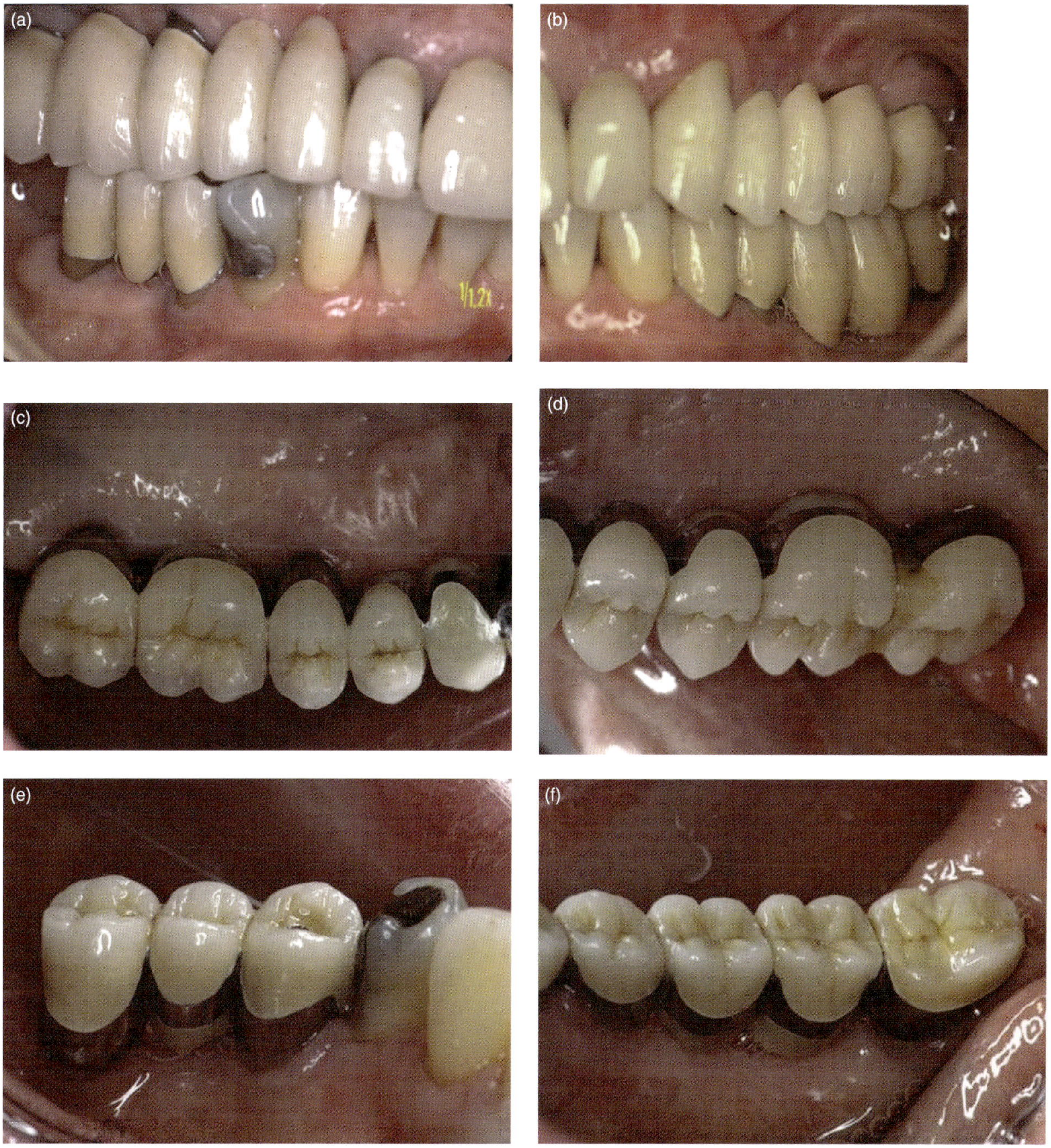

Figure 1.14 (a–f) Buccal and clinical views of the completed reconstruction after 10 years in function. Note the lack of a cuspid in the maxillary right quadrant. The patient's home care and soft tissue health are excellent.

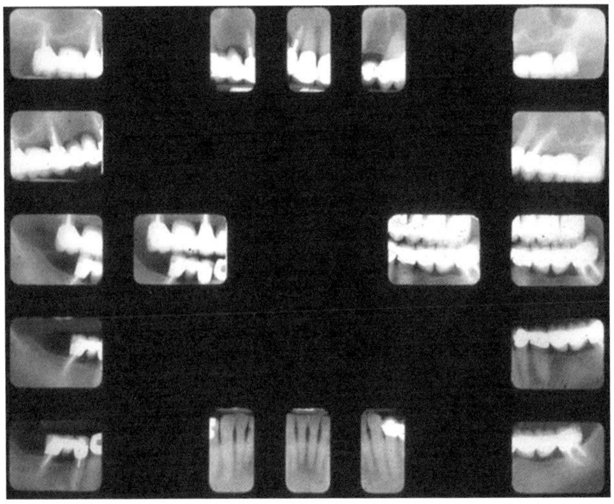

Figure 1.15 A full series of radiographs taken 10 years after completion of therapy demonstrate the stability of the periodontium and the prostheses which are in place.

core buildup if necessary, and the appropriate restoration: The predictability of crown-lengthening osseous surgery is well established. When performed appropriately, crown-lengthening surgery results in both adequate clinical crown for restoration of the tooth in a maintainable manner, and the development of a predictable attachment apparatus consisting of approximately 1 mm of connective tissue attachment, 1 mm of junctional adhesion, and a 1- to 1.5-mm-deep sulcus (Figure 1.16). It is imperative that such therapy be performed in a manner which ensures both the maintenance of the attained hard and soft tissue morphologies, and the ability of the patient to perform appropriate plaque control measures around the final restoration. Advocates of "minimal approach surgery," consisting of use of a laser or rotary instrumentation to "attain biologic width" only at the site of subgingival caries without ensuring a confluence with the adjacent hard and soft tissues, fail to understand the three-dimensional nature of tissue biodynamics and healing. Utilization of these limited access therapies results in eventual reformation of the presurgical soft tissue form and the presence of deep subgingival restorative margins. These problems

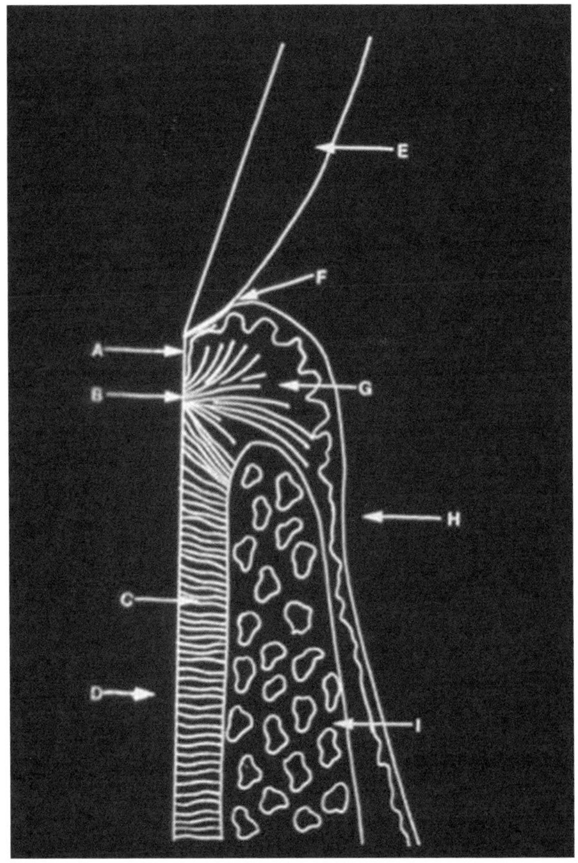

Figure 1.16 (A) Junctional epithelial adhesion; (B) connective tissue attachment; (C) periodontal ligament; (D) tooth root; (E) enanel; (F) gingival sulcus; (G) gingival connective tissue; (H) outer epithelium; (I) alveolar bone.

Table 1.1 Relative fees for various therapies.

Therapy	Fee
Endodontic—single root	0.9X
Endodontic—multiple root	1.3X
Core buildup—natural tooth	0.6X
Crown—natural tooth	1.4X
Pontic	1.4X
Crown-lengthening periodontal surgery	1.1X
Regenerative periodontal surgery	1.9X
Orthodontic supereruption	2.8X
Extraction	0.3X
Implant	2.1X
Implant abutment (stock) and crown	2.2X
Implant abutment (custom) and crown	2.7X
Regenerative therapy at tooth extraction	0.7–1.4X
Sinus augmentation	2.5X

are avoided through the employment of techniques which are well documented in the literature (146–149).

The precise position and extent of the carious lesion and/or tooth fracture to be uncovered through crown-lengthening osseous surgery must be assessed prior to initiation of surgery. The advisability of performing such treatment is directly dependent upon whether the lesion to be uncovered is buccally, lingually, or interproximally placed, and its proximity to adjacent roots and/or furcation entrances.

Prior to performing crown-lengthening osseous surgery, a number of factors must be considered including:

1. The effect of therapy on teeth adjacent to the tooth to be crown lengthened: Depending upon the tooth preparation technique to be employed, 3–4 mm of tooth must be exposed between the alveolar crest and the planned position of the final restorative margin. In situations where a patient presents with a short root form, or caries on the root surface which would require removal of extensive amounts of osseous support, the tooth may be unduly compromised following crown-lengthening osseous surgery. If such a procedure will result in periodontal instability, or the development of secondary occlusal trauma, crown-lengthening surgery should not be employed.
2. The effect of crown-lengthening osseous surgery on the entrance to a furcation of a multirooted tooth to be crown lengthened: If attainment of an adequate amount of exposed tooth structure for restorative intervention and development of a healthy attachment apparatus results in the development of an untreatable furcation involvement, such a therapeutic approach is ill advised. Should a Class I furcation involvement result following crown-lengthening osseous surgery, it is easily eliminated through odontoplasty, as will be discussed in Chapter 9. However, development of a furcation of any degree greater than Class I should be avoided at all costs.
3. The effect of crown-lengthening osseous surgery on the furcation entrances of adjacent teeth: As previously mentioned, if the necessary osseous resection will result in a significant furcation involvement on an adjacent tooth, it should be avoided. In addition, care must be taken to assess the extent of osseous support which will be removed from adjacent single- and multi-rooted teeth during the performance of crown-lengthening osseous surgery. It is illogical to significantly compromise the periodontal health of adjacent teeth so as to afford adequate clinical crown length for appropriate restoration of a severely decayed tooth.
4. The effect of crown-lengthening surgery on the patient's esthetics: While palatal caries on a maxillary anterior tooth may be safely exposed for restoration, the same procedure performed interproximally or buccally often results in an unacceptable esthetic treatment outcome. In such situations, other treatment options should be explored.

If a decayed single root tooth is to be crown lengthened and restored, the need for endodontic therapy, as well as the ease and predictability of such therapy, must be carefully considered prior to initiation of care. Should the clinician have any questions regarding these points, appropriate consultations should be sought.

It is also imperative that the ability to predictably restore a specific decayed tooth is assessed prior to the initiation of care. Both the extent and position of the carious lesion will be paramount in determining the feasibility of maintaining the tooth in question.

Clinical Example Three

A 51-year-old male presented with a buccal fracture on a mandibular left first molar (Figure 1.17). Radiographic examination demonstrated the short root trunk of the fractured tooth (Figure 1.18). Crown-lengthening osseous surgery would have led to significant invasion of the buccal furcation of the first molar, due to both its short root trunk and the position of the buccal fracture in relation to the furcation entrance. As a result, this tooth

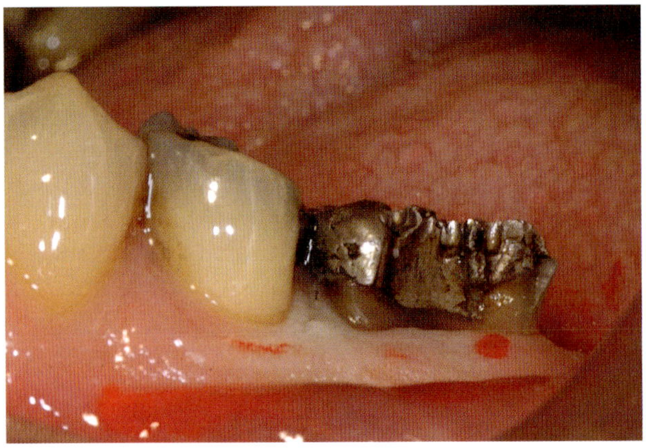

Figure 1.17 A patient presents with a subgingival buccal fracture of a mandibular first molar.

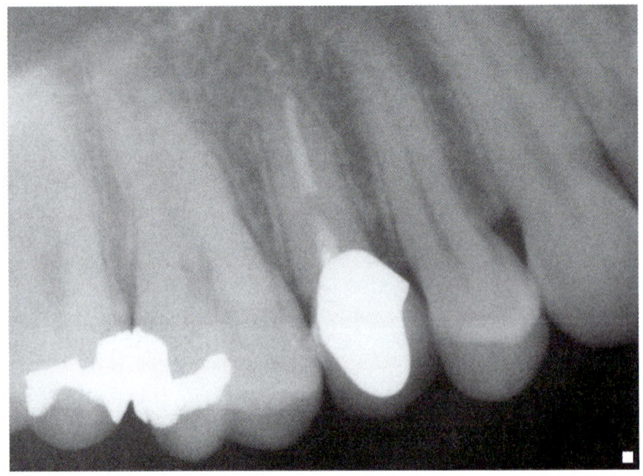

Figure 1.19 A patient presents with subgingival caries on the distal and palatal aspects of a maxillary right second bicuspid. Crown-lengthening osseous surgery would require removal of approximately 4 mm of bone at the area of the entrance to the mesial furcation of the first molar, and would unduly compromise the first molar.

must be removed and replaced with an implant at the time of tooth extraction, with concomitant regenerative therapy; this technique will be discussed in Chapter 9. Carious lesions which appear similar clinically often present with widely disparate prognoses when a radiographic examination is carried out.

Clinical Example Four

A 31-year-old female presents with subgingival caries on the distal and palatal aspects of her maxillary right secondary bicuspid (Figure 1.19). Appropriate crown-lengthening surgery would require removal of approximately 4 mm of bone at the area of the entrance to the mesial furcation of the first molar. Such therapy would compromise the prognosis of the first molar. Removal of 4 mm of bone from the distal aspect of the second bicuspid would also significantly alter its crown to root ratio and adversely affect the long-term prognosis of the tooth.

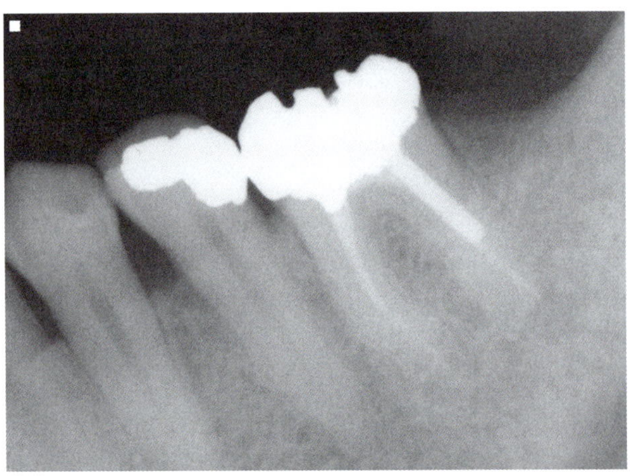

Figure 1.18 A radiograph demonstrates the short root trunk of the fractured mandibular first molar. Crown-lengthening osseous surgery would lead to invasion of the entrance to the buccal furcation and a compromised long-term prognosis for the tooth.

Due to these considerations, the maxillary second bicuspid was extracted and an implant was placed at the time of tooth removal. Following osseointegration, the implant is ready for restoration with a stock abutment and crown (Figure 1.20).

Figure 1.21 demonstrates a mandibular left first molar with caries on its distal aspect. The position of the caries with relation to both the interproximal osseous crest and the entrances to the furcations of the first molar renders it an excellent candidate for crown-lengthening osseous surgery and subsequent restoration.

In contrast, Figure 1.22 is a radiograph of another mandibular first molar which presents with distal subgingival caries. Both the more apical extent of the carious lesion interproximally and the fact that the mesial apical aspect of the lesion is approaching the entrance of the buccal furcation of the mandibular first molar render the tooth's

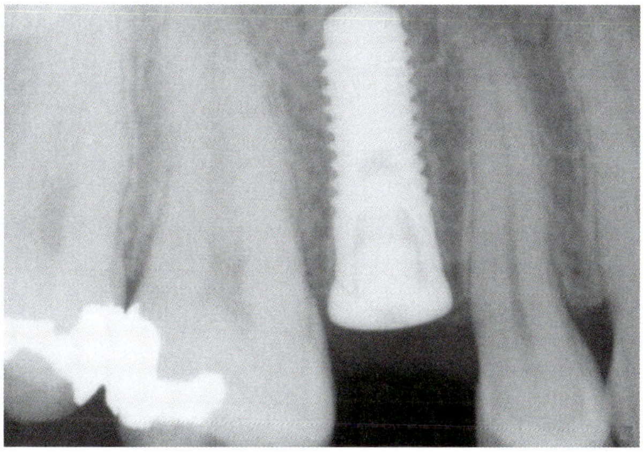

Figure 1.20 The decayed second bicuspid has been extracted and replaced with an implant at the time of tooth removal. Following completion of osseointegration, this implant is ready for restoration with a stock abutment and crown.

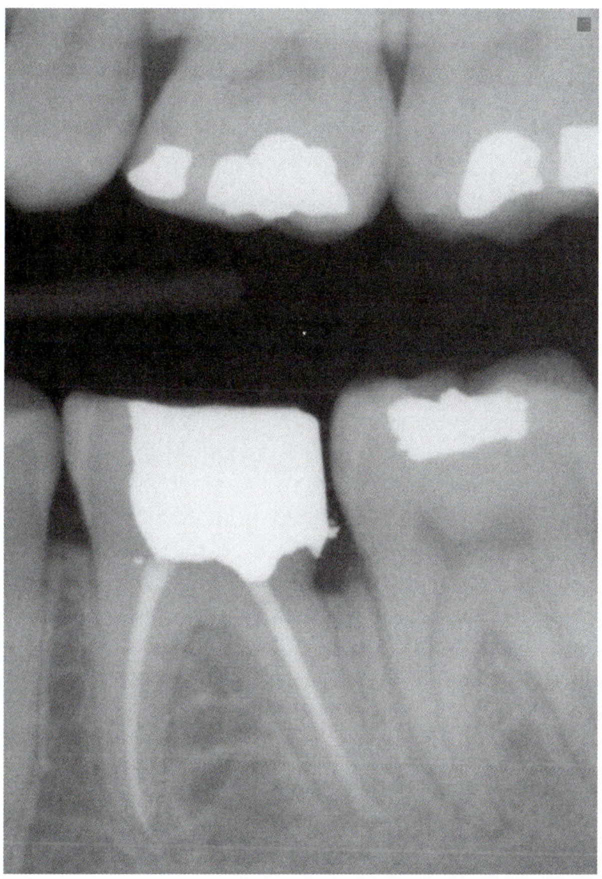

Figure 1.21 A patient presents with subgingival caries on the distal aspect of a mandibular first molar. The position and extent of this caries renders the tooth an excellent candidate for crown-lengthening osseous surgery and subsequent restoration.

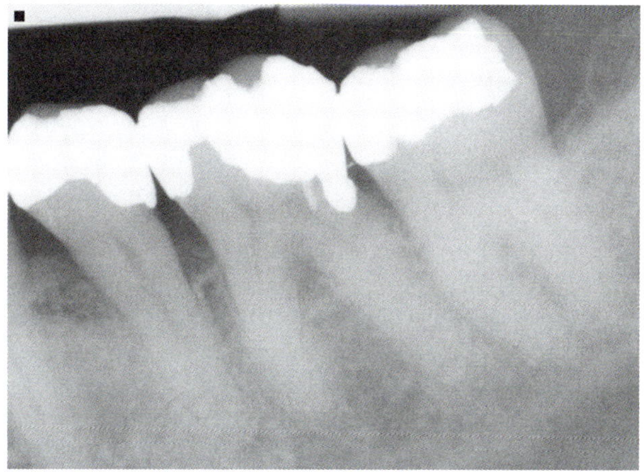

Figure 1.22 A patient presents with subgingival caries on the distal aspect of a lower first molar. The apical and buccal extents of the caries render this tooth a poor candidate for crown-lengthening osseous surgery. Such a procedure would unduly compromise the second molar and would invade the buccal furcation of the first molar.

prognosis poor. Attempts at crown-lengthening osseous surgery will unduly compromise the second molar and involve the entrance to the buccal furcation of the first molar. This tooth must be removed and replaced with an implant, abutment and crown.

The esthetic ramifications of crown-lengthening osseous surgery must be considered as well. Figure 1.23 demonstrates a fractured

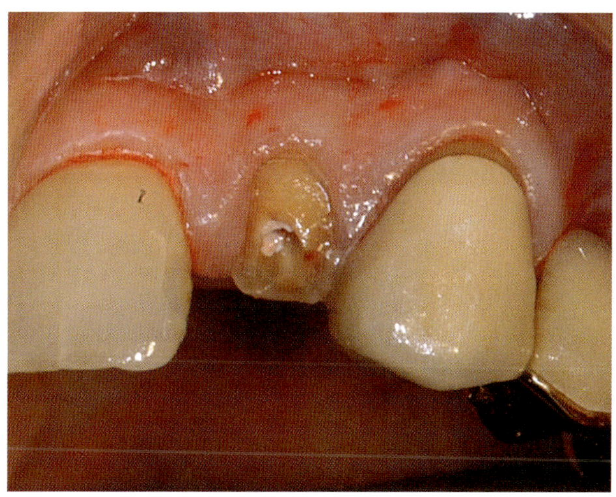

Figure 1.23 Attempts to crown lengthen the fractured lateral incisor would result in an esthetically unacceptable treatment result. If this tooth is to be maintained, orthodontic supereruption must first be carried out.

maxillary left lateral incisor. Appropriate crown-lengthening osseous surgery around this tooth would result in a highly unesthetic situation for the patient. If this tooth is to be maintained, orthodontic supereruption must be considered prior to crown-lengthening osseous surgery.

(b) Orthodontic supereruption with or without crown-lengthening osseous surgery: Super eruption of a decayed tooth affords the opportunity to minimize the removal of osseous support from adjacent teeth during crown-lengthening osseous surgery. In addition, the esthetic compromise of such surgery is significantly diminished. Finally, the need for crown-lengthening surgery may be obviated through severance of the periodontal ligament fibers at three-week intervals during the supereruption process. Such fiber separation often prevents the attachment apparatus from supererupting along with the orthodontically treated root, resulting in "nonsurgical crown lengthening."

When orthodontic supereruption is contemplated, it is imperative that a number of factors be considered including:

1. The effects of orthodontic supereruption and subsequent crown lengthening on the treated tooth: Appropriate assessment of the expected root length following active therapy is crucial prior to the initiation of orthodontic supereruption. The patient is ill served by a supererupted, crown lengthened, and restored tooth which is unstable due to a poor crown to root ratio.
2. The time involved in orthodontic supereruption: When assessing the advantages and disadvantages of various treatment approaches, the number of patient visits and the overall length of therapy must be openly discussed.
3. The cost of orthodontic supereruption: As noted in Table 1.1, the use of orthodontic supereruption prior to crown-lengthening surgery and tooth restoration, with or without endodontic intervention, significantly impacts the cost/benefit ratio to the patient.

(c) Tooth extraction, implant placement, and restoration: While this treatment approach eliminates the need for endodontic therapy and crown-lengthening osseous surgery, and theoretically addresses concerns regarding the effects of osseous resection on adjacent teeth, its utilization assumes a number of conditions. The tooth must be extracted in a minimally traumatic manner with as little bone removal as possible. In addition, it is highly advantageous to utilize extraction techniques which will result in the least postoperative bone resorption and remodeling. If high-speed rotary instrumentation is necessary to effect tooth extraction, the resorptive phase of bone remodeling will be significantly increased. In such a scenario, the clinician may contemplate a two-stage procedure, performing regenerative therapy at the time of tooth removal, and placing the implant at an additional visit. Such rotary instrumentation is ideally avoided at all times. If necessary, piezosurgery is employed to help effect minimally traumatic root removal. Single-rooted teeth are always removed with a flapless technique, as will be discussed in Chapters 10 and 11. A decision is made after tooth removal as to whether or not buccal and/or palatal/lingual flap reflection are necessary.

Prior to contemplating implant placement at the time of tooth removal, the patient's biotype and the esthetic risks involved must be diagnosed and considered, as will be discussed in detail in Chapters 10 and 11. The clinician must be familiar with various osteotomy preparation and implant insertion techniques that ensure ideal implant positioning at the time of removal of single-rooted teeth. Finally, the need or lack of need for concomitant regenerative therapy, must be considered, with regard to complexity, duration, and cost of care.

In the case of multirooted teeth, it is imperative that the clinician assesses the feasibility of placing an implant in an ideal restorative position at the time of tooth removal, the need for concomitant regenerative therapy, or the necessity of performing regenerative therapy and placing the implant at a second surgical visit. These considerations significantly impact the time and cost of therapy and the decision-making process regarding selection of the appropriate treatment modality. Chapters 8 and 9 will discuss these topics in depth.

Table 1.2 Treatment options for a decayed single-rooted tooth.

Treatment option	Advantages	Disadvantages
Crown-lengthening osseous surgery with endodontic therapy, if necessary, followed by restoration	1. Tooth retention 2. Lesser cost of therapy	1. Decreased periodontal support for the treated tooth 2. Possible decreased periodontal support for adjacent teeth 3. Possible esthetic compromise
Orthodontic supereruption with crown-lengthening osseous surgery followed by restoration	1. Tooth retention 2. Lessen effects on adjacent teeth 3. Ameliorate esthetic concerns	1. Reduced periodontal support around treated tooth 2. Protracted course of care 3. Greatest cost of therapy
Tooth removal, implant placement, and restoration	1. A high degree of predictability 2. No adverse effects on adjacent teeth	1. Tooth loss 2. Slightly greater potential cost of therapy than option 1
Tooth extraction, implant placement, concomitant regenerative therapy, and subsequent restoration	1. A high degree of predictability 2. No adverse effect on adjacent teeth	1. Tooth loss 2. Greater cost of therapy than option 1 3. Slightly protracted course of therapy

The advantages and disadvantages of each treatment approach are detailed in Table 1.2.

In addition to the clinical advantages and disadvantages of the above treatment approaches, a cost-benefit analysis must be carried out to help ensure appropriate patient care (Table 1.3). Interestingly, with the exception of the introduction of supereruption or significant regenerative therapy at the time of tooth removal, the differences in therapeutic costs are not enough to warrant selection of one treatment modality over the other. Rather, the site-specific considerations previously discussed are the overriding factors in the decision-making process in these situations.

Assessment of the aforementioned clinical, temporal, and financial variables affords the ability to construct a logical decision tree for therapy when faced with a single decayed tooth (Flow chart 1.1).

Table 1.3 Cost analysis of treatment options for a decayed single-rooted tooth.

Treatment option	Cost as a factor of "X"
Crown-lengthening osseous surgery followed by restoration	2.5X
Crown-lengthening osseous surgery followed by endodontic therapy and restoration, single-rooted tooth	4.0X
Crown-lengthening osseous surgery followed by endodontic therapy and restoration, multirooted tooth	4.4X
Orthodontic supereruption followed by crown-lengthening osseous surgery and restoration	5.3X
Orthodontic supereruption followed by crown-lengthening osseous surgery, endodontic therapy, and post and core buildup, single-rooted tooth	6.8X
Tooth extraction, implant placement, and restoration with a stock abutment	4.6X
Tooth extraction, implant placement, and restoration with a custom abutment	5.1X
Tooth extraction, implant placement, regenerative therapy, and restoration with a stock abutment	5.7X–6.0X
Tooth extraction, implant placement, regenerative therapy, and restoration with a custom abutment	6.2X–6.9X

If a tooth may be easily crown lengthened without unduly compromising either adjacent teeth, its own periodontal support, or the patient's esthetic profile, and no endodontic therapy is required; it is logical to perform crown-lengthening osseous surgery and restore the tooth appropriately.

However, if either the support of the tooth to be crown lengthened or the adjacent teeth will be unduly compromised, or the esthetic treatment outcome will be unsatisfactory, the tooth should be removed and replaced with an implant. Concomitant regenerative therapy is performed if necessary.

If a tooth may be safely crown lengthened without affecting its support or that of the adjacent teeth, and patient esthetics will not be unduly compromised, but endodontic therapy will be required, it is still more logical to remove the tooth and place a single implant, assuming significant regenerative therapy will not be necessary. In such a scenario, the patient is provided with a higher degree of long-term predictability without a significant increase in the overall cost of care.

Finally, if a tooth may be safely crown lengthened without affecting its support or that of adjacent teeth, the esthetic treatment outcome will be satisfactory, and tooth extraction and implant placement will require significant regenerative therapy, the patient may be logically treated by either of the aforementioned means. In such a situation, a clinician's understanding of therapeutic potentials and treatment philosophy will often be the determining factor in treatment selection. Nevertheless, it is logical, if all three therapies will be required around a natural tooth (i.e., crown-lengthening surgery, endodontic therapy, and subsequent restoration), to remove the tooth and replace it with an implant, due to both long-term predictability and cost considerations.

The use of orthodontic supereruption followed by crown-lengthening osseous surgery and restoration, with or without endodontic therapy, is rarely indicated. The significantly protracted course and increased cost of therapy make it hard to justify such a treatment approach. However, orthodontic supereruption is often indicated in cases where it is impossible to attain an acceptable esthetic treatment outcome through crown-lengthening osseous surgery and restoration, or tooth extraction, implant placement, and restoration without orthodontic intervention to "supererupt" the interproximal and/or buccal hard and soft tissues.

Scenario Two: A Single Missing Tooth

Nowhere has the paradigm shift brought about by the advent of predictable regenerative and implant therapies been felt as strongly as in the replacement of a single missing tooth with natural teeth on either side. Available treatment options are as follows:

(a) A three-unit fixed prosthesis: The advantages cited for such a treatment approach have traditionally included the alacrity of care and the ability to avoid surgical therapy. However, the introduction of newer implant surfaces has rendered the temporal differences meaningless. Implants placed in sites where regenerative therapy is not required can predictably be restored 2–4 weeks after insertion. In situations where a single tooth is replaced, the implant is often temporized at the time of placement. The time between implant placement, impressioning, and abutment and crown insertion is the same as the time between natural tooth preparation, impression taking, and fixed prosthesis insertion. The number of visits and overall time required for restoration of a single implant are less than those required for placement of a conventional three-unit fixed splint on natural teeth, as no framework try-in is required for single implant restoration.

Proponents of three-unit fixed bridges to replace a single tooth will often cite the conditions of the adjacent teeth as a determining factor in treatment selection. While at first glance it may appear that, if the single tooth edentulous site is bordered by restored teeth on one or both sides, it would be logical to place a three-unit fixed bridge, as "virgin" teeth are not being compromised. This philosophy would appear especially cogent if one or both of the adjacent teeth required restorations.

However, a close examination of the situation demonstrates that such thinking is inherently flawed. Teeth which have been restored, or which require restoration, exhibit a higher degree of probability to need endodontic intervention. Removal of older, large restorations and underlying tooth structure often mandates endodontic intervention and core buildup prior to restoration. In addition, teeth with significant carious lesions often require endodontic therapy. The argument could be made that such teeth should be treated prophylactically with endodontics if they are to serve as abutments for fixed prostheses, so as to avoid future problems.

Numerous studies have demonstrated the inadvisability of assuming that a three-unit fixed prosthesis will predictably remain intact for 20 years or more. Should one of the abutments of a fixed prosthesis become problematic, the entire prosthesis must be replaced. However, should a single implant or the crown it supports develop problems, this site may be addressed individually. From the point of view of predictability, it is more logical to place a three-unit fixed splint utilizing "virgin" teeth as abutments, than to depend upon the teeth which have been previously restored or exhibit active carious lesions.

Clinical Example Five

A 37-year-old male presented with a severely decayed mandibular left second bicuspid (Figure 1.24). The prognosis for this tooth was very poor.

Reasonable treatment options included tooth extraction with simultaneous implant placement and eventual restoration, or tooth extraction with fabrication of a three-unit fixed splint including the first molar and first bicuspid.

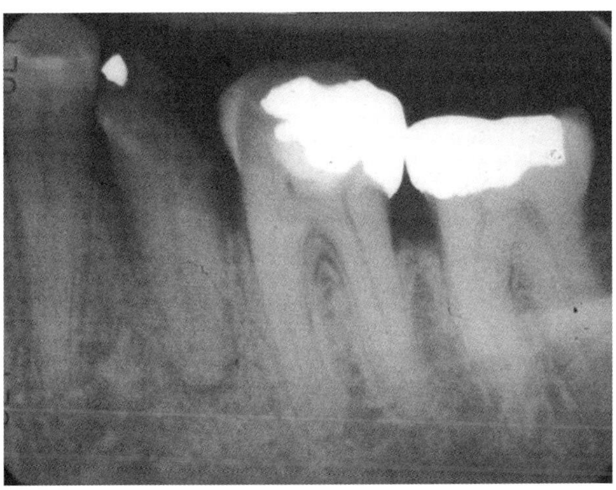

Figure 1.24 The mandibular second bicuspid is hopeless. It is best replaced with an implant abutment and crown. Placement of a three-unit fixed prosthesis would mandate endodontic therapy on the first molar.

The conventional argument would be that placement of a three-unit fixed bridge is indicated in this area, as the first molar presented with a significant amalgam restoration. However, because of this fact it is actually more logical to utilize a single implant, abutment and crown to replace the hopeless second bicuspid. Incorporation of the first molar into a three-unit fixed splint would undoubtedly result in the need for endodontic therapy on this tooth, thus increasing both the complexity and cost of care. In addition, the patient would be left with an area which would be more problematic with regard to appropriate plaque control measures.

Clinical Example Six

A 61-year-old male presented with recurrent decay around a crown on a maxillary right second bicuspid, the terminal abutment for a two-unit cantilevered fixed prosthesis (Figure 1.25). Significant osseous loss was noted around this bicuspid abutment which presented with a Class II mobility. In addition, the maxillary right first molar required crown-lengthening surgery and a new restoration.

Adequate bone remained around the maxillary right second bicuspid to maintain it following

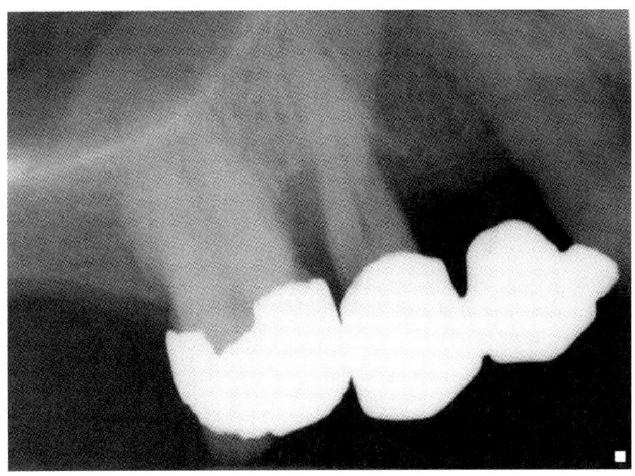

Figure 1.25 A patient presents with recurrent caries on the maxillary first molar and second bicuspid, and moderate periodontal destruction around the second bicuspid. The first bicuspid could be replaced with a fixed prosthesis. However, such therapy would almost certainly involve endodontic treatment of one or both abutments. Following periodontal therapy to rebuild damaged alveolar bone around the second bicuspid, an implant was placed in the first bicuspid position, and the implant, second bicuspid and first molar were restored with single crowns.

amelioration of excessive traumatic forces and performance of a conservative periodontal regenerative procedure. The question now became whether to replace the missing maxillary first bicuspid with an implant, abutment and crown, or through the use of a three- or four-unit fixed prosthesis including the second bicuspid and cuspid, and possibly the first molar.

If a three- or four-unit fixed prosthesis was utilized, the intact cuspid would be significantly involved. As a result, it was more logical to perform the aforementioned periodontal surgical therapy around the first molar and second bicuspid, place an implant in the position of the first bicuspid, and restore the implant, the second bicuspid and first molar with individual crowns. The end result will be greater ease of plaque control efforts and a highly predictable long-term prognosis.

From an ethical point of view, it is difficult to justify preparation of two adjacent "virgin" teeth to place a three-unit fixed splint when utilization of a single, implant abutment and crown will leave these teeth intact and uncompromised.

Patient hygiene capabilities are also enhanced when a single, implant abutment and crown are placed, as compared to a three-unit fixed splint. This fact once again offers a higher degree of long-term predictability to a single implant and crown as compared to a three-unit fixed bridge.

These rationales do not mean that implant placement is the ideal treatment of choice in all areas where a single tooth is missing and natural teeth are present on either side of the edentulous space. Specific site considerations must be assessed prior to committing to an implant therapeutic approach. The questions which must be asked include the following:

- Are the root angulations of the adjacent teeth appropriate for implant placement between them?
- Is adequate space available mesiodistally for retention of the bone and covering soft tissues between the implant and the adjacent teeth?
- Does the position of the inferior alveolar canal or the mental foramen preclude implant placement in the desired position?
- Will concomitant horizontal augmentation therapy be required to place the implant in the appropriate buccolingual position, and to ensure it is housed in bone of sufficient dimension to withstand functional forces over time?
- Can augmentation therapy be performed at the time of implant placement, or must the patient undergo two surgical sessions?
- Is sinus augmentation therapy necessary to effect appropriate implant placement?
- Can sinus augmentation therapy be performed at the time of implant placement, or must the patient undergo two surgical sessions?

The advantages and disadvantages of each treatment approach are outlined in Table 1.4.

Finally, financial assessment of each treatment option must be carried out to ensure the

Table 1.4 Treatment options for a single missing tooth in a tooth-bounded space.

Treatment option	Advantages	Disadvantages
Three-unit fixed bridge	1. Avoid surgical therapy 2. Avoid vital structures 3. Eliminate the need for regenerative therapy 4. Slightly lesser cost of therapy than implant placement and restoration, if no endodontic therapy is required on abutment teeth	1. Involvement of adjacent teeth 2. Potential for endodontic therapy 3. Greater cost of treatment if endodontic therapy is required 4. More difficult to perform adequate home care
Implant placement and restoration with a stock abutment and crown	1. No involvement of adjacent teeth 2. Greater ease of home care 3. Greater long-term predictability	1. Need to avoid vital structures 2. Potential need for regenerative therapy 3. Possibility of second surgical visit

Table 1.5 Cost analysis of treatment options for a single missing tooth in a tooth-bounded space.

Treatment option	Cost as a factor of "X"
Three-unit fixed bridge	4.1X
Three-unit fixed bridge with endodontic therapy and buildup on one abutment	5.6X–6.0X
Three-unit fixed bridge with endodontic therapy and buildups on two abutments	7.1X–7.5X
Implant placement with a stock abutment and crown	4.3X
Implant placement, regeneration, stock abutment and crown	5.0X–6.4X

patient is attaining the greatest monetary benefit from the care to be delivered (Table 1.5).

Once these factors have been taken into consideration, a simple, logical decision tree may be formulated (Flow chart 1.2).

Scenario Three: Multiple Missing Adjacent Posterior Teeth

A long span fixed prosthesis, defined as a prosthesis with more than one adjacent pontic, is rarely indicated due to the advent of predictable regenerative and implant therapies. Utilization of such a long span prosthesis represents a significant compromise in patient hygiene capabilities and long-term predictability of therapy. The increased stresses placed upon the abutment teeth in these scenarios result in an unacceptably high incidence of abutment and hence prosthesis failure. In addition, flexure of the prosthesis over time often leads to cement washout and recurrent caries beneath the crowns on the abutment teeth. As a result, the biomechanical prognosis is very poor.

The only indications for such a prosthesis are in situations where the positions of vital structures, combined with severe ridge atrophy, render appropriate implant placement impossible, even following extensive regenerative therapy. It must be cautioned that the clinician should not accept such a diagnosis too quickly. Simple, predictable regenerative techniques are available to sufficiently augment all but the most atrophic ridge. This fact, combined with the utilization of shorter implants with specific designs, makes it rare to encounter a site which may not be rendered suitable for implant reconstructive therapy, as will be seen in Chapters 2 and 7.

The only other rationale for placing a long-span fixed prosthesis instead of an implant-supported prosthesis is a patient who is medically unable to undergo any type of oral surgical procedure. Once again, such situations are rare.

Scenario Four: A Missing Maxillary First Molar, When the Second Molar Is Present

The reduced success rates of smooth surface threaded implants in the maxillary posterior region initially led clinicians to avoid such therapy, and place conventional fixed prostheses to replace missing maxillary first molars. However, rough surface implants of various topographies and formulations have demonstrated short- and long-term success rates equal to those of osseointegrated implants in other areas of the mouth. As a result, the maxillary posterior region must no longer be viewed as an undesirable site for implant reconstructive therapy. The decision as to whether to place a single implant abutment and crown or a three-unit fixed splint should be grounded in previously discussed considerations, including length and cost of therapy and long-term predictability of care.

As previously detailed, the belief that a three-unit fixed bridge is indicated over an implant abutment and crown when one or both of the adjacent teeth are either restored or require restoration, is a fallacy. The opposite is true. When the planned abutment teeth require removal of large older restorations, or treatment of significant caries lesions, the incidence of endodontic therapy increases dramatically, as do the complexity and cost of care. Significant involvement of the planned abutment teeth is actually an indication for placement of a single implant, abutment and crown rather than a three-unit fixed prosthesis.

In addition to the already discussed compromise of greater difficulty in performing adequate home care measures around a three-unit fixed bridge as compared to a restored implant, the suitability of a maxillary second molar to serve as a terminal abutment for a fixed prosthesis must be considered. The root morphology of the maxillary second molar is often conical and/or fused. In addition, care must be taken to ensure that a distal wedge periodontal surgical procedure is performed, if necessary, to eliminate redundant soft tissues on the distal aspect of the maxillary second molar. Failure to do so will result in a short preparation wall and a compromise in crown retention, and a milieu which will pose a further difficulty in plaque control efforts. When faced with such a short preparation wall, the clinician must choose between two unacceptable treatment options. Either the preparation extends further subgingivally, often encountering undercuts in the anatomy of the tooth, or the restoration ignores these undercuts as it extends subgingivally, resulting in a restorative overhang in the furcation area. If the preparation does not extend in this manner, the final restoration will have a short axial wall, resulting in cement washout and prosthetic failure.

The question of which therapeutic approach to adopt usually hinges upon the need or lack of need for concomitant or prior regenerative therapy, and the extent of the regenerative therapy which will be required. In order to fully address this topic, an in-depth discussion must be carried out regarding various treatment approaches for augmentation of the posterior maxilla, the indications for each treatment approach, and the minimum implant lengths suitable in maxillary posterior reconstructive scenarios. This discussion is the focus of Chapter 6.

In summary, the treatment options available for replacement of a missing maxillary first molar when the second molar is present are as follows:

(a) A three-unit fixed splint with endodontic therapy if required.
(b) Placement of a single implant without concomitant regenerative therapy. The implant is subsequently restored with a stock abutment and crown.
(c) Placement of a single implant with osteotome therapy. The implant is subsequently restored with a stock abutment and crown.
(d) Placement of a single implant with concomitant sinus augmentation therapy. The implant is subsequently restored with a stock abutment and crown.
(e) Placement of a single implant with concomitant sinus augmentation and buccal ridge augmentation. The implant is subsequently restored with a stock abutment and crown.
(f) Osteotome therapy followed by implant placement in a second stage surgery, and subsequent restoration with a stock abutment and crown.
(g) Sinus augmentation therapy, with concomitant buccal augmentation therapy if necessary, followed by implant placement at a second stage surgery, and subsequent restoration with a stock abutment and crown.

While the focus of the present discussion is not when to select a given regenerative therapy, the above outline allows comparisons to be made between three-unit fixed prostheses, implant placement and restoration, and regenerative and implant therapies followed by implant restoration (Tables 1.6 and 1.7).

A cost-benefit analysis of each treatment option is offered in Flow chart 1.3.

If no augmentation therapy is necessary, both clinical and financial determinants point to the most logical option as being that of implant placement and restoration with a stock abutment and crown. Even when an osteotome lift must be performed at the time of implant placement, it is inappropriate to look toward a three-unit fixed bridge. The performance of a concomitant osteotome procedure is atraumatic and adds at most 3–5 minutes to the overall time of the surgical visit.

Should simultaneous sinus augmentation therapy (with or without concomitant buccal ridge augmentation therapy) be required at the time of implant placement, the clinician's clinical philosophy and facility with various procedures will most likely dictate the chosen course of therapy. Performed appropriately, a sinus augmentation procedure takes 15–20 minutes and is not problematic for the patient either during the course of treatment or postoperatively. If such augmentation can be accomplished at the time of implant placement, the most ideal therapeutic approach is still implant utilization as opposed to a three-unit fixed bridge. However, if the treating clinician is not fluent in sinus augmentation procedures, and

Table 1.6 Treatment options for a missing maxillary first molar.

Treatment option	Advantages	Disadvantages
Three-unit fixed bridge	1. Avoid potential regenerative therapy 2. Slightly lesser cost of therapy 3. Significantly lesser cost of therapy if regenerative therapy is required for implant placement	1. Possible need for endodontic intervention 2. Greater difficulty in plaque control efforts 3. Potential need for periodontal surgical therapy on the second molar 4. Second molar is often ill suited to serve as a terminal abutment
Implant placement without regenerative therapy followed by restoration with a stock abutment and crown	1. No involvement of adjacent teeth 2. No need for endodontic therapy 3. Greater ease of plaque control efforts 4. Greater long-term predictability	1. Slightly higher cost of therapy than a three-unit fixed bridge without endodontic therapy
Implant placement with concomitant osteotome use followed by restoration with a stock abutment and crown	1. No involvement of adjacent teeth 2. No need for endodontic therapy 3. Greater ease of plaque control efforts 4. Greater long-term predictability	1. Slightly higher cost of therapy than a three-unit fixed bridge without endodontic therapy
Implant placement with concomitant sinus augmentation therapy followed by restoration with a stock abutment and crown	1. No involvement of adjacent teeth 2. No need for endodontic therapy 3. Greater ease of plaque control efforts 4. Greater long-term predictability	1. Greater cost of therapy than a three-unit fixed bridge without endodontic therapy
Sinus augmentation therapy followed by implant placement at a second surgical visit followed by restoration with a stock abutment and crown	1. No involvement of adjacent teeth 2. No need for endodontic therapy 3. Greater ease of plaque control efforts 4. Greater long-term predictability	1. Greater cost of therapy than a three-unit fixed bridge without endodontic therapy 2. Need for a second surgical visit

Table 1.7 Cost analysis of treatment options for a missing maxillary first molar.

Treatment option	Cost as a factor of "X"
Three-unit fixed bridge	4.1X
Three-unit fixed bridge with crown-lengthening surgery	5.2X
Three-unit fixed bridge with one endodontic therapy	5.0X–5.4X
Three-unit fixed bridge with two endodontic therapies	6.3X
Implant placement and restoration with a stock abutment and crown	4.3X
Implant placement with concomitant osteotome therapy and restoration with a stock abutment and crown	4.3X
Implant placement with concomitant sinus augmentation therapy and restoration with a stock abutment and crown	6.8X
Sinus augmentation therapy followed by implant placement at a second surgical visit and restoration with a stock abutment and crown	6.8X

views them as a major surgical event, a three-unit fixed bridge will be chosen as the appropriate therapy. Unfortunately, such an approach would leave the patient with the aforementioned compromises, and a lesser degree of long-term predictability than sinus augmentation, implant placement, and restoration.

Should endodontic therapy be required on one or more of the abutment teeth, sinus augmentation with simultaneous implant placement would be the appropriate course of therapy, from both clinical and financial points of view.

However, should sinus augmentation therapy have to be performed in a surgical visit prior to the time of implant placement, and should no endodontic therapy be required on the abutment teeth, a three-unit fixed splint is the therapeutic modality of choice, assuming the second molar is well suited to serve as a terminal abutment for a three-unit fixed bridge. Such an approach will eliminate the need for the patient to undergo two surgical sessions, and a protracted course of therapy. Before deciding upon this treatment approach, it is important to truly assess the need or lack of need for a separate sinus augmentation procedure, and to have a thorough understanding of the capabilities of implants of various lengths in replacing single missing maxillary posterior teeth.

Eliminating less predictable therapies through implant use

The predictability of regenerative and implant therapies affords the opportunity to avoid higher stress, less predictable treatment alternatives.

Long span fixed prostheses are rarely considered, and posterior cantilevers are never employed in fixed prosthetic situations. Distal cantilevers in posterior regions are only utilized when fabricating hybrid prostheses in edentulous arches.

Clinical Example Seven

A 36-year-old male presented with an inability to wear a maxillary removable partial prosthesis, and esthetic concerns regarding missing teeth in the maxillary bicuspid regions.

A full arch fixed splint was fabricated, employing two distal cantilevers in the maxillary right quadrant and one distal cantilever in the maxillary

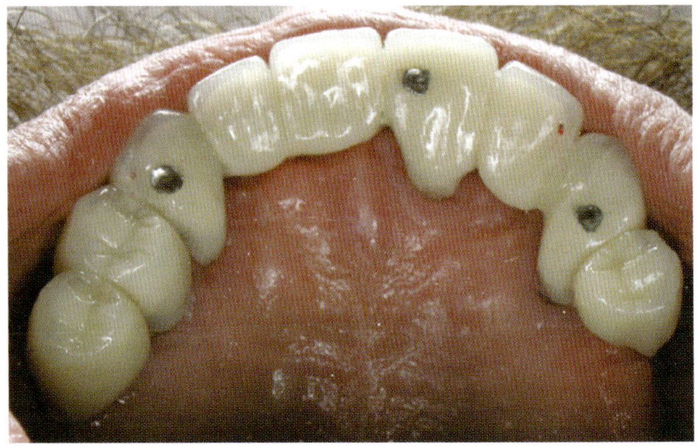

Figure 1.28 A temporary fixed prosthesis has been placed on three of the remaining maxillary teeth. Note the metal occlusal stops in the prosthesis, at the sites of the abutment teeth.

left quadrant. These cantilevers were not in contact with the opposing dentition and only served an esthetic purpose.

The patient was stable for over 10 years (Figure 1.26). Subsequently, the patient moved out of the area and another practitioner reconstructed the mandibular arch, with a cantilevered posterior fixed prostheses, which occluded with the maxillary cantilevers already in place (Figure 1.27). Within one year of this therapy being completed, accelerated bone loss and root fractures were noted around the maxillary abutments, undoubtedly due to the greater forces being placed upon them.

As the patient refused to wear a removable prosthesis at any time during therapy, treatment proceeded as follows: A maxillary temporary fixed splint was fabricated which was supported by three of the remaining maxillary teeth (Figure 1.28). Metal stops were evident on the temporary fixed prosthesis at the sites of the abutment teeth.

All other maxillary teeth were extracted and implants were placed. Subsequent to osseointegration of these implants, an impression was taken and an implant-supported temporary fixed prosthesis was fabricated. The remaining natural teeth were extracted, additional implants were placed, and the temporary prosthesis was inserted. Following completion of osseointegration, impressions were taken and a full arch, implant-supported fixed prosthesis was fabricated (Figure 1.29). No angled abutments were necessary, and all screw holes exited the prosthesis in ideal positions. A buccal clinical view of the prosthesis in place demonstrates the

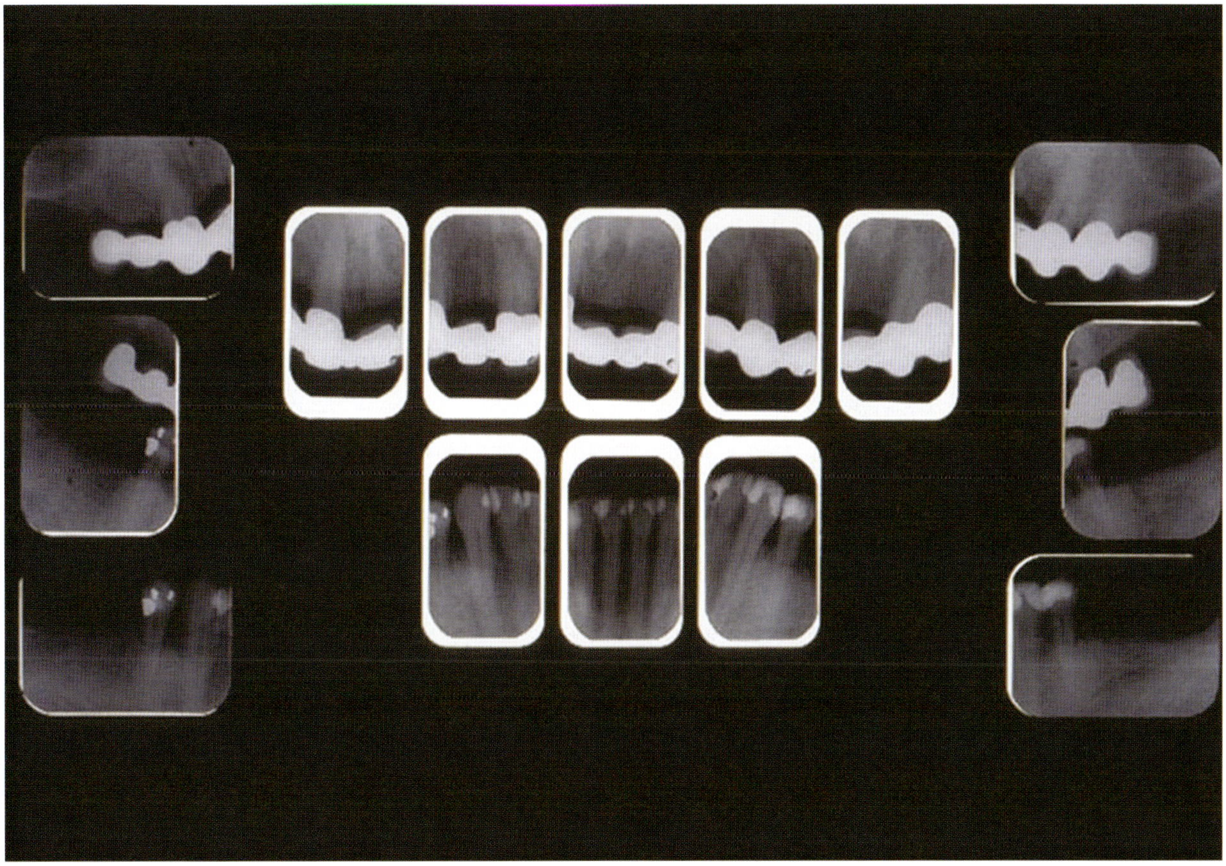

Figure 1.26 A patient has been reconstructed with a maxillary fixed prosthesis which includes two cantilevers in the maxillary right quadrant and one cantilever in the maxillary left quadrant. These cantilevers are not in function.

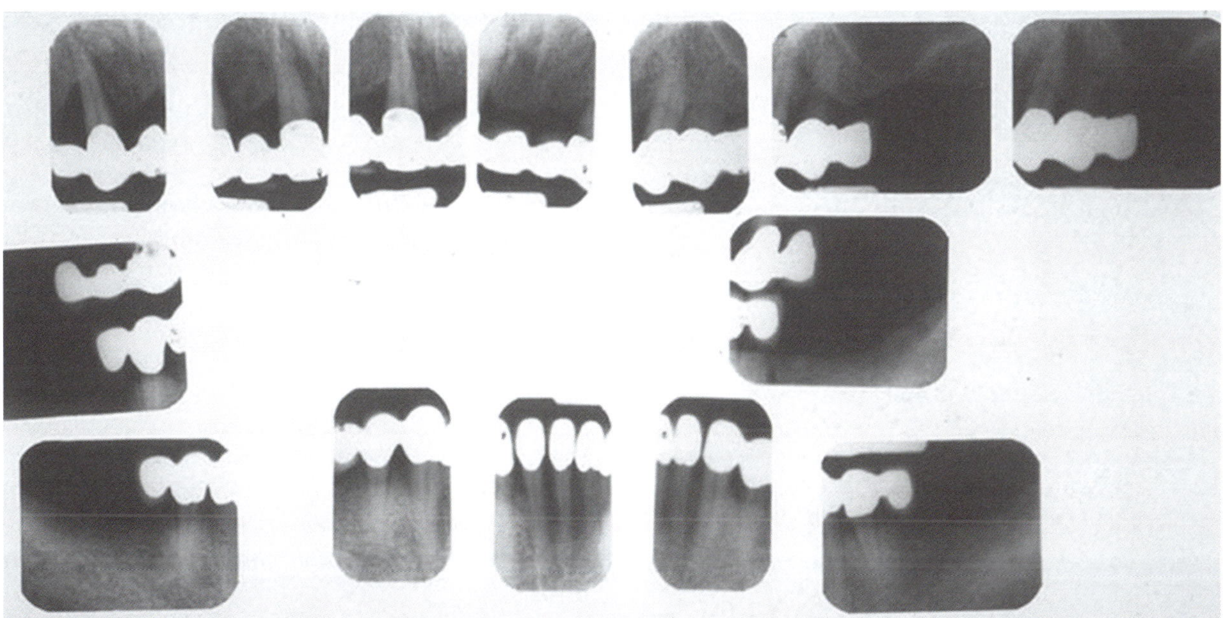

Figure 1.27 After more than 10 years of stability, a subsequent practitioner placed a mandibular fixed prosthesis with cantilevers which occluded with the maxillary cantilevers. Within one year of its placement, the maxillary abutments demonstrated accelerated periodontal destruction and root fractures.

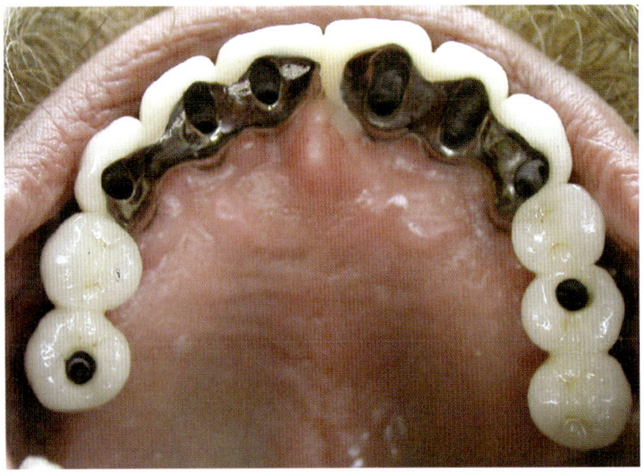

Figure 1.29 Following sequential implant placement and temporization, the final maxillary fixed prosthesis has been inserted. Note the ideal positions of the screw holes in the prosthesis.

patient's satisfaction with the esthetic outcomes of therapy (Figure 1.30).

The influence of patient health on treatment plan selection:

It is critical that the roles played by various systemic diseases and/or patient factors in the healing and long-term predictability of different treatment approaches be well understood. Should any questions arise, the patient's physicians must always be consulted.

Numerous comprehensive texts are available which discuss this topic in depth. There is no need to regurgitate the information here.

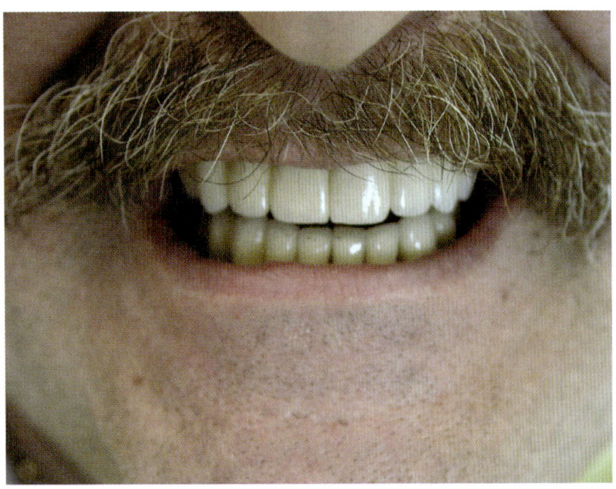

Figure 1.30 A buccal clinical view demonstrates the patient's esthetic satisfaction.

However, there are three common health concerns clinicians face every day, which are often misunderstood.

1. **Diabetes:** The presence of diabetes is not an absolute contraindication to therapy. The literature has demonstrated that success rates of regenerative and implant therapies in well controlled diabetics are essentially identical to those reported upon in nondiabetic patients (148). The problem arises in defining a controlled diabetic. Ideally, a consultation with the patient's physician should yield the information that the patient in question has had his or her diabetes under control for a minimum of one year. If this is not the case, it is prudent to have the patient demonstrate this level of control prior to the initiation of regenerative and/or implant therapies.
2. **Intravenous bisphosphonates:** Intravenous bisphosphonates (BIS), which are used to reduce bone pain and hypercalcemia of malignancy, have been linked with spontaneous bisphosphonate-associated osteonecrosis (BON). The ramifications of such problems are often severe and must be viewed as an absolute contraindication to periodontal or implant surgical therapy, unless the patient presents with an acute situation requiring intervention. Patients with a history of intravenous BIS therapy must be treated with care, as the potential for development of severe BON is significant. Current dental protocols suggested by Marx for patients who will receive or are receiving intravenous BIS therapy include:

   Before initiating intravenous BIS therapy:
   Due to the recognized high level of comorbidity of dental diseases with BIS therapy (84% of the patients followed by Marx and coworkers demonstrated periodontal disease, and 28.6% of these patients demonstrated dental caries), it is imperative that appropriate dental examination and diagnosis be carried out before the initiation of BIS therapy. Once a thorough examination with radiographs has been accomplished, necessary treatment is aimed at eliminating periodontal disease, active caries, and endodontic lesions, thus helping ensure that invasive dental procedures will not be

necessary in the near future. Dental implants should not be placed in these patients. The fit of all existing prostheses must be checked, and the prostheses adjusted or replaced as necessary to minimize trauma to underlying hard and soft tissues. Where possible, removable prostheses should be replaced with fixed appliances. Finally, a thorough prophylaxis should be performed before the initiation of BIS therapy, and the patient should be placed on a comprehensive four-month maintenance schedule to ensure their continued periodontal and restorative health.

During intravenous BIS therapy: Patients should be seen by their periodontist and restorative dentist so that the dental team can evaluate the oral cavity for the presence or absence of the aforementioned diseases and/or ill-fitting prostheses, and ensure that no exposed bone is present. A dental cleaning and fluoride treatment should be carried out, and the patient should be placed on a four-month maintenance schedule to ensure continued periodontal and restorative health. Teeth should only be extracted as a last resort. Nonrestorable teeth should be prepared to the gingiva and have their pulps extirpated, as such therapy is less risky than tooth extraction. Teeth with mild to moderate mobilities should be splinted together rather than removed. Teeth with extreme mobility should be extracted, as osteonecrosis is probably already present and merely hidden by the granulation tissue at the apex of the highly mobile tooth. Once extraction is carried out, appropriate measures must be taken with regard to debridement, tissue management, and antibiotic coverage to help minimize the risk of developing further osteonecrosis. Implants should not be placed in these patients. If BIS-induced osteonecrosis does occur, it is important to realize that such osteonecrosis may not be successfully treated by the modalities utilized for treatment of osteoradionecrosis, such as hyperbaric oxygen. Rather, efforts must be made to control infection and render palliative treatment to patients in the areas of the exposed bone.

3. **Oral BIS:** Oral BIS, which are utilized in the treatment of osteoporosis and osteopenia, are of relatively widespread use in postmenopausal females. Twenty-two million prescriptions for one of the oral BIS (Alendronate) were written between May 2003 and April 2004 alone.

   The question is whether or not oral BIS use predisposes a patient to the development of BON. This issue came to light following publications by Marx and coworkers (149) and Migliorati and coworkers (150). Each of these reports documented patients who had been taking oral BIS and demonstrated BON. It is important to realize that the patients in both of these studies had been referred to the institutions in question, thus making it impossible to assess the size of the patient pool taking oral BIS from which these patients were drawn. As a result, no statements could be made regarding the incidence of problems following tooth extraction in patients taking oral BIS, based wholly upon these studies.

   Jeffcoat (151), in a single masked controlled study, assessed the response of patients taking oral BIS for 1–4 years with a mean time of 3 years who received implant therapy, compared to age-matched controls taking no oral BIS. Three years postimplant placement, no implants had been lost and no BON had been reported in the 25 patients taking oral BIS. A recent study conducted in two private practices (152) evaluated 61 patients taking oral BIS for 1–5 years with a mean time of 3.3 years, who had implants placed in intact ridges or at the time of tooth extraction. None of these patients demonstrated complications post therapy. All implants were functioning successfully by the Albrektsson criteria 12–24 months postinsertion.

   Both of these studies seem to indicate that, in appropriately treated patients, a history of oral BIS does not increase the incidence of postoperative osteonecrosis or other complications. However, no definitive control studies have been published on this point. Naturally, prior to initiating therapy, patients must be informed of the likely risks and benefits of care. It is important to be cognizant of this history and to treat such patients in an appropriate manner.

Certain comorbidities may increase the chances of BON. Poor plaque control, a smoking habit, endodontic or carious pathologies, and overlying removable prostheses have all been implicated in the development of BON in patients with a history of oral BIS use. A recent article by Levin et al. (153) presented a patient with a history of oral BIS use who was wearing a maxillary removable partial prosthesis. This patient developed severe BON in the area of impingement of the prosthesis on the underlying hard and soft tissues.

In addition to eliminating the aforementioned pathological or habitual comorbidities, patients benefit greatly from removing the torqueing forces of distal extension removable prosthesis from underlying hard and soft tissues. This may be especially true in patients with a history or oral BIS use.

All too often implant therapies are viewed as an all or none scenario. A patient is either a "full implant patient" or is "not an implant patient." Such an artificial dichotomy does a disservice to our patients. Implants may be very predictably utilized to improve patient treatment plans without the substantial temporal and financial commitments commensurate with full mouth reconstructions.

Placement of individual implants in areas of a removable prosthesis' distal extensions affords a number of advantages:

- Prosthetic retention is improved.
- The need to clasp anterior teeth to provide retention is significantly decreased or eliminated, thus improving the prognoses of these teeth.
- The prosthesis rests upon the implants rather than the hard and soft tissues, thus lessening bone atrophy beneath the prosthesis.
- The lever arm of the prosthesis is significantly reduced both immediately and over time. The immediate reduction in lever arm forces is obvious. However, continued prosthesis use in a distal extension situation results in bone atrophy and further rotation and levering of the removable prosthesis in the absence of implants. Utilization of a single implant in each distal extension area significantly lessens this problem.

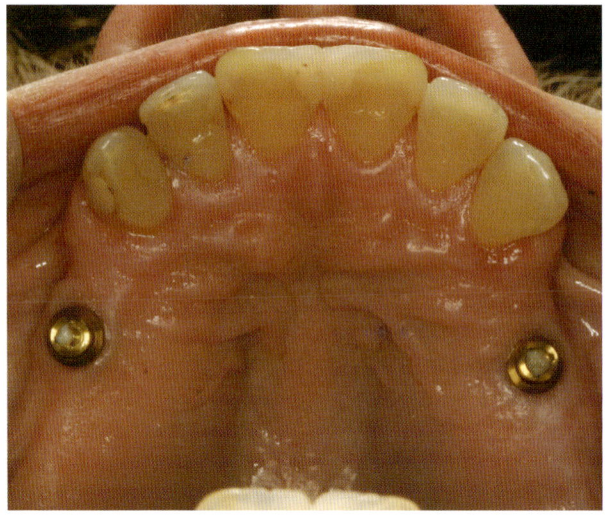

Figure 1.31 Implants have been placed in each distal extension area and restored with locator attachments.

A 51-year-old patient presented with a distal extension removable partial prosthesis. One implant was placed in each distal extension area. Locator attachments were utilized to help support the removable partial prosthesis, thus providing increased retention, and ameliorating the destructive lever arms of the distal extension prosthesis (Figures 1.31 and 1.32).

Early work suggests that the risk of development of BON may be assessed through a CTX blood test. Marx and coworkers (154) have noted a correlation between CTX blood test values and the development of postoperative complications in patients taking oral BIS.

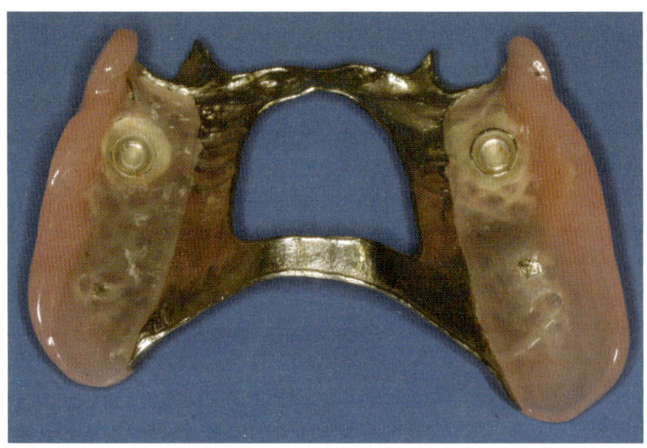

Figure 1.32 A view of the "female" components in the removable partial prosthesis.

They have proposed that a patient with a CTX value higher than 150 is at a minimal risk; a patient with a value between 100 and 150 is at moderate risk; and a patient with a CTX blood test value less than 100 is at a high risk for developing postoperative complications. However, the validity of this proposal has not yet been established through large-scale studies. While the need for further research and data regarding incidence of complications and suggested treatment protocols for intravenous and oral BIS patient is obvious, the available literature would point to the need for absolute care when treating patients with a history of intravenous BIS use, and comprehensive but undeterred care when treating patients with a history of oral BIS use.

4. **Smoking:** Smoking is not an absolute contraindication to regenerative or implant therapies. Nevertheless, the literature has demonstrated that various thresholds of smoking are more deleterious to short- and long-term treatment outcomes. A reasonable suggestion is that patients reduce their smoking habit to less than 10 cigarettes per day prior to any type of implant or regenerative therapy. No sinus augmentation, other than osteotome use, is carried out in patients who smoke. The desired level of smoking reduction or cessation must be attained and maintained for a minimum of three months prior to the initiation of therapy and a minimum of three months post-therapy.
5. **Parafunctional habits:** The forces generated from such habits significantly increase the chances of implant and/or prosthetic failure. The biological ramifications of such force application have been well established with regard to bone loss and eventual implant disintegration. Prosthetic failures as a result of biomechanical inability to withstand such excessive force application have been documented throughout the literature.

Significant time should be spent with the patient discussing concerns regarding uncontrolled diabetes, smoking, and other systemic conditions. Efforts should be made at behavioral modification rather than chastisement. It is illogical to tell a patient who has been smoking 20–30 cigarettes a day for decades that he or she "must stop completely." It is much more effective to work with this patient in an effort to decrease smoking to a level below 10 cigarettes per day. More often than not the clinician will find that the patient continues to decrease his or her smoking level until the habit ceases all together.

Conclusions

Claims of therapeutic success, regardless of the treatment modality employed, demand the ability to answer the following questions in the affirmative:

- Is the patient better off than before undergoing therapy?
- Has the longevity of the teeth been extended where practical and in the best interests of the patient?
- When natural teeth are to be maintained, has the longevity of the teeth been extended for as long as therapeutically possible?
- If regenerative and/or implant reconstructive therapies have been carried out, have they been utilized in the best interests of the patient, and in a manner by which to ensure maximization of long-term treatment outcomes?

Patients are human beings who have come to us and entrust us to provide appropriate care for them. The challenge facing the conscientious clinician today is not that of mastering available techniques. Such mastery is easily attained through education and practice. The challenge we all must meet is the determination of when to perform which therapy for an individual patient, in a given situation.

References

1. Fugazzotto PA. 1999. Guided tissue regeneration: Maximizing clinical results. *Compend Cont Dent Educ* 6(Suppl):1–42.
2. Caffesse RG. 1989. *Resective Procedures*. Chicago, IL: American Academy of Periodontology. Proceedings of the World Workshop in Clinical Periodontics.
3. Waerhaug J. 1978. Healing of the dento-epithelial junction following subgingival plaque control. II: As observed on extracted teeth. *J Periodontol* 49:119–134.

4. Stambaugh RV, Dragoo M, Smith DM, and Carosali L. 1981. The limits of subgingival scaling. *Int J Periodontics Restorative Dent* 1(5):30–42.
5. Buchanan S and Robertson P. 1987. Calculus removal by scaling/root planing with and without surgical access. *J Periodontol* 58:163.
6. Jones WA and O'Leary TJ. 1978. The effectiveness of root planing in removing bacterial endotoxin from the roots of periodontally involved teeth. *J Periodontol* 49:337–342.
7. Rabbani GM, Ash MM, and Caffesse RG. 1981. The effectiveness of subgingival scaling and root planing in calculus removal. *J Periodontol* 52:119–123.
8. Caffesse R, Sweeney PL, and Smith BA. 1986. Scaling and root planing with and without periodontal flap surgery. *J Clin Periodontol* 13:205–210.
9. Tabita PV, Bissada NF, and Maybury JE. 1981. Effectiveness of supragingival plaque control on the development of subgingival plaque and gingival inflammation in patients with moderate pocket depth. *J Periodontol* 52:88–93.
10. Waerhaug J and Steen E. 1952. The presence or absence of bacteria in the gingival pocket and the reaction in healthy pockets to certain pure cultures. *Odontol Tidsk* 60:1–24.
11. Stahl SS. 1965. Healing of gingival tissues following various therapeutic regimens—a review of histologic studies. *J Oral Ther Pharmacol* 2:145–160.
12. Morris M. 1954. The removal of pocket and attachment epithelium in humans: A histologic study. *J Periodontol* 25:7–11.
13. Smukler HM and Landsberg J. 1984. The toothbrush and gingival traumatic injury. *J Periodontol* 55:713–719.
14. Nevins M. 1982. Interproximal periodontal disease—the embrasure as an etiologic factor. *Int J Periodontics Restorative Dent* 2(6):9–27.
15. Fugazzotto PA. 1989. *Preparation of the Periodontium for Restorative Dentistry*. St Louis: Ishiyaku EuroAmerica, pp. 44–54.
16. Ochsenbein C. 1986. A primer for osseous surgery. *Int J Periodontics Restorative Dent* 6(1):8–46.
17. Johnson RL. 1979. Osseous surgery in periodontal therapy. In: Prichard JF (ed), *The Diagnosis and Treatment of Periodontal Disease in General Dental Practice*. Philadelphia: The W.B. Saunders.
18. Fugazzotto PA and Parma-Benfenati S. 1984. Preprosthetic periodontal considerations. Crown length and biologic width. *Quintessence Int* 15:1247–1256.
19. Gelfand HB, Tencate AR, and Freeman E. 1978. The keratinization potential of crevicular epithelium: An experimental study. *J Periodontol* 49:113–118.
20. Caffesse RG, Karring T, and Nasjleti CE. 1977. Keratinizing potential of sulcular epithelium. *J Periodontol* 48:140–146.
21. Caffesse RG and Nasjleti CE. 1976. Enzymatic penetration through intact sulcular epithelium. *J Periodontol* 47:391–397.
22. Thilander H. 1963. The effect of leukocytic enzymes activity on the structure of the gingival pocket epithelium in man. *Acta Odontol Scand* 21:431–451.
23. Rosenberg MM, Kay HB, Keough BE, and Holt RL. 1988. *Periodontal and Prosthetic Management for Advanced Cases*. Chicago: Quintessence, pp. 148–156.
24. Matherson DG. 1988. An evaluation of healing following periodontal osseous surgery in Rhesus monkeys. *Int J Periodontics Restorative Dent* 8(5):9–34.
25. Squier CA. 1981. Keratinization of the sulcular epithelium—a pointless pursuit. *J Periodontol* 52:426–429.
26. Schroeder HE and Munzel-Pedrazzoli S. 1970. Morphometric analysis comparing junctional and oral epithelium of normal human gingiva. *Helv Odontol Acta* 14:53–66.
27. Barnett ML. 1979. Letter to the editor. *J Periodontol* 50:154.
28. Saito I, Watanabe O, Kawahara H, Igarashi Y, Yamamura T, Shimono M. 1981. Intercellular junctions and the permeability barrier in the junctional epithelium. A study with freeze-fracture and thin sectioning. *J Periodontal Res* 16:467–480.
29. Shimono M and Clementi F. 1976. Intercellular junctions of oral epithelium. I. Studies with freeze-fracture and tracing methods of normal rat keratinized oral epithelium. *J Ultrastruct Res* 56:121–136.
30. Claude P and Goodenough DA. 1973. Fracture faces of zonulae occludentes from "tight" and "leaky" epithelia. *J Cell Biol* 58:390–400.
31. Shimono M, Yamamura Y, and Fumagalli G. 1980. Intercellular junctions in salivary glands: Freeze-fracture and tracer studies of normal rat sublingual gland. *J Ultrastruct Res* 72:286–299.
32. McDougall WA. 1971. Penetration pathways of a topically applied foreign protein into rat gingiva. *J Periodontal Res* 6:89–99.
33. McDougall WA. 1970. Pathways of penetration and effects of horseradish peroxidase in rat molar gingiva. *Arch Oral Biol* 15:621–633.
34. Tolo KJ. 1971. A study of permeability of gingival pocket epithelium to albumin in guinea pigs and Norwegian pigs. *Arch Oral Biol* 16:881–888.
35. Romanowski AW, Squier CA, and Lesch CA. 1988. Permeability of rodent junctional epithelium to exogenous protein. *J Periodontal Res* 23:81–86.
36. Neiders ME. 1972. Contact phenomena of epithelial cells. *Sci Rev* 1:69–101.
37. Listgarten MA. 1975. Similarity of epithelial relationships in the gingiva of rat and man. *J Periodontol* 46:677–680.

38. Listgarten MA. 1980. Periodontal probing: What does it mean? *J Clin Periodontol* 7:165–176.
39. Saglie R, Johansen JR, and Flotra L. 1975. The zone of completely and partially destructed periodontal fibers in pathological pockets. *J Clin Periodontol* 2: 198–202.
40. Spray JR, Garnick JJ, Doles LR, and Klawitter JJ. 1978. Microscopic demonstration of the position of periodontal probes. *J Periodontol* 49:148–152.
41. Silvertson JF and Burgett FG. 1976. Probing of pockets related to the attachment level. *J Periodontol* 47:281–286.
42. Powell B and Garnick JJ. 1978. The use of extracted teeth to evaluate clinical measurements of periodontal disease. *J Periodontol* 49:621–624.
43. Spray R and Garnick JJ. 1979. Position of probes in human periodontal pockets. *J Dent Res* 58(Special Issue A):176. Abstract No. 331.
44. Hancock EB, Wirthlin MR, and Ellingson J. 1978. Histologic assessment of periodontal probes in normal gingiva. *J Dent Res* 57(Special Issue A):239. Abstract No. 584.
45. Ezis I and Burgett F. 1978. Probing related to attachment levels on recently erupted teeth. *J Dent Res* 57(Special Issue A):307. Abstract No. 932.
46. Page RC and Schroeder HE. 1976. Pathogenesis of inflammatory periodontal disease. A summary of current work. *Lab Invest* 33:235–249.
47. Ruben MP, Schulman SM, and Kon S. 1973. Healing of periodontal surgical wounds. In: Goldman HM and Cohen DW (eds), *Periodontal Therapy*, 5th edn. St Louis: CV Mosby Company.
48. Parma-Benfenati S, Fugazzotto PA, and Ruben MP. 1985. The effect of restorative margins on the postsurgical development and nature of the periodontium. *Int J Periodontics Restorative Dent* 5(6):31–51.
49. Carnevale G, Sterrantino SF, and DiFebo G. 1983. Soft and hard tissue wound healing following tooth preparation to the alveolar crest. *Int J Periodontics Restorative Dent* 3(6):37–53.
50. Vieira E, O'Leary T, and Kafrawy A. 1982. The effect of sodium hypochlorite and citric acid solutions on healing of periodontal pockets. *J Periodontol* 53:71–80.
51. Caton J, Nyman S, and Zander H. 1980. Histometric evaluation of periodontal surgery. II. Connective tissue attachment levels after four regenerative procedures. *J Clin Periodontol* 7:224–231.
52. Kalkwarf K, Tussing G, and Davis M. 1982. Histologic evaluation of gingival curettage facilitated by sodium hypochlorite solution. *J Periodontol* 53:63–70.
53. Yukna R. 1976. A clinical and histologic study of healing following the excisional new attachment procedure in Rhesus monkeys. *J Periodontol* 47:701–709.
54. Yukna R and Lawrence J. 1980. Gingival surgery for soft tissue new attachment. *Dent Clin North Am* 24:705–718.
55. Bowen W, Bowers G, Bergquist J, and Organ R. 1981. Removal of pocket epithelium in humans utilizing an internally beveled incision. *Int J Periodontics Restorative Dent* 1(5):9–19.
56. Froum W, Coran J, Thaller B, et al. 1982. Periodontal healing following open debridement flap procedures. I. Clinical assessment of soft tissue and osseous repair. *J Periodontol* 53:8–14.
57. Caton J and Zander H. 1976. Osseous repair of an infrabony pocket without new attachment of connective tissue. *J Clin Periodontol* 47:54–62.
58. Hiatt W, Schallhorn R, and Aaronian A. 1978. The induction of new bone and cementum formation. IV. Microscopic examination of the periodontium following human bone and marrow allograft, autograft, and nongraft periodontal regeneration procedures. *J Periodontol* 49:495–512.
59. Egelberg J. 1987. Regeneration and repair of periodontal tissues. *J Periodontal Res* 22:233–242.
60. Wirthlin MR. 1981. The current status of new attachment therapy. *J Periodontol* 52:529–544.
61. Listgarten M and Rosenberg M. 1979. Histological study of repair following new attachment procedures in human periodontal lesions. *J Periodontol* 50:333–344.
62. Ellagaard B, Karring T, Listgarten M, and Loe H. 1973. New attachment after treatment of interradicular lesions. *J Periodontol* 44:209–217.
63. Stahl S, Froum S, and Kushner L. 1982. Periodontal healing following open debridement flap procedures. II. Histologic observations. *J Periodontol* 53: 15–21.
64. Frank R, Fiore-Donno G, Cimasoni G, and Matter J. 1974. Ultrastructural study of epithelial and connective tissue gingival reattachment in man. *J Periodontol* 45:626–635.
65. Stahl S. 1979. Repair or regeneration. *J Clin Periodontol* 6:389–396.
66. Magnusson I, Ronstad L, Nyman S, and Lindhe J. 1983. A long junctional epithelium—a locus minoris resistentiae in plaque infection? *J Clin Periodontol* 10:333–340.
67. Beaumont R, O'Leary T, and Kafrawy A. 1984. Relative resistance of long junctional epithelial adhesions and connective tissue attachments to plaque-induced inflammation. *J Periodontol* 55:213–225.
68. Caton J and Nyman S. 1980. Histometric evaluation of periodontal surgery. I. The modified Widman flap procedure. *J Clin Periodontol* 7:212–223.
69. Steiner S, Crigger M, and Egelberg J. 1981. Connective tissue regeneration to periodontally diseased teeth. II. Histologic observations of cases following replaced flap surgery. *J Periodontal Res* 16:109–116.
70. Ross I and Thompson R. 1980. Furcation involvement in maxillary and mandibular molars. *J Periodontol* 51:450–454.

71. Larato DC. 1975. Some anatomical factors related to furcation involvements. *J Periodontol* 46:608–609.
72. Ricchetti PA. 1982. A furcation classification based on pulp chamber–furcation relationships and vertical radiographic bone loss. *Int J Periodontics Restorative Dent* 2(5):51–59.
73. Sternlicht HC. 1963. New approach to the management of multirooted teeth with advanced periodontal disease. *J Periodontol* 34:150–158.
74. Karlsen K. 1970. Gingival reaction to dental restorations. *Acta Odontol Scand* 28:895–899.
75. Waerhaug J. 1953. Tissue reactions around artificial crowns. *J Periodontol* 24:172–185.
76. Newcomb GM. 1974. The relationship between the location of subgingival crown margins and gingival inflammation. *J Periodontol* 45:151–154.
77. Renggli HH and Regolati B. 1972. Gingival inflammation and plaque accumulation by well adapted supragingival and subgingival proximal restorations. *Helv Odontol Acta* 16:99–101.
78. Waerhaug J. 1956. Effect of rough surfaces upon gingival tissues. *J Dent Res* 35:323–325.
79. Silness J. 1970. Periodontal conditions in patients treated with dental bridges. II. The influence of full and partial crowns on plaque accumulation, development of gingivitis and pocket formation. *J Periodontal Res* 5:219–224.
80. Mormann W, Regolatti B, and Renggli HH. 1974. Gingival reaction to well fitted subgingival gold inlays. *J Clin Periodontol* 1:120–125.
81. Gilmore N and Sheiham A. 1971. Overhanging dental restorations and periodontal disease. *J Periodontol* 42:8–12.
82. Fugazzotto PA. 1985. Periodontal restorative interrelationships: The isolated restoration. *J Am Dent Assoc* 110:915–917.
83. Ramfjord S, Nissle R, Shick R, and Cooper H. 1968. Subgingival curettage vs. surgical elimination of periodontal pockets. *J Periodontol* 39:167–175.
84. Ramfjord S, Knowles J, Nissle R, Shick R, and Burgett F. 1973. Longitudinal study of periodontal therapy. *J Periodontol* 44:66–77.
85. Ramfjord S, Knowles J, Nissle R, Burgett F, and Shick R. 1975. Results following three modalities of periodontal therapy. *J Periodontol* 46:522–526.
86. Knowles J, Burgett F, Nissle R, Shick R, Morrison E, and Ramfjord S. 1979. Results of periodontal treatment related to pocket depth and attachment level. Eight years. *J Periodontol* 50:225–233.
87. Ramfjord S, Knowles J, Morrison E, et al. 1980. Results of periodontal therapy related to tooth type. *J Periodontol* 51:270–273.
88. Knowles J, Burgett F, Morrison E, Nissle R, and Ramfjord S. 1980. Comparison of results following three modalities of periodontal therapy related to tooth type and initial pocket depth. *J Clin Periodontol* 7:32–47.
89. Burgett F, Knowles J, Nissle R, Shick R, and Ramfjord S. 1977. Short term results of three modalities of periodontal treatment. *J Periodontol* 48:131–135.
90. Hill R, Ramfjord S, Morrison E, et al. 1981. Four types of periodontal treatment compared over two years. *J Periodontol* 52:655–662.
91. Ramfjord S, Caffesse R, Morrison E, et al. 1987. Four modalities of periodontal treatment compared over five years. *J Clin Periodontol* 14:445–452.
92. Becker W, Becker B, Ochsenbein C, et al. 1988. A longitudinal study comparing scaling and osseous surgery and modified Widman procedures—results after one year. *J Periodontol* 59:351–358.
93. Stahl S. 1974. Lecture given at Boston University School of Graduate Dentistry, Fall, 1981.
94. Ramfjord S and Nissle R. 1974. The modified Widman flap. *J Periodontol* 45:601–607.
95. Lindhe J, Socransky S, Nyman S, and Westfelt E. 1987. Dimensional alterations of the periodontal tissues following therapy. *Int J Periodontics Restorative Dent* 7: 9–21.
96. Attstrom A and Lindhe J. 1983. Pathogenesis of plaque associated periodontal disease. In: Lindhe J (ed), *Textbook of Clinical Periodontology*. Copenhagen: Munksgaard.
97. Egelberg J. 1989. The impact of regression towards the mean on probing changes in studies on the effect of periodontal therapy. *J Clin Periodontol* 16: 120–123.
98. Aeppli DM and Pihlstrom BL. 1989. Detection of longitudinal change in periodontitis. *J Periodontal Res* 24:329–334.
99. Sterne JAC, Johnson NW, Wilton JMA, Joyston-Bechal S, and Smales FC. 1988. Variance components analysis of data from periodontal research. *J Periodontal Res* 23:148–153.
100. Lindhe J and Nyman S. 1984. Long term maintenance of patients treated for advanced periodontal disease. *J Clin Periodontol* 11:504–514.
101. Saadoun A. 1985. Management of furcation involvement. *J West Soc Periodontol Abstr* 33:91–125.
102. Basaraba N. 1969. Root amputation and tooth hemisection. *Dent Clin North Am* 13:121–132.
103. Newell D. 1981. Current status of the management of teeth with furcation invasion. *J Periodontol* 52:559–568.
104. Rosenberg MM, Kay HB, Keough BE, and Holt RL. 1988. *Periodontal and Prosthetic Management for Advanced Cases*. Chicago: Quintessence, pp. 247–298.
105. Waerhaug J. 1980. The furcation problem. Etiology, pathogenesis, diagnosis, therapy and prognosis. *J Clin Periodontol* 7:73–95.
106. Everett F, Jump E, Holder T, and Wilson G. 1958. The intermediate bifurcational ridge: A study of the morphology of the bifurcation of the lower first molar. *J Dent Res* 37:162–169.

107. Gher M and Vernino A. 1981. Root anatomy: A local factor in inflammatory periodontal disease. *Int J Periodontics Restorative Dent* 1(5):53–63.
108. Bower R. 1979. Morphology relative to periodontal treatment: Furcation entrance architecture. *J Periodontol* 50:23–27.
109. Matia J, Bissada NF, and Maybury JE. 1986. Efficacy of scaling of the molar furcation area with and without surgical access. *Int J Periodontics Restorative Dent* 6(6):25–35.
110. Fleischer HC, Mellonig JT, Brayer WK, Gray JL, and Barnett JD. 1989. Scaling and root planing efficacy in multirooted teeth. *J Periodontol* 60:402–409.
111. Pihlstrom BL, Oritz-Campos C, and McHugh RB. 1981. A randomized four year study of periodontal therapy. *J Periodontol* 52:227–242.
112. Pihlstrom BL, McHugh RB, Oliphant TH, and Oritz-Campos C. 1983. Comparison of surgical and non surgical treatment of periodontal disease. A review of current studies and additional results after six and one half years. *J Clin Periodontol* 10:524–541.
113. Stern T, Everett F, and Robicsek KS. 1965. Robicsek: A pioneer in the surgical treatment of periodontal disease. *J Periodontol* 36:265–268.
114. Yukna R and Williams JE. 1980. Five year evaluation of the excisional new attachment procedure. *J Periodontol* 51:382–385.
115. Smith DH, Ammons WF, and van Belle G. 1980. A longitudinal study of periodontal status comparing flap curettage and osseous recontouring. I. Six month results. *J Periodontol* 51:367–375.
116. Olsen CT, Ammons WF, and van Belle G. 1985. A longitudinal study comparing apically repositioned flaps, with and without osseous surgery. *Int J Periodontics Restorative Dent* 5:11–33.
117. Lindhe J and Nyman S. 1980. Alterations of the position of the marginal soft tissue following periodontal surgery. *J Clin Periodontol* 7:525–530.
118. Lindhe J, Haffajee AD, and Socransky SS. 1983. Progression of periodontal disease in adult subjects in the absence of periodontal therapy. *J Clin Periodontol* 10:433–442.
119. Nabers CL, Stalker WH, Esparza D, et al. 1988. Tooth loss in 1535 treated periodontal patients. *J Periodontol* 59:297–300.
120. McFall WT. 1982. Tooth loss in 100 treated patients with periodontal disease—a long term study. *J Periodontol* 53:539–549.
121. Goldman MJ, Ross IF, and Goteiner D. 1986. Effect of periodontal therapy on patients maintained for 15 years or longer. A retrospective study. *J Periodontol* 57:347–353.
122. Kaldahl WB, Kalkwarf KL, Kashinath DP, Molvar MP, and Dyer JK. 1996. Long term evaluation of periodontal therapy: I. Response to four therapeutic modalities. *J Periodontol* 67:93–102.
123. Kaldahl WB, Kalkwarf KL, Kashinath DP, Molvar MP, and Dyer JK. 1996. Long term evaluation of periodontal therapy: II. Incidence of sites breaking down. *J Periodontol* 67:103–108.
124. Lindhe J, Okamoto H, Yoneyama T, Haffajee A, and Socransky SS. 1989. Longitudinal changes in periodontal disease in untreated subjects. *J Clin Periodontol* 16:662–670.
125. Badersten A, Nilveus R, and Egelberg J. 1984. Effect of nonsurgical periodontal therapy. II. Severely advanced periodontitis. *J Clin Periodontol* 11:63–76.
126. Badersten A, Nilveus R, and Egelberg J. 1984. Effect of nonsurgical periodontal therapy. III. Single versus repeated instrumentation. *J Clin Periodontol* 11:114–124.
127. Waite IM. 1976. A comparison between conventional gingivectomy and a nonsurgical regime in the treatment of periodontitis. *J Clin Periodontol* 3:173–185.
128. Buchanan SA and Robertson PB. 1987. Calculus removal by scaling/root planing with and without surgical access. *J Periodontol* 58:159–163
129. Rabbani GM, Ash MM, and Caffesse RG. 1981. The effectiveness of subgingival scaling and root planing in calculus removal. *J Periodontol* 52:119–123.
130. Jeffcoat MK and Reddy MS. 1991. Progression of probing attachment loss in adult periodontitis. *J Periodontol* 62:185–189.
131. Badersten A, Nilveus R, and Egelberg J. 1985. Effect of non-surgical periodontal therapy. VII. Bleeding, suppuration and probing depth in sites with probing attachment loss. *J Clin Periodontol* 12:432–440.
132. Grbic JT and Lamstr IB. 1992. Risk indicators for future clinical attachment loss in adult periodontitis. Tooth and site variables. *J Periodontol* 63:262–269.
133. Haffajee AD, Socransay SS, Smith C, and Divart S. 1991. Microbrial risk indicators for periodontal attachment loss. *J Periodontal Res* 26:293–296.
134. Vanooteghem R, Hutchenes LH, Garrett S, Kiger R, and Egelberg J. 1987. Bleeding on probing and probing depth as indicators of the response to plaque control and root debridement. *J Clin Periodontol* 14:226–230.
135. Nyman S, Gottlow J, Karring T, et al. 1982. The regenerative potential of the periodontal ligament. An experimental study in the monkey. *J Clin Periodontol* 9:257–265.
136. Gottlow J, Nyman S, Karring T, et al. 1984. New attachment formation as the result of controlled tissue regeneration. *J Clin Periodontol* 11:494–503.
137. Nyman S, Lindhe J, Karring T, et al. 1982. New attachment following surgical treatment of human periodontal disease. *J Clin Periodontal* 9:290–296.
138. Gottlow J, Nyman S, Lindhe J, et al. 1986. New attachment formation in the human periodontium by guided

tissue regeneration. Case reports. *J Clin Periodontol* 13:604–616.
139. Schallhorn RG, Hiatt WH, and Boyce W. 1970. Iliac transplants in periodontal therapy. *J Periodontol* 41:566–580.
140. Hiatt WH and Schallhorn RG. 1973. Intraoral transplants of cancellous bone and marrow in periodontal lesions. *J Periodontol* 44:194–208.
141. Froum SJ, Ortiz M, Witkin RT, et al. 1976. Osseous autografts. III. Comparison osseous coagulum-bone blend implants with open curettage. *J Periodontol* 47:287–294.
142. Renvert S, Garrett S, Schallhorn RG, et al. 1985. Healing after treatment of periodontal intraosseous defects. III. Effect of osseous grafting and citric acid conditioning. *J Clin Periodontol* 12:441–455.
143. Quintero G, Mellonig JT, Gambil VM, et al. 1982. A six month clinical evaluation of decalcified freeze-dried bone allografts in periodontal osseous defects. *J Periodontol* 53:726–730.
144. Fugazzotto PA. 2001. A comparison of the success of root resected molars and molar position implants in function in private practice: Results of up to 15-plus years. *J Periodontol* 72:1113–1123.
145. Fugazzotto PA and Hains F. 2009. The effect of therapeutic costs on development of treatment algorithms in the partial edentulous patient. A comparative fee survey and treatment planning philosophy. *J Acad Gen Dent* (submitted for publication).
146. Fugazzotto PA. 1985. *Preparation of the Periodontium for Restorative Dentistry*. St Louis: Ishiyaku Euro America.
147. Fugazzotto PA. 1998. Comprehensive surgical management of the embrasure space in the prosthetic patient. *J Mass Dent Soc* 46:18–22.
148. Bakhshandeh S, Murtomaa H, Mofid R, Behkalahti MM, and Suomalainen K. 2007. Periodontal treatment needs of diabetic adults. *J Clin Periodontol* 1:53–57.
149. Marx R, Sawatari Y, Fortin M, and Broumand V. 2005. Bisphosphonate induced exposed bone of the jaws: Risk factors, recognition, prevention, and treatment. *J Oral Maxillofac Surg* 63:1567–1575.
150. Migliorati CA, Schubert MM, Peterson DE, and Seneda LM. 2005. Bisphosphonate associated osteonecrosis of mandibular and maxillary bone: An emerging complication of supportive cancer therapy. *Cancer* 104:89–93.
151. Jeffcoat MK. 2006. Safety of oral bisphosphonates: Controlled studies on alveolar bone. *Int J Oral Maxillofac Implants* 21:349–353.
152. Fugazzotto PA, Lightfoot WS, Jaffin R, and Kumar A. 2007. Implant placement with or without simultaneous tooth extraction in patients taking oral bisphosphonates: Post-operative healing, early follow-up, and the incidence of complications of two private practices. *J Periodontol* 78:1664–1669.
153. Levin A, Aviv A, and Schwartz-Arad D. 2007. Denture related osteonecrosis of the maxilla associated with oral bisphosphonate treatment. *J Am ENT Assoc* 138:1218–1220.
154. Marx RE, Cillo JE, Jr, and Uloa JJ. 2007. Oral bisphosphonate induced osteonecrosis: Risk factors, prediction of risk using serum CTX testing, prevention, and treatment. *J Oral Maxillofac Surg* 65:2397–2410.

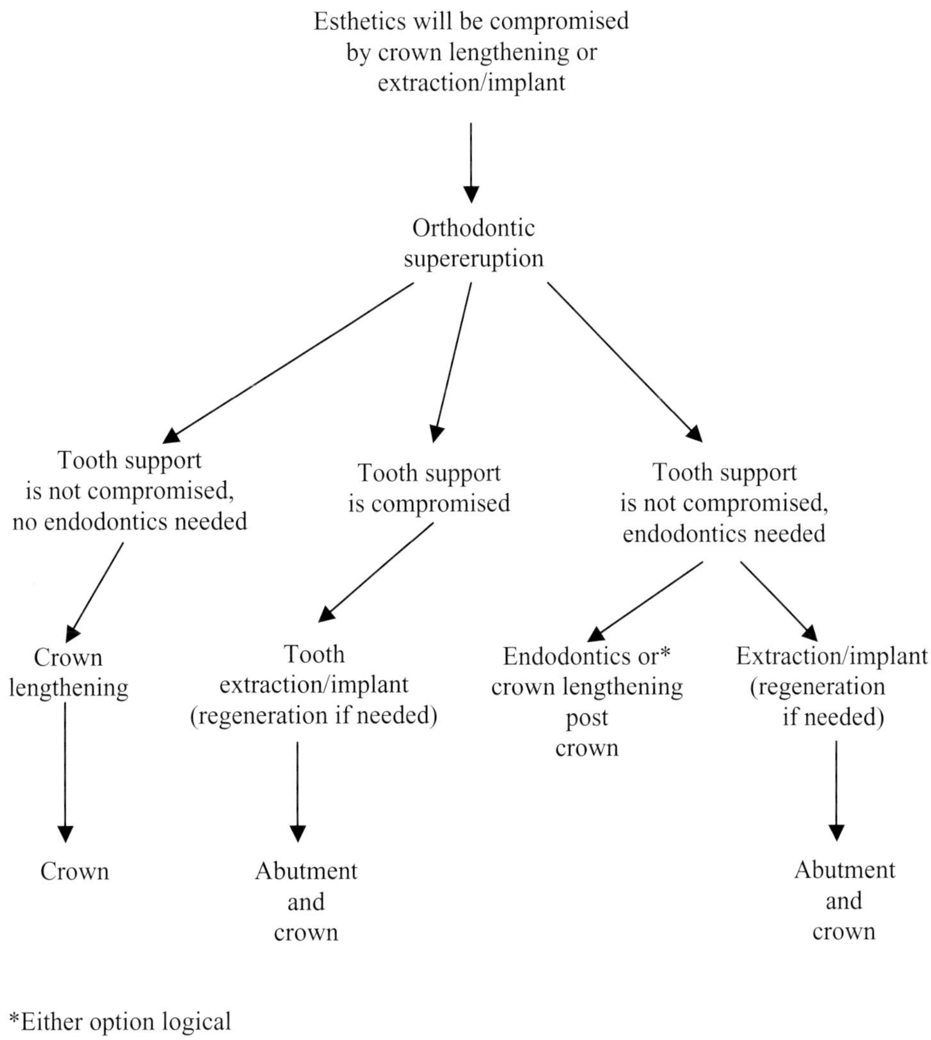

Flow chart 1.1 Treating a decayed single tooth (Part 1 of 3).

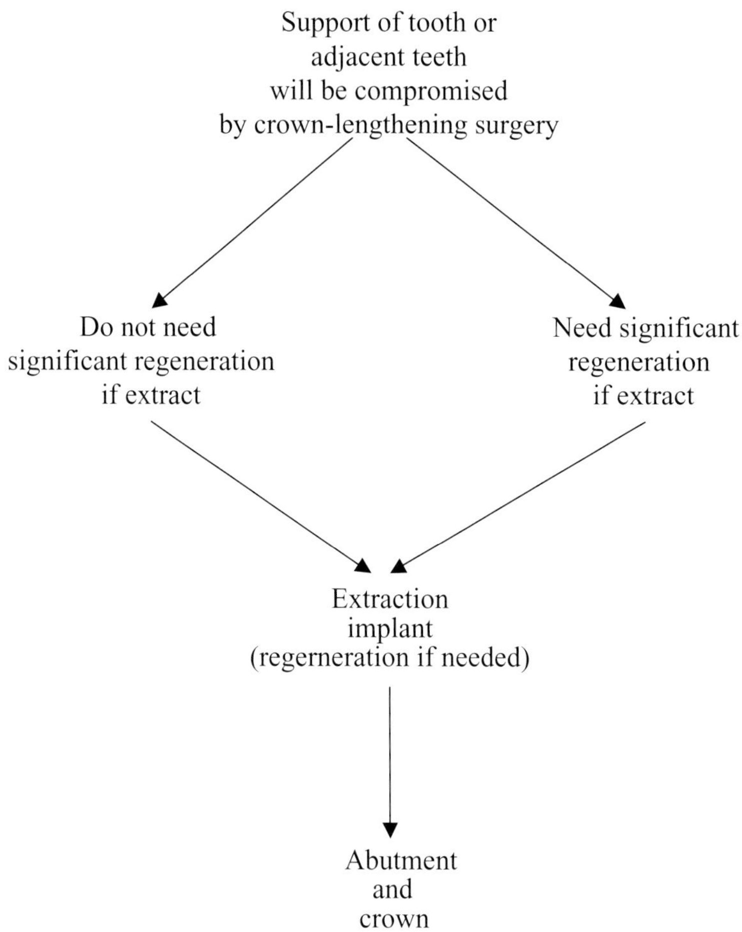

Flow chart 1.1 Treating a decayed single tooth (Part 2 of 3).

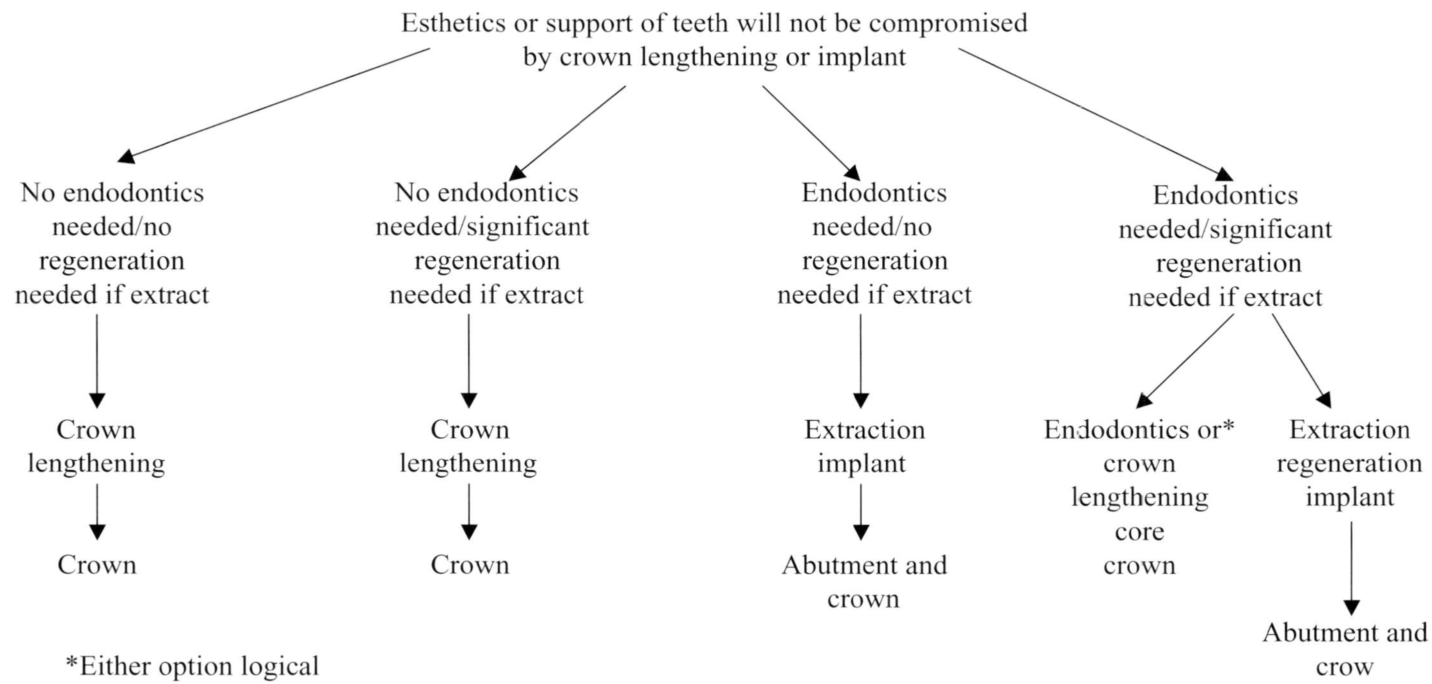

Flow chart 1.1 Treating a decayed single tooth (Part 3 of 3).

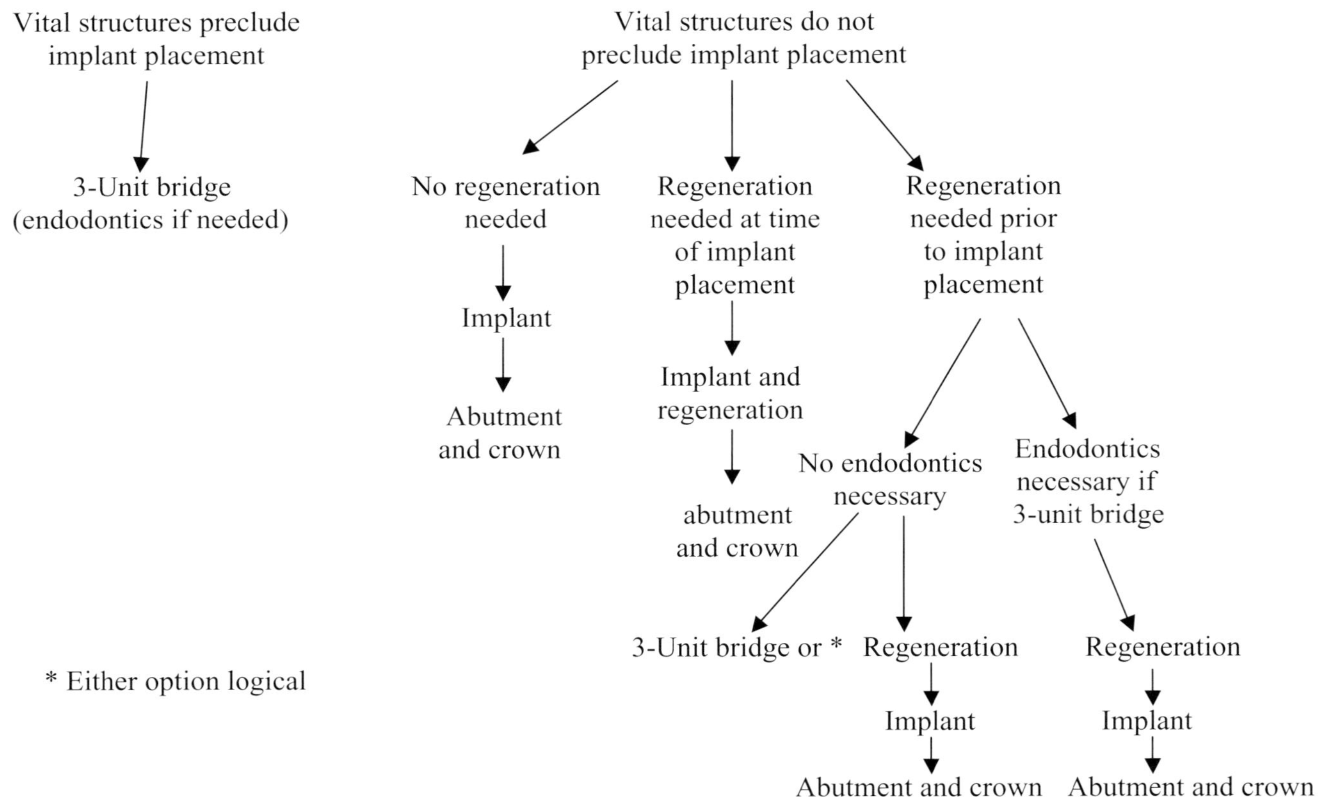

Flow chart 1.2 Replacing a single missing tooth in a tooth-bounded space.

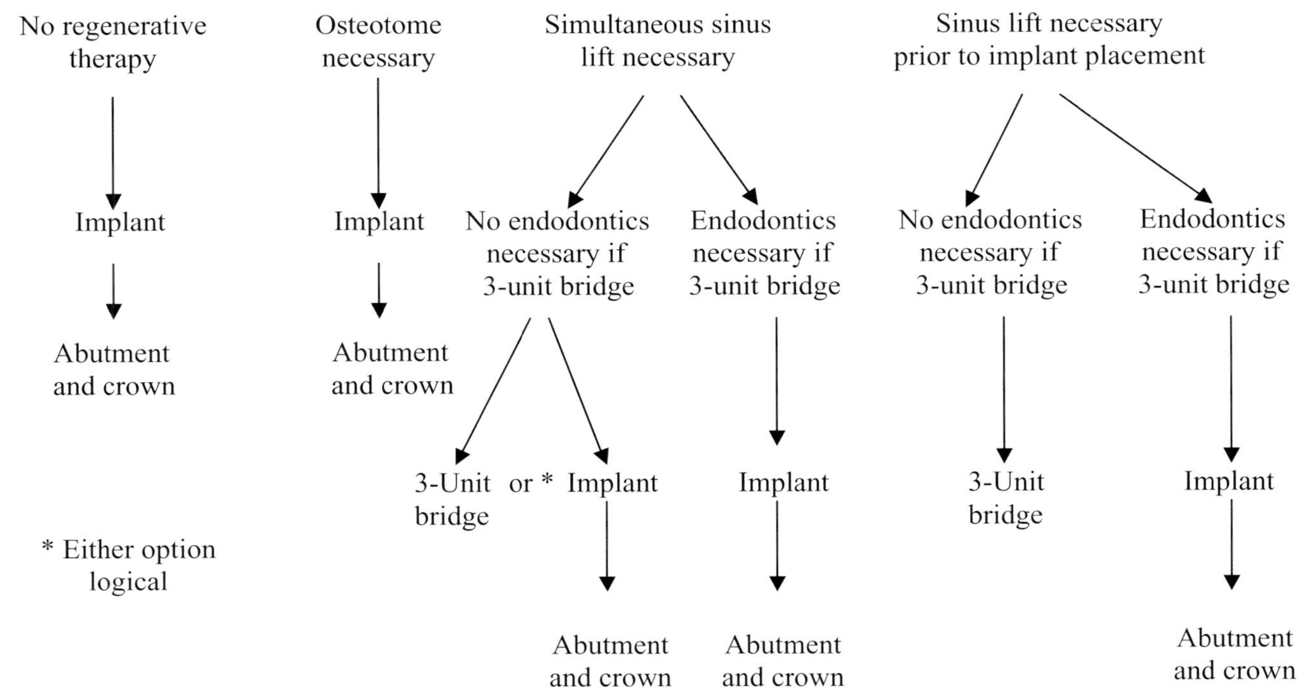

Flow chart 1.3 Replacing a maxillary first molar when the second molar is present.

Chapter 2

Guided Bone Regeneration

Paul A. Fugazzotto, DDS

Outline

The introduction of guided bone regeneration therapy to clinical practice affords a means of provided previously undreamt-of treatment results (1–9). As a result, guided bone regeneration therapy has changed the framework within which the conscientious clinician practices, through the modification of both treatment expectations, and the definition of a successful treatment outcome. Unfortunately, because guided bone regeneration does not always yield optimal treatment outcomes due to inappropriate execution of therapy, guided bone regeneration is often utilized as a means to a compromised treatment end point.

It has long been recognized that three seminal questions must be answered to justify a given guided bone regeneration treatment protocol:

- Does it work: Is the treatment approach outlined highly predictable in a variety of clinical situations?
- Is it bone: Will the guided bone regeneration treatment approach employed and the materials utilized result in predictable regeneration of bone, and not of a dense nonosseous structure?
- Will it last: Will regenerated bone around implants, whether it is generated around implants already placed, or is generated to serve as a receptor for implants placed at the second stage, withstand function forces over time in a manner comparable to that of nonregenerated bone?

While there is widespread agreement regarding the need to answer the above three questions in the affirmative before accepting any treatment modality as an everyday component in the clinician's armamentarium, such agreement is all too often based upon vague definitions of success. Is success to be defined merely as covering of a dehisced or fenestrated implant surface with regenerated hard tissues, or the ability to place an implant in regenerated bone without generating a fenestration or dehiscence? Should any consideration be given to the dimension of the regenerated bone and its ability to withstand functional forces over time? Should the morphology of the regenerated bone be considered?

The initial definition of success following guided bone regeneration therapy, as proposed by Mellonig and Triplett (10), was the ability to completely cover a dehisced or fenestrated implant surface with regenerated hard tissue. While certainly useful at the time of its introduction, such a definition of success, which will be called the **first-generation definition of success**, is no longer sufficient. At the minimum, bone of an adequate dimension must be regenerated to withstand functional forces over time. Generation of a thin, translucent patina of hard tissues as a covering over an implant surface will not add appreciatively to the long-term stability of the implant, as this bone may be expected to resorb under function over time. The regeneration of a sufficient dimension of bone to withstand functional forces over time will be called the **second-generation definition of success**. Is this definition of success adequate today? This question will be explored below.

Diagnostic Requirements

PATIENT EXAMINATION AND DIAGNOSIS

This discussion will assume a noncontributory medical history. Medical contraindications to guided bone regeneration therapy will be discussed at a later point in the chapter.

A thorough clinical examination must be carried out to assess both the patient's regenerative needs and the feasibility of performing the proposed regenerative therapy. This examination should be grounded in the overall patient treatment plan, and must consider all planned surgical, restorative and orthodontic (if applicable) treatments to be carried out.

The components of such an examination include clinical appraisal of not only the sites that are to be regenerated, but also of all other aspects of the patient's oral cavity, with appropriate measurements and record taking. There is no need to itemize the components of a thorough clinical examination, including the status of remaining teeth, periodontal health, malpositioned teeth, etc. However, it should be stressed that care must be taken to accurately assess the condition of the soft tissues not only over the site to be regenerated but also throughout the mouth; the quantities of the remaining soft tissues in the area to be regenerated; and both the shape and position of the residual alveolar ridge. A full occlusal examination must also be carried out.

It is imperative that, at the very least, a set of digital clinical photographs be taken which include photographs of the jaw in various lateral and protrusive positions. A full series of radiographs must include the use of number zero-size films in the maxillary and mandibular anterior regions if teeth are present, so as to help ensure appropriate film angulations and the elimination of distortion of alveolar crest position and tooth root length. Ideally, these films will be digital in format.

A formatted CAT scan study may also be necessary, depending on the therapy planned, and the need to assess the presence or absence of various pathologies.

Facebow-mounted models are a key component of any treatment plan involving more than the most isolated of therapies. These facebow-mounted models serve multiple purposes, including:

- Diagnostic: Tooth position, maxillary and mandibular occlusal interrelationships, wear facets, tooth drifting and/or supraeruption, and the need for orthodontic therapy are but a few of the important diagnostic elements which are best assessed through a combination of clinical examination, clinical photographs, and facebow-mounted models.
- Fabrication of accurate implant placement stents: The usefulness of surgical implant stents is compromised when they are fabricated on handheld or inappropriately articulated models. If care is to be taken to fabricate such stents, it is only logical to render them as accurate as possible in a given clinical situation.
- Fabrication of regeneration stents: It is foolhardy to believe that regeneration stents may be accurately fabricated if the appropriate maxillomandibular interrelationship of the two arches has not been established through proper record taking and mounting of models.

The above stents are often combined into one guide, or incorporated into a metal frame temporary fixed prosthesis, both to ensure accuracy and to lessen the financial impact of therapy to the patient.

Technical Considerations in Guided Bone Regeneration Therapy (GBR)

Guided bone regeneration is potentially one of the most misused, poorly understood therapies in the field of implant dentistry. Clinicians often exclude various materials from consideration due to perceived technical difficulties in handling, and complications in postoperative care. Manufacturers champion materials which are meant to succeed in the face of such complications, stating that "It doesn't matter if this membrane becomes uncovered"; "This membrane is meant to stay uncovered"; "When you use this bone graft material you don't need a membrane"; "This material works as well as X (fill in any name), and is easier to use"; "This material is cheaper than X and works just as well."

The maximization of treatment outcomes following guided bone regenerative therapy does not begin with the selection of graft materials, nor the utilization of various membranes. As with all other treatments, GBR therapy is highly diagnosis dependent. Once the appropriate diagnosis is carried out, the results of guided bone regenerative therapy are directly attributable to appropriate incision design and flap management.

More than adequate data exists for us to understand both what ideal treatment outcomes are following guided bone regeneration therapy, and how best to achieve these treatment outcomes. All conscientious clinicians must choose materials and techniques that help ensure the attainment of such ideal treatment outcomes.

Such a philosophy demands a reworking of the conceptual framework utilized by many clinicians when carrying out guided bone regeneration therapy. There are essentially two frameworks within which to work.

The first is to accept the inability to overcome many of the bandied about limitations in guided bone regeneration therapy, and choose the materials to be utilized, and hence the potential of treatment outcomes, accordingly. Such an approach, while it will result in regeneration of some lost bone, will never predictably yield optimal treatment outcomes.

The second conceptual framework to work within is one which strives to develop an understanding of techniques which will overcome the supposed technical problems when performing guided bone regeneration therapy, and thus afford the opportunity to choose between all available materials. When utilizing such an approach, the clinician chooses the materials to be utilized by the specific case in question, rather than fitting the patient's needs into a limited framework of therapeutic capabilities. In this way, treatment outcomes are consistently maximized.

When assessing the literature to determine the capabilities of guided bone regeneration therapy, it is important to do so with a critical eye and a reasonable dose of skepticism. While certainly important, the available literature is limited in guiding the clinician on a daily basis because of a number of factors:

- The definitions of success are variable from author to author, as already discussed. Definitions of success must be clearly defined, and must be clinically applicable. For example, a definition of success of ridge augmentation therapy that includes nothing more than the ability to place an implant within a regenerated ridge is not instructive. Did a reduced diameter implant have to be placed due to a compromised regenerative result? If a standard or wide diameter implant was able to be placed, what was the width of the residual regenerated bone on the buccal and lingual/palatal aspects of the implant? What was the width of the residual regenerated bone, not only in the apical area of the implant, where the ridge would be expected to be thicker in many situations, but also in the crestal area of the regenerated ridge? Was adequate bone regenerated to allow ideal implant positioning? In situations where bone was regenerated over an implant fenestration or dehiscence, what was the width of the regenerated bone? These are examples of some of the questions which must be answered to appropriately assess the regenerative results of a championed treatment approach.
- An adequate number of consecutively treated cases must be documented to assess the success and failure rates of a given therapy.
- What types of cases were treated and documented? If implants were placed in extraction sockets wholly within the three-dimensional confines of the alveolus, and the attendant dehiscence or fenestration defects were rebuilt

with regenerative materials, such treatment outcomes are not useful when assessing a specific regenerative approach in more severe situations. As will be explained, different materials and techniques are often required when guided bone regeneration must occur around an implant whose body is at least partially outside of the confines of the residual alveolar ridge. Unfortunately, limitations in available journal space often preclude the inclusion of numerous clinical pictures which would be instructive to readers. As a result, the precise types of defects treated must be clearly elucidated in all publications dealing with guided bone regeneration.

For example, Figure 2.1 demonstrates a titanium plasma-sprayed implant placed at the time of tooth removal, which resides wholly within the confines of the alveolus. As a result, essentially any resorbable graft materials covered by a membrane, and subsequently protected by appropriate soft tissue closure, will demonstrate complete regeneration of the damaged alveolar bone at the six-month reentry visit (Figure 2.2). The implant, following restoration with a single crown, should hold up well under function (Figure 2.3). Treatment of such a defect is not helpful in determining either the appropriate surgical approach to be employed, or the regenerative graft and membrane materials to be chosen, for treatment of more challenging areas.

Figure 2.4 demonstrates an 11-mm-long titanium plasma-sprayed surface implant placed in the area of a maxillary cuspid. A 10.9-mm buccal

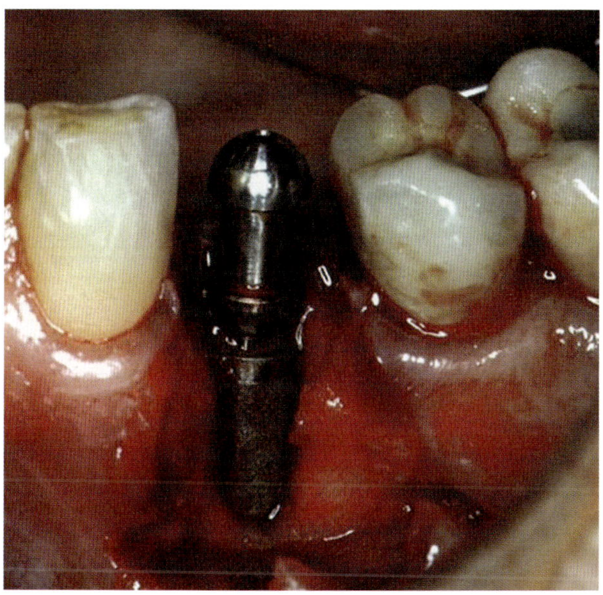

Figure 2.1 A 4-mm-wide titanium plasma-sprayed IMZ implant has been placed following tooth removal. The implant is within the confines of the residual alveolar ridge. The area will be treated with particulate material and a covering membrane.

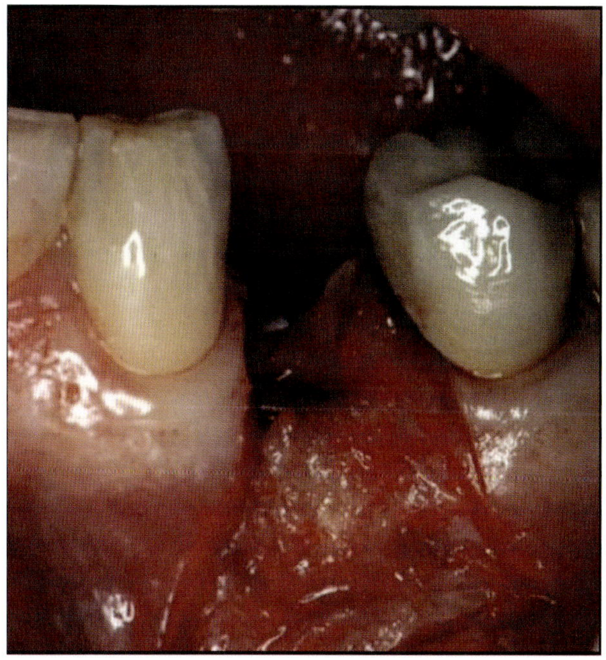

Figure 2.2 Following flap reflection and membrane removal six months postregenerative therapy, complete regeneration of the alveolar bone over the previously exposed implant surface is evident.

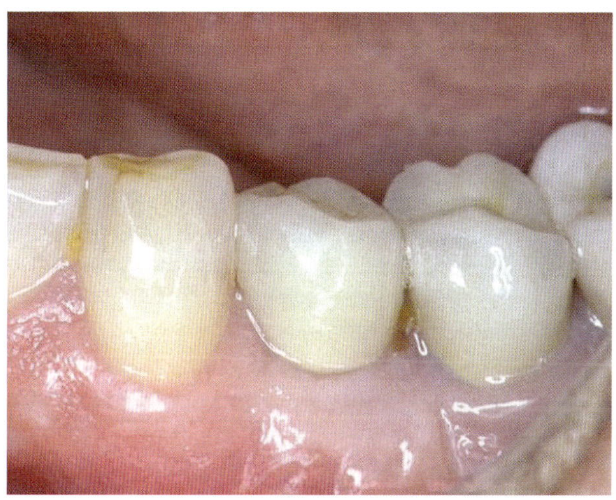

Figure 2.3 The implant is restored with a single crown.

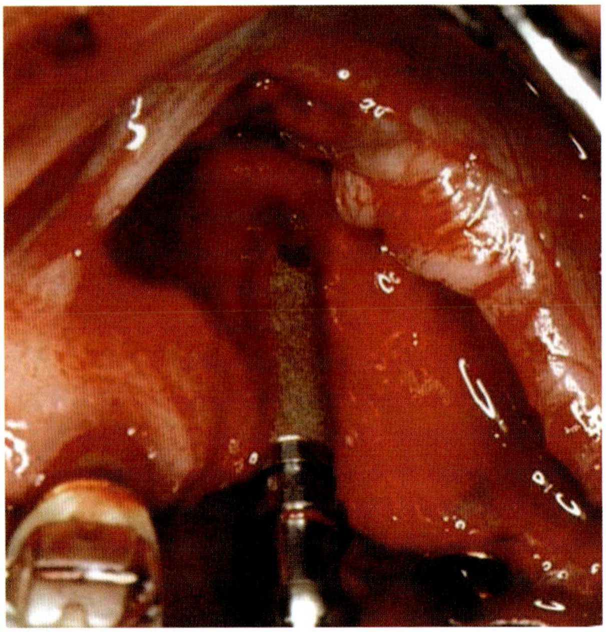

Figure 2.4 A 4-mm-wide and 11-mm-long titanium plasma-sprayed IMZ implant has been placed in the cuspid position in an atrophic alveolar ridge. Approximately 160° of the implant circumference is outside of the confines of the residual alveolar bone.

dehiscence is noted, which extends mesially and distally around approximately 160° of the circumference of the implant. The dehisced buccal aspect of the implant is outside of the confines of the residual alveolar ridge. Nevertheless, following utilization of the appropriate graft materials and covering membrane, and assurance of maintenance of soft tissue primary closure throughout the course of regeneration, complete coverage of the previously exposed root surface with regenerated hard tissues is evident at the eight-month clinical reentry (Figure 2.5). Note both the thickness of the bone attained on the buccal aspect of the implant, and the concomitant lateral ridge augmentation achieved. This implant has now been in function for over 15 years and demonstrates no radiographic loss of supporting bone around the implant (Figure 2.6). The space noted between the marginal area of the prosthesis and the osseous crest is due to a combination of the implant having been placed in a noncountersunk manner, and various components (a transmucosal extension and an intramobile element) having been stacked on top of the implant prior to prosthesis placement. Such results are predictably attainable regardless of implant type or position relative to the alveolar crest (Figures 2.7 and 2.8).

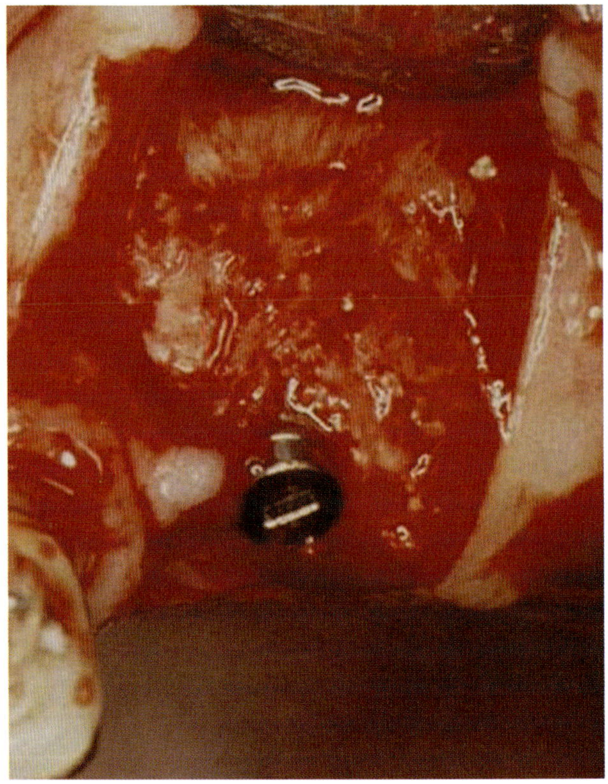

Figure 2.5 Following flap reflection and membrane removal six months postregenerative therapy, extensive alveolar bone regeneration is noted, covering the previously exposed implant surface.

- Reporting of appropriate parameters to assess regenerative success: Figure 2.6 demonstrates an apparently radiographically successful implant under function for 15 plus years. However, because regeneration was performed on the buccal aspect of the implant, the radiograph offers no evidence of maintenance or loss of the regenerated hard tissues. Such assessment can only be carried out through bone sounding. Any literature reporting upon success or failure of regenerated bone on the buccal aspect of implants over time must include both only radiographic assessment and clinical bone sounding.

Much of the literature assessing success and failure of guided bone regeneration therapy in terms of rebuilding bone in implant defects present at the time of implant insertion unfortunately utilizes either the first- or second-generation

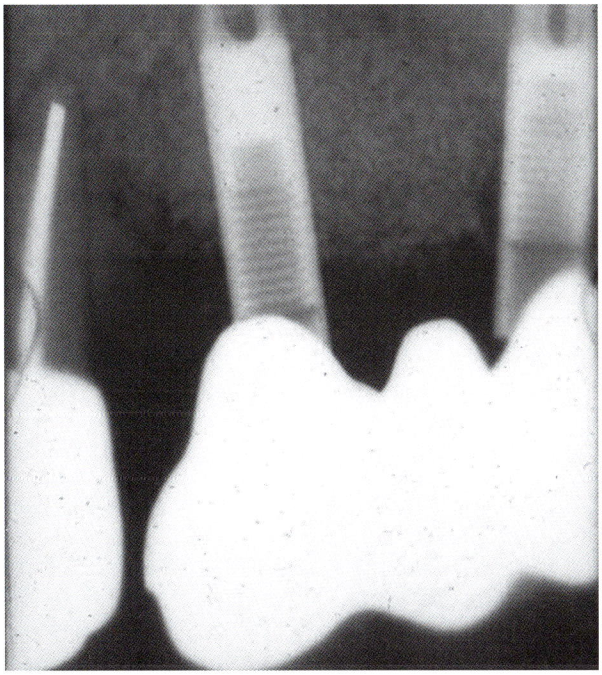

Figure 2.6 A radiograph taken 14-plus years post-bone regeneration demonstrates the stability of the regenerated peri-implant bone. The space between the bone crest and the crown margin is not representative of progressive bone loss. Rather, it is due to the noncountersunk nature of the implant, and the presence of components stacked on top of the implant (a TIE and an IME).

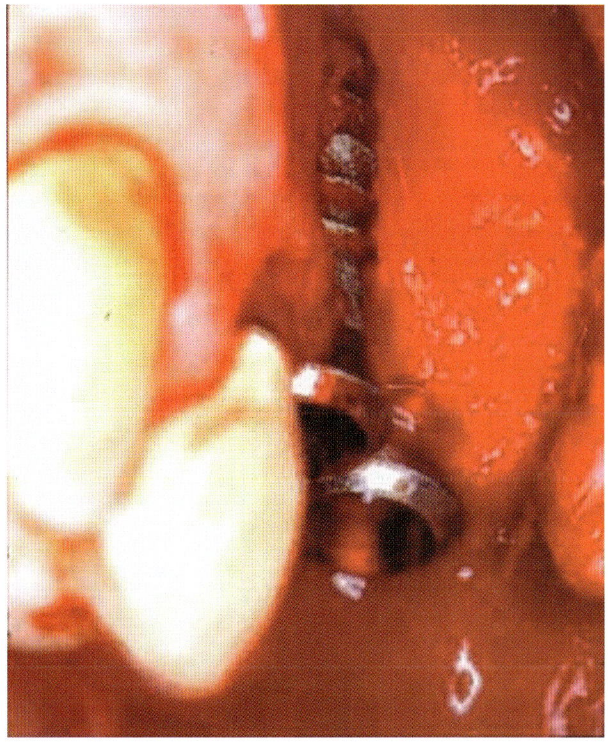

Figure 2.7 Two 4.1-mm-wide titanium plasma-sprayed Straumann implants have been placed. Approximately 140° of the circumference of the anterior implant is outside of the confines of the residual alveolar bone. The area will be treated with particulate material and a reinforced Gore-Tex membrane.

definition of success of guided bone regeneration. Fugazzotto et al. (11) documented success and failure rates of guided bone regeneration around 1,503 implants, when the guided bone regeneration therapy was performed at the time of implant placement. Implants were placed in extraction sockets at the time of tooth removal (581 cases); or bone was rebuilt at the sites of dehiscence (613 cases) or fenestration (209 cases) defects present at the time of implant placement. The definition of success was covering of all exposed implant surfaces with regenerated hard tissues. Utilizing this first-generation definition of success, the success rate of guided bone regeneration on implants placed in extraction sockets was 96.7%; in treatment of implant dehiscences, the success rate was 97.2%; and in treatment of implant fenestrations, the success rate was 97.6%. While these success rates are not as high as they would undoubtedly be today, the cases treated and reported upon in this paper included the first cases managed by the authors. A significant evolution in the understanding of soft tissue flap designs and the prerequisites for successful guided bone regeneration treatment outcomes, as well as the availability of newer materials including various graft materials, reinforced membranes, and fixation tacks, have significantly impacted success rates with such therapies.

Because the definition of success utilized in this paper, which was prevalent at the time of publication, was the first-generation definition of success, the data are of limited values when striving to maximize treatment outcomes when faced with a wide spectrum of patient problems and challenges.

SOFT TISSUE MANAGEMENT

The sine qua non of successful guided bone regeneration therapy is appropriate flap management. While there is no doubt that bone regeneration can be achieved without attaining and maintaining passive soft tissue primary closure over the regenerating site, the extent and morphology of the

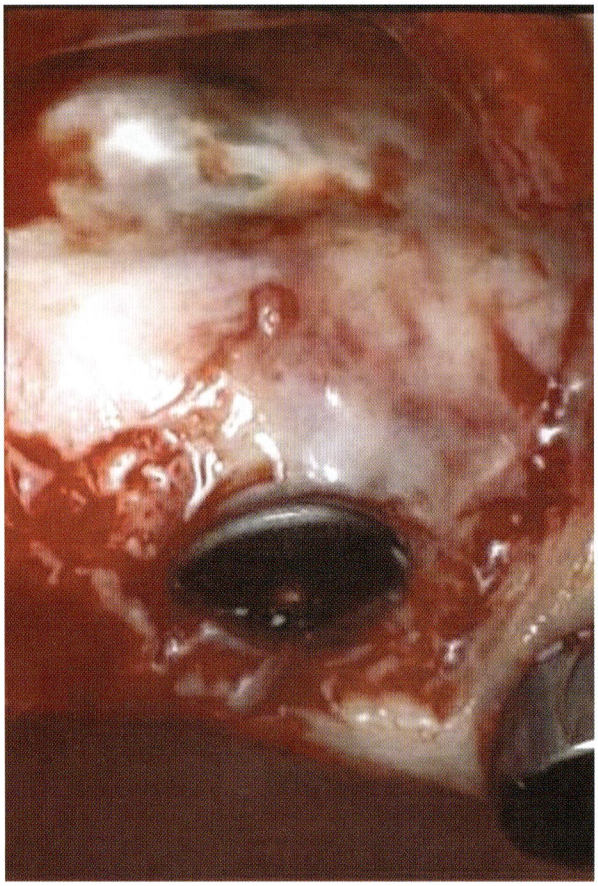

Figure 2.8 Following flap reflection and membrane removal six months postregenerative therapy, extensive bone regeneration over the previously exposed implant surface is evident.

regenerated hard tissues will often fall short of the desired ideal treatment outcome. In addition, the resultant soft tissue covering when passive soft tissue primary closure is not maintained is usually thinner than desired, and represents a potential esthetic compromise (12–16). Any discussion of graft material selection or options in membrane utilization is inherently flawed if it is not conducted within the therapeutic envelope of predictably attaining and maintaining passive soft tissue primary closure throughout the course of regeneration, over the regenerating site.

As with all surgical procedures, soft tissue manipulation must be as gentle and atraumatic as possible. In addition, incisions should be made within keratinized tissue so as to ensure keratinized margins to the mucoperiosteal flaps, both to enhance soft tissue manipulation and to help avoid fraying of the mucoperiosteal flap margins.

The basic components of incision design are as follows:

- A horizontal mid-crestal incision within keratinized tissue: In all areas except the maxillary anterior region, this incision is made along the crest of the ridge. When treating edentulous posterior areas, this incision is carried at least 6–8 mm distal to the area to be augmented, so as to provide appropriate access to the underlying atrophic ridge. The incision is carried to within 1–2 mm of the tooth anterior to the edentulous posterior region. However, the incision does not reach the adjacent tooth, so as to preserve a portion of the papilla and thus a soft tissue cover over the supporting bone on the distal aspect of the tooth.

In the maxillary anterior region, two options are feasible. If the teeth bordering the area to be augmented demonstrate periodontal loss and/or infrabony defect formation, the horizontal incision is placed palatal to the papillae rather than mid-crestally. This design will allow reflection of the papillae as unaffected units along with the buccal flap, and provides access to the roots adjacent to the site to be regenerated. The clinician may then perform debridement, periodontal regeneration, etc. as necessary in conjunction with the ridge augmentation therapy.

If the teeth bordering the area to be regenerated are periodontally sound on their aspects facing the edentulous region, the horizontal incision is placed mid-crestally, and stops short of the adjacent teeth so as to preserve the papillae.

- Releasing incisions: In the mandible, four releasing incisions are utilized. They are placed at the mesiobuccal, distobuccal, mesiolingual, and distolingual aspects of the mid-crestal horizontal incision. These releasing incisions extend beyond the mucogingival junction well into the mucosa, and are crucial if appropriate flap reflection and defect visualization are to be achieved. When placing a releasing incision in the vicinity of the mental foramen, the initial releasing incision is extended approximately 2 mm beyond the mucogingival junction. The flap is then held with a tissue forcep, and blunt dissection is carried out internally, until the foramen is visualized. Once this visualization has been accomplished, the releasing incision is extended at such an angle as to avoid the mental foramen. If the clinician is concerned about placing lingual releasing incisions, they should initially extend approximately 2 mm beyond the mucogingival junction. The lingual mucoperiosteal flap is then held with a tissue forcep and the releasing incision is continued as the clinician visualizes the internal aspect of the flap. Such an approach will help allay any fears the clinician may have regarding impingement upon structures such as the lingual nerve, lingual artery, etc. If a clinician is wary of placing lingual releasing incisions, examination of dry skull specimens, and cadaver specimens if available, will demonstrate the margin of safety between where the releasing incisions are to be placed and the vital structures in question, except in the most atrophic of situations.

When guided bone regenerative therapy is to be performed in the maxilla, the positions of the releasing incisions will be dependent upon the type of area to be augmented. If the ridge to be augmented is bounded by natural teeth, the palatal releasing incisions are placed one tooth mesial and distal to the edentulous area. The reason for this placement will become evident. Should guided bone regeneration be planned in the edentulous maxilla, the releasing incisions should be placed at least 10 mm away from the anticipated site of augmentation.

All palatal releasing incisions are placed obliquely. An oblique incision may be placed approximately 30% less deeply into the palatal vault than a straight releasing incision, while still retaining the same degree of flap reflection and defect visualization.

- Horizontal extensions of the releasing incisions: Horizontal releasing incisions are placed at the most apical extents of all buccal vertical releasing incisions in the maxilla and mandible. These horizontal releasing incisions should extend at least 3–4 mm, and may extend up to 10 mm, depending upon the need for greater flap mobility. Such horizontal extensions are not required in mandibular posterior regions, and are of no use throughout the palate, as the palatal flap cannot be coronally positioned. Horizontal extensions at the apices of the vertical releasing incisions are very often necessary in the mandibular anterior region to help counteract the pull of the tongue, which will result in flap tension and subsequent retraction following suturing (see Figures 2.9 and 2.10).
- Full thickness flap reflection: All flaps are reflected in a full thickness manner, including the horizontal extensions at the apices of the vertical releasing incisions. No periosteal fenestration is employed at any time. The use of adequate full thickness flap reflection following appropriate releasing incision design results in greater flap mobility than periosteal fenestration. In addition, postoperative morbidity (i.e., swelling) is much less when full thickness reflection is utilized as compared to periosteal fenestration. However, it must be noted that, if extension of full thickness reflection is insufficient, inadequate flap mobility will result (see Figure 2.11). A useful rule of thumb is the following: If the clinician thinks that adequate flap mobility has been attained, it has not. If the clinician is sure that adequate flap mobility has been attained, it has.

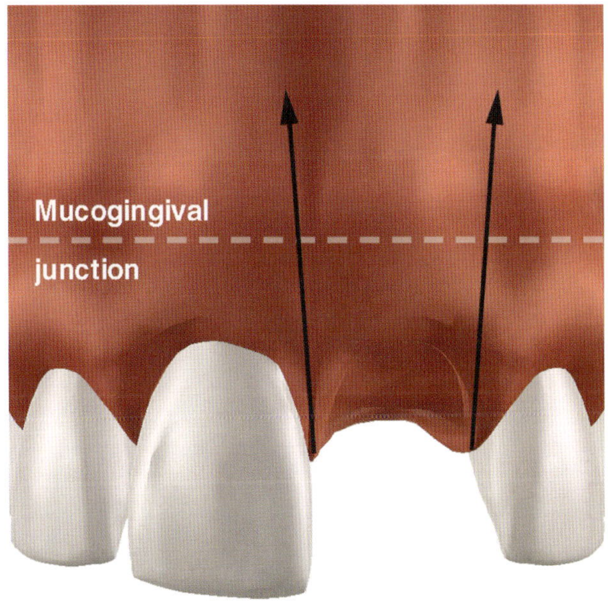

Figure 2.9 Vertical releasing incisions extend beyond the mucogingival junction, well up into the buccal fold. Note that the integrity of the adjacent soft tissue papillae has not been compromised.

The above outlined flap designs will provide adequate flap mobility to attain and maintain passive soft tissue primary closure

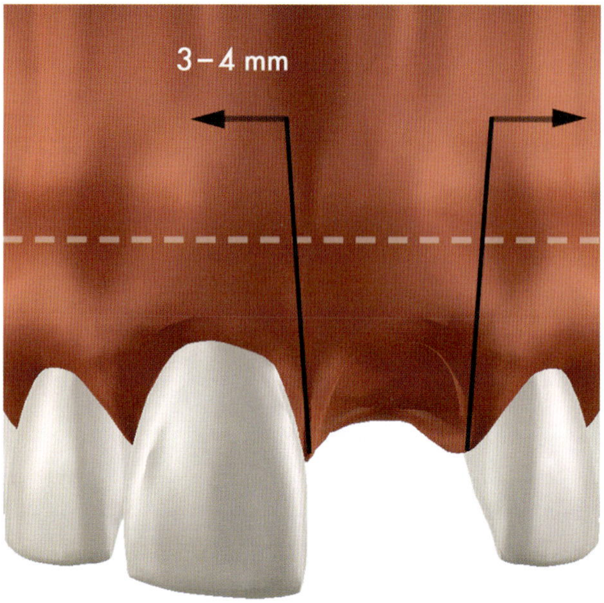

Figure 2.10 Horizontal releasing incisions are placed at the most apical extents of the vertical releasing incisions. These horizontal extensions will be carried for a distance of 3–4 mm initially. The need or lack of need for further extension is decided upon following flap reflection and assessment of the area to be regenerated.

throughout the course of regeneration, following mandibular guided bone regeneration procedures, and the majority of maxillary guided bone regeneration procedures. When the previously outlined flap designs are not adequate to attain passive primary closure following placement of regenerative materials in the maxilla, a rotated palatal pedicle is employed. Designed and published by Fugazzotto et al. (16), the rotated palatal pedicle flap is carried out as follows (Figures 2.12–2.15).

A full thickness palatal mucoperiosteal flap is reflected. An incision is then made with a 15 blade mesiodistally on the internal aspect of the palatal flap, approximately 3–4 mm from the base of the mucoperiosteal flap. Utilizing a tissue forcep and a 15 blade, the flap is split internally toward its crestal aspect. The internal aspect of the flap is filleted, and rotated crestally so as to lengthen the palatal flap by approximately 70%.

Care is taken neither to perforate the flap at its most crestal aspect, nor to render the residual isthmus of tissue so thin as to be in danger of sloughing during healing.

Figures 2.16–2.33 provide a clinical demonstration of the utilization of this flap during guided bone regeneration surgery. A 19-year-old patient presented with significant ridge atrophy in the area

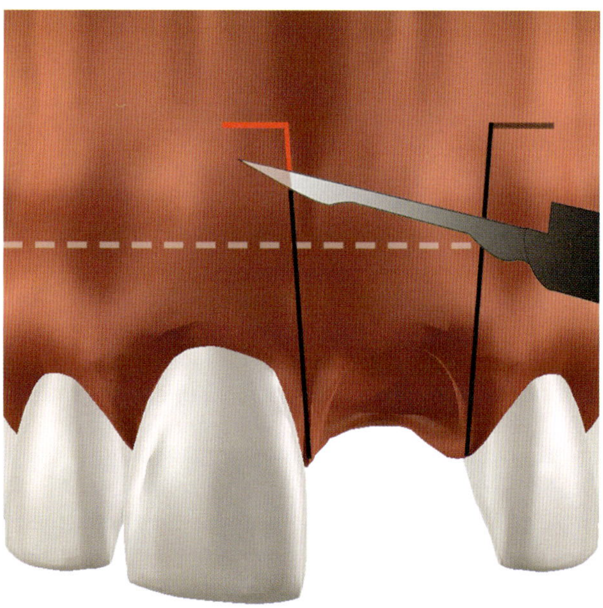

Figure 2.11 All flap reflection is carried out in a full thickness manner.

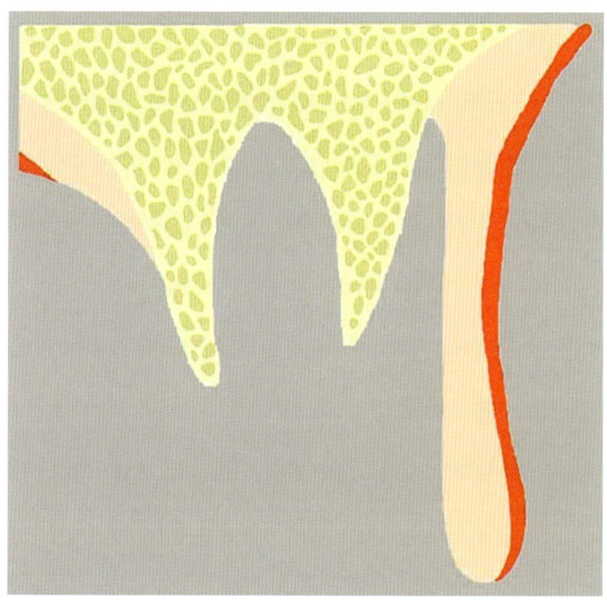

Figure 2.12 A palatal flap has been reflected.

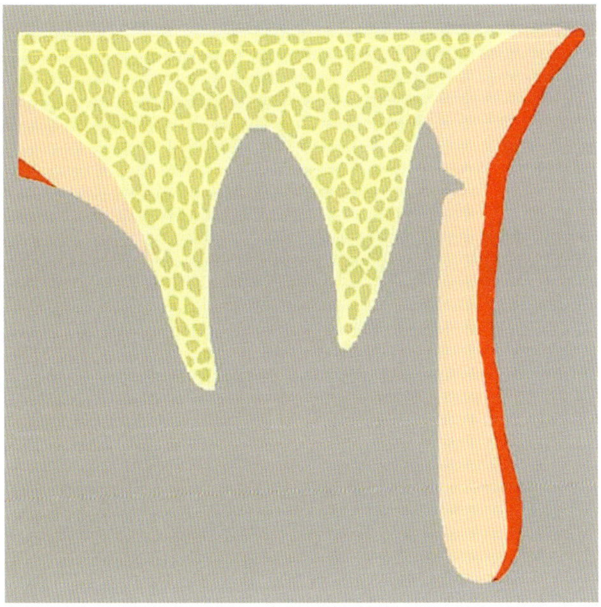

Figure 2.13 An incision is made on the internal aspect of the palatal flap approximately 3–4 mm from the base of the flap. This incision extends mesiodistally over the area to be regenerated.

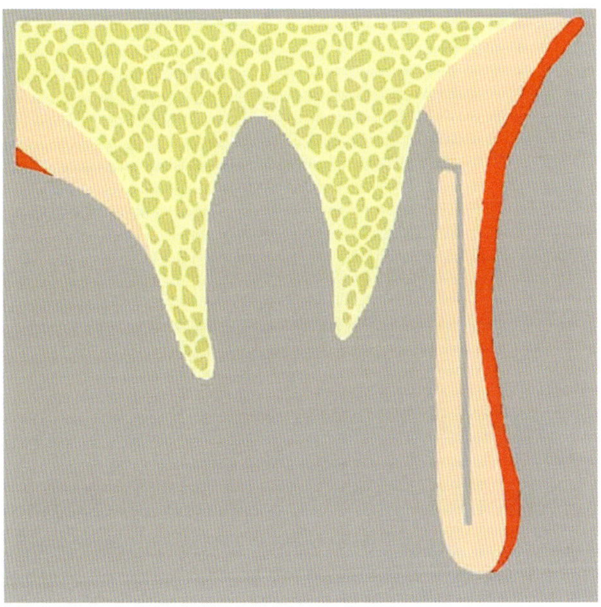

Figure 2.14 Utilizing a tissue forcep and a 15 blade, the internal aspect of the palatal flap is split, extending toward its crestal aspect. Care is taken not to excessively thin the isthmus of soft tissue remaining at the crestal aspect of the flap.

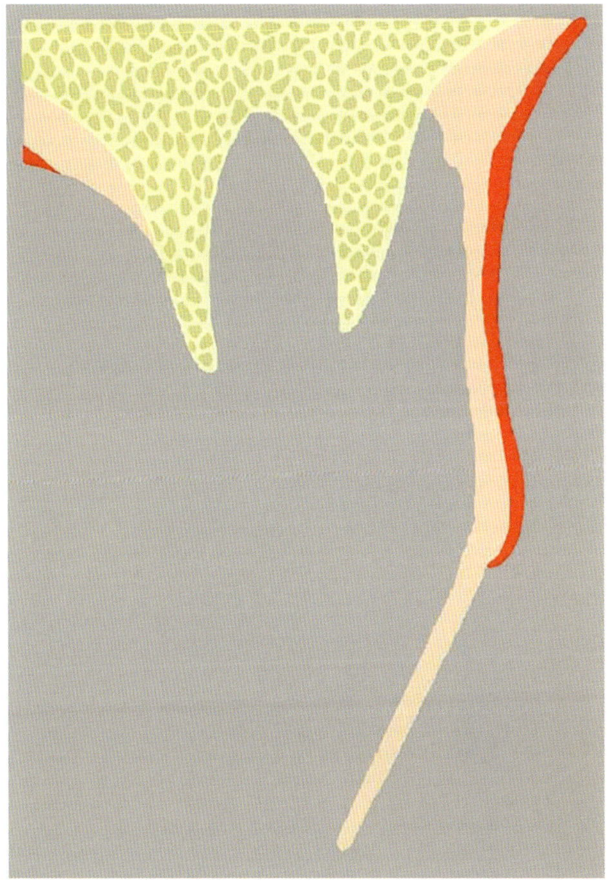

Figure 2.15 Utilizing a tissue pickup and a 15 blade, the flap is filleted, rotating a palatal pedicle from its internal aspect, and extending the flap length by approximately 70%.

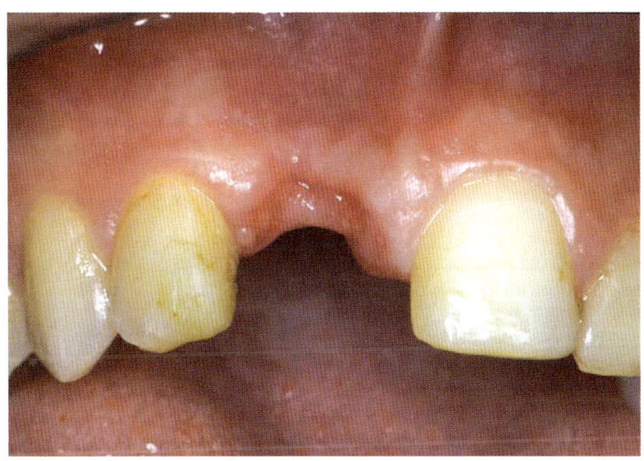

Figure 2.16 A buccal view demonstrates both the loss of the maxillary right central incisor and the atrophic nature of the residual alveolar ridge.

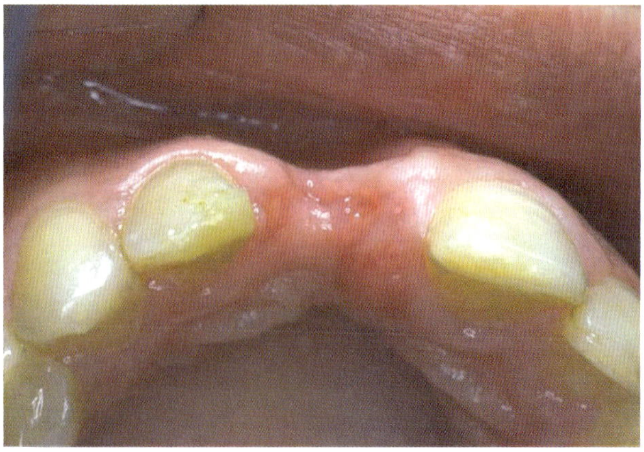

Figure 2.17 A crestal view demonstrates the severe buccal ridge atrophy which has occurred.

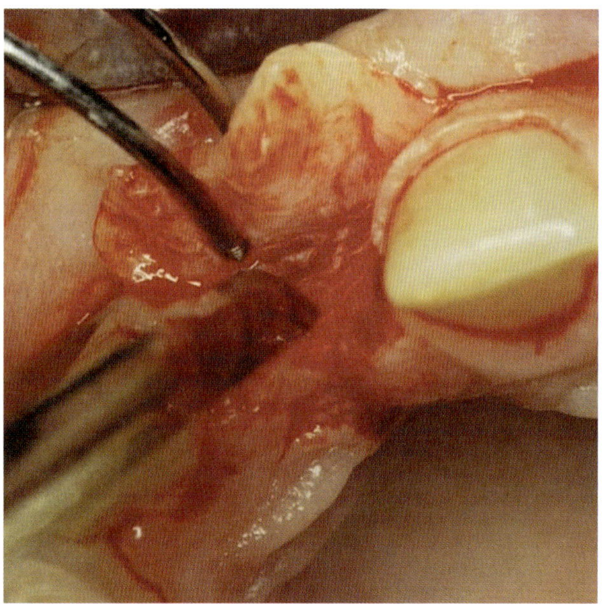

Figure 2.18 A horizontal releasing incision is made 8 mm palatal to the crest of the ridge, and carried buccally in a split thickness manner.

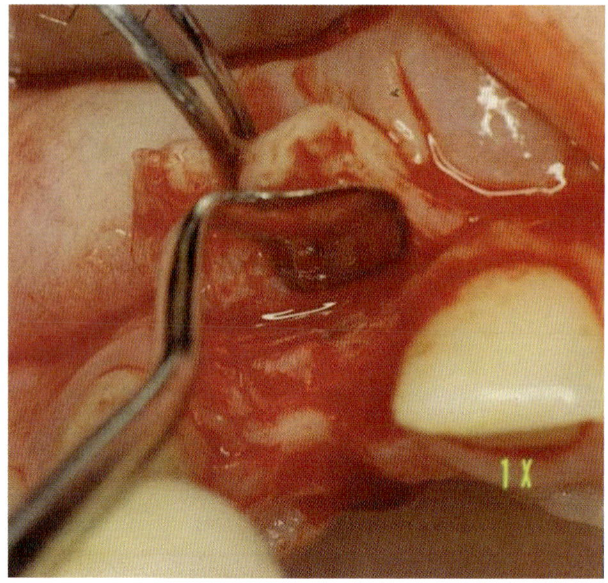

Figure 2.19 At the buccal line angle of the ridge, a Goldman-Fox 7 knife is utilized to score the flap, transforming the reflection from a partial thickness reflection into a full thickness reflection.

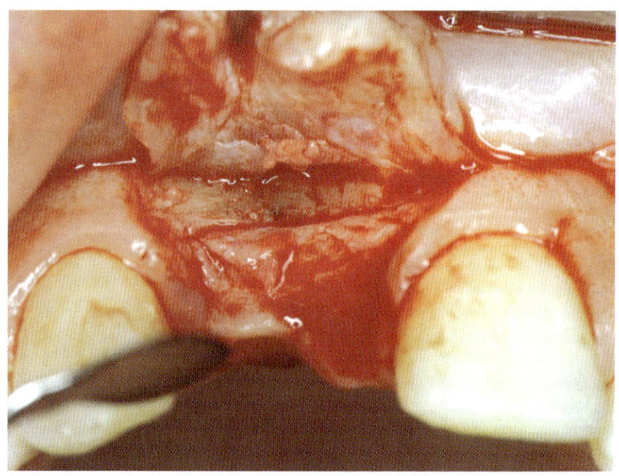

Figure 2.20 Following reflection of the buccal mucoperiosteal flap, the residual soft tissue covering the alveolar ridge is evident.

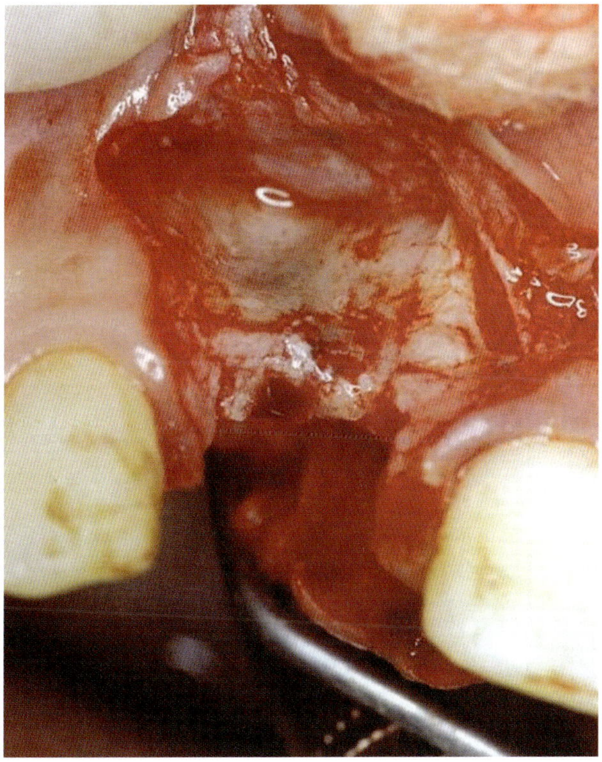

Figure 2.21 Buccal flap reflection reveals a significant buccal ridge defect.

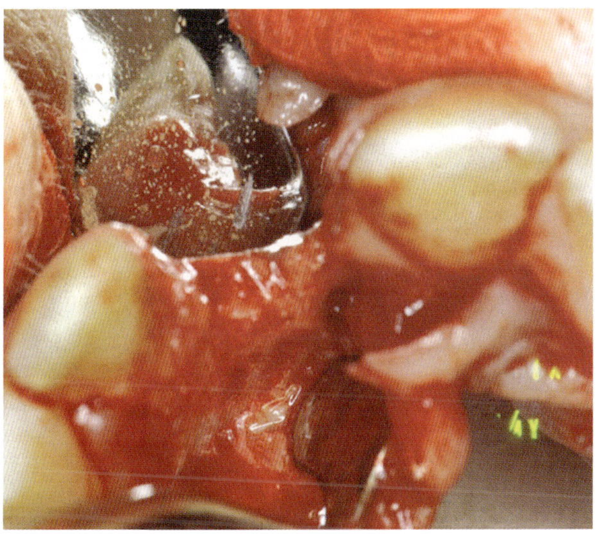

Figure 2.22 A crestal view demonstrates the severe ridge atrophy which has occurred.

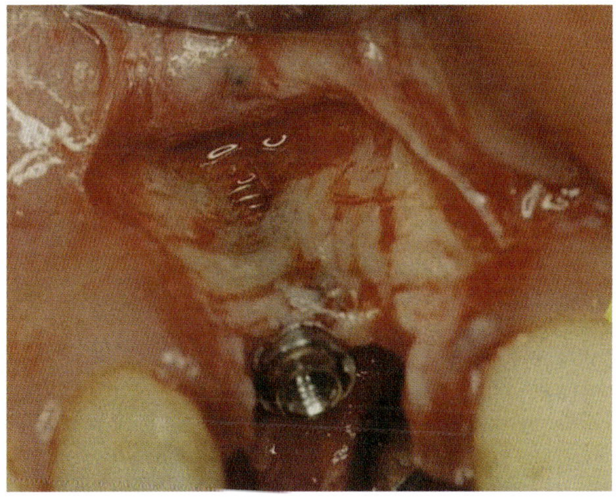

Figure 2.23 Following implant placement a minor buccal fenestration is noted.

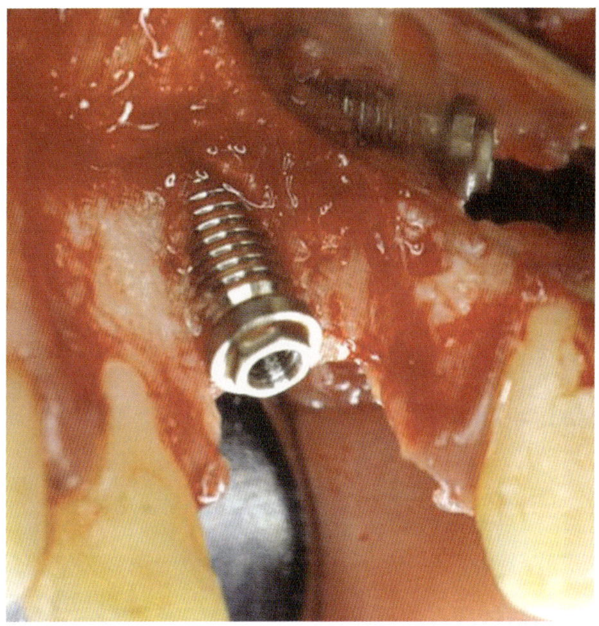

Figure 2.24 A palatal view demonstrates a moderate alveolar bone dehiscence.

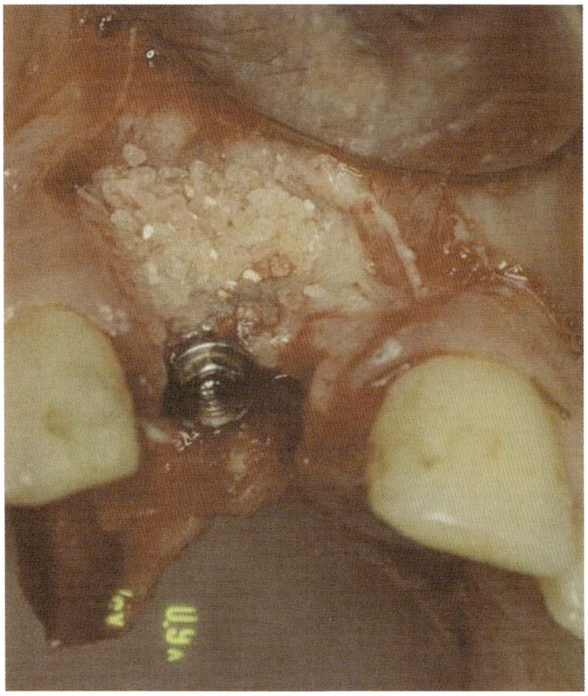

Figure 2.25 A combination of demineralized freeze-dried bone allograft and resorbable hydroxyapatite are placed around the implant.

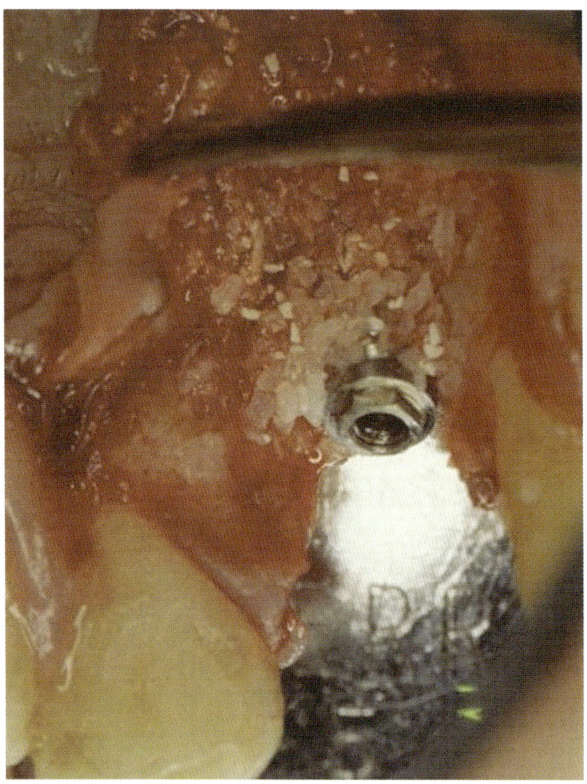

Figure 2.26 The palatal dehiscence is covered with the aforementioned particulate graft mixture.

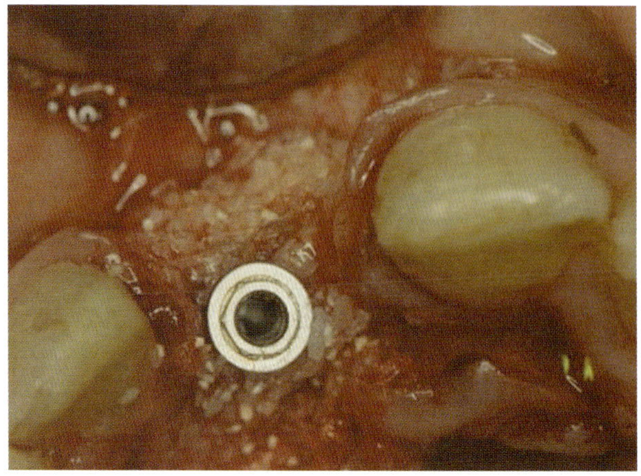

Figure 2.27 A crestal view demonstrates the palatal implant position which was dictated by the position of the residual alveolar ridge, and limitations in performing ridge augmentation therapy at the time of treatment. Such a therapeutic approach would not be utilized today.

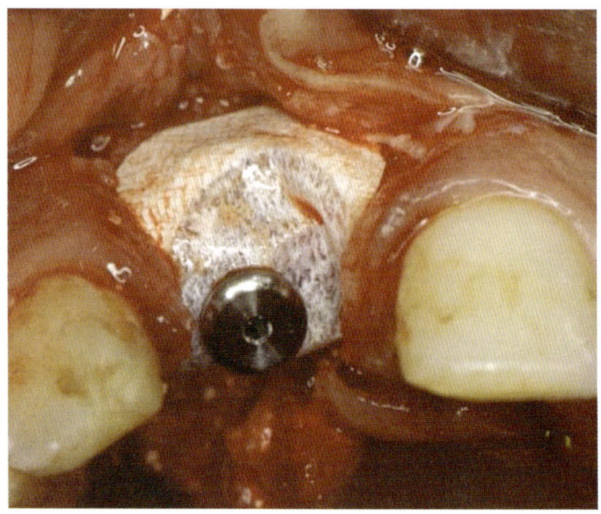

Figure 2.28 A Gore-Tex membrane is shaped and secured with a first-stage implant surgical sealing screw.

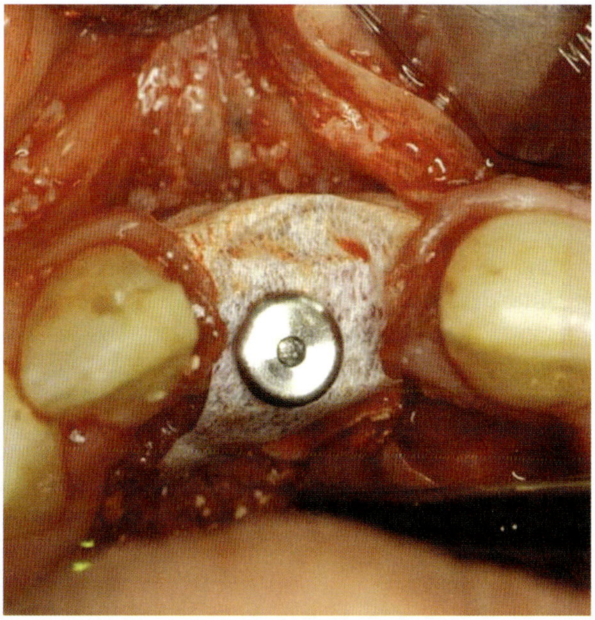

Figure 2.29 A crestal view demonstrates reestablishment of ideal ridge contours with the Gore-Tex membrane.

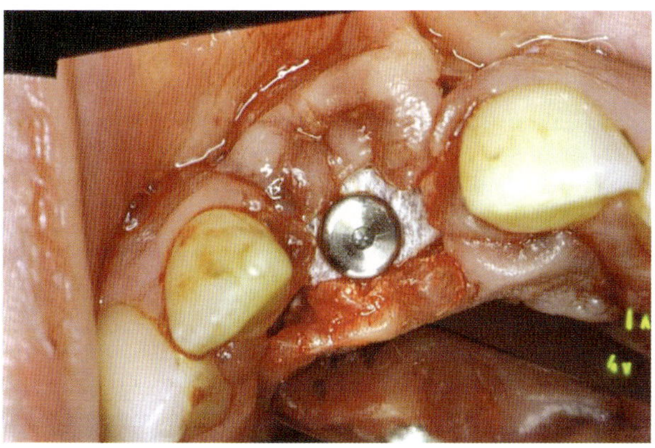

Figure 2.30 Inadequate soft tissue is present to attain passive soft tissue primary closure. A small amount of soft tissue extension of the palatal flap has been gained through the use of the split thickness approach previously described. Note the palatal vertical releasing incisions at a distance one tooth mesial and distal from the site to be regenerated.

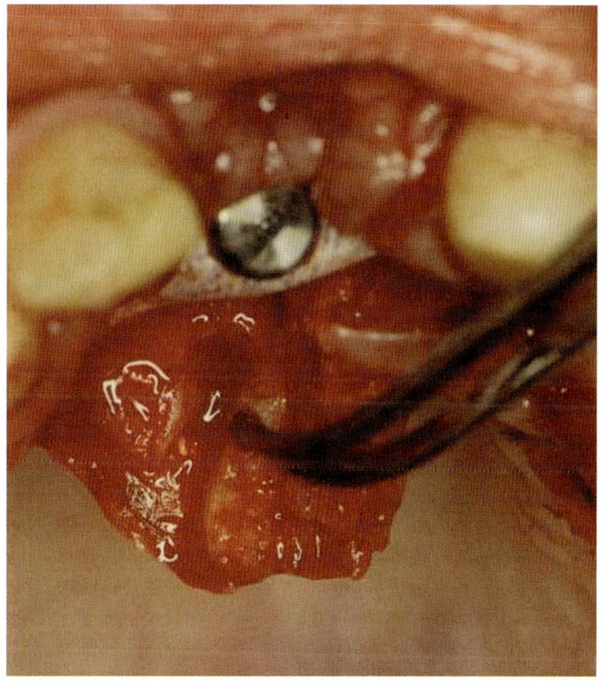

Figure 2.31 Following placement of an incision on the internal aspect of the palatal flap approximately 3–4 mm from the base of the flap, the internal aspect of the flap is held with a tissue forcep. A 15 blade will now be utilized to fillet this internal aspect of the palatal flap.

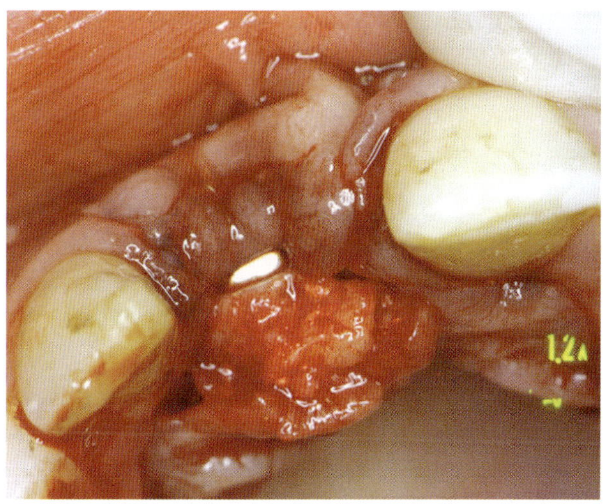

Figure 2.32 A palatal pedicle is rotated from the internal aspect of the palatal flap.

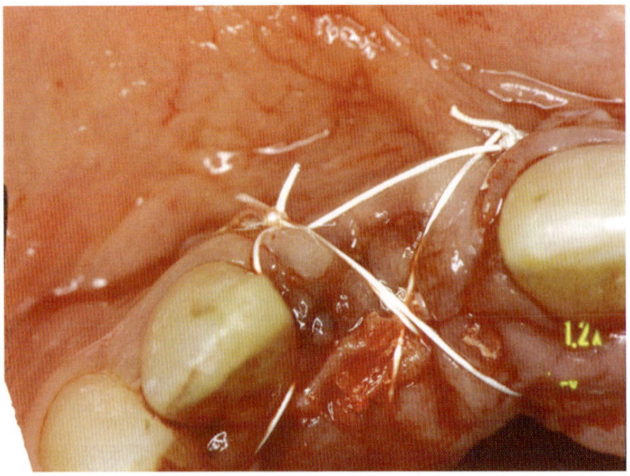

Figure 2.33 The rotated pedicle is tucked beneath the buccal flap and the mucoperiosteal flaps are sutured with interrupted Gore-Tex sutures.

of her missing maxillary central incisor. Preoperative clinical examination demonstrated that regenerative therapy would be necessary to maximize the esthetic outcomes of treatment.

Mesial and distal releasing incisions were placed, taking care to preserve the papillae against the adjacent teeth.

A horizontal incision was made approximately 8 mm palatal to the crest of the ridge. This incision was carried buccally in a split thickness manner, until the buccal line angle of the ridge was reached. A Goldman-Fox 7 was utilized to score the underlying soft tissue at this point, changing the split thickness reflection into a full thickness reflection. The buccal flap was reflected in a full thickness manner. Following buccal flap reflection, soft tissue remains covering the crest of the ridge, which will be reflected as part of the palatal flap, as previously described by Langer and Langer (Figures 2.18–2.20).

Following buccal and palatal mucoperiosteal flap reflection, the atrophic nature of the residual alveolar ridge was evident (Figures 2.21 and 2.22). Due to limitations of when the patient was treated, the implant was placed within the residual alveolar ridge, and regenerative therapy was performed around the implant. As will be demonstrated through examination of subsequent cases, the treatment approach employed today would be to rebuild an ideal ridge form and place the implant in the most ideal prosthetic position. This approach was not considered predictable at the time the patient in question was treated.

Following implant placement, a minor buccal fenestration and a moderate palatal dehiscence were present (Figures 2.23 and 2.24). Note that a smooth surface, hex-headed, screw type Branemark implant was utilized. This implant type would not be employed today.

A combination of demineralized freeze-dried bone and resorbable hydroxyapatite were placed around the implant to rebuild the desired ridge contours (Figures 2.25 and 2.26). The theory at the time of treatment was that the resorbable hydroxyapatite would maintain space beneath the membrane and slowly resorb, while the bone morphogenic proteins in the demineralized freeze-dried bone allograft would facilitate conversion of pluripotential mesenchymal cells into bone forming cells, and thus enhance bone regeneration. As the new bone formed it would replace the resorbing, space maintaining hydroxyapatite. Subsequent research has demonstrated the fallacy of this approach. It has been demonstrated that hydroxyapatite does not resorb at a predictable rate. Furthermore, the osteoinductive capabilities of powdered freeze-dried bone allograft vary widely, not only between companies but also from vial to vial, and cannot be depended upon to predictably induce the necessary regenerative activity.

A crestal view made demonstrates the palatal position of the implant, due to its having been placed in the residual alveolar ridge (Figure 2.27). Subsequent cases will demonstrate that such an approach would not be acceptable today.

Because neither titanium-reinforced membranes nor fixation tacks were available at the time treatment was carried out, a conventional e-PTFE (Gore-Tex) membrane was shaped to the desired ridge contours, placed over the site to be regenerated, and secured with a first-stage implant surgical sealing screw (Figures 2.28 and 2.29). Flap replacement demonstrated that, while some additional soft tissue had been gained by utilizing the split crest Langer and Langer approach, additional soft tissue was required to attain passive soft tissue primary closure (Figure 2.30). Following placement of oblique palatal releasing incisions one tooth mesial and distal to the site to be regenerated, a horizontal incision was made on the internal aspect of the flap, as previously described. Figure 2.31 demonstrates utilization of the 1–2 tissue pickup to hold this internal aspect of the flap, which was to be rotated. A 15 blade was utilized to fillet the internal aspect of the flap (Figure 2.32), resulting in a significant rotated palatal pedicle flap, which was tucked underneath the buccal mucoperiosteal flap. Following suturing, the importance of this rotated palatal pedicle in attaining passive soft tissue primary closure was evident (Figure 2.33).

The efficacy of the aforementioned flap designs in the attainment and maintenance of soft tissue primary closure throughout the course of regeneration was assessed through the examination of 723 consecutive guided bone regeneration cases (17). The following therapies were carried out:

- Tooth extraction with concomitant ridge preservation/regeneration (161 cases).
- Tooth extraction with simultaneous implant placement and regeneration (136 cases).
- Regenerative therapy over implant dehiscences (180 cases).
- Apico-occlusal and/or buccal lingual ridge augmentation (246 cases).

All sites were treated utilizing particulate graft materials and either resorbable Resolut or titanium-reinforced Gore-Tex membranes. Therapy was effected in all areas of the mouth. It is important to realize that regenerative therapy was aimed at reattainment of the prepathologic alveolar ridge morphology. Regenerative therapy in extraction socket areas, with or without concomitant implant placement, was not carried out in conjunction with "crushing" of the walls of the extraction socket defects so as to help attain passive primary closure. Rather, all extraction socket walls were left intact, and efforts were made to regenerate bone within them.

The definition of success was the maintenance of passive soft tissue primary closure for at least six months postregenerative therapy. If a site demonstrated any membrane exposure it was classified as a failure, even if eventual implant placement and restoration were effected.

Utilizing these criteria for success, passive soft tissue primary closure was maintained 96.1% of the time six months postoperatively (Table 2.1).

While the ability to maintain passive soft tissue primary closure throughout the course of regeneration in 96.1% of the cases is encouraging, the fact remains that the 3.9% of the sites that demonstrated membrane exposure did not yield ideal treatment outcomes. There is no doubt that bone regeneration will occur in the face of membrane exposure. However, the morphology of the regenerated bone, and the thickness and quality of the covering soft tissues in such an instance, are not conducive to maximization of esthetic treatment outcomes. Figures 2.34 through 2.46 demonstrate such a situation.

A patient presented with a hopeless prognosis for a maxillary central incisor (Figure 2.34). Following tooth extraction, flap reflection, and defect debridement, the alveolar ridge defect is evident (Figure 2.35). Unfortunately, the buccal releasing incisions which have been employed are inadequate in their apical extension. As a result, two compromises will be encountered. The first is that the titanium-reinforced membrane which is placed over the particulate graft materials will have to be secured in a more crestal position than ideal (Figure 2.36), resulting in less available space for regenerating bone, and creating an undercut in the regenerated bone. In addition, the flaps will be sutured under tension (Figure 2.37).

Table 2.1 Maintenance of soft tissue primary closure after GBR procedures.

Type of therapy	Number of cases	Primary closure maintained	Primary closure lost	Percentage primary closure maintained
Tooth extraction with concomitant ridge preservation/regeneration	161	155	6	96.3
Tooth extraction with simultaneous implant placement and regeneration	136	130	6	95.6
Treatment of implant dehiscences	180	176	4	97.8
Apico-occlusal and/or buccal lingual ridge augmentation	246	234	12	95.1
Total	723	695	28	96.1

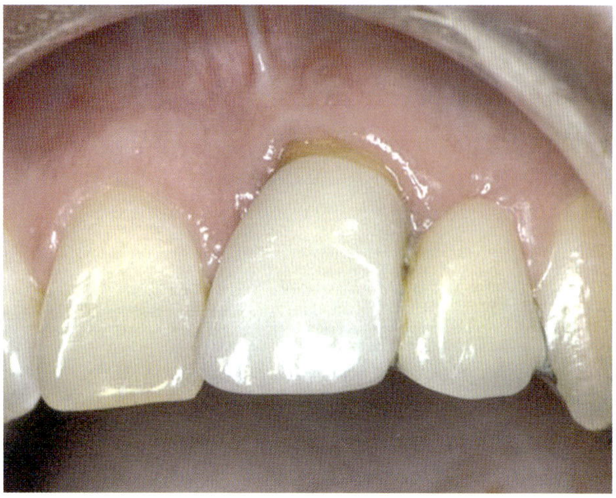

Figure 2.34 The patient presents with a hopeless prognosis for a maxillary central incisor.

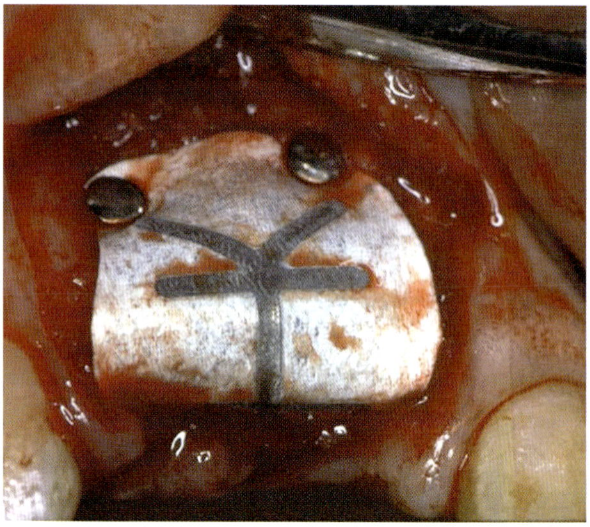

Figure 2.36 A titanium-reinforced membrane is secured with fixation tacks over particulate graft material. Because of the inadequate apical flap reflection which has occurred, the membrane is secured in a position which is too far crestal and will decrease the space available for bone regeneration.

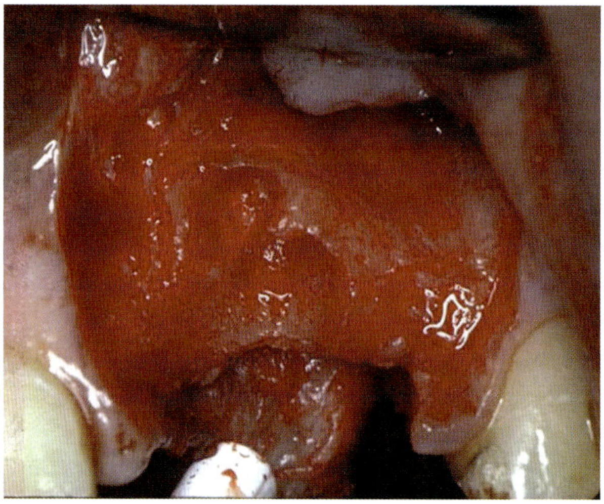

Figure 2.35 Following flap reflection and tooth extraction, a significant alveolar ridge defect is evident. Note the inadequate apical extensions of the releasing incisions.

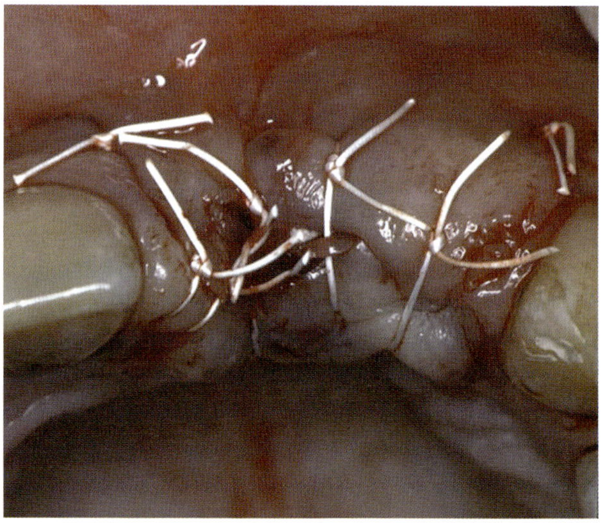

Figure 2.37 The mucoperiosteal flaps are sutured with Gore-Tex sutures. The aforementioned inadequate flap reflection has resulted in the flaps being sutured under tension.

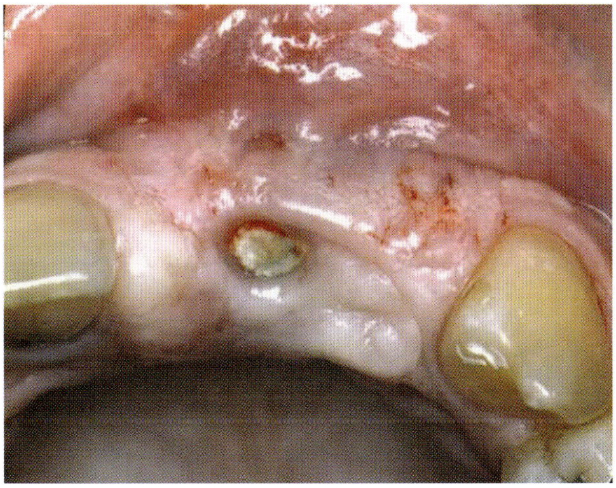

Figure 2.38 Membrane exposure is evident approximately five weeks after regenerative therapy has been performed.

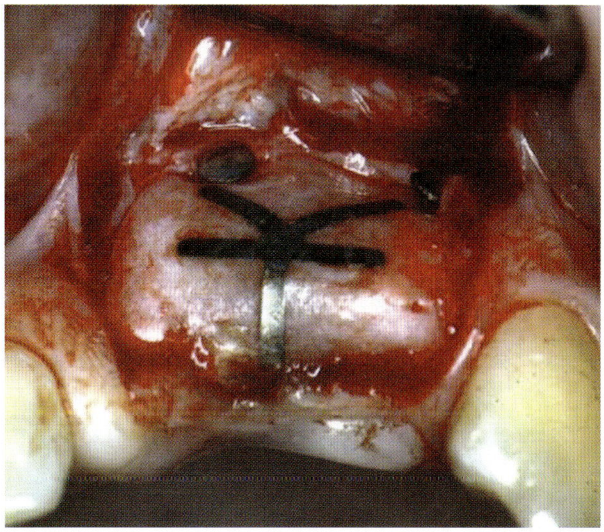

Figure 2.40 A buccal view demonstrates the undercut which has been created in the regenerating ridge, due to the need to secure the membrane with fixation tacks in a position which is too far crestal.

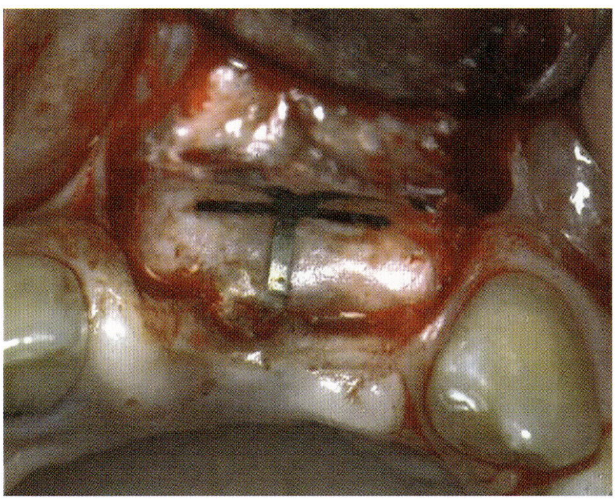

Figure 2.39 The area of previous membrane exposure is evident following flap reflection six months post-regenerative therapy.

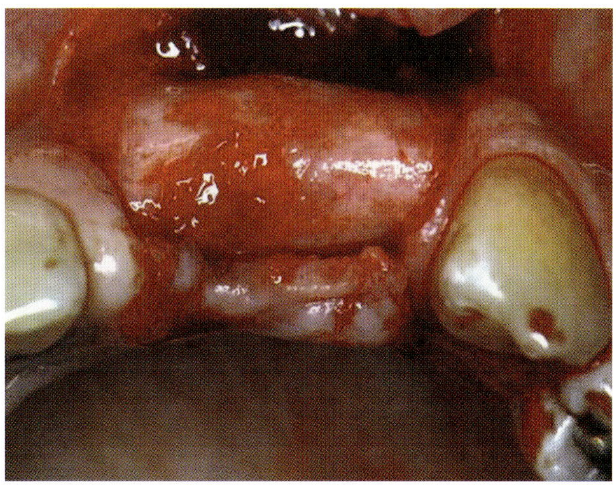

Figure 2.41 Following membrane removal, the area of previous membrane exposure is evident.

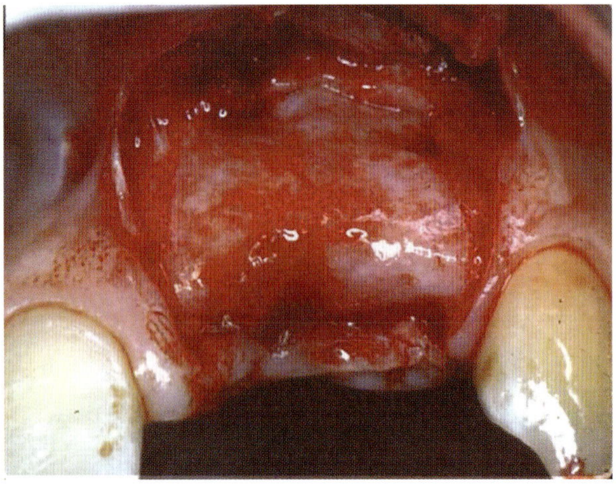

Figure 2.42 A buccal view demonstrates the severe undercut created in the regenerated alveolar bone.

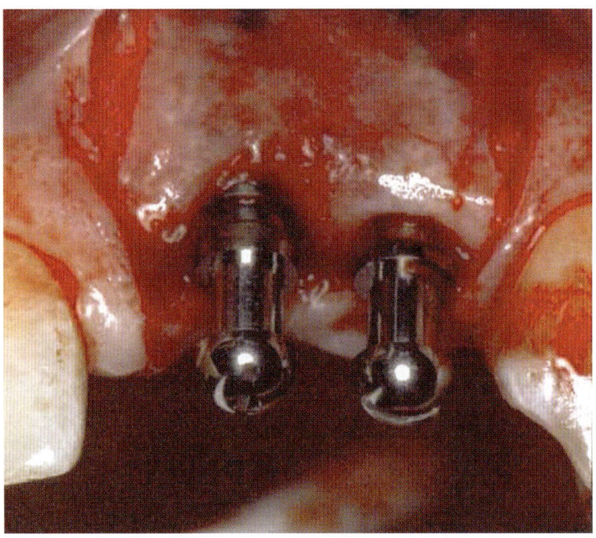

Figure 2.43 Following implant placement, fenestrations are noted at the "apices" of the implants.

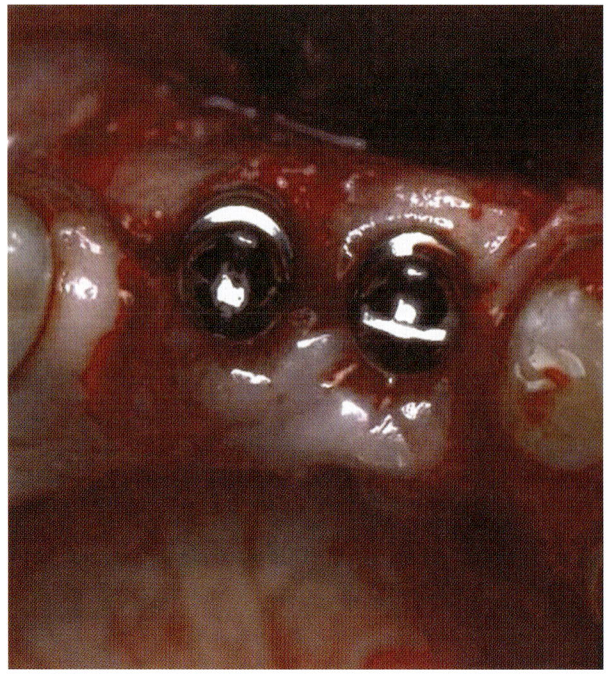

Figure 2.44 A nonresorbable membrane is placed over the fenestrated areas. This membrane will be subsequently removed.

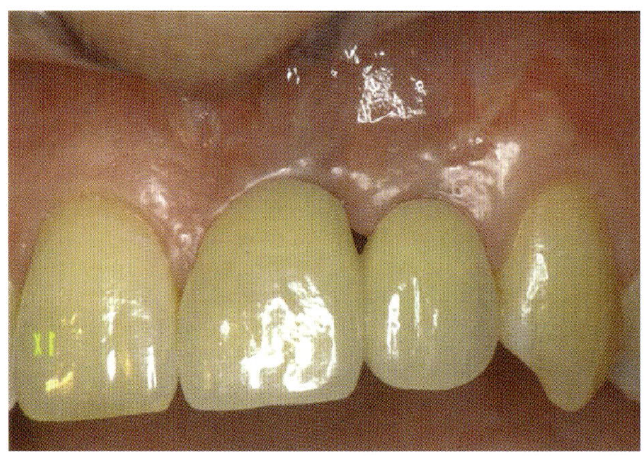

Figure 2.45 Following implant restoration, the lack of a soft tissue papilla between the implants, which corresponds to the site of previous membrane exposure, is evident.

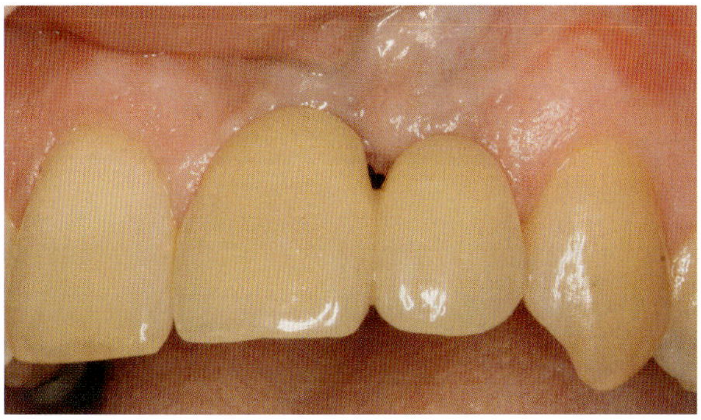

Figure 2.46 Fifteen plus years postoperatively, the peri-implant soft tissues are stable. However, the soft tissues have not regenerated in the area of the missing papilla.

This tension under suturing resulted in membrane exposure approximately five weeks post-regenerative therapy (Figure 2.38). Following flap reflection six months postregenerative therapy and membrane removal, both the lesser bone regeneration at the site of membrane exposure, and the undercut created in the regenerated alveolar bone, are evident (Figures 2.39–2.42). Following placement of titanium plasma-sprayed IMZ implants, a fenestration was evident at the "apex" of the implant in the central incisor position. The limited selection of implant diameters and configurations at the time this patient was treated precluded implant selection would have avoided such a fenestration (Figure 2.43). A nonresorbable membrane was placed over the fenestrated area (Figure 2.44), and removed at a later date. Following implant restoration, the lack of an interimplant papilla is evident (Figure 2.45), and is due at least in part to the loss of soft tissue primary closure and subsequent membrane exposure in this site. While a 15-plus postoperative view demonstrated stability of the peri-implant soft tissues, no regeneration of soft tissue in the papillary area has occurred.

Membrane exposure posttherapy; a compromise in the volume and morphology of regenerated bone; the need to perform additional therapies; an increase in the complexity and postoperative morbidity of therapy; protraction of the length of therapy; and a nonideal esthetic result are all attributable to the use of inadequate buccal releasing incisions.

Assessment of the surgical photographs of the sites that exhibited membrane exposure postoperatively in the previously quoted study demonstrated three contributing factors to such exposure:

- Inadequate horizontal releasing incisions: If the extent of the horizontal releasing incisions is not appropriate, adequate flap mobility will not occur, and the mucoperiosteal flaps will be sutured under tension.
- The need for secondary reflection: Following membrane placement and securing with an appropriate fixation system, a secondary full thickness flap reflection must be carried out, to ensure that no flap fibers are attached to the bone within 3 mm of the most apical border and the apical "corners" of the membrane. Failure to carry out this secondary reflection will result in the flap becoming caught on the borders of the membrane, leading to additional tension on the flap and an increased incidence of membrane exposure postoperatively.
- Performance of regeneration with or without simultaneous implant placement in maxillary molar sites where the presence of an extensive palatal torus results in soft tissues which are too thin to afford the opportunity for palatal pedicle flap rotation: Recognition of this problem led to the creation of a new flap design (Figures 2.47–2.52), described below.

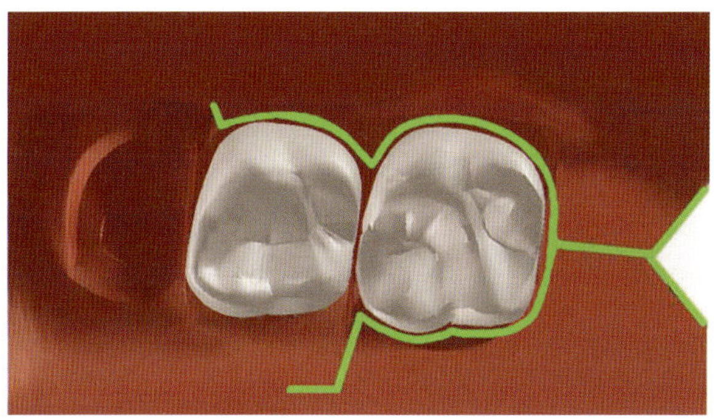

Figure 2.47 A sulcular incision is placed on the buccal aspect of the second molar. This incision is extended over the tuberosity. Distal to the tuberosity, an oblique buccal releasing incision is placed. A buccal vertical releasing incision is placed on the mesial aspect of the second molar. A horizontal releasing incision is placed at the apex of the vertical releasing incision, as previously described. A sulcular incision is placed on the palatal aspects of the first and second molars. This incision continues along the crestal incision on the tuberosity area, and ends with an oblique palatal releasing incision in the mucosa distal to the tuberosity. An oblique releasing incision is placed on the mesial aspect of the first molar.

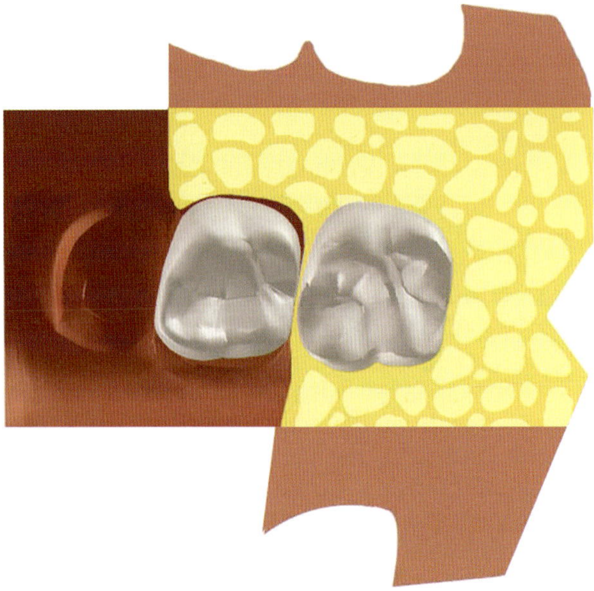

Figure 2.48 The buccal and palatal mucoperiosteal flaps are reflected in a full thickness manner.

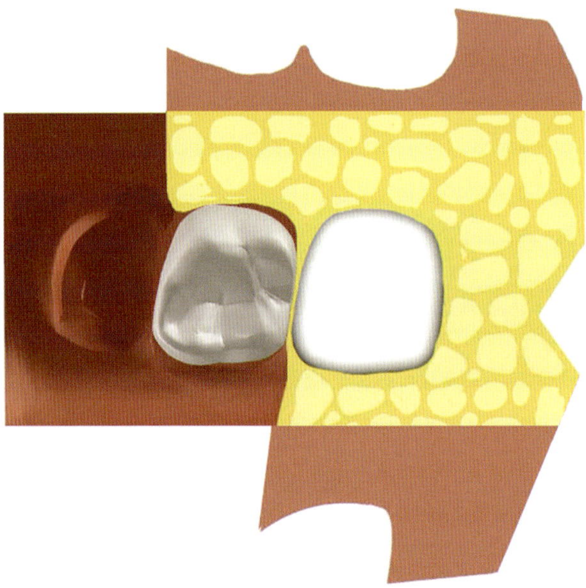

Figure 2.49 The second molar is extracted, following tooth sectioning to preserve the residual alveolar bone.

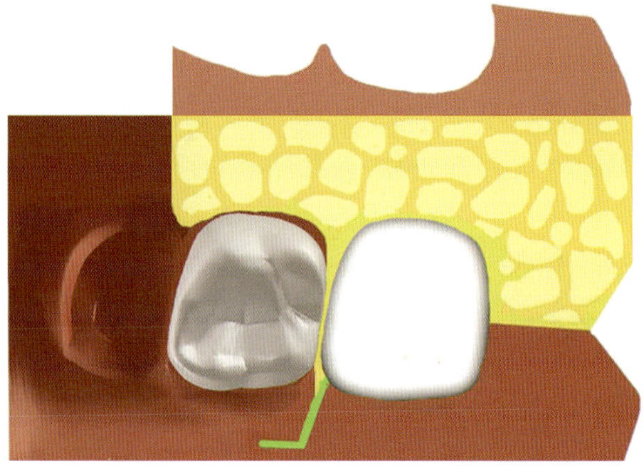

Figure 2.50 Following tooth removal and placement of regenerative materials, inadequate soft tissues are present for attainment of passive primary closure over the treated site, without flap repositioning and pedicle rotation.

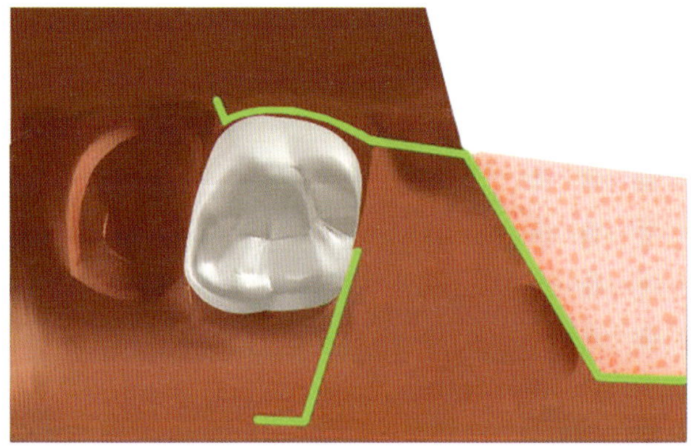

Figure 2.51 The buccal flap is rotated mesially and crestally to cover the treated site. The most mesiocrestal aspect of the buccal flap will contact the distopalatal line angle of the adjacent tooth. A palatal pedicle flap is now rotated from the area palatal to the tuberosity to cover any bone which has been exposed following buccal flap rotation.

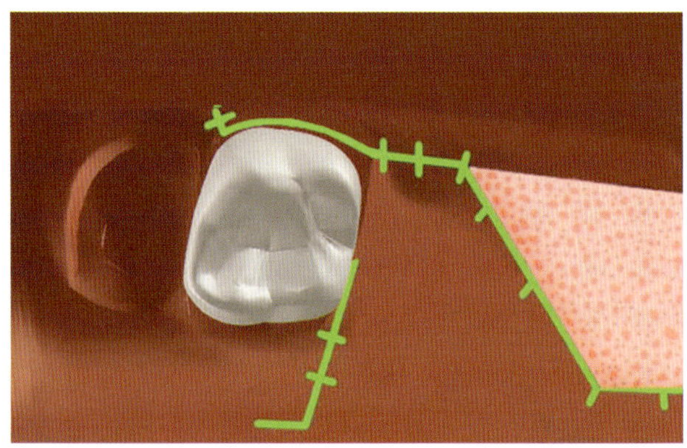

Figure 2.52 The flaps are sutured with interrupted sutures.

A buccal sulcular incision is performed around the tooth to be extracted. This incision is carried distally across the tuberosity, into the mucosa distal to the tuberosity. An oblique buccal releasing incision is placed in the mucosa distal to the tuberosity. A vertical releasing incision is placed at the mesial aspect of the tooth to be extracted, and a horizontal releasing incision is placed at the base of the mesiobuccal releasing incision, as previously described. A sulcular incision is placed palatally around the tooth to be extracted and the tooth mesial to the tooth to be extracted. This palatal sulcular incision joins the tuberosity incision which has already been created. A palatal oblique releasing incision is placed in the mucosa distal to the tuberosity. An oblique releasing incision is placed at the most mesial extent of the palatal sulcular incision. The buccal and palatal mucoperiosteal flaps are reflected in a full thickness manner.

The maxillary molar to be extracted is sectioned and removed, with care being taken to preserve all remaining alveolar bone. Following placement of graft materials and the appropriate secured covering membrane, the buccal mucoperiosteal flap is rotated mesially and crestally. This rotation is easily effected, as this flap is highly mobile once adequate full thickness reflection is carried out into the mucosa distal to the tuberosity. The flap is rotated to such an extent as to cover the site treated with regeneration. The most mesiocrestal aspect of the buccal mucoperiosteal flap should contact the distopalatal line angle of the adjacent tooth. Such flap reflection often results in bone exposure in the tuberosity area.

A rotated palatal pedicle flap is now carried out in the soft tissues palatal to the tuberosity. Adequate soft tissue thickness is almost always present in this area to effect such therapy. While a significant incidence of tori on the palatal aspects of maxillary molars has been reported in the literature, such tori are rarely found palatal to the tuberosity area. The mucoperiosteal flaps are sutured with interrupted Gore-Tex and 4-0 plain gut sutures.

The efficacy of these flap designs was examined in a publication reporting upon 173 consecutive guided bone regeneration procedures (18). Case types treated included tooth extraction with regeneration; tooth extraction with implant placement and regeneration; implant dehiscences; and apical occlusal and or buccal lingual ridge augmentation procedures. The techniques utilized to attain soft tissue primary closure included both those reported upon in the previously cited publication, and utilization of longer horizontal releasing incisions at the apical extents of the buccal vertical releasing incisions; "secondary reflection" around the apical border and corners of the membranes; and the incorporation of the flap designs specifically created for utilization when extracting molars in areas with large palatal tori. Any membrane exposure within six months after regeneration had been performed was classified a failure, even if the regenerative therapy was successful. Utilizing these criteria, primary closure was maintained in 171 of 173 cases, yielding a success rate of 98.8% (Table 2.2).

SUTURING MATERIALS AND TECHNIQUES

All mucoperiosteal flaps are sutured with individual interrupted sutures. Releasing incisions are always sutured with 4-0 plain gut sutures. Crestal

Table 2.2 Maintenance of soft tissue closure after GBR procedures utilizing technical modifications.

Type of therapy	Number of cases	Primary closure maintained	Primary closure lost	Percentage primary closure maintained
Extraction with concomitant regeneration	73	72	1	98.6
Extraction with simultaneous implant placement and regeneration	47	46	1	97.9
Apico-occlusal and/or buccal lingual ridge augmentation	53	53	0	100
Total	173	171	2	98.8

incisions are sutured with Gore-Tex sutures on the mesial and distal extensions of the mucoperiosteal flaps, and mid-flap. Additional Gore-Tex sutures may be utilized in flaps of wide expanses. The 4-0 plain gut interrupted sutures are employed between the interrupted Gore-Tex sutures. No continuous sling sutures or other suturing materials are utilized. The Gore-Tex sutures are placed as mentioned to hold the flap positions passively attained through appropriate design and reflection. The plain gut sutures, which resorb at 3–6 days postoperatively, are employed to minimize patient discomfort due to sutures "tightening up" in mucosal areas.

DECORTICATION

All mandibular sites to be regenerated are decorticated with a piezo surgery tip under copious irrigation. Maxillary ridges are not decorticated, as a cortex is rarely present. The purpose of decortication is to open the marrow spaces, provide bleeding to the site, and afford a path of ingress for endothelial and blood cells.

Graft material must always be placed beneath a covering membrane, to stabilize the blood clot necessary to effect bone regeneration. Failure to place graft material will result in clot shrinkage of up to 15–20%, yielding a lesser volume of regenerated bone.

MEMBRANE SELECTION

Ideally, membrane utilization in guided bone regeneration therapy should accomplish a number of goals, including:

- graft containment
- defect and graft isolation from overlying soft tissue cells
- assistance in underlying clot stabilization
- space maintenance in non-space-maintaining defects to help maximize the volume of regenerated bone

While a variety of resorbable and nonresorbable membranes are available for clinical use, membrane selection should not be dependent upon cost or ease of implementation. Rather, membranes should be chosen in accordance with the aforementioned membrane functions.

All membranes should be biocompatible, and nonallergenic. In addition, resorbable membranes should resorb at a predictable rate, and should not release byproducts during resorption which are deleterious to bone growth or overlying soft tissue healing. Nonresorbable membranes should be conducive to the maintenance of soft tissue primary closure, and should not initiate a reaction in the soft tissues which hastens membrane exposure. Reinforced membranes must provide adequate reinforcement to maintain the desired space in individual clinical situations.

Inadequacies in clinical acumen or chosen technique should not be offered as an excuse for limiting the type of membrane utilized. If a clinician is unable to predictably attain and maintain soft tissue primary closure, nonresorbable titanium-reinforced membranes will rarely be employed, as the postoperative sequellae would be highly problematic. Rather than eliminating such membrane use from the clinical practice, efforts should be made to seek the appropriate education and to master techniques to properly manage soft tissues and ensure the maintenance of passive soft tissue primary closure over regenerating sites.

MEMBRANE FIXATION

All membranes are fixated. Failure to secure membranes with fixation tacks or screws results in the following complications:

- A greater incidence of loss of soft tissue primary closure: A membrane which is not secured with fixation tacks, and thus is able to move beneath the covering mucoperiosteal flaps, will often institute an inflammatory process in the soft tissues and result in an increased incidence of membrane exposure.
- Membrane movement beneath the mucoperiosteal flaps, even if membrane exposure does not occur, will result in a thicker connective tissue interposed between the covering flaps and the underlying membrane, thus lessening the volume of regenerated bone.
- The precise quantity and morphology of regenerating bone is not predictable beneath an unsecured membrane. In contrast, when a membrane is secured over appropriately chosen graft materials, beneath passively closed covering soft tissues, the morphology of the regenerated bone is highly predictable.

Table 2.3 Membrane fixation options.

Fixation system	Advantages	Disadvantages
Titanium screws	• Ease of use in dense bone	• Need to predrill the site • Length of time involved in use • Need to remove*
Titanium tacks	• Predictability in dense bone • No need to predrill the site • Ease and speed of use	• Need to remove*
Resorbable screws	• Do not have to be removed	• Need to predrill the site • Prone to fracture in dense bone
Resorbable tacks with air gun insertion	• Do not need to be removed • Ease and speed of use	• Problematic in delicate bone • Potentially disconcerting to the patient

*Because the tacks are titanium, many clinicians elect to leave them in place.

Any fixation system utilized during guided bone regeneration should meet the following criteria:

- It must be simple to utilize.
- Tack or screw placement must be rapid. If tack or screw utilization requires a great amount of time, the clinician will often find excuses not to utilize the appropriate number of tacks and/or screws.
- Tack or screw removal must be easily and quickly accomplished.

The systems available for membrane fixation fall into four basic categories (Table 2.3). When examining the advantages and disadvantages of each fixation technique, it becomes evident that employment of a simple nonresorbable tack system offers the greatest number of advantages and the highest degree of clinical applicability.

Figures 2.53–2.57 demonstrate tack placement in an edentulous mandibular model. The tack is picked up in a holder (Figure 2.53). While the assistant reflects the mucoperiosteal flap, the clinician holds the membrane in place and brings the tack to the mouth, laying the tip of it against the membrane (Figure 2.54). Care must be taken to ensure that the tack holder is perpendicular to the plane of the membrane. Failure to accomplish this will result in a large number of tacks "skipping off" the membrane and bone surface as malleting begins. Such off-angle malleting may also result in tack fracture. A tack is gently malletted to place with 3–4 taps (Figure 2.55). The carrying instrument is not removed from the tack at this point. Such removal will often result in removal of the tack in type 3 or 4 bone. A 23 explorer is placed so that its end passes through the prongs at the head of the tack holder (Figure 2.56). The end of the 23 explorer is now held against the tack head. The carrying instrument is removed from the tack head in a turning motion, while the 23 explorer holds the head of the tack in place. The result is fixation of the membrane in the desired position (Figure 2.57). The total elapsed time from engaging the tack in the carrying instrument, to removal of the carrying instrument from the head of the placed tack, is approximately 30–40 seconds.

Appropriately employed guided bone regeneration therapy affords the opportunity to predictably

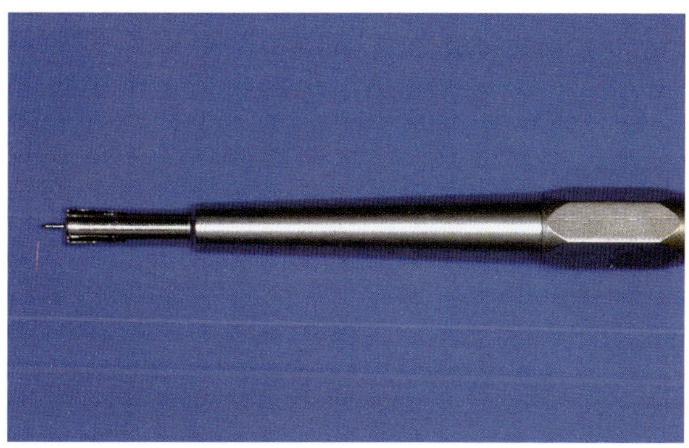

Figure 2.53 A fixation tack is picked up with the carrying instrument.

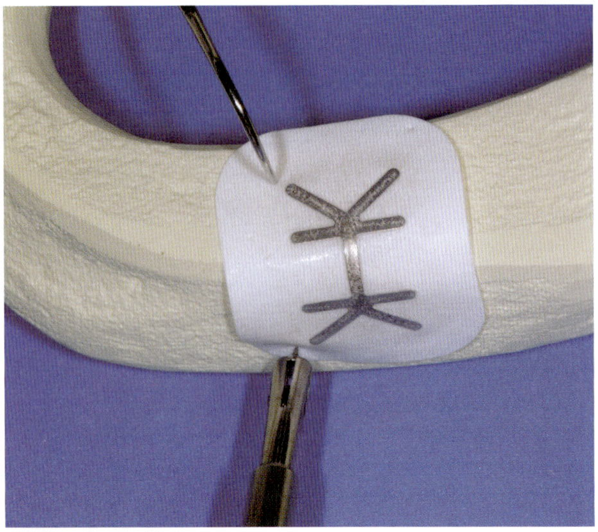

Figure 2.54 While the assistant holds the membrane in place, the tack is placed against it. Care is taken that the carrying instrument is perpendicular to the alveolar ridge.

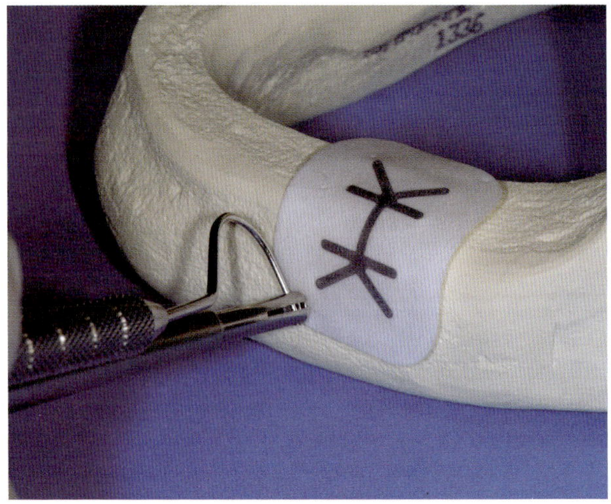

Figure 2.56 The head of the explorer is placed beneath the tines of the tack and held against the head of the tack. The carrying instrument is removed from the head of the tack in a turning motion.

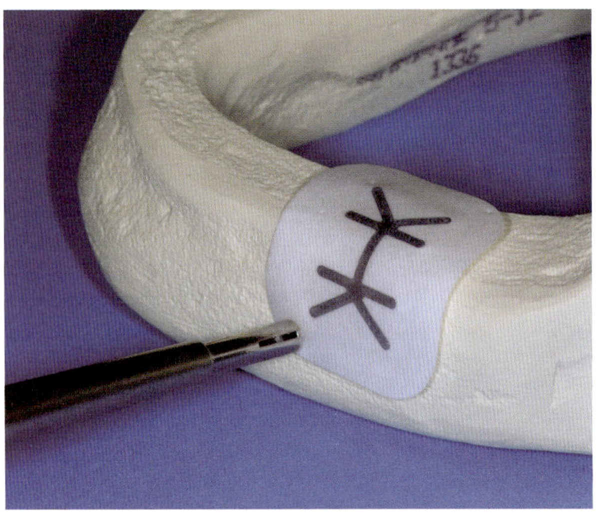

Figure 2.55 A tack is gently malletted to place.

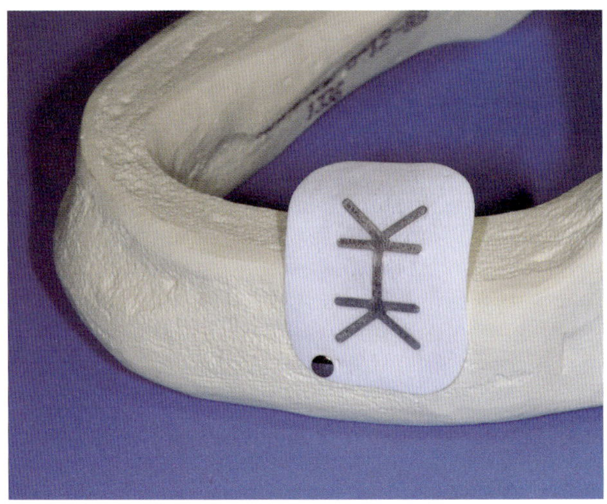

Figure 2.57 The membrane has been secured with a fixation tack.

manage a number of clinical challenges, including regeneration of bone over dehisced or fenestrated implants; regeneration of bone in extraction socket defects surrounding immediately placed implants; and regeneration of atrophic alveolar ridges in bucco lingual/palatal and apio occlusal directions in anticipation of implant placement, or to improve the esthetics of edentulous ridges. It is important to utilize the aforementioned techniques to comprehensively manage such scenarios.

A crucial element of successful guided bone regeneration therapy is membrane selection. Not all membrane types will afford comparable treatment outcomes in all situations.

Clinical Example One

Figure 2.58 demonstrates a dehisced implant in a maxillary bicuspid position. This dehiscence defect is not space maintaining. While the residual mesial alveolar bony wall could support a membrane in the appropriate position, the damage to the alveolar bone on the distal aspect of the implant has resulted in a lack of necessary bone for membrane support. If a resorbable membrane is placed over graft material, regardless of the consistency of the graft material, there is no assurance that appropriate space will be maintained to effect bone regeneration of sufficient dimension to withstand functional forces over time. As a result, a titanium-reinforced Gore-Tex membrane was placed over bovine bone matrix (Bio-Oss) graft material and secured with fixation tacks. Six months postoperatively (Figure 2.59) extensive regenerated bone in this region is evident following membrane removal. The thickness of the regenerated bone must at least be sufficient to withstand functional forces over time, thus fulfilling the second-generation definition of success for guided bone regeneration therapy.

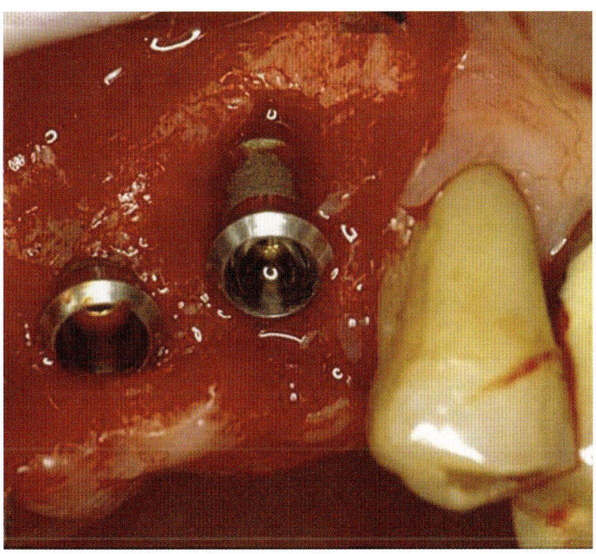

Figure 2.58 Following implant placement, a non-space-maintaining buccal dehiscence defect is noted around the implant in the bicuspid position. This area will be treated with particulate material and a secured titanium-reinforced membrane.

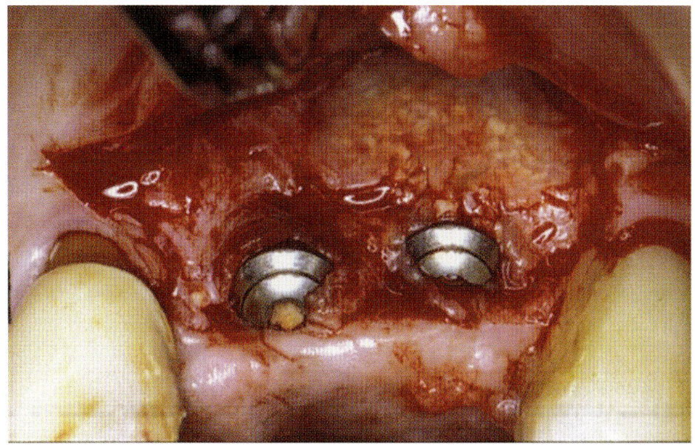

Figure 2.59 Following flap reflection and membrane removal six months postregenerative therapy, significant alveolar ridge regeneration is evident.

Clinical Example Two

A severely atrophic maxillary edentulous ridge is evident in Figure 2.60. Following placement of three 4-mm-wide cylindrical implants, extensive fenestration and dehiscence defects were noted (Figure 2.61). Prior to placement of regenerative materials, the mesial and distal vertical releasing incisions were extended. Horizontal releasing incisions were placed at the most apical extents of the vertical releasing incisions. Due to the non-space-maintaining nature of the dehiscence and fenestration defects, a titanium-reinforced Gore-Tex membrane was trimmed to shape and secured with four apical fixation tacks. Fixation tacks were placed at the mesial and distal corners of the membrane, and "between" the implants apically. The membrane was placed far enough apically to ensure that adequate space remained for placement of graft materials beyond the apices of the implants. Once the

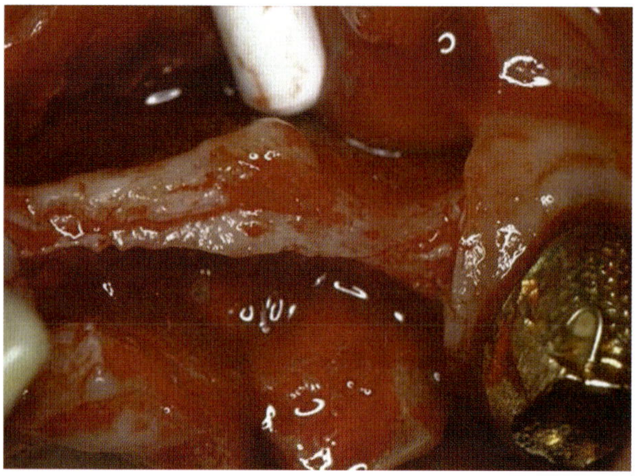

Figure 2.60 The patient presents with a severely atrophic maxillary alveolar ridge.

membrane had been secured, Bio-Oss graft material was placed beneath it.

Care is taken to always secure the implant prior to graft placement. If the graft material is placed first, membrane fixation is difficult, as the graft material may interpose itself between the membrane and the bone in the area where the securing tack is being placed.

Once the graft material had been placed beneath the membrane, the membrane was secured crestally with a single fixation tack. Passive soft tissue primary closure was attained and maintained throughout the course of regeneration.

Eight months postregenerative therapy (Figure 2.62), extensive bone regeneration is evident

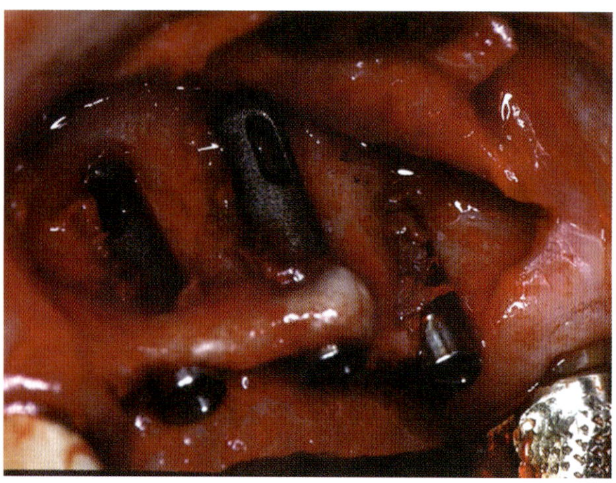

Figure 2.61 Following placement of 4-mm wide IMZ implants, severe fenestration and dehiscence defects are noted. This area will be treated with a Bio-Oss and a secured titanium-reinforced membrane.

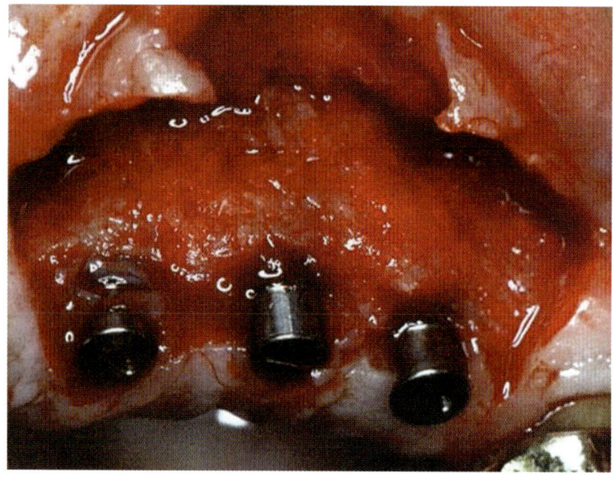

Figure 2.62 Following flap reflection and membrane removal eight months postregenerative therapy, extensive alveolar bone regeneration is noted around the implants.

following membrane removal. This result could not be predictably obtained utilizing a resorbable membrane over particulate graft material.

IMPLANT PLACEMENT IN ATROPHIC RIDGES

Placement of implants in ridges which demonstrate severe bucco lingual/palatal atrophy may prove challenging. The tendency is for the bur to move along the ridge as pressure is applied, resulting in osteotomy preparation in a nonideal position. Such a problem is easily overcome utilizing a specific osteotomy preparation technique (19) designed for atrophic ridges (Figure 2.63–2.67). A 2- or

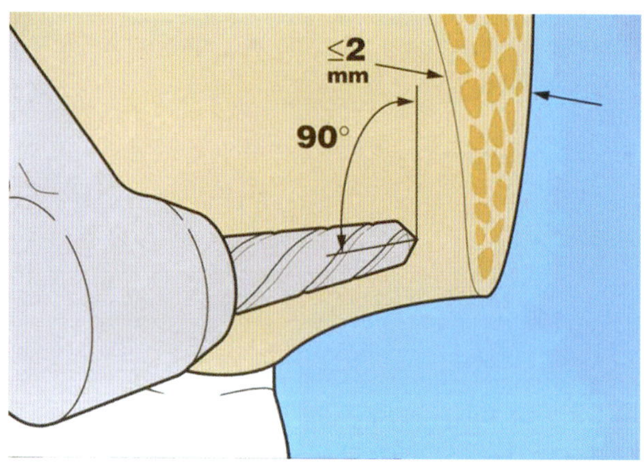

Figure 2.63 A 2.2-mm wide bur is placed perpendicular to the residual alveolar ridge and utilized at a speed of 1000 RPMs.

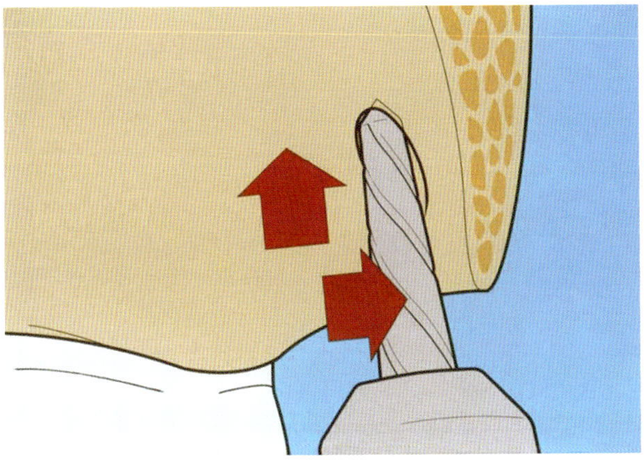

Figure 2.64 Both lateral and vertical pressures are applied with the bur, creating a notch in the alveolar ridge, which will stabilize the bur during osteotomy preparation.

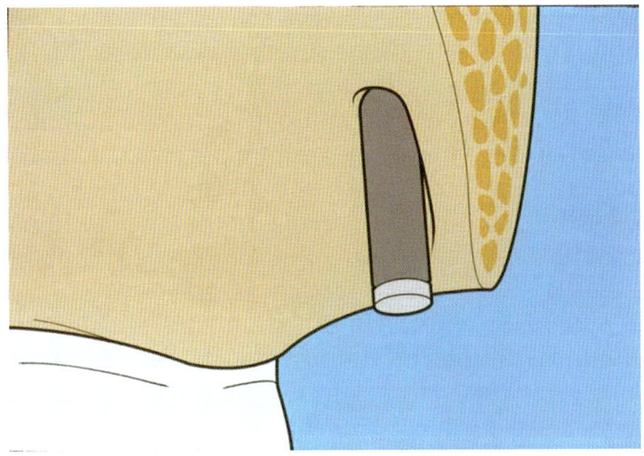

Figure 2.66 The implant is inserted following tapping of the osteotomy site.

2.2-mm-wide twist drill (depending upon the implant system to be utilized) is placed perpendicular to the residual alveolar ridge. Its precise position on the alveolar ridge is dependant upon the desired position of final implant placement. The bur is employed at a speed of 1,000 RPMs. As the bur enters the ridge, pressure is applied laterally and vertically. The result is that the bur creates a "notch" in the ridge. The bur is straightened up gradually as it proceeds more apically. Once the bur has attained its appropriate vertical position, the side of the bur will prepare the previously uncut alveolar ridge crestal to the initial point of entry. Sequentially sized burs are utilized as suggested for the given implant to be placed. Each bur entry is made at a lesser angle to the ridge, until the final bur enters the osteotomy site at close to conventional angulation.

Prior to implant placement the site is tapped, even if a self-tapping implant is to be utilized. Placement of an implant in such a situation often results in only 2–3 threads of the implant securing the fixture in the osteotomy. As a result, it is imperative that the site first be tapped, as adequate bone is not present to allow movement and "wobbling" of the implant as it engages the compromised walls of the osteotomy.

Once the implant has been secured in the appropriate position, a titanium-reinforced Gore-Tex membrane is secured with fixation tacks. Graft material is placed beneath the membrane and

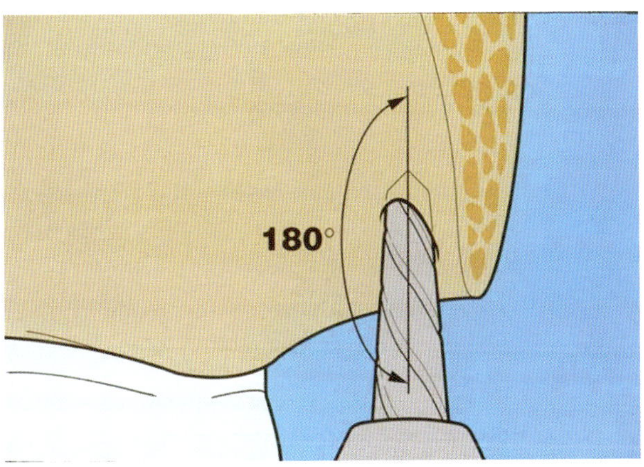

Figure 2.65 Each sequentially sized bur enters the osteotomy at a lesser angle, until the final bur insertion approaches that of conventional osteotomy site preparation. The side of the bur prepares the previously unprepared alveolar bone crestal to the initial point of bur entry.

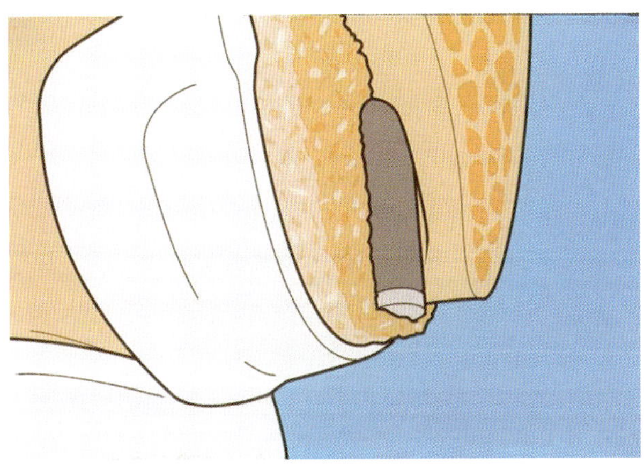

Figure 2.67 Regenerative materials are placed beneath a secured titanium-reinforced membrane.

an additional crestal tack is placed, if necessary. Attainment of soft tissue primary closure proceeds as previously described.

Although such an approach affords the ability to predictably place implants in severely atrophic ridges and attain primary stability at the time of the insertion, with the confidence that sufficient bone may be regenerated to cover all exposed implant surfaces, such an approach is not always the treatment of choice. Because implant positioning is limited by the location of the residual alveolar ridge, implants placed in severely atrophic ridges often must be placed in a position palatal to the ideal prosthetic position which would help ensure maximum esthetics of the final treatment outcome. In addition, narrower implants will often have to be placed in severely atrophic ridges, as compared to the diameters of implants which could be placed in ideally regenerated alveolar ridges. Such a quandary is underscored in the examination of the following patient.

Clinical Example Three

A 19-year-old girl presented following trauma in which she had avulsed her maxillary and mandibular incisors, as well as having lost significant portions of her maxillary and mandibular anterior alveolar ridges.

Examination of the residual maxillary anterior alveolar ridge demonstrated that inadequate bone remained for ideal implant positioning, which would be necessary to afford appropriate implant restoration and esthetics (Figures 2.68 and 2.69). Due to the morphology of the residual alveolar bone, a titanium-reinforced Gore-Tex membrane was chosen. This membrane was shaped with a 15 blade in such a manner as to preserve its space maintaining capabilities where regeneration was required, while not impinging upon either the nasal spine or the nasopalatine foramen (Figure 2.70–2.74). The mucoperiosteal flaps were passively sutured utilizing interrupted Gore-Tex and 4-0 plain gut sutures (Figure 2.75).

Six months postregenerative therapy, passive soft tissue primary closure had been maintained (Figure 2.76). A CAT scan taken at that time demonstrated the extensive buccal ridge regeneration which had occurred. The buccal palatal dimension of the alveolar ridge had been increased two- to threefold (Figure 2.77). Flap reflection and membrane removal confirmed the extensive bone regeneration which had taken place (Figure 2.78).

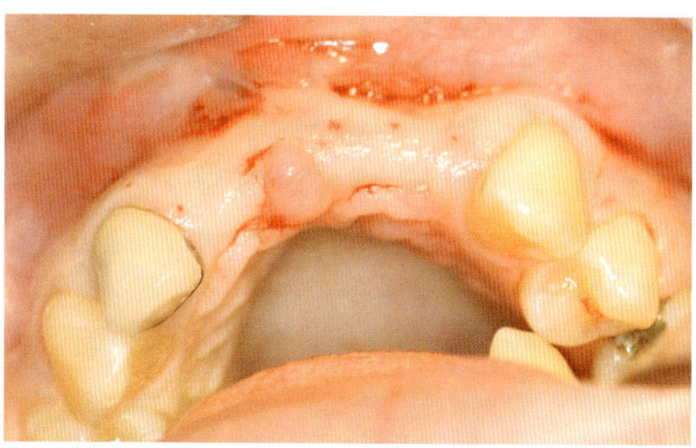

Figure 2.68 A 19-year-old girl presents having avulsed her maxillary anterior teeth.

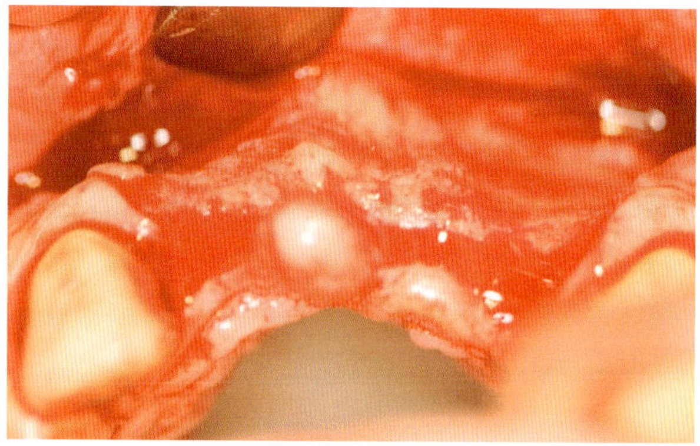

Figure 2.69 Flap reflection reveals the damaged nature of the buccal alveolar bone, and a ridge morphology which precludes ideal implant positioning.

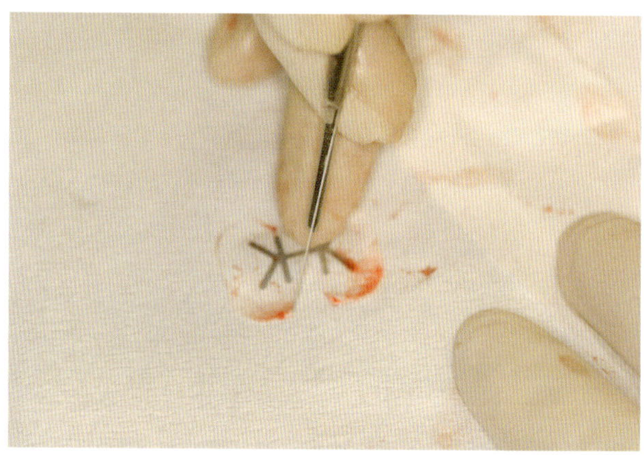

Figure 2.70 A titanium-reinforced Gore-Tex membrane is trimmed with a 15 blade, so as not to impinge upon the nasal spine or the nasopalatine foramen.

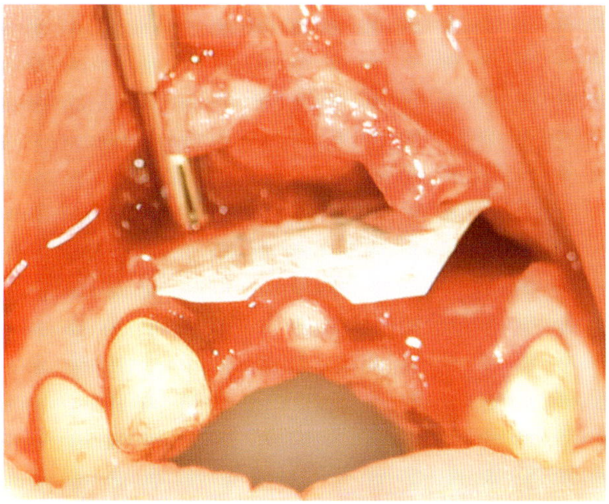

Figure 2.71 The membrane is secured with fixation tacks.

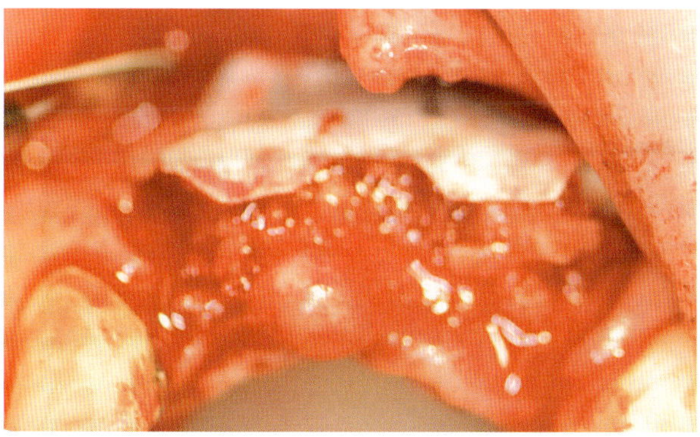

Figure 2.72 The horizontal releasing incisions are extended to increase flap mobility.

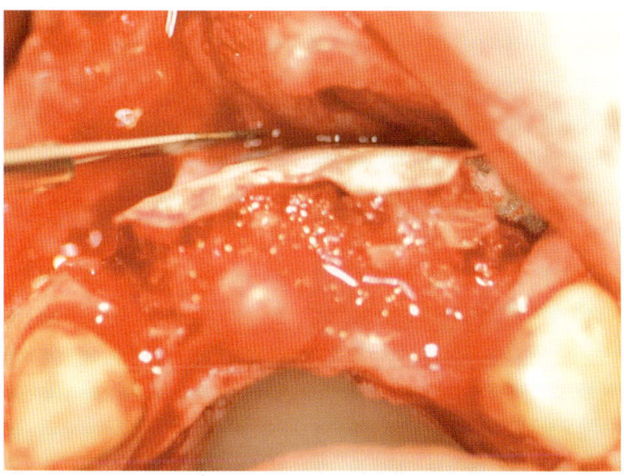

Figure 2.73 Additional flap reflection is carried out over the nasal spine area. Blunt, full thickness dissection will now be accomplished to a distance of 3 mm from the apical border and corners of the membrane.

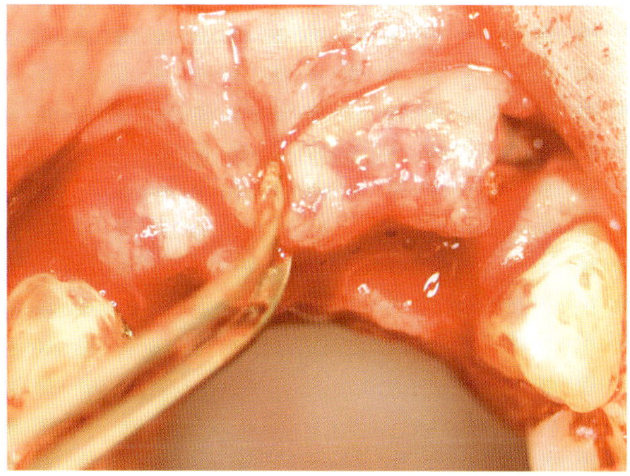

Figure 2.74 Flap mobility is tested to ensure that the flap may be brought to a position equal to the levels of the marginal ridges of the adjacent teeth.

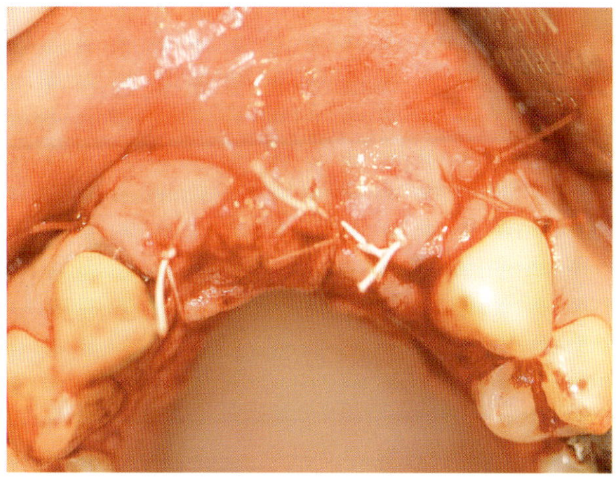

Figure 2.75 The flaps are sutured with interrupted Gore-Tex and 4-0 plain gut sutures.

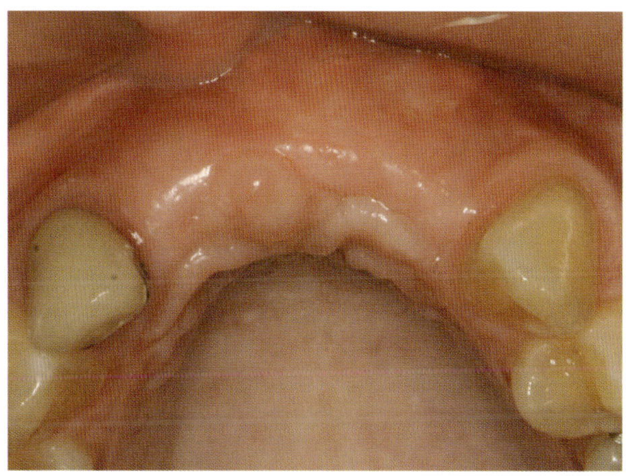

Figure 2.76 Six months postregenerative therapy, passive soft tissue primary closure has been maintained.

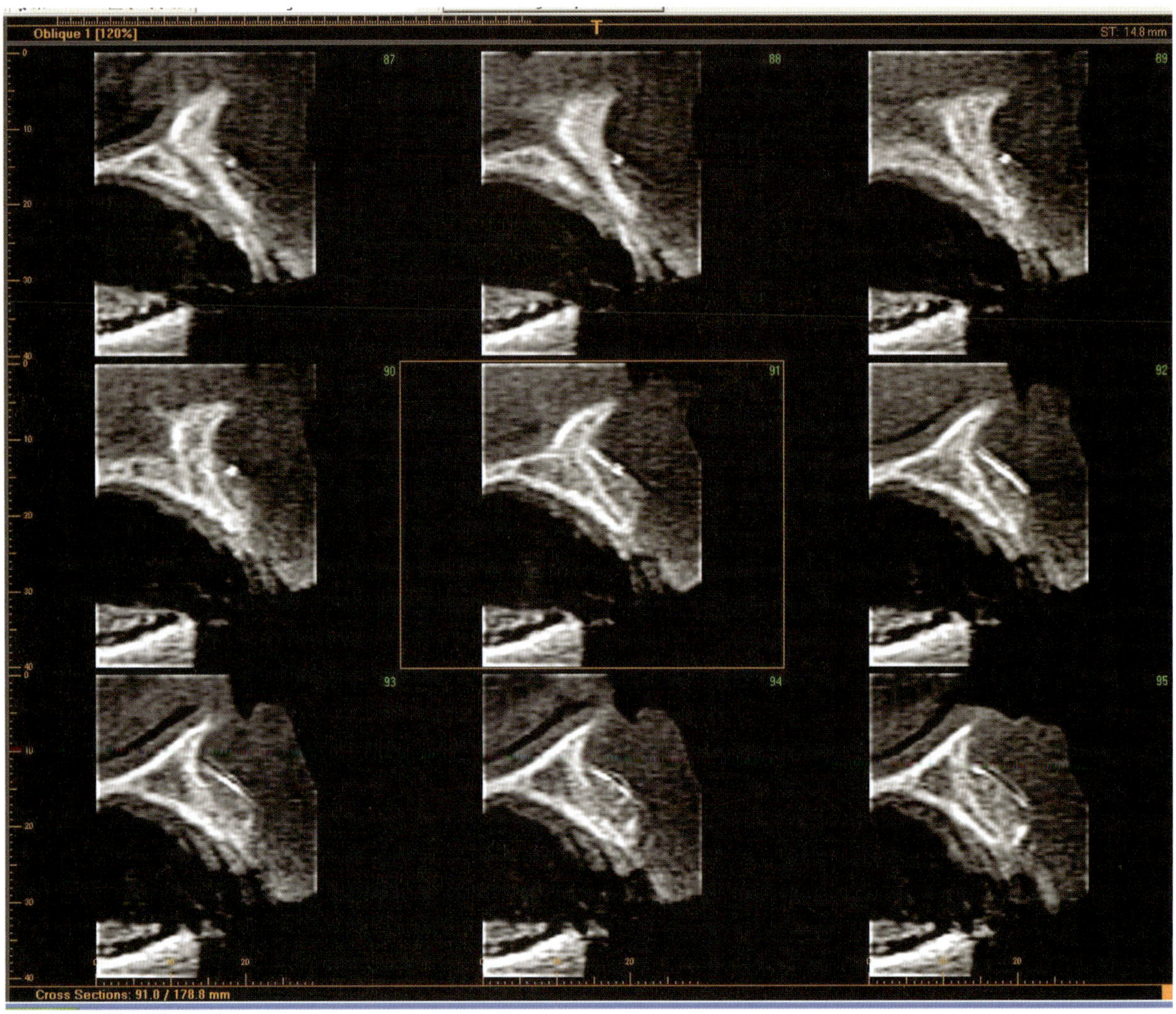

Figure 2.77 A six-month postoperative CAT scan demonstrates the extensive buccal ridge regeneration which has occurred. The buccopalatal width of the ridge has been increased two- to threefold.

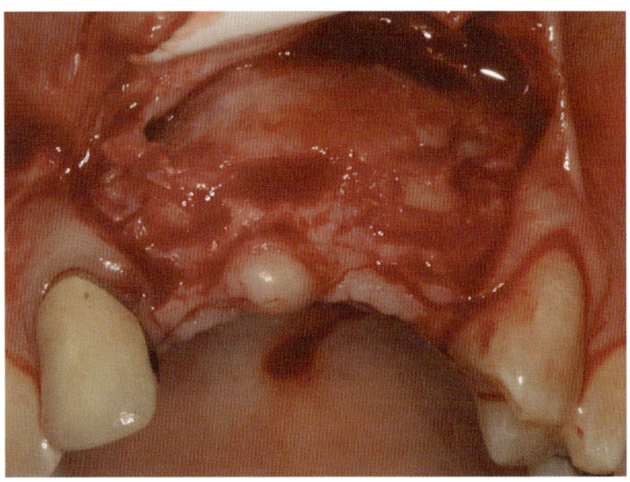

Figure 2.78 Six months postoperative, flap reflection and membrane removal confirms extensive regenerated bone. Implants may now be placed in ideal positions.

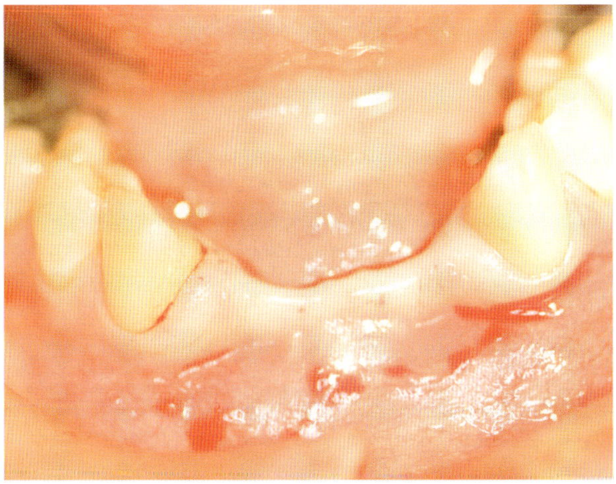

Figure 2.79 The same patient presents having avulsed her mandibular anterior teeth.

Implant may now be placed in ideal prosthetic positions.

The same patient's mandibular arch demonstrated similar alveolar bone loss in conjunction with tooth avulsion (Figures 2.79 and 2.80). A Gore-Tex membrane was trimmed and secured with fixation tacks, and graft material was placed beneath it (Figure 2.81). Following confirmation of adequate buccal and lingual mucoperiosteal flap mobility, the soft tissue flaps were sutured with interrupted Gore-Tex and 4-0 plain gut sutures (Figure 2.82). Flap reflection and membrane removal six months postregenerative therapy demonstrated extensive alveolar ridge regeneration, which will allow implant placement in ideal prosthetic positions (Figure 2.83).

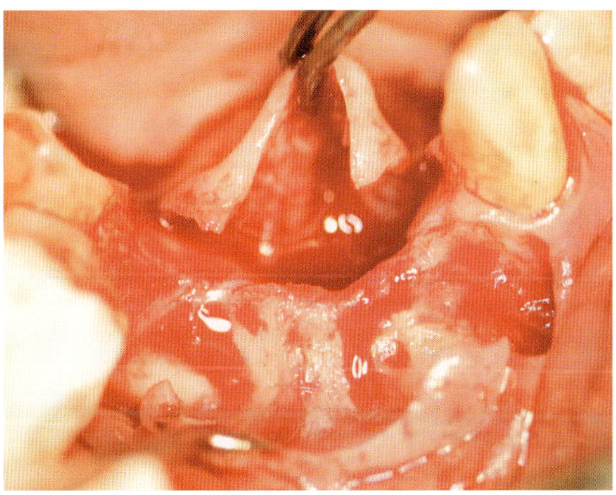

Figure 2.80 Flap reflection demonstrates the damaged alveolar ridge.

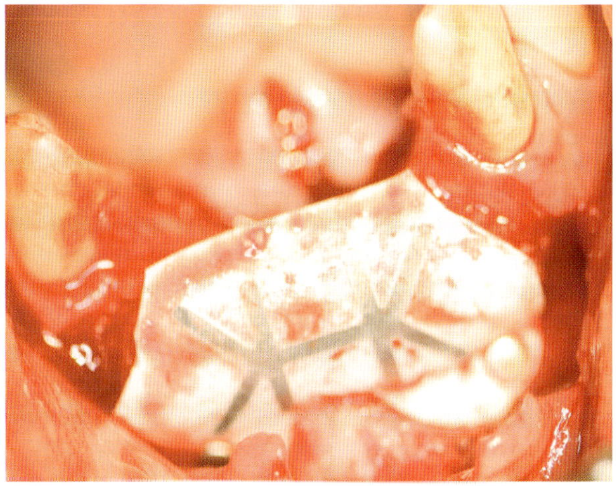

Figure 2.81 Following appropriate contouring, the membrane is secured with fixation tacks.

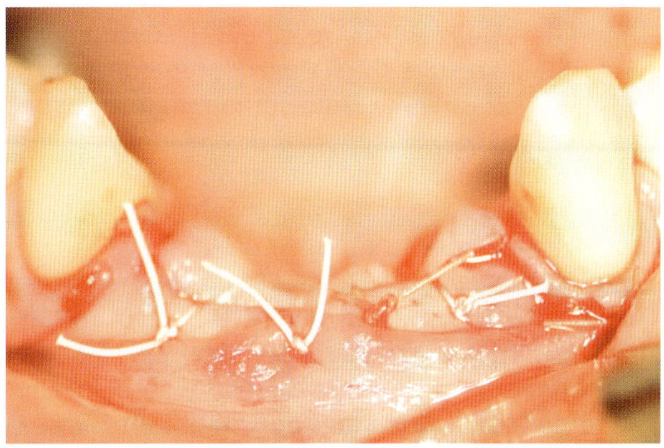

Figure 2.82 Particulate materials are placed, flap mobility is ensured, and the mucoperiosteal flaps are sutured with interrupted Gore-Tex and 4-0 plain gut sutures.

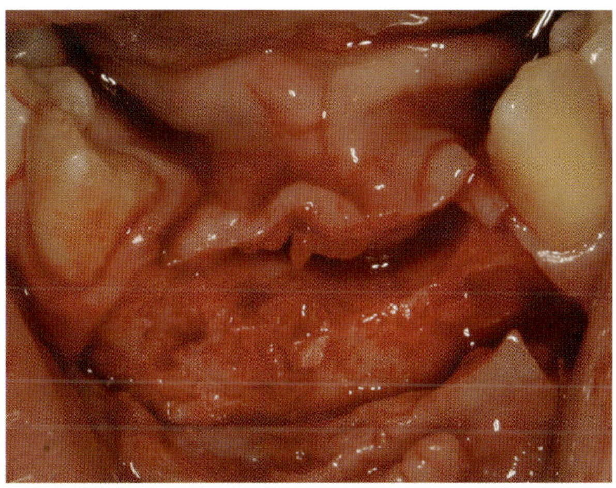

Figure 2.83 Following six months reentry and membrane removal, extensive alveolar ridge regeneration is noted.

THE INFLUENCE OF INFLAMMATION AND INFECTION ON GUIDED BONE REGENERATION THERAPY

The ability to effect guided bone regeneration, with or without simultaneous implant placement, in the face of an active inflammatory lesion is often called into question. The advent of osseointegrated implant utilization in North America was accompanied by the warning that all "infected teeth" should be extracted, defects should be debrided, and sites should be allowed to heal for approximately one year before placing implants. Such caution was meant to ensure that no active inflammatory lesions were present in the bone receptor sites. Numerous authors have demonstrated the ability to place implants and predictably attain osseointegration at the time of extraction of periodontically and/or endodontically involved teeth. Such results challenged the concept of having to definitively resolve inflammatory lesions prior to implant placement.

A previously reported upon case demonstrates the envelope of possibility when considering implant placement in the face of an active inflammatory lesion (Figures 2.84–2.91).

A patient presented with a fractured and fistulating mandibular right first bicuspid. Following tooth removal, the defect was debrided, and a 3.3-mm-wide and 8-mm-long titanium plasma-sprayed IMZ implant was placed. One half of the extraction socket was filled with Interpore 200. No graft materials were placed in the other half of the extraction socket. The area was covered

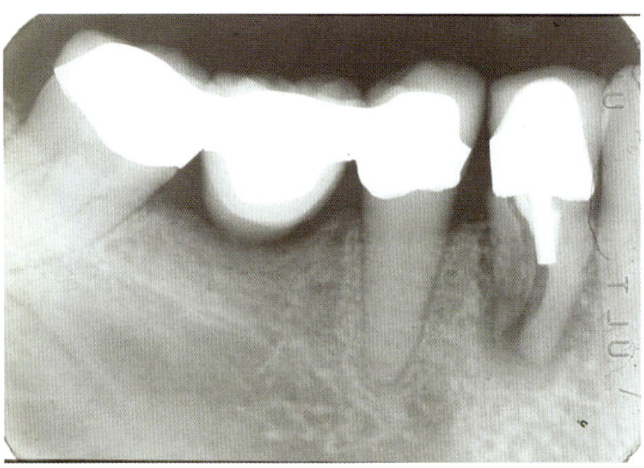

Figure 2.84 A patient presents with a fractured and fistulating mandibular first bicuspid.

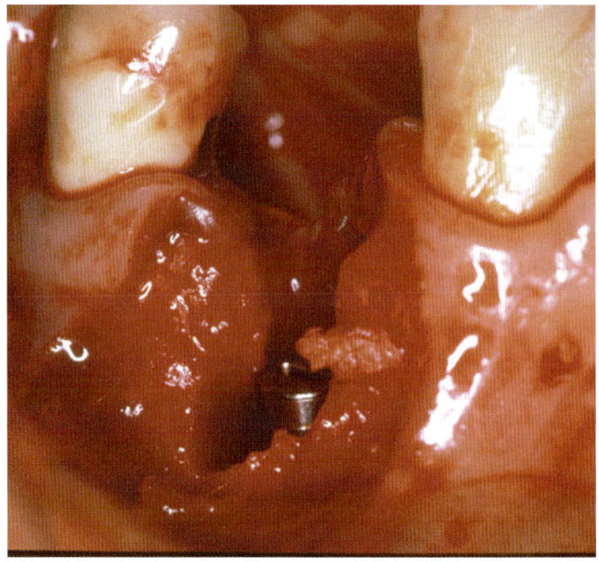

Figure 2.85 Following tooth removal and defect debridement, a 3.3-mm-wide and 8-mm-long titanium plasma-sprayed IMZ implant has been placed. One half of the socket will be filled with Interpore 200. No graft material will be placed in the other half of the socket. The area will be covered with a nonreinforced Gore-Tex membrane.

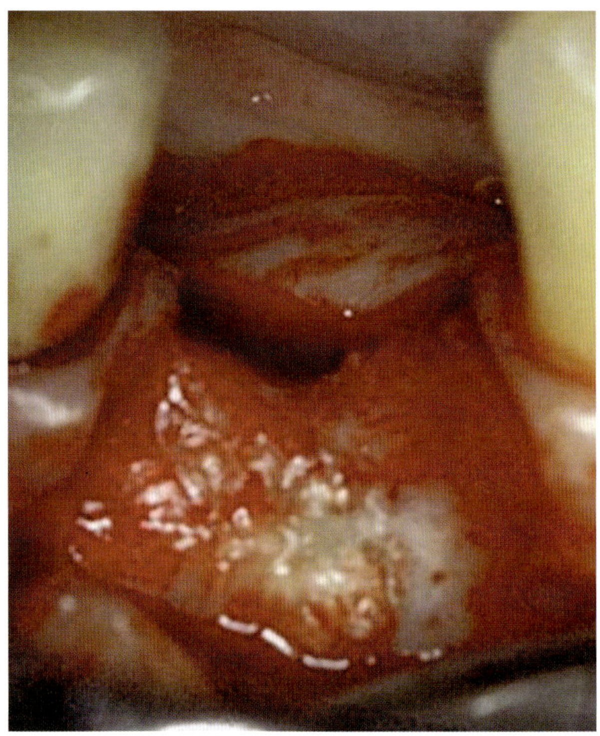

Figure 2.86 Eight months posttherapy flap reflection and membrane removal demonstrate complete bone regeneration in the area.

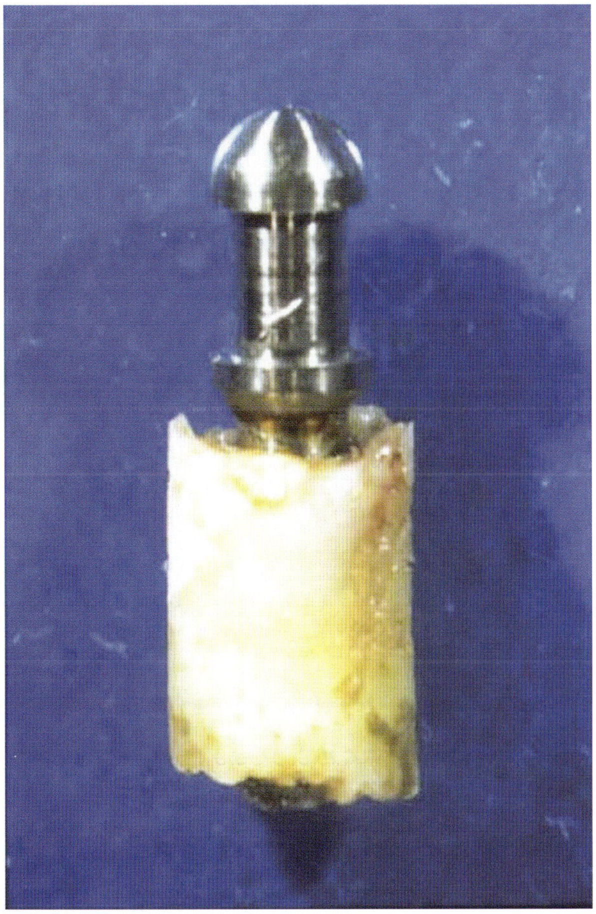

Figure 2.87 The implant and surrounding bone are removed with a trephine bur.

with a nonresorbable, nonreinforced Gore-Tex membrane. Flap reflection and membrane removal eight months postoperatively demonstrated complete regeneration of the alveolar ridge in the treated area (Figure 2.86). A block section was taken utilizing a trephine (Figure 2.87). A longer, wider implant was placed at this time. Following implant uncovery, the patient received an abutment and implant crown. All therapy was performed for the patient at no charge.

The block section was prepared, stained, and processed by Dr Donath of Germany. Figure 2.88 demonstrates a gross section of the histological specimen. Figure 2.89 is a view of the base of the implant in prior host bone.

New bone regeneration and attainment of osseointegration are evident on the side of the implant where Interpore 200 was placed prior to membrane utilization (Figure 2.90).

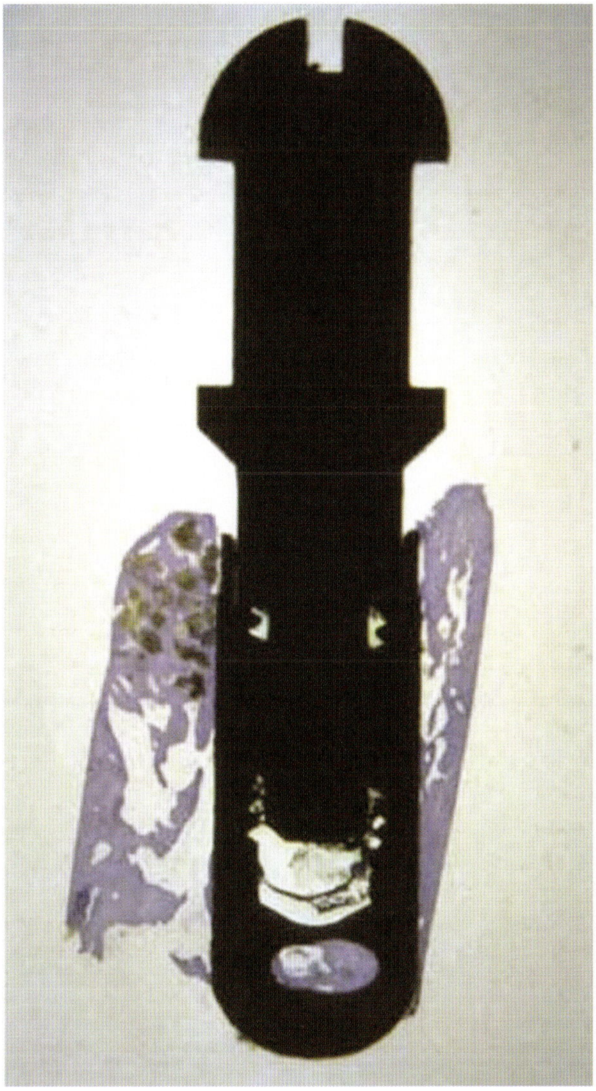

Figure 2.88 A gross histologic section demonstrates the implant and residual Interpore 200 particles.

New bone formation and osseointegration are also present on the side of the implant where only a membrane had been placed (Figure 2.91).

Three important facts were demonstrated by this histological study:

- Guided bone regeneration may be accomplished in the face of an active inflammatory lesion.
- Osseointegration may be attained when an implant is placed in an "infected site."
- Bone regenerated at the time of implant placement in an "infected site" will attain osseointegration to the implant.

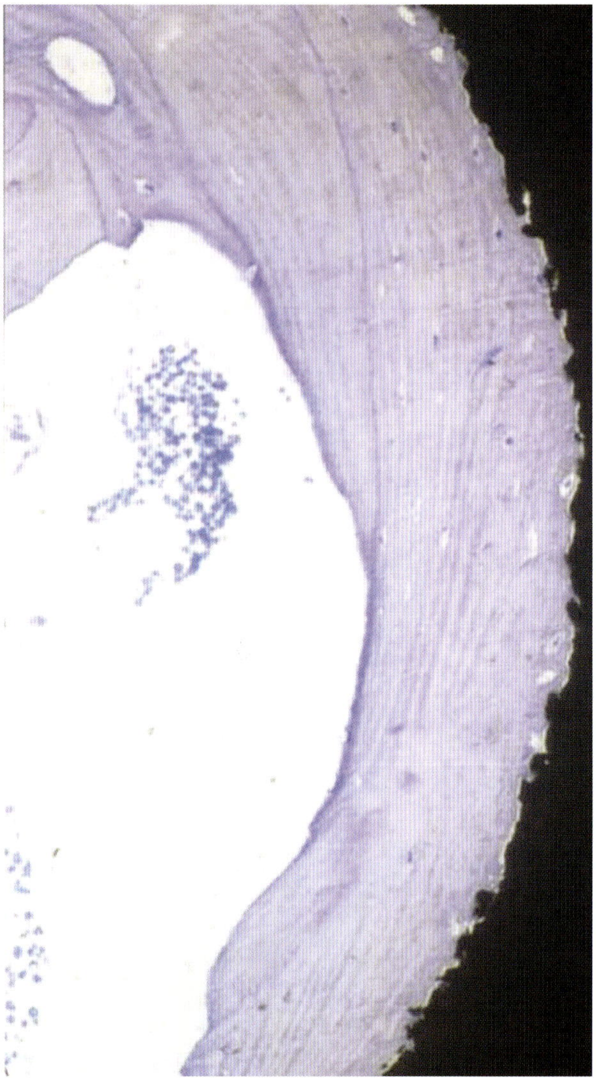

Figure 2.89 A histologic view of the base of the implant which had been placed in the residual host bone.

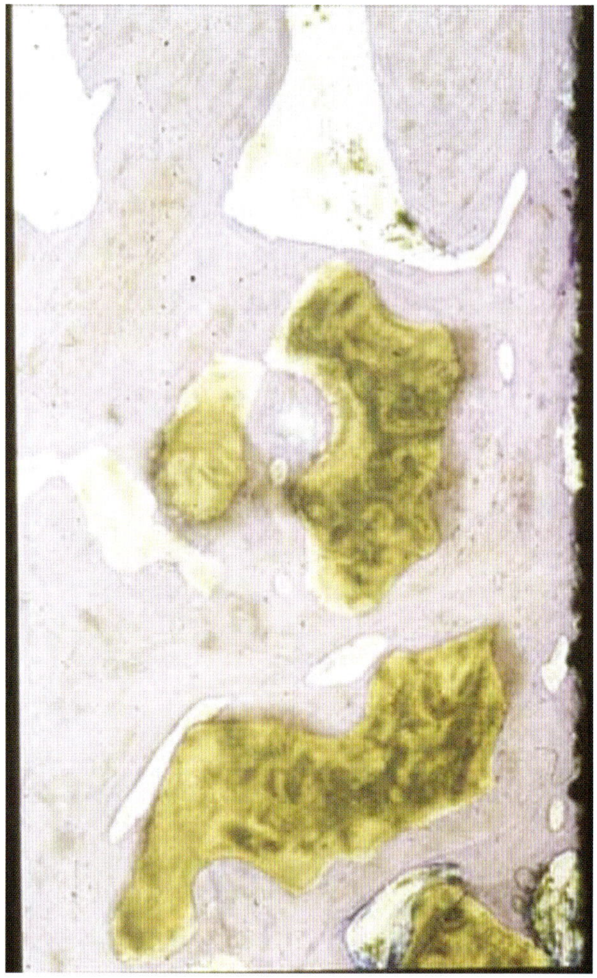

Figure 2.90 A histologic view of the side of the socket treated with Interpore 200 and the covering Gore-Tex membrane demonstrates regeneration of healthy, viable bone, attainment of osseointegration, and residual Interpore 200 particles.

Tooth Extraction as a Reconstructive Event

The aforementioned three facts significantly impact treatment planning and patient care. The realization that guided bone regeneration, with or without simultaneous implant placement, may be predictably and successfully performed in the areas of active inflammation represents a significant paradigm shift. No longer must teeth be extracted, and ridges be allowed to resorb during healing, resulting in esthetic and morphologic challenges. No longer must a patient undergo multiple procedures as teeth are extracted, sites are allowed to heal, resorbed ridges are rebuilt, and implants are eventually placed. No longer must significant hard and soft tissue augmentation procedures be performed in pontic areas following post-extraction resorption prior to prosthetic reconstruction.

Tooth extraction should be viewed as an opportunity to perform the necessary reconstructive therapy, whether it be hard tissue augmentation, or implant placement with concomitant guided bone regenerative treatment.

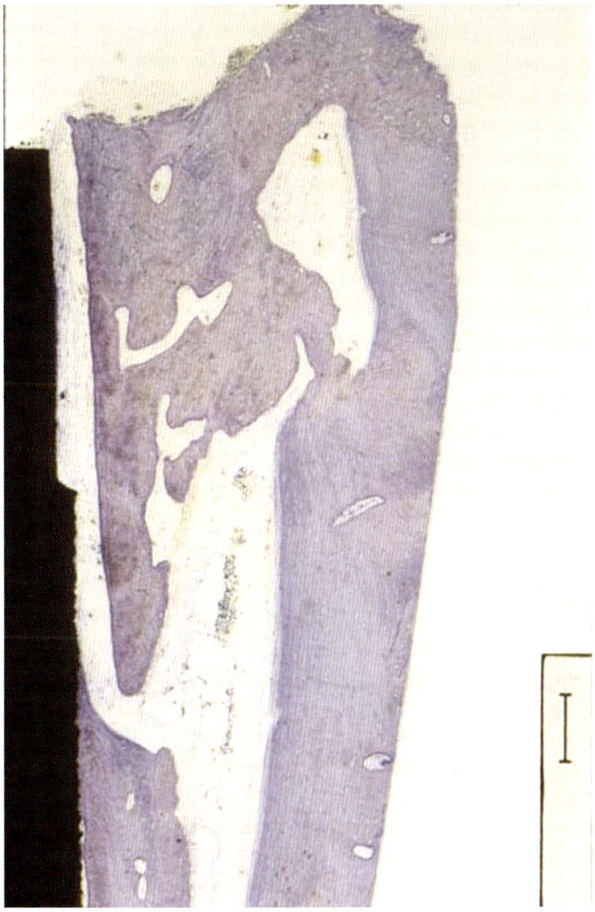

Figure 2.91 A histologic view of the site treated only with a covering membrane demonstrates regenerated viable bone and osseointegration.

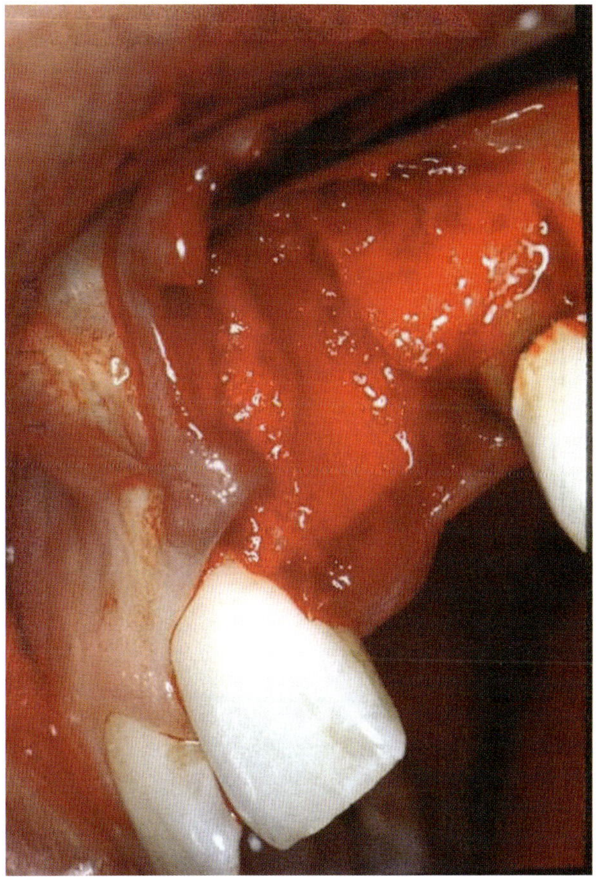

Figure 2.92 A significant ridge defect is evident following removal of a vertically fractured maxillary central incisor. Failure to perform regeneration at the time of tooth removal would result in marked alveolar ridge resorption with its attendant compromises.

Clinical Example Four

However, Figure 2.92 details a more significant guided bone regeneration result. A 26-year-old young male presented with a vertically fractured maxillary central incisor. Flap reflection revealed complete dehiscence of the buccal surface of the fractured root. A significant defect was evident following tooth extraction. If no regenerative therapy was performed in this region, unpredictable ridge resorption would have occurred, leading to esthetic disfiguration, inadequate bone for ideal implant positioning, and potential bone loss on the interproximal surfaces of the adjacent teeth. As a result of these concerns, graft material was placed beneath a nonresorbable titanium-reinforced membrane. Following membrane removal six months postregeneration, an ideal ridge form was evident (Figure 2.93). An implant may now be placed in an ideal restorative position.

Clinical Example Five

A patient treated in 1989 demonstrates the potential advantages of reconstructive therapy at the time of tooth removal. This 41-year-old female presented with two fractured and fistulating maxillary cuspids (Figure 2.94). The four maxillary incisors were missing and had been replaced by pontics in her fixed reconstruction. Due to a less complete understanding of regenerative and implant treatments in 1989, the patient's therapy would entail a number of phases. The maxillary cuspids

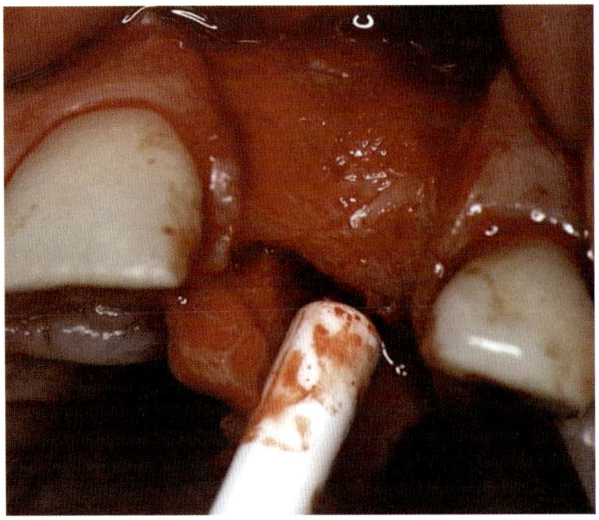

Figure 2.93 Flap reentry six months following regenerative therapy with particulate material and a covering membrane demonstrates reattainment of an ideal ridge form in anticipation of implant placement.

would first be extracted, the defects debrided, and regenerative therapy performed. Once this regeneration was complete, the atrophic ridge in the incisor region would be rebuilt through guided bone regeneration. Finally, a series of implants would be placed in the maxillary arch which would eventually be restored with fixed prosthetics.

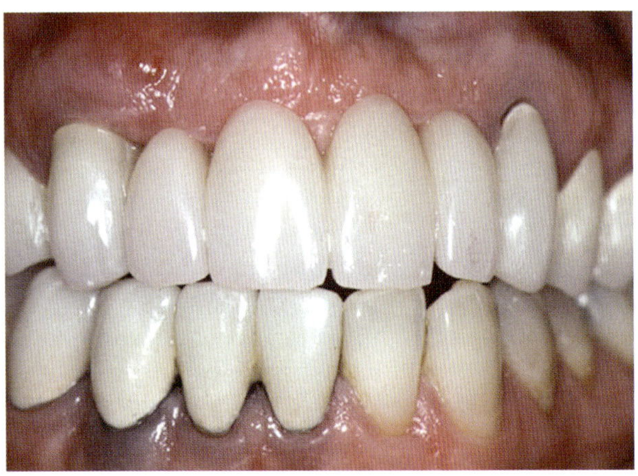

Figure 2.94 The patient presented with fractured and fistulating maxillary cuspids, which were helping to support a full arch fixed reconstruction. Due to limitations in therapy in the late 1980s, treatment was to be performed in three distinct stages.

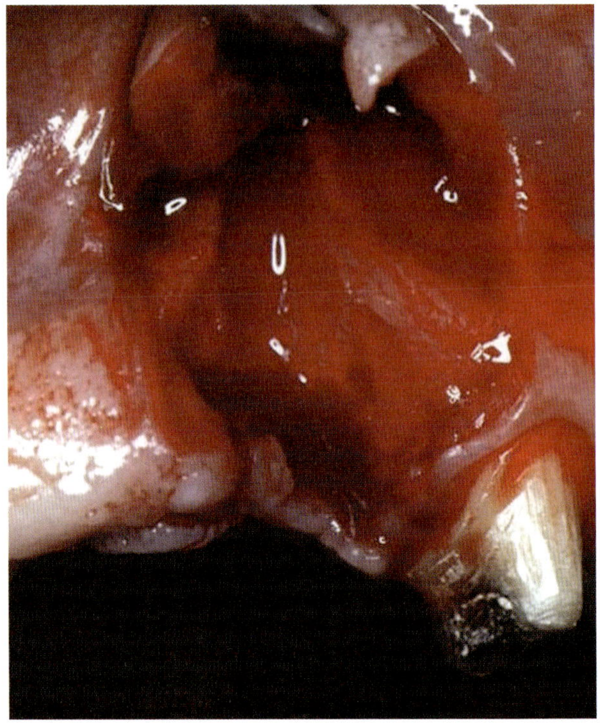

Figure 2.95 Following flap reflection, tooth extraction, and defect debridement, a severe osseous defect was evident in the area of the maxillary left cuspid. This region was treated with particulate graft material and a nonreinforced covering membrane.

Figure 2.95 demonstrates the alveolar ridge defect present following removal of the maxillary left cuspid. Due to the limitations of available materials at the time, demineralized freeze-dried bone allograft and a nonresorbable nonreinforced covering membrane were utilized to effect bone regeneration.

Six months posttherapy, mucoperiosteal flaps were reflected in anticipation of performing guided bone regeneration in the maxillary incisor region. Flap reflection demonstrated the difference in alveolar ridge morphology in the area of the missing cuspid, where regenerative therapy was performed in the presence of a severe defect at the time of tooth removal, and in the area of the lateral incisor where no regenerative therapy had been performed when the tooth was removed. The difference in ridge morphology was dramatic (Figure 2.96).

It could be contended that the morphology demonstrated in the incisor region was the result of disuse atrophy over time. However, the dental literature has never demonstrated such disuse atrophy to occur. It is well documented that ridge

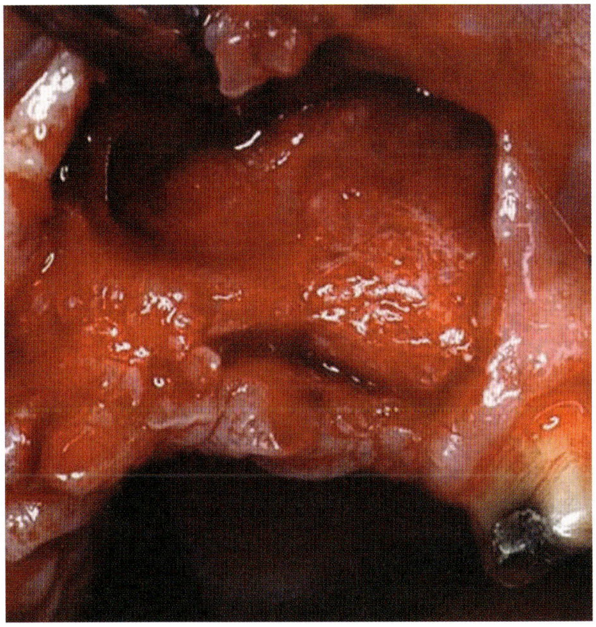

Figure 2.96 Following flap reflection and membrane removal six months postregenerative therapy, the dramatic difference in alveolar ridge morphology between the infected site treated with regeneration at the time of tooth removal, and the adjacent alveolar ridge where no regenerative therapy was performed at the time of tooth removal, is dramatic. The difference between destructive (tooth extraction) and reconstructive (tooth extraction with concomitant regeneration) has been underscored.

resorption and bone loss will occur up to one year post-tooth extraction if regenerative therapy is not performed at the time of tooth removal. The literature has also documented continued ridge atrophy beneath removable prostheses, or beneath fixed prostheses that impinge on the ridge either at rest or through flexure during function. The literature has never demonstrated continued ridge atrophy beneath well fitting fixed prostheses over time. The difference in ridge morphologies between the augmented cuspid site and the nonaugmented lateral incisor site represents the difference between destructive (tooth extraction) and reconstruction (tooth extraction with concomitant regeneration) therapies.

Considering the abilities of talented clinicians to restore teeth in such a manner as to render them indistinguishable from their natural counterparts, it is illogical not to regenerate the hard tissue scaffold of the soft tissue drape of esthetics whenever teeth are removed.

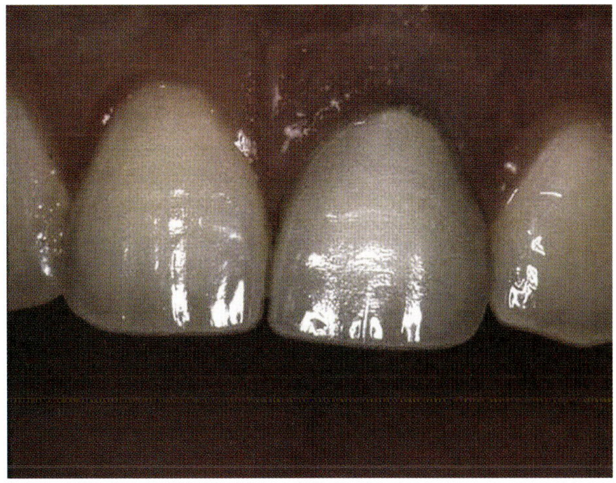

Figure 2.97 A patient presents with a vertically fractured and fistulating maxillary central incisor.

Clinical Example Six

Performance of regenerative therapy at the time of tooth removal has the potential to rebuild the prepathologic ridge morphology, or to extend beyond the original confines of the alveolar ridge. A 31-year-old female (Figure 2.97) presented with a vertically fractured maxillary central incisor. Following tooth extraction (Figure 2.98), an extensive

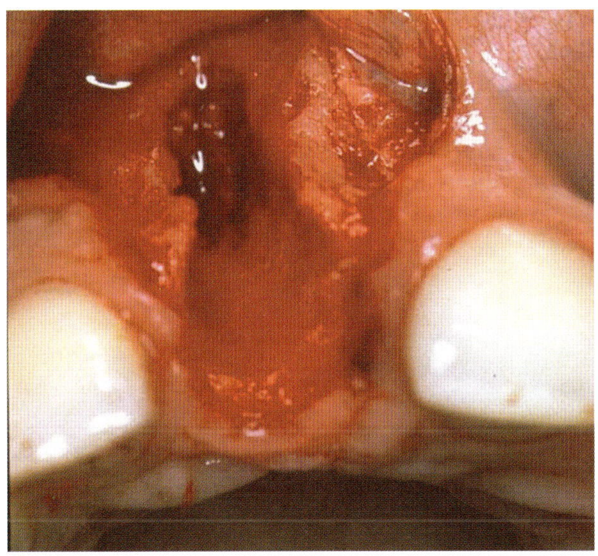

Figure 2.98 Following flap reflection, tooth extraction, and defect debridement, a severe alveolar defect is evident. Failure to perform regeneration at the time of tooth removal will result in extensive bone loss and ridge collapse.

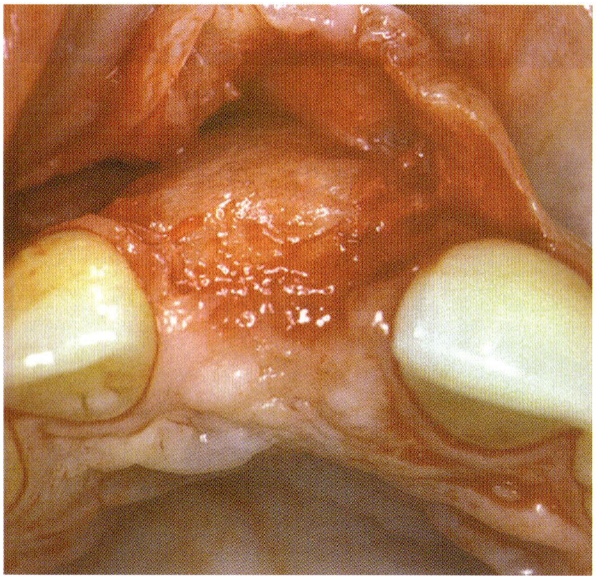

Figure 2.99 Following flap reflection and membrane removal six months after regenerative therapy has been performed, extensive alveolar bone regeneration is evident beyond the original confines of the alveolus.

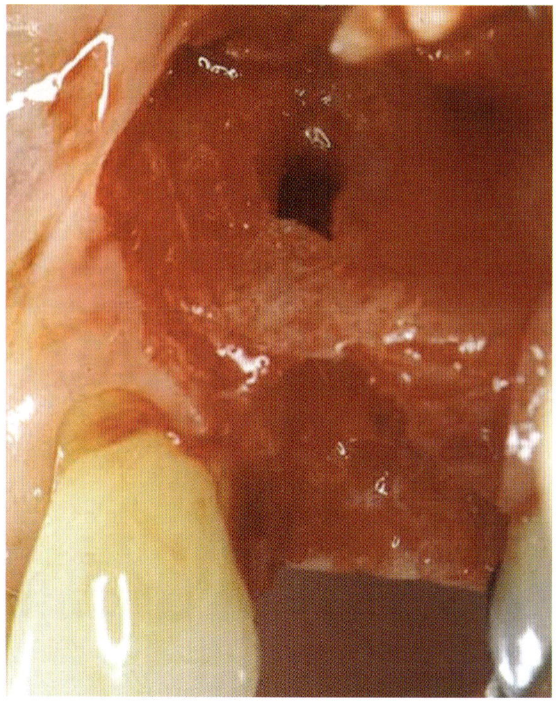

Figure 2.100 Following tooth removal and defect debridement, a buccal fenestration is evident in the alveolar ridge.

ridge defect was evident. Failure to perform appropriate regenerative therapy at this time would result in severe ridge collapse, an esthetic deformity, inadequate bone for implant placement, and compromise of the interproximal bone of the adjacent teeth. As a result, Bio-Oss was placed beneath a covering titanium-reinforced Gore-Tex membrane, secured with fixation tacks. Passive soft tissue primary closure was attained and maintained throughout the course of regeneration.

Flap reflection and membrane removal six months postregenerative therapy demonstrated regeneration of all lost alveolar bone, as well as generation of bone beyond the original confines of the alveolus (Figure 2.99). This excess bone was removed at the time of implant placement, so as to provide a more natural ridge form.

The inability to predictably maintain passive soft tissue primary closure following tooth removal and placement of regenerative materials has directly contributed to the development of a number of proposed alternative therapies. Such approaches include:

- Tooth extraction without concomitant regenerative therapy. The site is allowed to heal for 5–6 weeks, allowing soft tissues to migrate over the extraction socket, providing adequate soft tissue to effect passive primary closure following placement of regenerative materials. Proponents of this approach state that by reentering the area six weeks postextraction, only minimal bone resorption has occurred. While this statement may be true if a patient presents with an intact, thick buccal alveolar plate, such a scenario is not always encountered. Figures 2.100 and 2.101 demonstrate a compromised site following extraction of a maxillary first bicuspid. The combination of a buccal fenestration and a thin residual buccal alveolar ridge would lead to extensive alveolar resorption following tooth removal if regenerative therapy was not performed during the same visit, regardless of whether an implant was placed at the time of tooth removal. Passive soft tissue primary closure is easily attained over the site in question through the utilization of one of two approaches. Either the buccal flap is coronally positioned following placement of appropriate vertical releasing incisions with horizontal releasing incision extensions and full thickness reflection, or a rotated palatal pedicle is utilized to attain soft tissue closure over

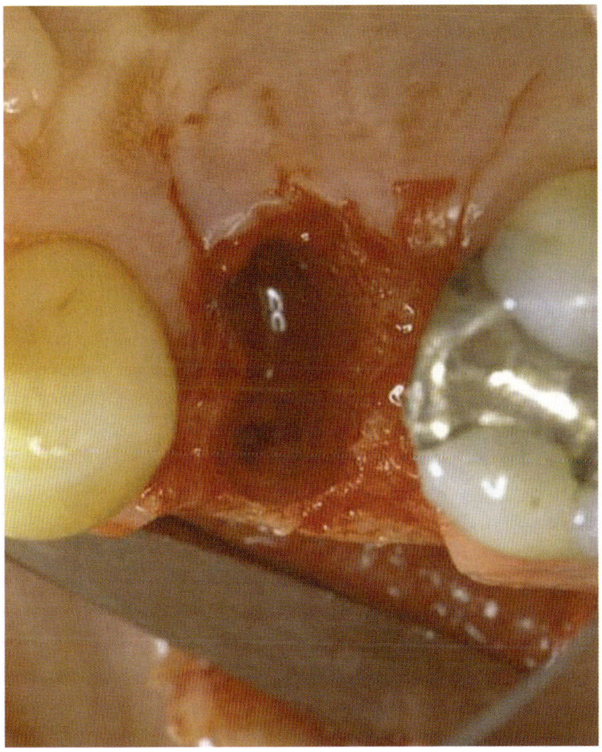

Figure 2.101 A crestal view demonstrates the thin labile nature of the buccal alveolar plate. Failure to perform regenerative therapy at the time of tooth removal, either alone or in conjunction with implant placement, will result in severe ridge resorption and the attendant compromises.

the extraction socket without crestal repositioning of the buccal flap and the attendant compromise to the buccal vestibule.

- Various authors have also proposed that the tooth to be extracted be prepared to osseous crest. The soft tissue is then allowed to granulate over the root for approximately 6–8 weeks, providing adequate soft tissue to effect passive primary closure following tooth extraction and regenerative therapy with or without simultaneous implant placement. Such an approach represents two compromises. The first is that the patient must undergo two procedures, one to prepare the root to osseous crest and one to extract the root and proceed with regenerative therapy and possible implant placement. The second compromise is that the clinician is now faced with having to extract a root which has been prepared to osseous crest. Such an extraction often leads to additional bone removal to gain access to the root in question.

The utilization of well-thought-out innovative flap designs eliminates the need to employ such therapies in the quest to attain and maintain passive soft tissue primary closure throughout the course of regeneration.

MEMBRANE SELECTION

Membrane selection must be driven by the morphology of the defect to be treated. Resorbable membranes should not be employed over non-space-maintaining defects, as their ability to maintain space and ensure a precise morphology to the regenerated hard tissues when placed over graft materials is not predictable (Flow Chart 2.1).

With the advent of preparations rich in growth factors (PRGFs), which offer a fibrin membrane derived from the patients' own blood impregnated with platelets and growth factors which are time released over 10–12 days, the indications for resorbable membranes are few.

As will be discussed in Chapter 3, PRGF offers a bioactive alternative to resorbable membranes. However, PRGF does not have space maintaining capabilities, for use alone as a membrane to effect guided bone regeneration in non-space-maintaining defects.

Clinical Example Seven

Figures 2.102 and 2.103 offer two views of an alveolar defect following extraction of a maxillary central incisor. Due to the loss of a significant amount of buccal alveolar bone, the defect is not space maintaining. Following placement of bovine bone matrix, a resorbable membrane was placed over the graft material, and secured with two fixation tacks. Passive soft tissue primary closure was attained and maintained throughout the course of regeneration. Two views of the area at the six-month reentry demonstrate that, while significant bone regeneration has occurred, the prepathologic ridge morphology has not been reattained (Figures 2.104 and 2.105). Where the initial alveolar defect was not space maintaining, membrane collapse led to a diminution of the quantity of regenerated bone. In addition, the buccal line angle of the alveolar ridge was not regenerated, and cannot provide the necessary support to the covering soft tissues. In order to maximize esthetic treatment outcomes following implant placement, either

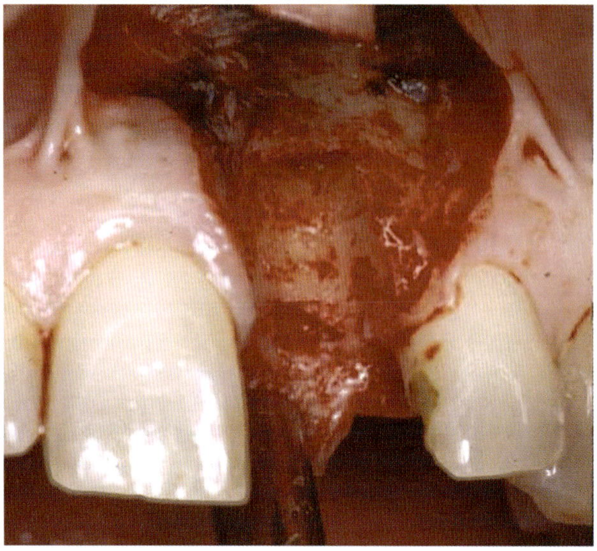

Figure 2.102 Following removal of a fractured maxillary central incisor, the damaged buccal alveolar plate is evident.

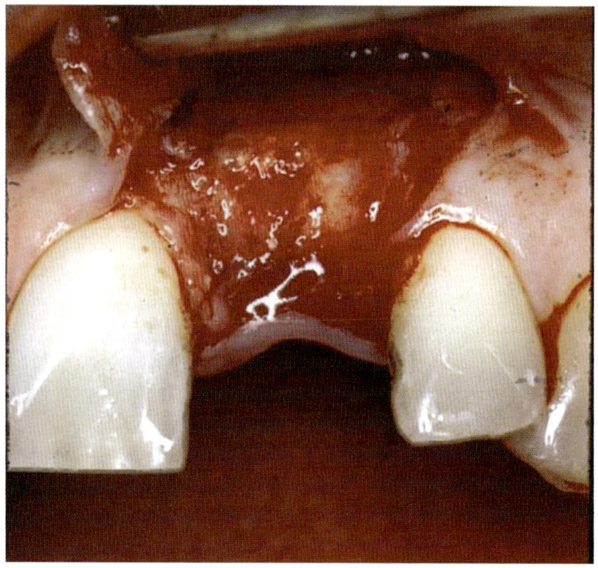

Figure 2.104 Following flap reflection six months post-regenerative therapy, bone regeneration in the extraction socket defect is evident. However, an ideal alveolar ridge bone has not been regenerated.

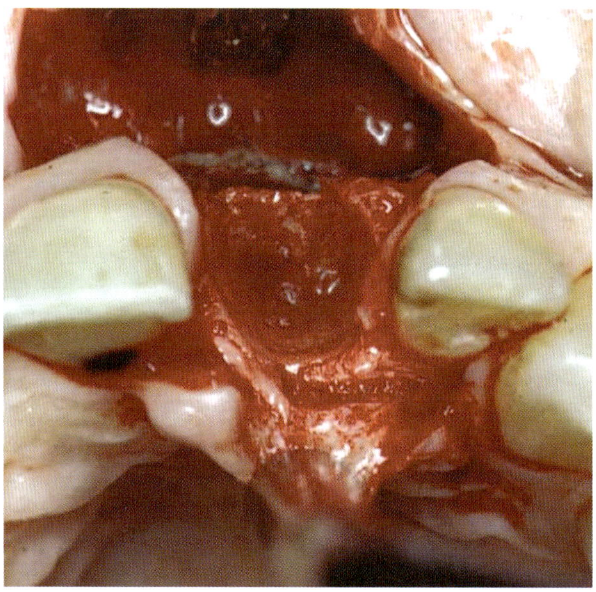

Figure 2.103 A crestal view demonstrates the non-space-maintaining nature of the residual extraction socket defect. The area was treated with Bio-Oss and a fixated resorbable covering membrane.

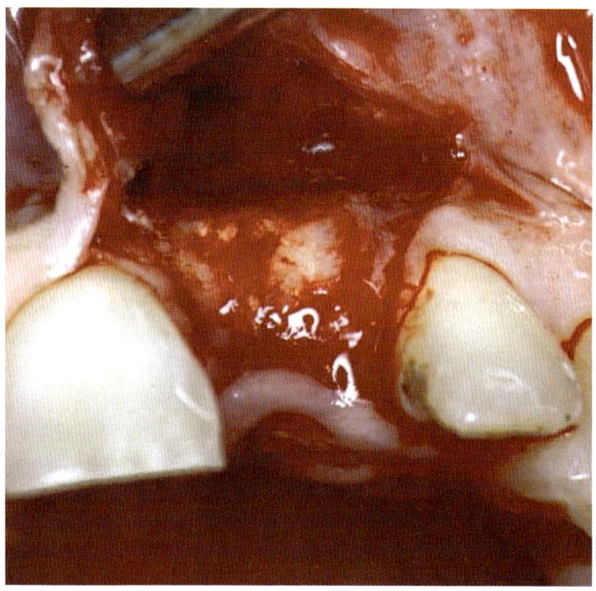

Figure 2.105 A crestal view demonstrates a failure to regenerate the buccal line angle of the alveolar ridge. Additional regenerative therapy or connective tissue graft placement will be required to maximize the esthetic outcomes of treatment.

additional regeneration will have to be performed, or a connective tissue graft will have to be placed.

Clinical Example Eight

Figures 2.106 and 2.107 demonstrate a defect in another patient, following extraction of a hopeless maxillary central incisor. At first glance, this defect appears to have greater space maintaining capabilities than the previous case. However, the buccal alveolar walls required for membrane support are only present in the apical 2/3 of the defect. The crestal area of the defect is devoid of buccal alveolar support, and is not space maintaining. The defect was treated with bovine bone matrix and a covering resorbable membrane which was secured with two fixation tacks. Passive soft tissue primary closure was attained and maintained throughout the course of regeneration.

The six-month reentry (Figures 2.108 and 2.109) demonstrates significant bone regeneration. However, the prepathologic ridge morphology has only been reestablished where adequate buccal bone remained to support the membrane appropriately. Once again, the crestal area of the alveolar ridge is compromised with regard to both quantity of regenerated bone and ridge morphology. Following implant placement, a connective tissue graft will have to be placed to maximize the esthetic outcomes of therapy.

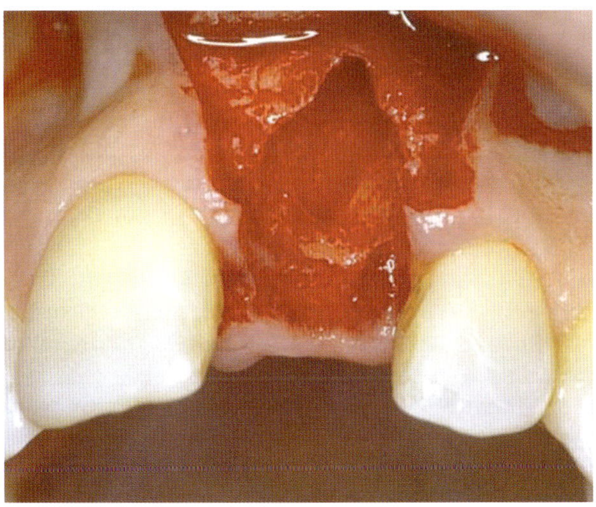

Figure 2.106 Following extraction of a fractured maxillary left central incisor, the morphology of the residual extraction socket defect is evident. Buccal walls remain at the apical half of the defect, to help afford membrane support.

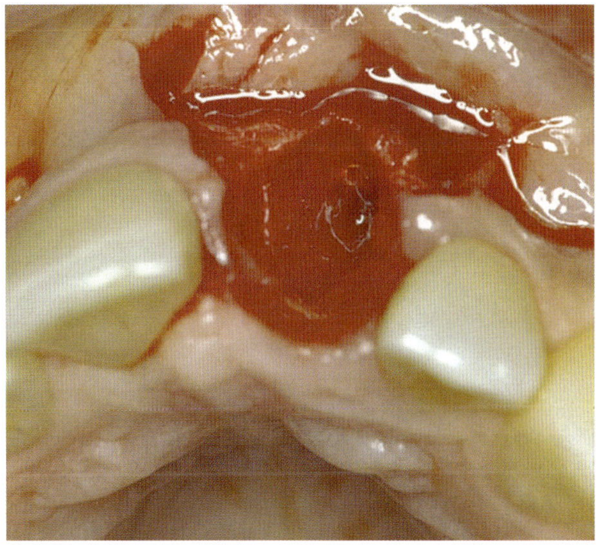

Figure 2.107 A crestal view demonstrates the lack of supporting buccal alveolar walls in the extraction socket at its most crestal aspect. The defect was treated with Bio-Oss and a fixated resorbable covering membrane.

Clinical Example Nine

Following loss of a hopeless maxillary central incisor in another patient, an extensive buccal alveolar ridge defect is noted which presents with

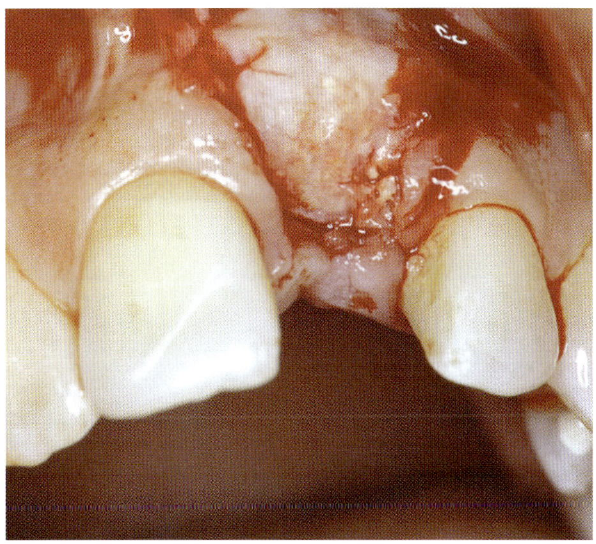

Figure 2.108 Following flap reflection six months post-regenerative therapy, extensive bone regeneration in the previous extraction socket defect is evident. Note the ideal ridge form in the apical half of the prior defect.

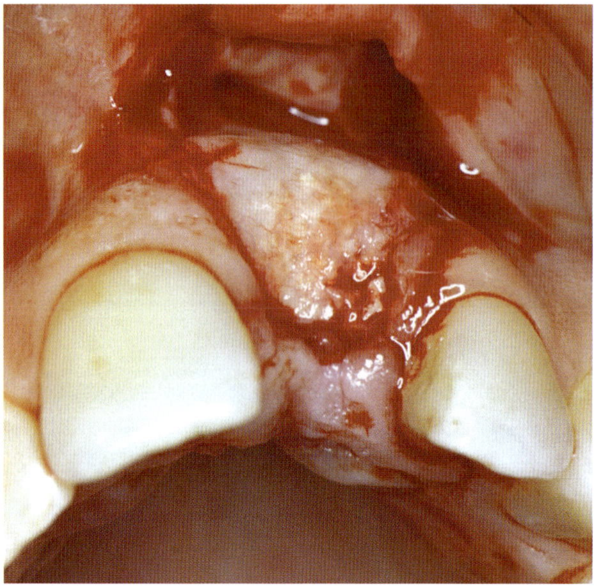

Figure 2.109 A crestal view demonstrates a failure to regenerate a buccal alveolar ridge line angle, due to the lack of supporting buccal walls of the extraction socket defect in this region. Further regenerative therapy, or connective tissue grafts, will have to be employed to maximize esthetic treatment outcomes.

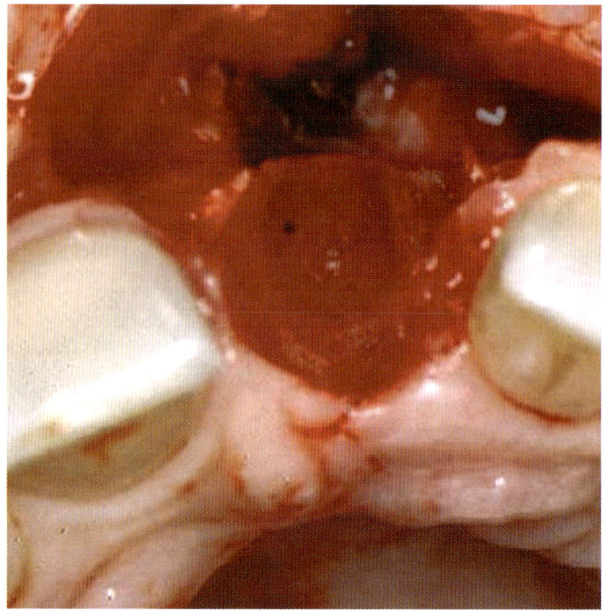

Figure 2.111 A crestal view demonstrates the lack of buccal supporting walls around the complete extent of the extraction socket defect. The defect was treated with Bio-Oss and a fixated titanium-reinforced Gore-Tex covering membrane.

no buccal alveolar walls to help maintain space beneath a covering membrane (Figure 2.110 and 2.111). As a result of the defect morphology, a titanium-reinforced Gore-Tex membrane was utilized over a Bio-Oss graft. The membrane was secured with two fixation tacks, and passive soft tissue primary closure was attained and maintained throughout the course of regeneration.

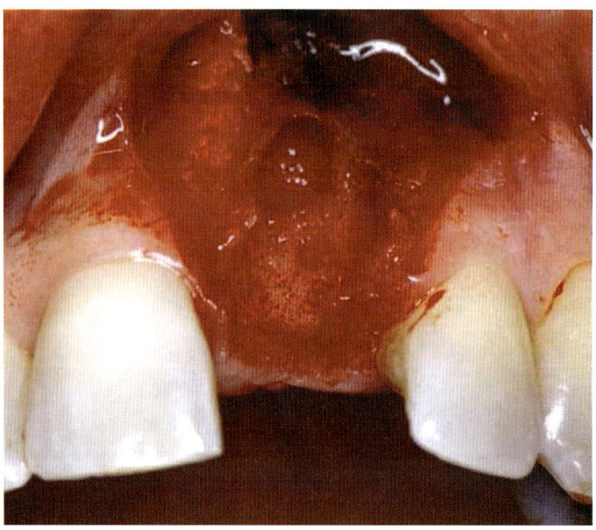

Figure 2.110 Following removal of a fractured maxillary left central incisor, an extensive ridge defect is noted.

Following flap reflection and membrane removal six months postoperatively, regeneration of an ideal alveolar ridge form was evident (Figures 2.112 and 2.113). Note the reattainment of a buccal alveolar ridge line angle in the appropriate position to support the overlying soft tissues. No additional hard or soft tissue augmentation therapy will be necessary at the time of implant placement to maximize the esthetic outcomes of therapy. Free floating Bio-Oss graft particles were noted at the clinical reentry, and the regenerated bone demonstrated evidence of nonresorbed bone graft particles imbedded within it. Such a finding is a result of clinical mishandling of the Bio-Oss graft material. Bio-Oss graft material placed beneath a covering membrane resorbs over time following the ingress of blood cells through its "trabeculae." The graft is resorbed from all aspects, as the trabeculae are surrounded by blood cells. If the Bio-Oss graft is packed too tightly, the graft particles are crushed and the trabecular morphology is lost. As a result, the graft becomes more of an amorphous mass which may only be resorbed from the outside,

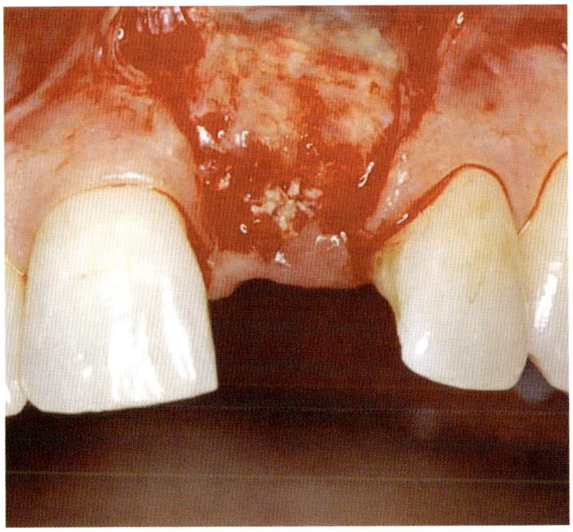

Figure 2.112 Following flap reflection and membrane removal six months postregenerative therapy, significant bone regeneration is evident in the previous ridge defect area. Note the free floating Bio-Oss particles at the most crestal aspect of the regenerated ridge.

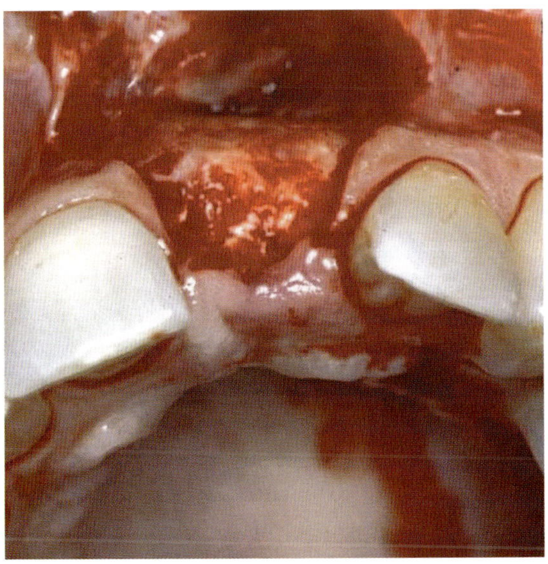

Figure 2.113 A crestal view demonstrates regeneration of the buccal line angle of the damaged alveolar ridge. The morphology of the regenerated alveolar bone will support the covering soft tissues and help idealize the final esthetic treatment outcome.

rather than from outside and within the trabeculae. In such situations, graft resorption is significantly delayed and may take 18–24 months.

Utilization of Bio-Oss grafts in over 3,000 cases has resulted in less than 20 sites which demonstrated significant residual bone particles 8 months postregenerative therapy. Each of these sites was reentered 14–20 months after initial graft placement. No residual graft particles were encountered at that time. All of these sites occurred within a specific time frame of therapy, indicating operator error with regard to graft compression.

Nonautogenous bone graft selection will be discussed in Chapter 6. Appropriate utilization of titanium-reinforced Gore-Tex membranes offers the opportunity to attain regenerative results which are unmatched by those possible through the use of particulate grafts and covering resorbable membranes, and result in significantly less postoperative morbidity than the utilization of autogenous block grafts with covering membranes.

TREATMENT PLANNING EXERCISE # 1

A 49-year-old male presented with a highly atrophic alveolar ridge in the area of tooth # 9 (Figure 2.114). The tooth had been extracted 20 years previously and no regenerative therapy had been performed at the time of tooth removal. The available treatment options included the following:

- Placement of a narrow implant in the residual alveolar ridge.

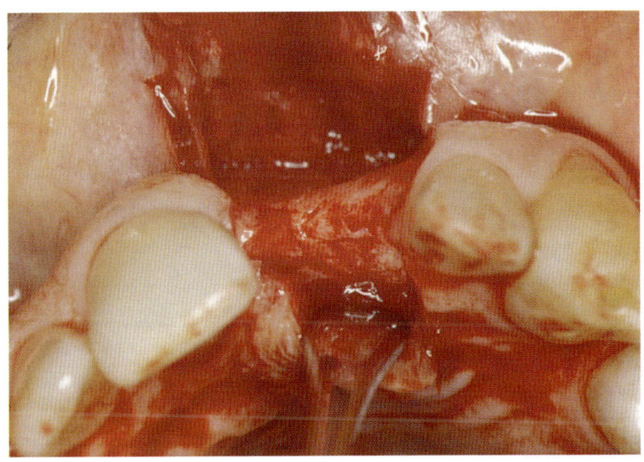

Figure 2.114 The patient presents with a severely atrophic alveolar ridge in the area of a missing central incisor. The region was treated utilizing Bio-Oss and a fixated titanium-reinforced covering membrane.

- Placement of an implant of ideal width in the residual alveolar ridge with concomitant regenerative therapy.
- Ridge augmentation utilizing particulate or block nonautogenous graft material and a resorbable covering membrane, followed by implant placement at a second-stage surgery.
- Placement of particulate or block nonautogenous graft material beneath a titanium-reinforced membrane, followed by implant placement at a subsequent surgery.
- Ridge augmentation therapy utilizing an autogenous block graft without a covering membrane, followed by implant placement at a second surgical visit.
- Ridge augmentation utilizing an autogenous block with a resorbable or nonresorbable covering membrane, followed by implant placement at a second surgical visit.

The advantages and disadvantages of each treatment approach are summarized in Table 2.4.

A bovine bone matrix graft was placed beneath a titanium-reinforced membrane which had been secured with two fixation tacks. Six months postoperative, passive soft tissue primary closure has been maintained (Figure 2.115).

Flap reflection and membrane removal six months postoperative (Figure 2.116) demonstrates regeneration of an ideal alveolar ridge form. An implant with the desired dimensions may now be placed in an ideal prosthetic position.

TREATMENT PLANNING EXERCISE # 2

A 28-year-old female presented having lost her maxillary central incisor at age 16. She has been wearing a removable partial prosthesis since this time. Flap reflection (Figures 2.117 and 2.118) demonstrated a severely atrophic residual alveolar ridge. The buccopalatal dimension of the ridge was approximately 1–1.5 mm.

Possible treatment approaches included:

- Placement of a connective tissue graft to help improve the soft tissue profile, followed by fabrication of either a three-unit Maryland splint, or a three-unit fixed prosthesis.
- Placement of a narrow implant in the residual alveolar ridge.
- Placement of an implant of desired width in the residual alveolar ridge, with concomitant regenerative therapy.
- Ridge augmentation utilizing particulate or block nonautogenous graft material and a resorbable covering membrane, followed by implant placement at a second-stage surgery.
- Placement of particulate or block nonautogenous graft material beneath a titanium-reinforced membrane, followed by implant placement at a subsequent surgery.
- Ridge augmentation therapy utilizing an autogenous block graft without a covering membrane, followed by implant placement at a second surgical visit.
- Ridge augmentation utilizing an autogenous block graft with a resorbable or nonresorbable

Table 2.4 Treatment options for implant placement in an atrophic ridge (Treatment Planning Exercise # 1).

Treatment modality	Advantages	Disadvantages
Placement of a narrow implant in the residual alveolar ridge	• Requires no concomitant regenerative therapy	• Significantly decreases available surface area for osseointegration as compared to a wider implant • Represents a potential esthetic compromise in therapy
Placement of a wider implant in the residual alveolar ridge with concomitant augmentation therapy	• Greater implant surface area is available for potential osseointegration • Implant neck width is better suited to accept the planned restoration • All therapy is performed in one visit	• The implant is placed in a nonideal, more palatal position • A ridge lap restoration may be required, representing an esthetic compromise

Table 2.4 (*Continued*)

Treatment modality	Advantages	Disadvantages
Ridge augmentation utilizing particulate or block nonautogenous graft material and a resorbable covering membrane or PRGF followed by implant placement at a second-stage surgery	• Depending upon the extent of bone regeneration, the implant may be placed in a more ideal buccal palatal position • No need for membrane removal	• The extent of bone regeneration is unpredictable • The morphology of the regenerated bone is unpredictable • A secondary soft tissue procedure may be required to help idealize the esthetic outcome
Placement of particulate or block nonautogenous graft material beneath a titanium-reinforced membrane, followed by implant placement at a subsequent surgery	• Ridge augmentation will allow placement of the implant in a more ideal buccal palatal position • The precise extent of bone regeneration is predictable • The precise morphology of regenerated bone is predictable • No need for secondary procedures to help maximize esthetic outcomes	• The need to master appropriate soft tissue techniques to prevent premature membrane exposure • The need to remove the membrane
Ridge augmentation utilizing an autogenous block graft with no covering membrane	• The potential to place the implant in a more ideal buccal palatal position following bone regeneration • No membrane removal is required • No membrane expenses entailed	• The need to procure graft material from a second surgical site • The precise quantity of regenerated bone is not predictable • The precise morphology of the regenerated bone is not predictable • May require a secondary soft tissue procedure to help maximize treatment outcomes
Ridge augmentation utilizing an autogenous block graft with a resorbable or nonresorbable covering membrane or PRGF, followed by implant placement at a second surgical visit	• The ability to place the implant in a more ideal buccal palatal position following regenerative therapy • The quantity of regenerated bone is predictable • The quality of regenerated bone is predictable	• The need to procure the graft material from a second surgical site • The need to remove the membrane if a nonresorbable membrane is utilized

PRGF, preparations rich in growth factor.

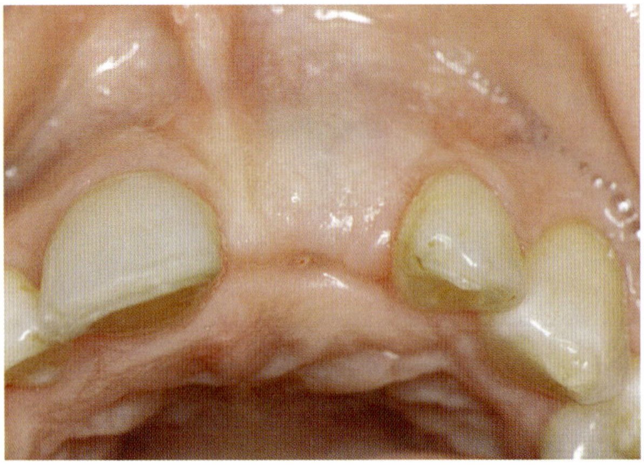

Figure 2.115 Six months following regenerative therapy, soft tissue passive primary closure has been maintained.

covering membrane, followed by implant placement at a second surgical visit.

The advantages and disadvantages of each treatment approach are summarized in Table 2.5.

Bio-Oss was placed beneath a titanium-reinforced membrane which was secured with three fixation tacks. Soft tissue passive primary closure was attained and maintained throughout the course of regeneration.

Following flap reflection and membrane removal eight months postregenerative therapy, the ideal alveolar ridge form which has been attained is evident. An implant of the appropriate dimension may now be placed in a prosthetically driven position. In addition, due to regeneration of the buccal line angle of the alveolar ridge, no soft tissue grafting will be necessary to help maximize the esthetic outcomes of therapy.

It is well recognized that failure to regenerate bone of sufficient dimension to withstand functional forces over time can lead to clinical disasters (Figure 2.119).

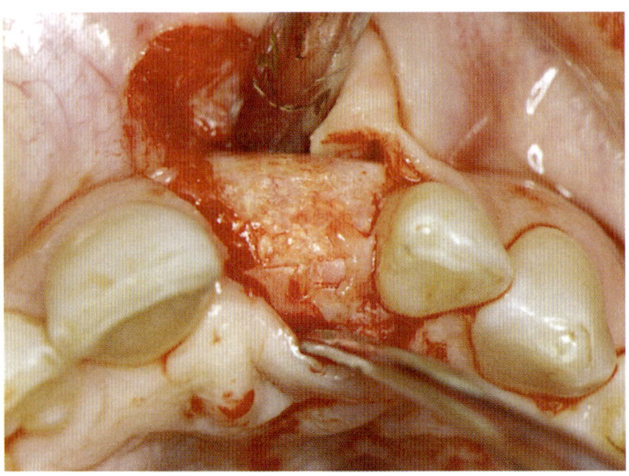

Figure 2.116 Following flap reflection and membrane removal, the ideal contours of the regenerated alveolar ridge are evident. An implant of the desired dimensions may now be placed in a perfect, prosthetically driven position.

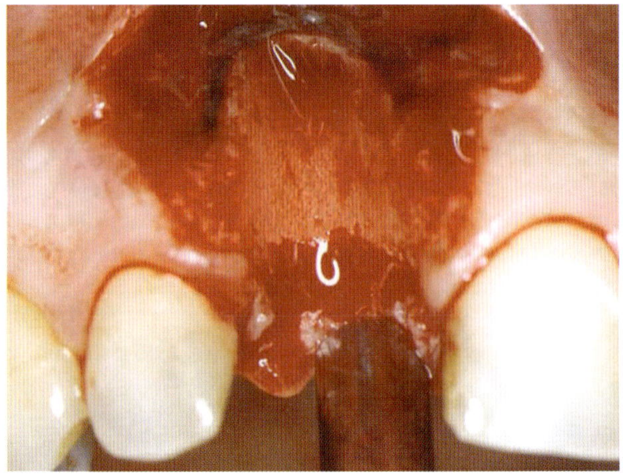

Figure 2.117 Flap reflection demonstrates a highly deficient alveolar ridge in the area of the missing maxillary right central incisor.

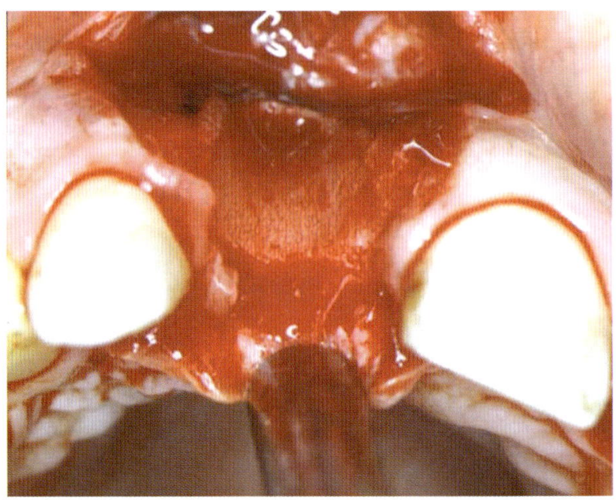

Figure 2.118 A crestal view underscores the highly atrophic nature of the residual alveolar ridge. The area was treated with Bio-Oss and a fixated titanium-reinforced covering membrane. Passive soft tissue primary closure was maintained throughout the course of regeneration.

Table 2.5 Treatment options for Treatment Planning Exercise # 2.

Treatment modality	Advantages	Disadvantages
Placement of a connective tissue graft to help improve the soft tissue profile, followed by fabrication of either a three-unit Maryland splint, or a three-unit fixed prosthesis	• No need to remove a membrane postoperatively	• An implant is not placed • Adjacent teeth are involved in restorative dentistry • Patient expectations are not met
Placement of a narrow implant in the residual alveolar ridge	• Requires no concomitant regenerative therapy	• Significantly decreases available surface area for osseointegration as compared to a wider implant • Represents a potential esthetic compromise in therapy
Placement of a wider implant in the residual alveolar ridge with concomitant regenerative therapy	• Greater implant surface area is available for potential osseointegration	• Implant is placed in a nonideal, more palatal position
	• The implant neck width is better suited to accept the planned restoration • All therapy is performed in one visit	• A ridge lap restoration may be required, representing an esthetic compromise
Ridge augmentation utilizing particulate or block nonautogenous graft material and a resorbable covering membrane or PRGF, followed by implant placement at a second-stage surgery	• Depending upon the extent of bone regeneration, the implant may be placed in a more ideal buccal palatal position	• Extent of bone regeneration is unpredictable
	• No need for membrane removal	• Morphology of the regenerated bone is unpredictable • Secondary soft tissue procedure may be required to help idealize the esthetic outcome
Placement of particulate or block nonautogenous graft material beneath a titanium-reinforced membrane, followed by implant placement at a subsequent surgery	• Ridge augmentation will allow placement of the implant in a more ideal bucco palatal position	• Need to master appropriate soft tissue techniques to prevent premature membrane exposure
	• The precise extent of bone regeneration is predictable • The precise morphology of regenerated bone is predictable • No need for secondary procedures to help maximize esthetic outcomes	• Need to remove the membrane

(*Continued*)

Table 2.5 (*Continued*)

Treatment modality	Advantages	Disadvantages
Ridge augmentation utilizing an autogenous block graft with no covering membrane	• The potential to place the implant in a more ideal buccopalatal position following bone regeneration • No membrane removal is required • No membrane expenses entailed	• The need to procure graft material from a second surgical site • The precise quantity of regenerated bone is not predictable • The precise morphology of the regenerated bone is not predictable • May require a secondary soft tissue procedure to help maximize treatment outcomes
Ridge augmentation utilizing an autogenous block graft with a resorbable or nonresorbable covering membrane or PRGF, followed by implant placement at a second surgical visit	• The ability to place the implant in a more ideal bucco palatal position following regenerative therapy • The quantity of regenerated bone is predictable • The quality of regenerated bone is predictable	• The need to procure the graft material from a second surgical site • The need to remove the membrane if a nonresorbable membrane is utilized

PRGF, preparations rich in growth factor.

However, regeneration of bone to cover an exposed implant surface, or regeneration of covering bone of sufficient thickness to withstand function forces over time are no longer adequate definitions of success following guided bone regeneration therapy. In the esthetic zone, any definition of success must include regeneration or prepathologic alveolar ridge morphology, to ideally support the covering soft tissues and help maximize treatment outcomes. Such a definition represents the **third-generation definition of success** of guided bone regeneration therapy.

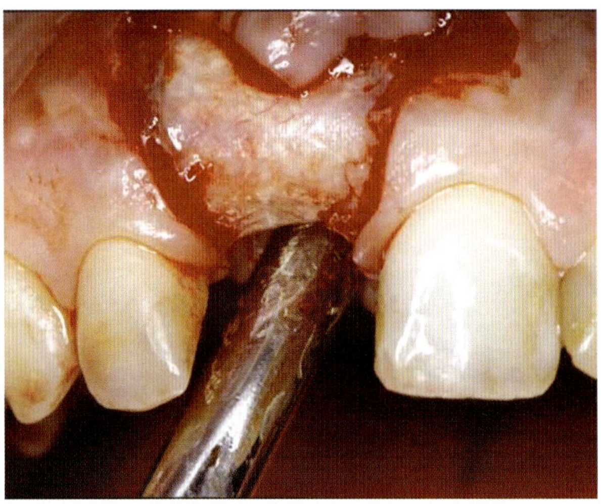

Figure 2.119 Following flap reflection and membrane removal eight months postregenerative therapy, extensive bone regeneration is evident.

TREATMENT PLANNING EXERCISE # 3

A 67-year-old female presented having lost her maxillary left posterior teeth approximately 20 years previously. She has been wearing a removable partial prosthesis to replace these teeth for over 20 years. At the time of flap reflection, significant ridge atrophy was noted, as the ridge progressed apically (Figure 2.120). Two, 8-mm-long Straumann implants were placed in the ideal prosthetic positions (Figure 2.121). The most anterior Straumann implant demonstrated fenestration of its apical aspect. While it would have been possible to place this implant at approximately a 30–35° angle and lessen or eliminate this fenestration, such

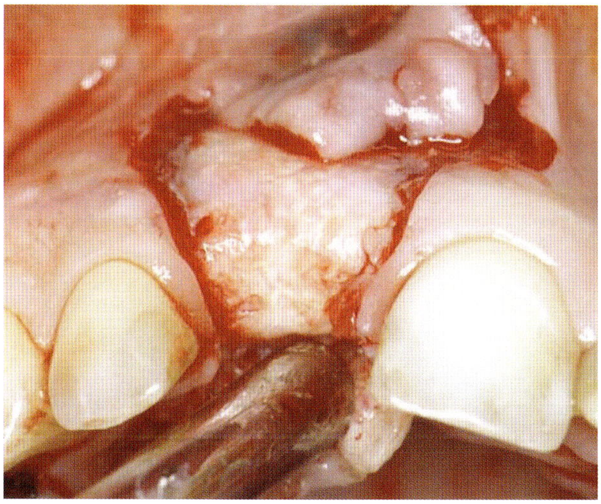

Figure 2.120 A crestal view demonstrates regeneration of an ideal alveolar ridge form including a perfectly shaped alveolar crest and buccal line angle. No soft tissue procedures will be required to help maximize esthetic treatment outcomes.

a treatment approach was never considered due to its inherent prosthetic compromises.

It must now be determined whether or not regenerative therapy should be performed over the fenestrated portion of the implant. While no data exist which document success and failure rates in such situations when these fenestrations are not covered by regenerated bone as compared to when they are covered by regenerated bone, it would seem most prudent to maximize the bone support around the implants, so as to help improve their long-term prognoses.

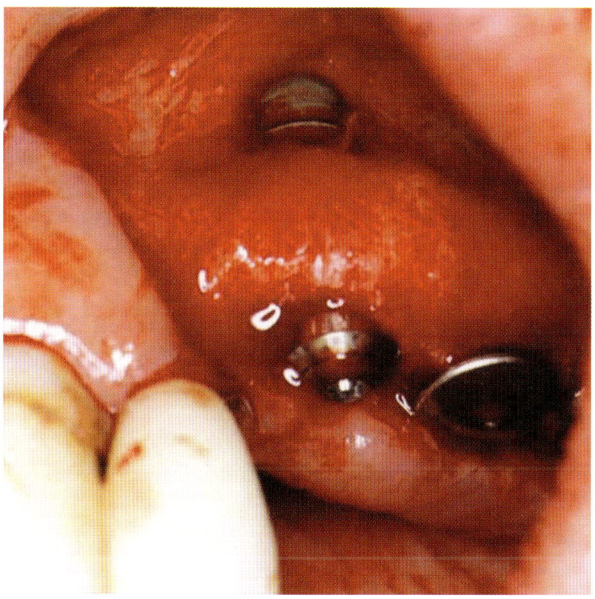

Figure 2.121 Two implants have been placed in a compromised maxillary alveolar ridge. Note the significant apical fenestration of the most anterior implant, extending around the "apex" of the fixture.

Treatment options for regeneration of the bone around the apical third of the implant, including its "apex", are as follows:

- Placement of a shorter implant in the residual alveolar ridge without concomitant regenerative therapy.
- Augmentation around the exposed implant surface utilizing particulate or block nonautogenous graft material and a resorbable covering membrane.
- Placement of particulate or block nonautogenous graft material around the exposed implant surface beneath a titanium-reinforced membrane.
- Augmentation therapy utilizing an autogenous block graft without a covering membrane around the exposed implant surface.
- Augmentation utilizing an autogenous block graft with a resorbable or nonresorbable covering membrane around the exposed implant surface.
- Placement of autogenous or nonautogenous particulate graft material around the exposed implant surface without use of a membrane.

The advantages and disadvantages of each treatment approach are summarized in Table 2.6.

A titanium-reinforced Gore-Tex membrane was trimmed, inserted, and secured with three apical fixation tacks. Following placement of a Bio-Oss graft beneath the membrane, an additional tack was placed at the most crestal extent of the membrane, to ensure its immobility. The graft material had been placed beneath the membrane in such a manner so as to cover the previously exposed implant surface, and extend approximately 3 mm apical to the apex of the implant. Note the morphology of the covering membrane (Figure 2.122).

Following flap reflection and membrane removal six months postregenerative therapy, extensive bone regeneration was evident. The morphology of the regenerated bone mimicked the space created beneath the covering titanium-reinforced membrane. The implant body was wholly ensconced in thick alveolar bone (Figure 2.123).

Table 2.6 Treatment options for Treatment Planning Exercise # 3.

Treatment modality	Advantages	Disadvantages
Placement of a shorter implant in the residual alveolar ridge without concomitant regenerative therapy	• No need for regenerative therapy	• Limitation in available implant designs of a 5-mm length • Lesser amount of implant surface available for potential osseointegration
Augmentation around the exposed implant surface utilizing particulate or block nonautogenous graft material and a resorbable covering membrane, or PRGF	• No need to procure graft material from a second surgical site • No need to perform membrane removal at a later date	• Unpredictability of the quantity of regenerated bone • Tendency of the resorbable membrane to collapse under pressure during healing, lessening the amount of regenerated bone
Ridge augmentation utilizing particulate or block nonautogenous graft material and a titanium-reinforced covering membrane	• Predictability of quantity of regenerated bone • Predictability of morphology of regenerated bone • No need to procure graft material from a second surgical site	• Need to remove the membrane at a second stage
Placement of particulate or block autogenous graft material around the exposed implant surface without a covering membrane	• No need for membrane removal • No additional cost of membrane use	• Unpredictability of regenerated bone quantity • Unpredictability of regenerated bone morphology • Need to procure the graft from a second surgical site
Ridge augmentation utilizing and autogenous block graft around the exposed implant surface with a resorbable or nonresorbable covering membrane, or PRGF	• Predictability of quantity of regenerated bone • Predictability of the morphology of the regenerated bone	• Need to procure graft material from a second surgical site • Need for membrane removal for nonresorbable membranes utilized
Placement of autogenous or nonautogenous particulate graft material around the exposed implant surface without use of a membrane	• No need for membrane removal • No cost to membrane use	• Highest degree of unpredictability of regenerated bone quantity and morphology

PRGF, preparations rich in growth factor.

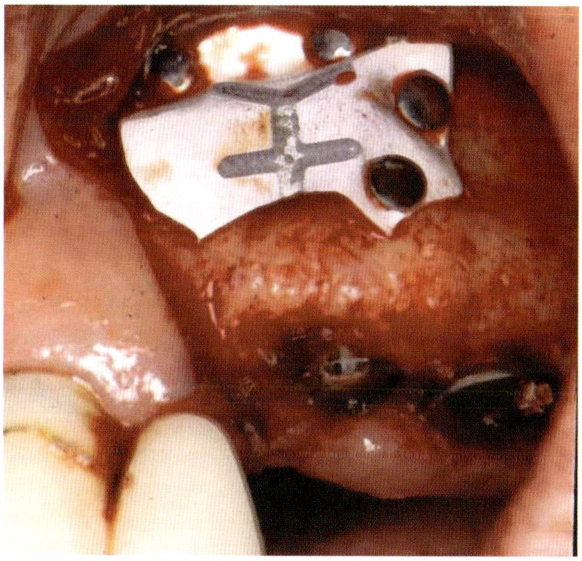

Figure 2.122 A titanium-reinforced Gore-Tex membrane has been placed over a Bio-Oss graft, and secured with four fixation tacks. Note the morphology of the membrane.

Ridge Augmentation Therapy

Numerous authors have demonstrated high levels of success following ridge augmentation through guided bone procedures, utilizing a variety of autogenous and nonautogenous materials. While claims are still made that autogenous bone represents the "gold standard" in guided bone regeneration therapy, the success and failure rates quoted following ridge augmentation utilizing autogenous or nonautogenous materials are comparable. A report of 302 consecutive ridge augmentation procedures which eventually accepted 574 implants, utilizing various allografts and xenografts beneath covering resorbable, nonresorbable, and nonresorbable titanium-reinforced membranes, reported an overall success rate of 96.0% (Table 2.7). The definitions of success utilized in the cited paper were as follows. If implants of 4 mm or greater diameter could be placed in the augmented ridges without generation of fenestrations or dehiscences, the augmentation procedures were deemed successes. If placement of 4 mm or wider diameter implants resulted in any implant fenestrations or dehiscences, the treatment outcome was classified as a partial success, even if the areas were regrafted, and the implants were restored and functioning successfully by the Albrektsson criteria. Any buccolingual ridge augmentation procedure that required placement of an implant of a lesser diameter than 4.0 mm was deemed a failure, despite the fact that narrower implants were placed and successfully restored.

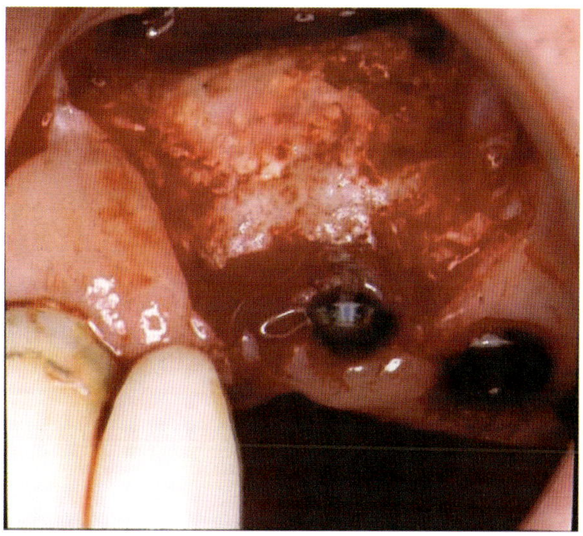

Figure 2.123 Following flap reflection and membrane removal six months postregenerative therapy, alveolar bone regeneration is noted which precisely mimics the morphology of the space created beneath the covering membrane. The "apex" of the implant is ensconced in thick alveolar bone.

Table 2.7 Success and failure rates of ridge augmentation therapy.

Type of therapy performed	Success	Partial success	Failure	Total
Buccolingual ridge augmentation	246	32	11	289
Apico-occlusal ridge augmentation	9	3	1	13

Apicocrestal ridge augmentation procedures were considered successful if a 10-mm implant could be placed which was wholly ensconced in bone following augmentation therapy. If up to 2 mm of the 10 mm or longer implant was exposed crestally following insertion, the apicocrestal ridge augmentation was deemed a partial success. The one failure in this group represented an early case in which primary closure was lost, and the regenerative procedure failed.

Crestal Augmentation

Crestal augmentation of up to 3 mm of lost hard tissues is predictably attainable through the utilization of the described materials and approaches. If simultaneous implant placement is to be carried out, the implant is placed so that 3 mm of the implant body is crestal to the residual ridge crest. Graft materials are packed around the implant, and the implant helps to further support the covering titanium-reinforced, secured membrane. Should greater than 3 mm of crestal augmentation be desired, augmentation of 3 mm of crestal bone is first accomplished utilizing fixated titanium-reinforced membranes. Implants are then placed after completion of regeneration, with their necks once again extruding 3 mm from the regenerated ridge crest. These implants help to support the covering reinforced membrane, as already described. The net result of this two-stage procedure is up to 6 mm of regenerated crestal bone.

While these definitions of success are not as stringent as the second- and third-generation definitions of success for guided bone regeneration therapy, the definitions utilized in the publication exceeded the standards employed at that time.

Despite the acceptable success rate of the performed therapy, various limitations at the time of treatment prevented an even higher success rate from being attained. These limitations included:

- The relatively primitive state of guided bone regenerative therapy at the time that the earliest cases were treated. The publication under discussion documented all cases treated up to that time in a single private practice, including the first efforts at guided bone regeneration therapy. As a result, an appropriate understanding of flap designs and other technical considerations had not yet fully evolved.
- Limitations in available membrane configurations: A number of the augmentation procedures reported upon were performed prior to the advent of titanium-reinforced Gore-Tex membranes. Various screws were utilized in attempts to support the membranes, thus providing space for the ingress of regenerative cells, and maximization of the volume of regenerated bone.
- No membrane fixation systems were readily available at the time of treatment of the earliest cases: As previously discussed, membrane fixation is crucial to the maximization of treatment outcomes following guided bone regeneration therapy. Failure to attain such stabilization will predictably lead to a diminution in the quantity of regenerated bone.

Clinical Example Ten

A 21-year-old patient, who presented in 1988 following trauma in which she had avulsed her mandibular incisors and a significant portion of the buccal aspect of the alveolar ridge (Figure 2.124), underscores these limitations. Following flap reflection utilizing relatively primitive incision designs, the residual buccal alveolar plate was tapped and first-stage implant healing screws were inserted in an attempt to provide support for the covering membrane. A mixture of resorbable tricalcium phosphate (Augmen) and demineralized freeze-dried bone allograft were placed and covered with a nonresorbable, nonreinforced Gore-Tex membrane. Soft tissue primary closure was attained and maintained throughout the course of regeneration. Flap reflection five and a half months postregenerative therapy (Figure 2.125) demonstrated significant enhancement of the residual

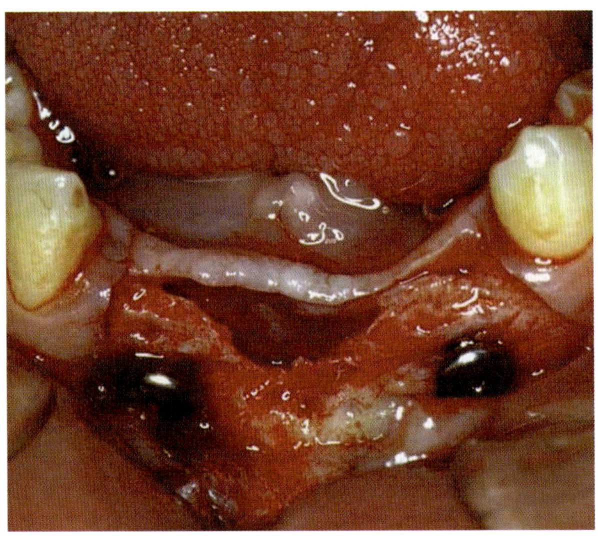

Figure 2.124 The residual alveolar crest has been tapped and first-stage surgical sealing screws have been inserted to help afford membrane support during regeneration. The area was treated with resorbable tri-calcium phosphate and a nonreinforced Gore-Tex membrane. Passive primary closure was maintained throughout the course of regeneration.

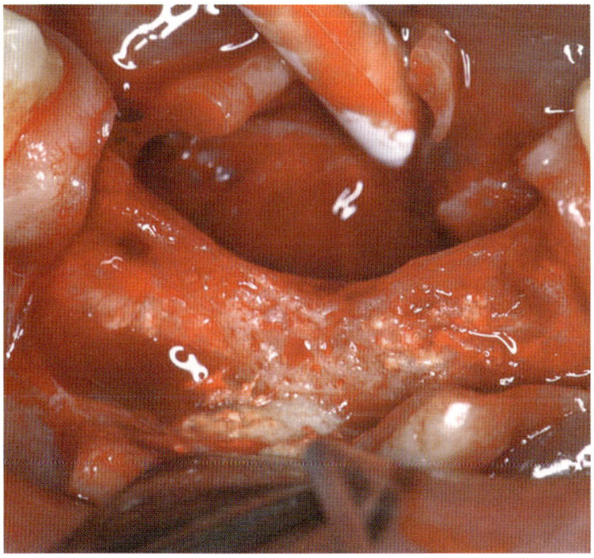

Figure 2.125 Six months postregenerative therapy, extensive ridge augmentation is noted. However, an ideal ridge form has not been regenerated.

alveolar ridge. However, the ridge form was far from ideal, and was less abundant than would be deemed acceptable today. Three titanium plasma-sprayed IMZ implants were inserted and restored (Figure 2.126). Due to the limited crestal bone regeneration which had occurred, the implants were placed in a position which resulted in approximately a 7-mm pocket between the implants and the adjacent teeth. Seventeen years postoperatively, the implants continue to function successfully with no evidence of peri-implant bone loss. As already discussed, the goals of guided bone regeneration therapy in such an area today are not simply the ability to place implants. Rather, the prepathologic ridge morphology must be regenerated, including significant crestal regeneration, allowing ideal implant placement and ease of maintenance for the patient.

When crestal augmentation therapy was carried out in the mid- to late-1980s prior to the advent of titanium-reinforced Gore-Tex membranes, support screws were placed to help effect such regeneration. A 61-year-old female patient presented with a failed mandibular second bicuspid, which was the terminal abutment for a three-unit fixed splint. Following sectioning of the splint, removal of the second bicuspid and the pontic in the first molar position, flap reflection and defect debridement, a significant alveolar ridge defect was evident. A screw was inserted into the ridge that protruded crestally, in an effort to attain membrane support at the ideal position (Figure 2.127). At flap reentry and membrane removal six months postregenerative therapy, significant crestal ridge augmentation was evident (Figure 2.128). Implants may now be placed in ideal positions in the second bicuspid and first molar areas.

The use of screws to support nonreinforced membranes represents a compromise in treatment

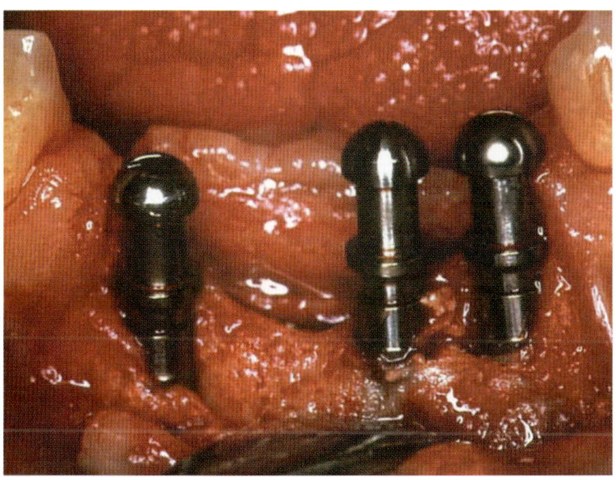

Figure 2.126 Three titanium plasma-sprayed IMZ implants have been placed in the regenerated bone. Note the height discrepancy between the implants and the cementoenamel junctions of the adjacent teeth.

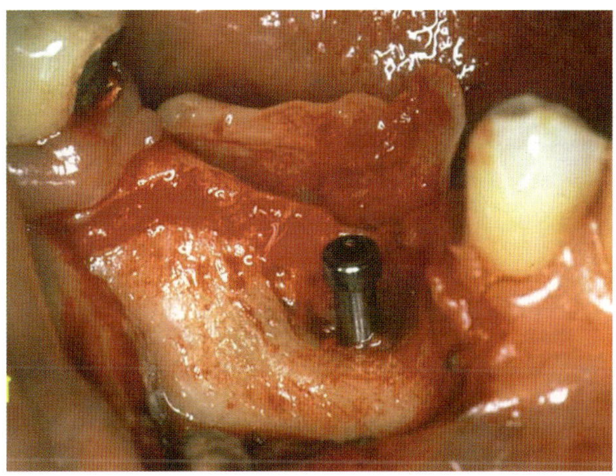

Figure 2.127 A titanium support screw has been placed in an alveolar ridge defect in an attempt to prevent collapse of the covering membrane. The area was treated with resorbable tri-calcium phosphate and a nonreinforced Gore-Tex membrane.

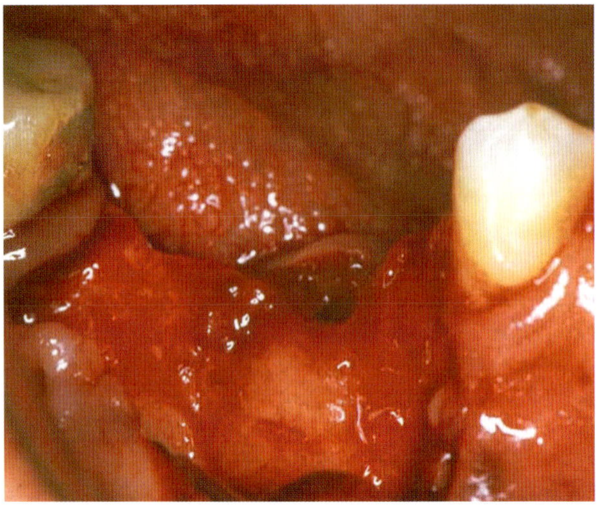

Figure 2.128 Following flap reflection and membrane removal six months postregenerative therapy, extensive buccal lingual and crestal bone regeneration are evident. Implants may now be placed in prosthetically driven positions.

outcomes following guided bone regeneration therapy. While these screws will provide support at their point of contact with the membrane, the extent of support afforded lessens as the distance from the support screw increases. Figure 2.129 demonstrates a severely damaged alveolar ridge following removal of two hopeless maxillary anterior teeth and debridement of the periodontal and periapical lesions which were present. Following insertion of a support screw in the buccal aspect of the residual alveolar ridge (Figure 2.130), resorbable tri-calcium phosphate and demineralized

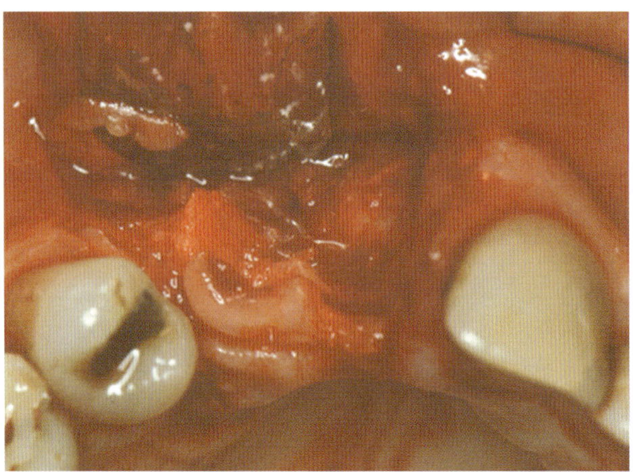

Figure 2.129 A severe alveolar ridge defect is noted following tooth removal and defect debridement.

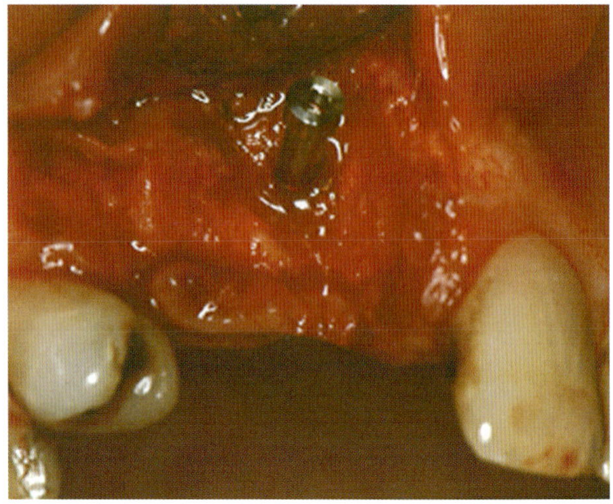

Figure 2.130 A support screw has been placed in an effort to prevent membrane collapse during regeneration. The area was treated with demineralized freeze-dried bone allograft and a covering nonreinforced Gore-Tex membrane.

freeze-dried bone allograft were placed. A nonreinforced Gore-Tex membrane was employed over the graft material, and passive soft tissue primary closure was attained and maintained throughout the course of healing. At flap reflection and membrane removal six months postoperatively, bone augmentation was evident. However, note the decreased buccopalatal width of the regenerated bone at sites more distant from the position of the support screw, when compared to the ridge width at the support screw's location (Figure 2.131).

When non-space-maintaining defects are treated, the clinician cannot depend on the underlying graft materials to predictably maintain space beneath the membrane and ensure the morphology of the regenerated bone, regardless of the configurations or consistencies of the graft materials employed. Some proponents of mineralized or demineralized bone blocks or bone substitutes contend that the "firmness" of the graft materials obviates the need for placement of a nonresorbable titanium-reinforced covering membrane. Despite these claims, no publications to date have demonstrated the ability to predictably rebuild prepathologic ridge morphologies when treating non-space-maintaining defects in such a manner. Only the appropriate utilization of titanium-reinforced membranes over graft materials, in the presence of proper flap management to ensure maintenance of soft tissue primary closure, will predictably yield such treatment outcomes.

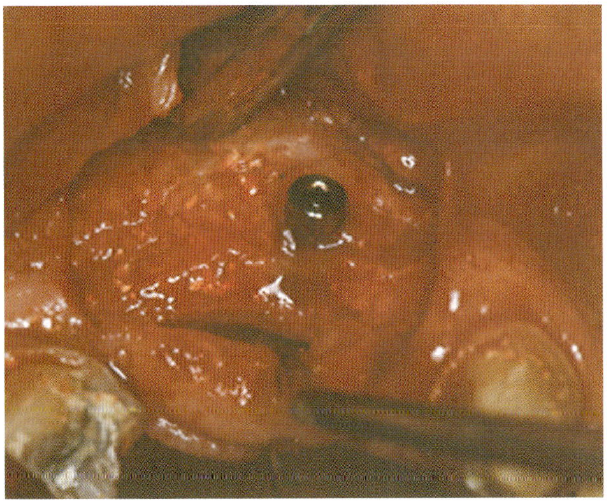

Figure 2.131 Following flap reflection and membrane removal six months postregenerative therapy, bone regeneration is evident. However, note the decrease in the buccopalatal width of the regenerated bone at sites more distant from the support screw.

Clinical Example Eleven

Figures 2.132 and 2.133 demonstrate a severely damaged alveolar ridge following removal of two fractured maxillary central incisors and debridement of the periodontal and periapical lesions which were present. The defect was treated through the use of a demineralized bone

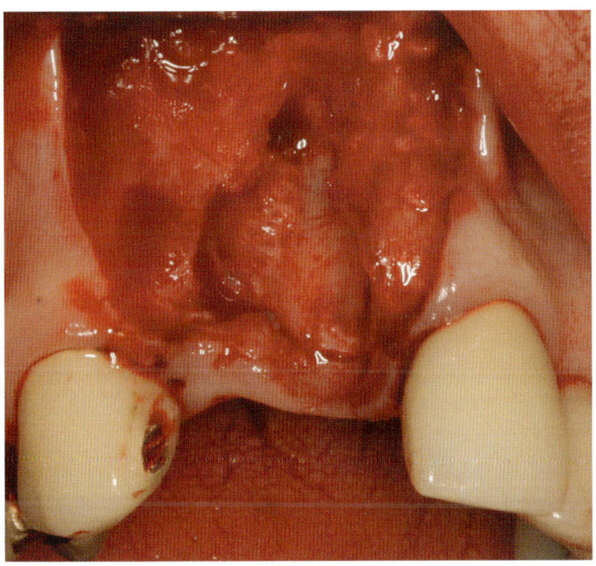

Figure 2.132 A severe alveolar ridge defect is evident following tooth removal and defect debridement.

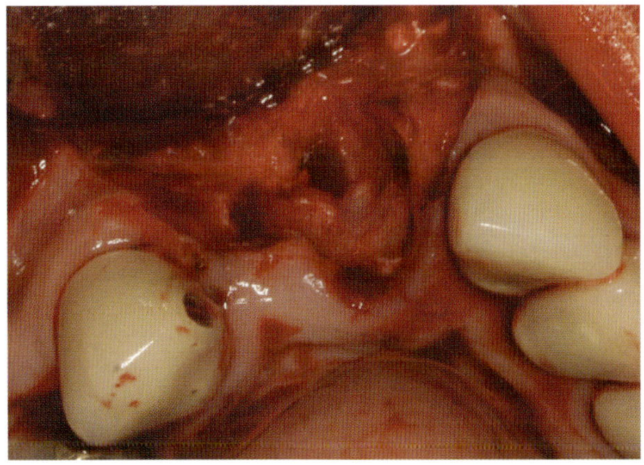

Figure 2.133 A crestal view demonstrates the extent of the damage which has occurred to the alveolar ridge. The area is treated with a Regenaform bone matrix block impregnated with cortical chips and a secured resorbable membrane.

matrix putty impregnated with cortical chips (Regenaform) and a covering Resolut membrane secured with fixation tacks, in the hope that the combination of the relative firmness of the graft material and the relative stiffness of the Resolut membrane would maintain the space created at the time of treatment. However, while the six-month surgical reentry demonstrates extensive ridge regeneration, the previous buccal line angle of the alveolar ridge has not been rebuilt (Figure 2.134).

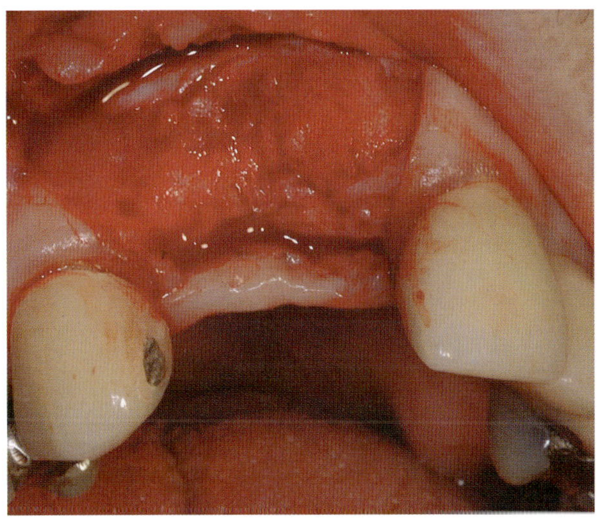

Figure 2.134 Flap reflection six months postregenerative therapy demonstrates significant alveolar bone regeneration. However, prepathologic alveolar ridge morphologies have not been reattained. Soft tissue grafting will have to be performed to help idealize esthetic treatment outcomes.

As a result, a soft tissue augmentation procedure will have to be performed at the time of implant placement to help maximize the esthetic outcomes of therapy. Such a treatment outcome should not be deemed a success.

TREATMENT PLANNING EXERCISE # 4

A 48-year-old female presented with a severely atrophic mandibular posterior alveolar ridge. The teeth in this area had been missing for approximately 35 years. Following flap reflection, the atrophic nature of the ridge was evident (Figure 2.135). Treatment options to effect regeneration included the following:

- Procurement of an autogenous bone block and its placement beneath the mucoperiosteal flaps without utilization of a covering membrane.
- Procurement of an autogenous bone block and its placement beneath the mucoperiosteal flaps with utilization of a covering membrane.
- Placement of a nonautogenous particulate or block graft beneath a covering resorbable membrane.
- Placement of a nonautogenous particulate or block graft beneath a covering titanium-reinforced membrane.

The advantages and disadvantages of each approach have been previously discussed. Failure to place a covering membrane over an autogenous block graft will lead to unpredictable resorption of up to 25–30% of the graft during healing and remodeling. Such remodeling of the block graft is avoidable if a covering, fixated membrane is utilized. The disadvantage of this approach is the need to procure the graft from a second surgical site, thus increasing the length of the procedure and postoperative morbidity.

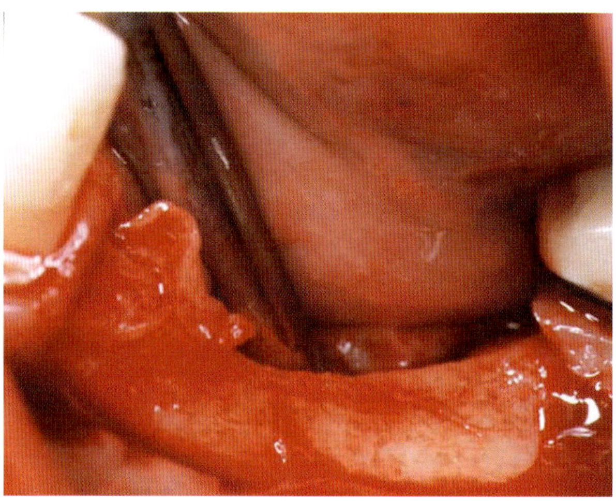

Figure 2.135 Flap reflection reveals a severely atrophic alveolar ridge. Implants may not be placed in an ideal position.

Employment of nonautogenous graft materials beneath a resorbable membrane will lead to an unpredictable regenerative result. Although there is no doubt that, if soft tissue primary closure is maintained throughout the course of regeneration, ridge augmentation will be effected, the precise quantity and morphology of the regenerated bone cannot be ascertained until the time of surgical reentry. As discussed, there is no literature to support the contention that the morphology created through the use of graft material of choice and a covering resorbable membrane at the time of surgery will be maintained throughout the course of regeneration. Rather, literature demonstrates precisely the opposite results upon reentry.

Utilization of nonautogenous graft material beneath a fixated titanium-reinforced membrane offers significant advantages over the other treatment approaches. If passive soft tissue primary closure is maintained throughout the course of regeneration, the quantity and morphology of regenerated bone will be that created at the time of the surgery through the shaping, positioning, and fixating of the titanium-reinforced membrane over the graft materials. In addition, the procedure is less lengthy, and the postoperative morbidity less severe, than if a membrane is utilized over an autogenous graft which must be procured from a second surgical site.

Unfortunately, the description of the treatment options, which is carried out above, mimics the manner in which conversations seem to proceed during clinicians' discussion of treatment options when faced with such defects. All too often, the focus is immediately placed upon the type of graft material and membrane to be utilized, without first discussing appropriate incision and flap designs.

The case presented above was treated utilizing the following flap designs:

- **A crestal incision** was placed within 1.5 mm of the teeth adjacent to the defect, bisecting the papillae.

- **Four releasing incisions** were placed on the mesiobuccal, distobuccal, mesiolingual, and distolingual corners of the crestal incision: When faced with ridge atrophy, clinicians are often hesitant to place lingual releasing incisions for fear of compromising vital structures. Such a concern is easily overcome as follows: The lingual vertical releasing incision extends 2 mm beyond the mucogingival junction. Except in the cases of the most severe ridge atrophy, which may very well not be candidates for this type of regenerative therapy and implant placement, no vital structures will be encountered at this point. The corner of the flap is engaged with a tissue forcep, blunt dissection is carried out, and the lingual releasing incision is extended through sharp dissection as the clinician visualizes the area from the internal aspect of the flap, ensuring that no vital structures are compromised.
- **Horizontal releasing incisions** were placed at the most apical extents of the buccal vertical releasing incisions: These horizontal extensions are crucial to the attainment of passive soft tissue primary closure following placement of regenerative materials. Concern is often voiced regarding placement of either a vertical releasing incision or its horizontal extension in the area of the mental foramen. If the clinician feels that the mental foramen may be in the area of planned incision design and flap reflection, he or she should proceed as follows. The buccal vertical releasing incision extends approximately 2 mm beyond the mucogingival junction. A tissue forcep is used to reflect the flap which has been created, and a blunt dissection is carried out with a periosteal elevator, until the entrance to the mental foramen is visualized. This area can now be isolated, and both the vertical releasing incision and its horizontal extension may be angled appropriately to avoid any vital structures in this area.
- **Full thickness flap reflection** was carried out buccally and lingually. Periosteal fenestrations were not utilized.
- **The degree of buccal and lingual flap mobility which had been attained was tested**. Using a tissue forcep, both the buccal and lingual flaps should be able to be lifted to the levels of the marginal ridges of the adjacent teeth. If they cannot be so displaced, the horizontal releasing incisions and full thickness reflections must be continued until adequate flap mobility is attained.

Following appropriate flap design and reflection, the ridge was decorticated utilizing a piezo surgery tip under copious irrigation. A titanium-reinforced membrane was trimmed and secured with fixation tacks. The membrane was trimmed in a specific manner to include the following characteristics:

- The apical extent of the membrane demonstrated two wings mesially and distally. These "wings" allowed the membrane to be secured with fixation tacks lateral to the planned site of augmentation therapy. If a membrane is secured with fixation tacks apical to the site of planned augmentation, the result is often diminution of the space available beneath the membrane for placement of regenerative materials, and hence for attainment of regenerated bone.
- The membrane was shaped to avoid the mental foramen and any other vital structures of concern.
- The rest of the membrane extended beyond the mesial, distal, and lingual aspects of the defect by only 1–2 mm. Because the membrane was secured with fixation tacks, and the soft tissue flaps will be successfully closed and soft tissue primary closure will be maintained throughout the course of regeneration, there is no need to extend the membrane further beyond the defect peripheries. Such extension may impinge upon adjacent teeth or vital structures. In addition, there is no reason to ask the soft tissue flaps to tolerate the presence of a greater amount of foreign material than is necessary
- The position of the membrane relative to the releasing incisions is of no concern. Once again, because the membrane is secured with fixation tacks, and the flaps will be closed in a passive manner so as to maintain soft tissue primary closure throughout the course of regeneration, placement of a membrane margin within a millimeter of a releasing incision does not represent a compromise.

Following flap reflection and membrane removal six months postregenerative therapy, both the extent of the ridge augmentation procedure and the ideal shape of the regenerated bone were evident

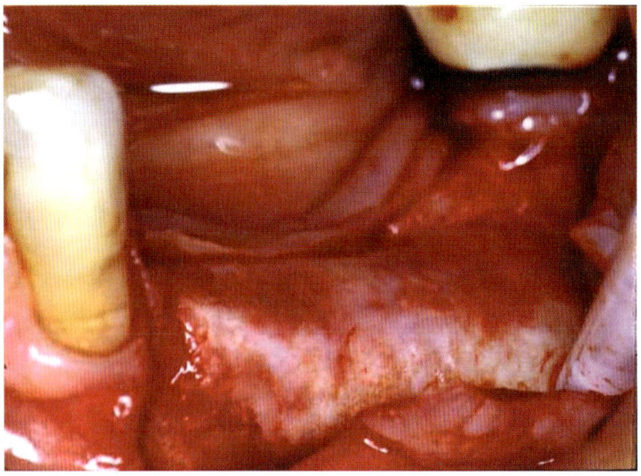

Figure 2.136 Six months after treatment with Bio-Oss and a secured titanium-reinforced Gore-Tex membrane, regeneration of prepathologic ridge morphology is evident. Implants may now be placed in prosthetically driven positions.

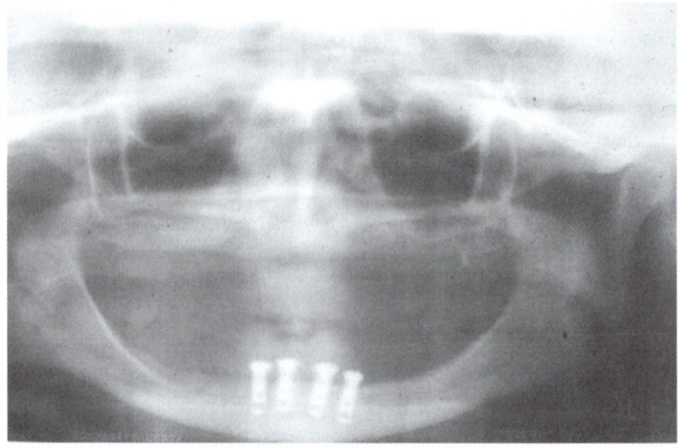

Figure 2.138 Nine months after treatment with Bio-Oss and multiple secured titanium-reinforced Gore-Tex membranes, extensive bone regeneration in the premaxillary area is evident radiographically.

(Figure 2.136). Implants of sufficient diameters to withstand functional forces over time may now be placed in ideal positions, without the need for additional regenerative treatments.

The appropriate utilization of the above concepts and techniques affords the opportunity to treat a variety of cases previously considered too advanced for such an approach. For example, a patient presented with clinical and radiographic evidence of severe maxillary and mandibular ridge atrophy following 40 plus years of denture use (Figure 2.137). The premaxillary bone had resorbed to the level of the nasal spine. Such a scenario is often treated through the use of an iliac crest graft, due to its extent and severity. However, the patient refused such therapy. Sinus augmentation therapy could not be carried out due to a significant history of chronic sinusitis. Bio-Oss was placed beneath three covering, titanium-reinforced Gore-Tex membranes which were secured with fixation tacks. Nine months postoperatively, significant ridge regeneration was evident radiographically (Figure 2.138). While awaiting regeneration in the premaxillary area, four titanium plasma-sprayed IMZ implants were placed in the mandibular anterior region. These implants will eventually support an over denture appliance.

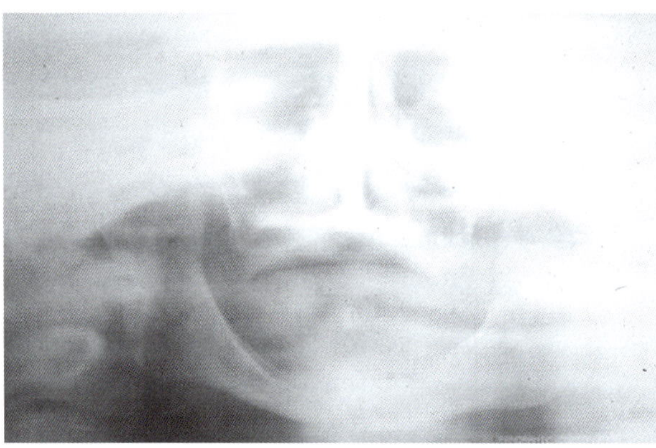

Figure 2.137 A patient who has been edentulous for over 30 years presents with severe maxillary atrophy. Sinus augmentation therapy cannot be performed due to history of chronic sinusitis.

Six titanium plasma-sprayed IMZ implants were placed in the regenerated maxillary bone (Figure 2.139). These implants were restored with a milled bar palateless removable prosthesis. The prosthesis has been functioning successfully for 17 years with no evidence of peri-implant bone loss.

The Stability of Regenerated Bone

While dramatic regenerative results may be attained without the use of autogenous bone grafts, such bone regrowth is meaningless unless implants placed in the regenerated bone demonstrate success rates under function comparable to those of implants placed in native host bone. The first paper published on this topic documented the success and failure rates of 626 implants either placed in regenerated alveolar ridges, inserted in extraction sockets at the time of tooth removal, or treated

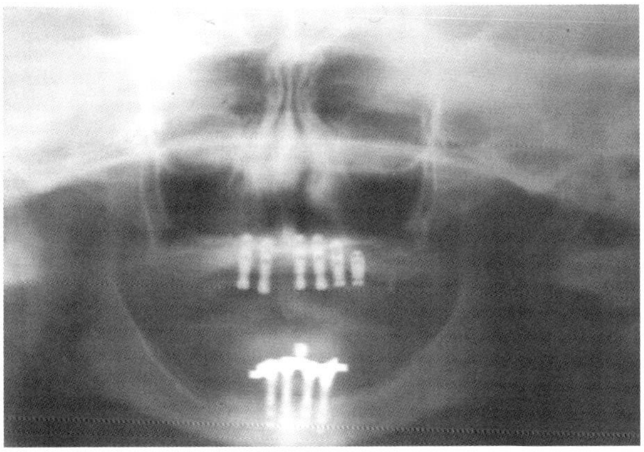

Figure 2.139 Eight titanium plasma-sprayed IMZ implants have been placed in the regenerated maxillary bone.

with guided bone regeneration to rebuild bone over implant fenestrations and/or dehiscences (20). The reported cumulative success rate was 93.8%. The definition of success for this paper was not the Albrektsson et al.'s criteria alone. The widely accepted success criteria of Albrektsson et al. do not address the stability of regenerated bone on the buccal and/or lingual/palatal aspects of implants, as such bone levels are not assessable radiographically. As a result, the paper expressed success in terms of both the aforementioned criteria and bone sounding at the sites of regeneration. Each implant was bone sounded under anesthesia at the site(s) where regenerative therapy had been carried out, to document the level of the regenerated bone. Subsequent publications have confirmed the high success rates of implants functioning in regenerated bone which were reported in this paper.

An additional paper published in 2005 documented the success and failure rates of 1,233 implants in regenerated bone after 78–123 months in function (21). These implants included those reported upon in the previous publication, and followed for a greater length of time, and implants placed since the previous publication. Utilizing the success criteria previously described, an overall cumulative success rate of 97.3% was reported. Cumulative success rates of 97.2% and 97.4% were reported in the maxilla and mandible, respectively.

Of note is a comparison between the more recently placed implants reported upon in the study, which had been in function for up to six years, and the implants which were followed for a longer period of time and had been reported upon in the previous study. The implants reported upon in the previous study, and followed for a longer time in the second study, included the first implants placed in regenerated bone. As a result, three potential compromises were present at the time of implant insertion. First, the quantity of regenerated bone was less than it would have been if the areas had been treated with materials that later became available (i.e., titanium-reinforced membranes, fixation tacks, etc.). Second, many of the initial implants were placed at an earlier time in the evolution of understanding of the capabilities of the implants to support force loads in various situations. There is no doubt that the "engineering" of implant reconstructive cases has evolved significantly since the 1980s. Finally, the implants which were available for use in the 1980s represented a compromise when compared to their current counterparts. Implant morphology, implant diameter, implant abutment design, and implant surfaces have all progressed dramatically over the past two decades, yielding significantly higher success rates in both host and regenerated bone.

Despite these compromises, the success rates reported upon for implants in regenerated bone easily matched those for implants functioning in native host bone.

Maintenance of Regenerated Bone Without Implant Placement

The literature does not demonstrate consistent evidence of the loss of residual alveolar bone beneath a well-fitting fixed prosthesis longer than one year after tooth removal. Rather, clinical observation would indicate the reverse. If no forces are placed upon this alveolar bone, it does not continue to atrophy beneath well-fitting fixed prostheses. The question is whether regenerated bone demonstrates the same stability in a similar situation.

Clinical Example Twelve

A 51-year-old male presented with a hopeless prognosis for his central incisor, which was part of a three-unit fixed splint. Flap reflection revealed a severe osseous defect around the root of this tooth, which had adversely effected the mesial aspect of the adjacent lateral incisor (Figure 2.140).

Following removal of the root from beneath the fixed splint and debridement of the defect,

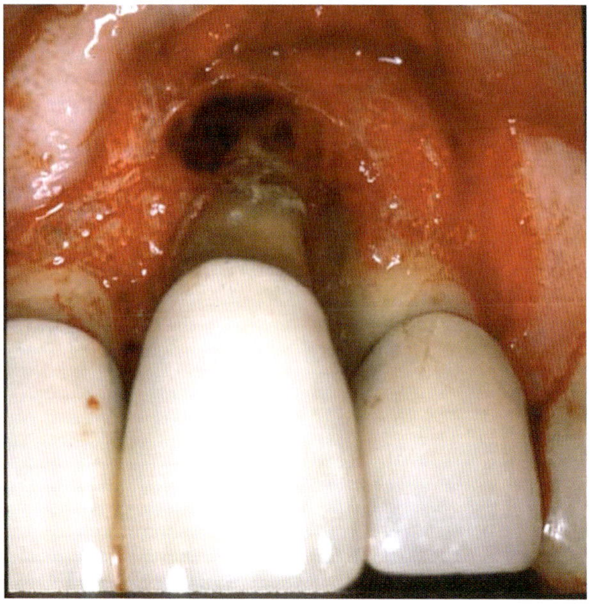

Figure 2.140 A patient presents with a hopeless prognosis for a maxillary central incisor, and significant osseous loss on the mesial aspect of the adjacent lateral incisor.

Bio-Oss was placed, and a titanium-reinforced membrane was secured over the graft material (Figure 2.141). The rotation of a palatal pedicle flap, and its placement beneath the created pontic of the three-unit fixed splint, afforded the opportunity to attain and maintain passive soft tissue primary closure throughout the course of regeneration.

Following flap reflection and membrane removal six months postregenerative therapy (Figure 2.142), significant ridge regeneration was evident beneath the created pontic. Bone had also been regenerated on the mesial aspect of the adjacent lateral incisor.

Sixteen years posttherapy, no recession on ridge atrophy has occurred in the area of regeneration (Figure 2.143). Does this bone maintain itself over time?

In an attempt to answer this question, 43 cases of ridge augmentation were assessed. Following ridge augmentation therapy (Figure 2.144), and fixed prosthesis reconstruction, measurements were taken as follows. Impressions of the final fixed prostheses were made, and vacuform stents were fabricated over the areas of the prostheses. Buccal and palatal holes were made in the stents and calipers were utilized to measure the buccopalatal width of the regenerated

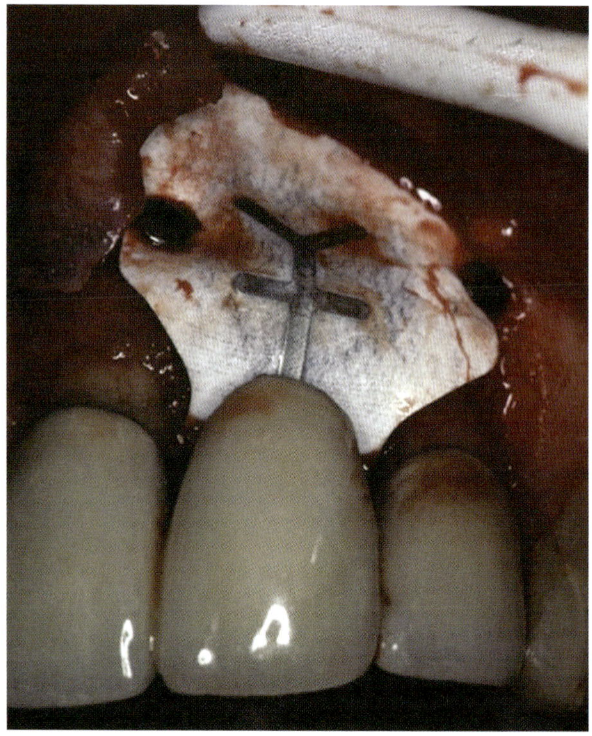

Figure 2.141 Following root removal from beneath the three-unit fixed splint, the area is treated with Bio-Oss and a secured, titanium-reinforced Gore-Tex membrane. A rotated palatal pedicle flap is utilized to attain and maintain soft tissue primary closure throughout regeneration.

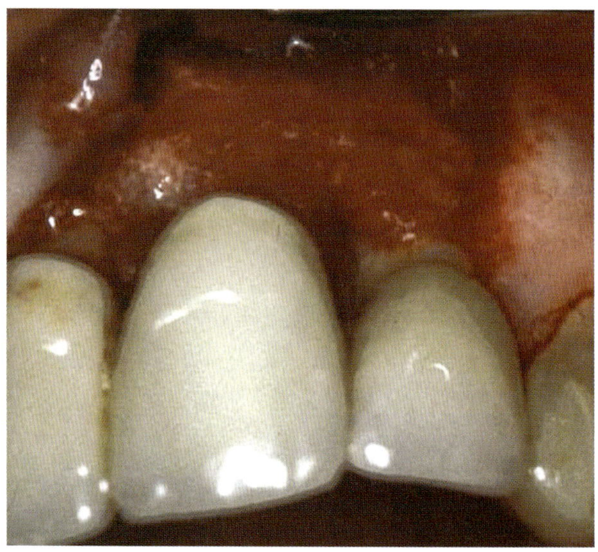

Figure 2.142 Flap reflection and membrane removal six months posttherapy demonstrates significant regeneration of the damaged alveolar bone. This bone should remain stable beneath the fixed prosthesis, as no pressure is being placed upon it.

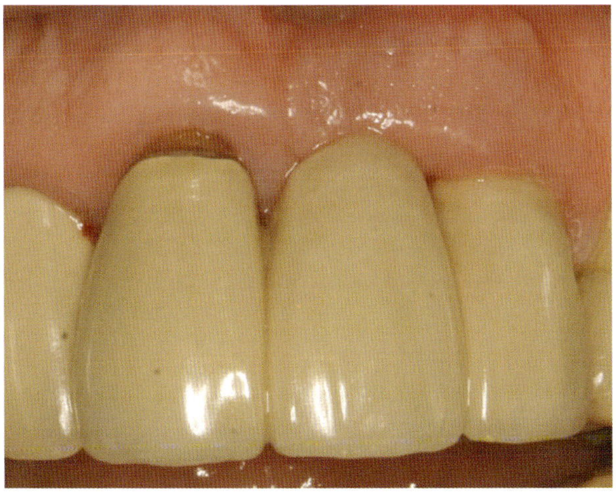

Figure 2.143 Sixteen years after regenerative therapy was performed at the time of tooth extraction, the stability of the soft tissues in the area, and the underlining bone, is noted.

alveolar bone, under anesthesia, immediately following prosthesis insertion.

A mean time of 28.6 months after the initial measurements were taken, the stents were reinserted and the same calipers were utilized to measure the buccopalatal dimension of the regenerated ridge in the pontic area, under anesthesia. An average change in the buccolingual dimension of the regenerated alveolar ridge of less than 0.1 mm was noted. Therefore, it may be stated that regenerated alveolar bone beneath pontics is stable for at least 28.6 months postrestoration. There would

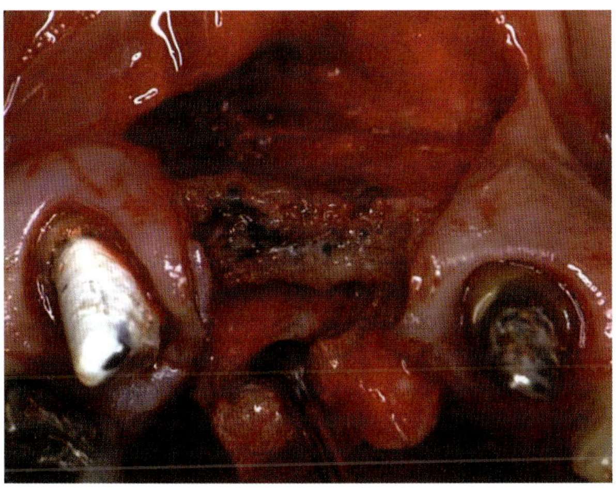

Figure 2.144 A patient presents with the need for both preprosthetic periodontal surgery and ridge augmentation in the pontic area to help idealize the final esthetic treatment outcomes.

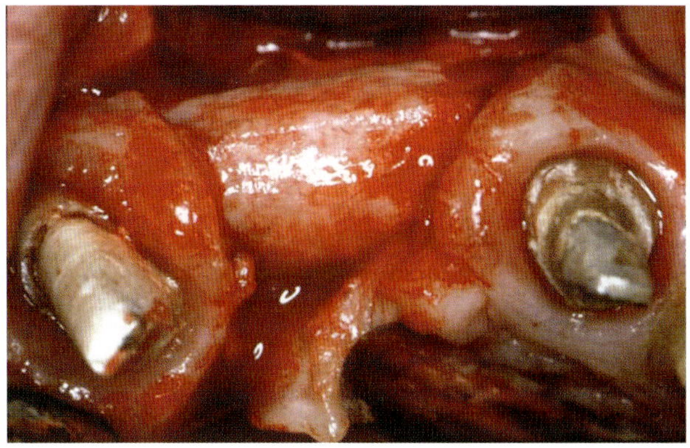

Figure 2.145 Six months following reconstructive therapy, extensive bone regeneration is evident. As this regenerated bone will be beneath a fixed prosthesis and free of overlying pressures, it should remain stable over time.

be no reason to expect this bone to subsequently resorb, as it had been stable for over two years (Figure 2.145).

THE QUESTION OF AUTOGENOUS BONE

Autogenous bone has long been referred to as the "gold standard" of regenerative graft materials. It has been cited as such due to both its ability to effect regeneration, and the rapidity of such regeneration. Numerous reports document the placement of implants in autogenous bone block grafts 4–5 months post-regenerative therapy, as compared to the 6–9 months often reported when various allografts or xenografts have been employed.

There is no doubt that autogenous bone offers significant advantages when compared to nonautogenous alternatives, if regenerative therapy is performed in the absence of covering membranes. The failure of other graft materials to demonstrate predictable and acceptable regenerative results when placed without covering membranes must lead one to conclude that their utilization in such situations represents a significant compromise to treatment outcomes, and thus to the patient.

However, when utilized in conjunction with appropriately employed membrane therapy, does autogenous bone offer significant advantages over its allograft or xenograft counterparts?

Assuming appropriate incision designs and flap reflections to ensure attainment and maintenance of the soft tissue primary closure;

complete defect debridement; decortication when necessary; selection of a reinforced or nonreinforced membrane as dictated by defect morphology; fixation of the membrane; passive suturing to attain soft tissue primary closure; maintenance of soft tissue closure; and control of overlying forces; what advantages does autogenous bone afford the clinician and ultimately the patient? An in-depth analysis of available literature, coupled with clinical expertise, leads to the indisputable fact that the only advantage autogenous bone offers in such a situation, when compared to predictably resorbable allografts and xenografts, is that of speed. Rather than having to wait 6–7 months to reenter an area treated with nonautogenous grafts and covering membranes, the clinician can reenter a site grafted with autogenous bone and covering membranes 4–5 months postoperatively to effect implant placement.

This fact mandates a paradigm shift when selecting a graft material to be utilized beneath an appropriately employed membrane. If the speed to be gained from the use of autogenous bone is justified by the additional time and morbidity inherent in graft procurement, autogenous bone should be employed. For example, if augmentation is to be carried out in the area of teeth numbers 12 and 13, and autogenous bone may be easily obtained from the tuberosity region in the same sextant, its use is logical, as there is little increase in either operating time or postoperative morbidity (Flow Chart 2.2).

However, if procurement of autogenous bone requires the involvement of a second, distant surgical site, it becomes difficult if not impossible to justify its utilization in the majority of situations, with the attendant increase in operating time and postoperative morbidity.

The fourth generation definition of success is therefore simplification of therapy for the patient without compromising treatment outcomes.

Controlling Overlying Forces

Failure to control forces on regenerating sites generated by overlying prostheses will result in an increase in postoperative complications, including loss of soft tissue primary closure, soft tissue abscesses, and a decrease in the volume of regenerated bone. It is imperative that a treating clinician stand firm in the face of patient requests and concerns when considering the use of overlying prostheses throughout the course of regeneration.

Naturally, if the patient can be temporized with a fixed prosthesis, whether it be to reestablish an appropriate occlusion or for other reasons, the question of controlling forces from an overlying prosthesis is easily solved. However, in situations where a temporary fixed prosthesis will not be employed, controlling overlying forces on graft sites is of paramount importance.

When the bone in a single- or two-tooth site is to be regenerated, numerous simple temporization options present themselves. An Essex retainer may be employed. It affords the advantages of an inexpensive, easy to fabricate temporary solution which will not impinge upon the underlying regenerative site. The limitations to Essex retainer utilization include the need to use it in only one- or two-tooth sites, as its employment over greater edentulous spans will result in retainer flexure and impingement upon the regenerating area. In addition, a patient's occlusion may preclude Essex retainer utilization if adequate interocclusal space is not present to allow its placement. Finally, an Essex retainer is an esthetic compromise in the best of situations.

A Monodent bridge or a Maryland bridge may also be employed if temporization is to be carried out in a one- or two-tooth site. While a Maryland bridge is less invasive to the adjacent teeth, it is more expensive and requires additional visits, when compared to a Monodent bridge. The Monodent bridge is minimally invasive (not noninvasive) to adjacent teeth, and often represents a viable treatment option, especially if the adjacent teeth already present with Class III restorations.

If an anterior area of greater than two teeth in width is to be treated with regeneration, and the patient is not having a fixed temporary prosthesis placed for other reasons, a removable partial prosthesis must be utilized. In such a situation, it is imperative that the buccal flange of the prosthesis be removed to the level of the cementoenamel junctions of the acrylic teeth, and that the undersurface of the prosthesis be hollowed out where it overlays the regenerating site. The patient is allowed to wear the prosthesis for esthetic reasons, but is admonished not to eat with the prosthesis in place at any time throughout the course of regeneration. It is critical that this point is underscored to the patient by explaining that if the patient does eat with the prosthesis in place, the regenerative therapy will fail, and the patient will have to incur both the expense and the discomfort of undergoing the treatment a second time. Failure to provide such severe admonishments often results in patient misuse of the prosthesis once the soft tissues have healed, with a resultant compromise in the regenerative outcomes of therapy. When a removable prosthesis is being utilized by the patient over a posterior site which will be regenerated, one of two approaches is always employed. If the prosthesis is not in an esthetic area, it is taken from the patient so that it cannot be utilized inappropriately.

If the patient insists on retaining the prosthesis, it is adjusted as previously described, removing the buccal flange and hollowing out the prosthesis where it overlays the regenerating site. The same admonishments are given to the patient as already explained.

The most potentially difficult situation is that of a patient who is wearing a full maxillary denture. Such a scenario will be discussed in a subsequent chapter, when various therapeutic options are explored.

Conclusions

The maximization of treatment outcomes following guided bone regenerative therapy does not begin with the selection of graft materials, nor the utilization of various membranes. As with all other treatments, GBR therapy is highly diagnosis dependent. Once the appropriate diagnosis is carried out, the results of guided bone regenerative therapy are directly attributable to appropriate incision design, flap management, membrane selection, and ultimately the individual clinician's inflexibility when defining success (Table 2.8).

Table 2.8 Definitions of success following guided bone regeneration.

	Buccolingual ridge augmentation	Implant dehiscences fenestrations	Extraction socket reconstruction	Apico-occlusal ridge augmentation
First generation	Adequate bone to place an implant	Coverage of exposed implant surface with regenerated hard tissues	Adequate bone to place an implant	Adequate bone to place a 10-mm-long implant
Second generation	Adequate bone to withstand functional forces over time	Adequate bone to withstand functional forces over time	Adequate bone to withstand functional forces over time	Adequate bone to place a 10-mm-long implant and adequate bone to withstand functional forces over time
Third generation	All of the above plus regeneration of prepathologic alveolar morphology, allowing placement of an ideally sized implant in a perfect prosthetic position, and maximum esthetic support for covering tissues	All of the above plus regeneration of prepathologic alveolar morphology, and maximum esthetic support for covering soft tissue	All of the above plus regeneration of prepathologic alveolar morphology, allowing placement of an ideally sized implant in a perfect prosthetic position, and maximum esthetic support for covering soft tissues	All of the above plus regeneration of prepathologic alveolar morphology, allowing placement of an ideally sized implant in a perfect prosthetic position, and maximum esthetic support for covering soft tissues
Fourth generation	Simplification of therapy as much as possible, without compromising treatment outcomes	Simplification of therapy as much as possible, without compromising treatment outcomes	Simplification of therapy as much as possible, without compromising treatment outcomes	Simplification of therapy as much as possible, without compromising treatment outcomes

References

1. Buser D, Dula K, Belser U, Hirt H-P, and Berthold H. 1993. Localized ridge augmentation using guided bone regeneration. 1. Surgical procedure in the maxilla. *Int J Periodontics Restorative Dent* 13:29–45.
2. Bahat O, Fontanesi RV, and Preston J. 1993. Reconstruction of the hard and soft tissues for optimal placement of osseointegrated implants. *Int J Periodontics Restorative Dent* 13:255–275.
3. Nevins M and Mellonig JT. 1994. The advantages of localized ridge augmentation prior to implant placement: A staged event. *Int J Periodontics Restorative Dent* 14:96–111.
4. Simion M, Trisi P, and Piatelli A. 1994. Vertical ridge augmentation using a membrane technique associated with osseointegrated implants. *Int J Periodontics Restorative Dent* 14:497–511.
5. Buser D, Dula K, Hirt H-P, and Schenk RK. 1996. Lateral ridge augmentation using autografts and barrier membranes: A clinical study with 40 partially edentulous patients. *J Oral Maxillofac Surg* 54:420–432.
6. Fugazzotto PA. 1998. Report of 302 consecutive ridge augmentation procedures: Technical considerations and clinical results. *Int J Oral Maxillofac Implants* 13:358–368.
7. Bahat O and Fontanessi RV. 2002. The efficacy of implant placement after bone grafting for three-dimensional reconstruction of the posterior jaw. *Int J Periodontics Restorative Dent* 22:109–117.
8. Fiorellini JP and Nevins ML. 2003. Localized ridge augmentation/preservation. A systematic review. *Ann Periodontal* 8:321–327.
9. Park SH and Wang HL. 2006. Management of localized buccal dehiscents defect with allografts and a cellular dermal matrix. *Int J Periodontal Restorative Dent* 26:589–595.
10. Mellonig JP and Triplett RG. 1993. Guided tissue regeneration and osseous dental implants. *Int J Periodontal Restorative Dent* 13:109–119.
11. Fugazzotto PA, Shanaman R, Manos T, and Shectman R. 1997. Guided bone regeneration around titanium implants: Reports of the treatment of 1503 sites with clinical re-entries. *Int J Periodontal Restorative Dent* 17:292–299.
12. Lekholm U, Becker W, Dahlin C, Becker B, Donath K, and Morrison E. 1993. The role of early versus late removal of GTAM membranes on bone formation at oral implants placed into immediate extraction sockets. An experimental study in dogs. *Clin Oral implants Res* 4:121–129.
13. Shanaman RH. 1994. A retrospective study of 237 sites treated consecutively with guided tissue regeneration. *Int J Periodontal Restorative Dent* 9:31–40.
14. Simion M, Baldoni M, Rossi P, and Zaffe D. 1994. A comparative study of the effectiveness of e-PTFE membranes with and without early exposure during the healing period. *Int J Periodontics Restorative Dent* 14:166–180.
15. Machtei EE. 2001. The effect of membrane exposure on the outcome of regenerative procedures in humans: A meta-analysis. *J Periodontol* 72:512–516.
16. Fugazzotto PA, DePaoli S, and Parma-Benfenati S. 1993. Flap design considerations with implant placement in the maxillary anterior region. *Implant Dent* 2:93–96.
17. Fugazzotto PA. 1999. Maintenance of soft tissue closure following guided bone regeneration: Technical considerations and report of 723 cases. *J Periodontol* 70:1085–1097.
18. Fugazzotto PA. 2006. Maintaining primary closure after guided bone regeneration procedures: Introduction of a new flap design and preliminary results. *J Periodontol* 77:1452–1457.
19. Fugazzotto PA. 1998. Implant placement in atrophic ridges: A simplified technique. *Implant Dent* 7:193–197.
20. Fugazzotto PA. 1997. Success and failure rates of 626 osseointegrated implants in function in regenerated bone for 6–51 months: A preliminary report. *Int J Periodontics Restorative Dent* 7:293–299.
21. Fugazzotto PA. 2005. Success and failure rates of osseointegrated implants in function regenerated bone for 72–133 months. *Int J Oral Maxillofac Implants* 20: 77–83.

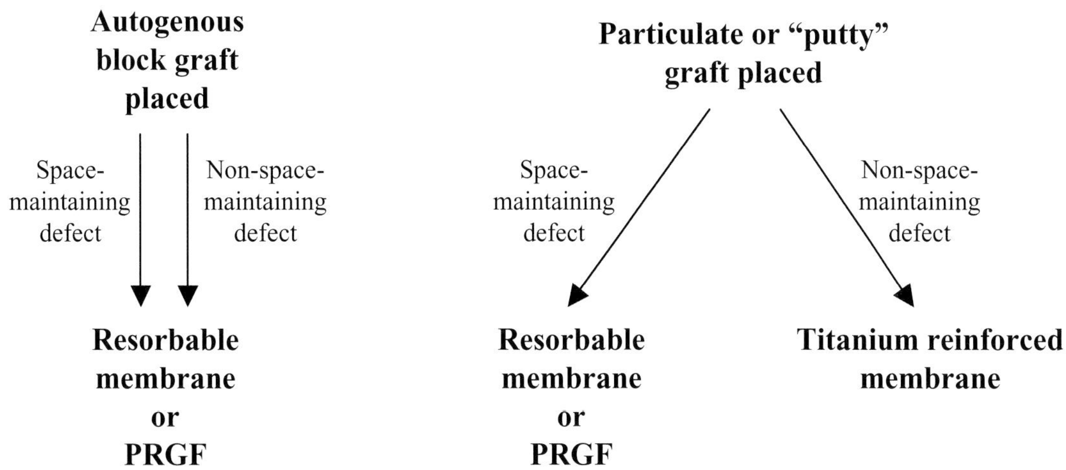

Flow chart 2.1 Membrane selection (all membranes are secured with fixation tacks).

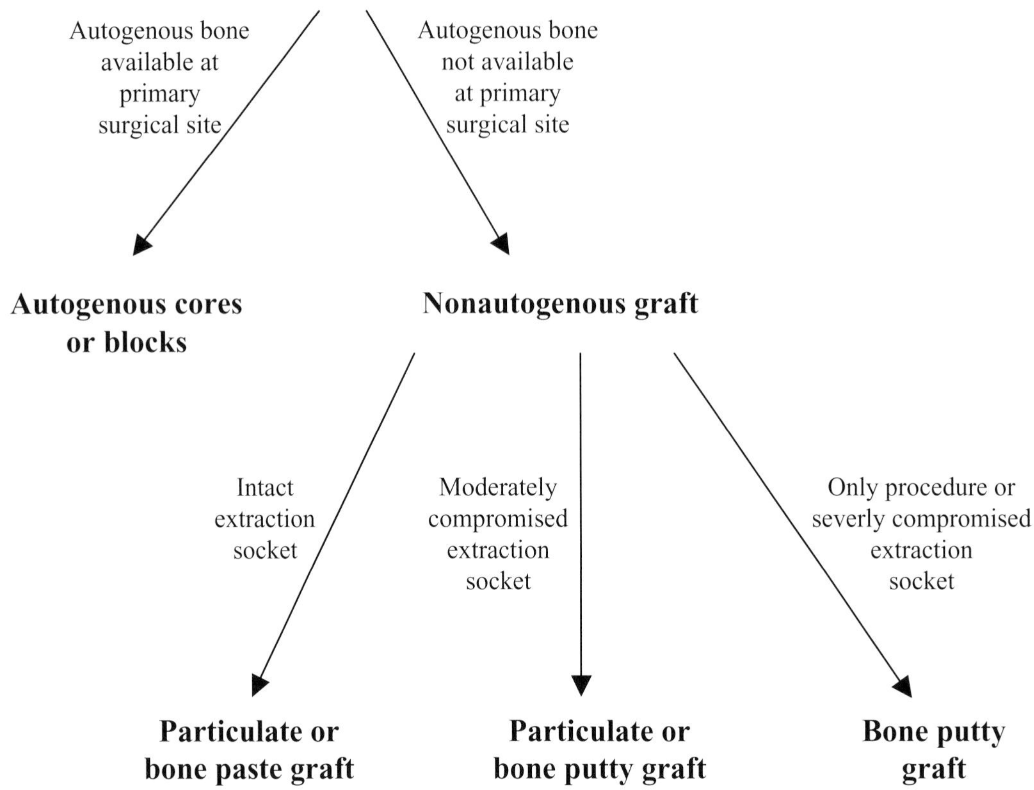

Flow chart 2.2 Graft selection (osseous coagulum is collected, if possible).

Chapter 3

The Therapeutic Potential of PRGF in Dentistry and Oral Implantology

Eduardo Anitua, DDS, MD, Gorka Orive, PhD, and Isabel Andía, PhD

Outline

Introduction

The process of tissue repair involves a complex cascade of biological events in which a large list of cytokines and growth factors provide signals at local injury sites, regulating the mechanisms and pathways that govern wound healing and tissue regeneration (1). Although each tissue has its own specific characteristics and properties, most of them share common steps and pathways. One critical point is the implication of a wide range of biological mediators in the spatiotemporal control of the processes that govern tissue regeneration including chemotaxis, cell proliferation and differentiation, angiogenesis and extracellular matrix formation among others. In the process of bone regeneration, locally produced growth factors initially mediate the migration of osteoprogenitor cells to the defect site, and later mediate the direct differentiation of the osteoprogenitors toward specific cell lineages. Growth factors also control cell proliferation, bone revascularization, and extracellular matrix production (2).

Successful restoration of tissue functions depends upon a sequence of steps regulated by multiple bioactive growth factors and proteins that unfold over time through an orchestrated sequence of spatial changes (3). The progressive understanding of these facts at a basic level provides a more sophisticated, knowledge-based approach to help develop technologies that allow controlled spatiotemporal release of bioactive factors (4, 5). One major breakthrough in the last few years has been the discovery that platelets may have important therapeutic roles apart from their physiologic role in hemostasis. Recently, the therapeutic potential of platelets in promoting and accelerating tissue regeneration has gained the interest of the scientific and medical community (6, 7). This interest is in part because platelets, once activated, secrete a large pool of proteins such as fibrinogen, fibronectin and vitronectin, and growth factors including platelet-derived growth factor (PDGF), transforming growth factor-β (TGF-β), vascular endothelial growth factor (VEGF), insulin-like growth factor (IGF-I), hepatocyte growth factor (HGF), angiopoietins, platelet factor-4 (PF-4), and thrombospondin among others to the local milieu, which may drive tissue regeneration mechanisms (8, 9). Assuming the potential of platelets as biological systems for growth factor delivery, much effort has been devoted to properly formulate platelets into "therapeutic preparations" that could be clinically tested and utilized in the treatment of numerous medical disorders.

PRGF: An Optimized Platelet-Rich Plasma

The concept of platelet-rich plasma is relatively new in biomedicine and biotechnology. In the pioneering studies of Marx et al. and Anitua (6, 7), a preparation rich in platelets, or platelet-rich plasma, was reported as a new therapeutic tool to promote bone and soft tissue regeneration. This approach used platelets as growth factor reservoirs with the aim of releasing biological mediators and proteins close to the injured tissues.

Numerous research groups have produced their own platelet-rich plasmas using different protocols and techniques, leading to a large list of experimental data which has provoked discrepancies and controversies, especially regarding the potential benefits of this biotechnological procedure. In the field of bone regeneration, some authors have reported significant improvements in tissue healing and bone formation using platelet-rich plasma (10, 11), while others did not observe any benefit (12, 13). This controversy is the consequence of the lack of suitable qualitative and quantitative standardization of different platelet-rich preparations, and great variation in the processes for producing them. Unfortunately, there is a trend to condense all reported results, and consider all products as one platelet-rich plasma.

Preparation rich in growth factor (PRGF) follows the philosophy of classical platelet-rich products. However, it represents an alternative method by which to formulate and use platelets in a 100% autologous and biocompatible product that circumvents some of the limitations reported for other platelet-rich plasma preparations. PRGF is an autologous plasma product enriched in platelets which, after activation, release multiple growth factors and bioactive proteins locally that modulate the processes of wound healing and tissue engineering (14). This type of preparation is easily and rapidly obtained from the patient's blood. Because the donor and receptor are the same, the immunological concerns are circumvented. PRGF is obtained from a simple spin method and utilizes small and variable blood volumes depending upon the type of surgery. Sodium citrate and calcium chloride are used as anticoagulant and clot activator, respectively. The former protects the platelets from fragmentation, helping to avoid the loss of growth factor content; while the latter enables a safer and more sustained physiological release of the stored growth factors (15). The potential risks associated with the bovine thrombin are avoided with this approach (16). PRGF contains a moderate elevated platelet concentration of approximately 600×10^3 platelets/μL, which has been reported to induce optimal biological benefit (17). PRGF does not contain neutrophils, which express matrix-degrading enzymes, such as matrix metalloproteinases-8 (MMP-8) and MMP-9, and release reactive oxygen species that destroy surrounding injured or healthy cells (18). As a result, a more homogeneous and reproducible preparation is obtained. In addition, the collection and fractionation tubes employed in PRGF elaboration are accepted by the European regulatory agency to be used in the field of tissue engineering, which represents a significant step in reinforcing the biosafety and standardization of this technology.

Developing the Concept of PRGF Technology

PRGF is a technology that enables the formation of different autologous and biocompatible formulations. By controlling the elaboration protocol and coagulation degree of the samples, it is possible to obtain different formulations with therapeutic potential (19) (Figure 3.1). In addition, the combination of these formulations with biomaterials increases the versatility of the approach (4). For example, a liquid supernatant enriched in proteins and growth factors can be easily obtained from the patient's blood after platelet activation and retraction. This PRGF supernatant might be used as conventional eyedrop and cell culture media (20, 21). The activated liquid PRGF is a formulation utilized to bioactivate dental implant surfaces, creating a biologically active nanomembrane on the titanium surface (22). This approach potentially accelerates dental implant osseointegration, improving the initial stability of the implant and helping ensure success.

In order to maintain the growth factors at the site of implantation, retain them from excessive initial burst release, and provide a scaffold that promotes tissue regeneration, the scaffold-like PRGF might be utilized. By controlling the activation process of the platelets, it is possible to obtain a three-dimensional fibrin scaffold, from which a more controlled growth factor delivery is achieved. Control over growth factor pharmacokinetics and biodistribution is obtained by combining the scaffold-like preparation with different natural and synthetic biomaterials including collagen, calcium sulfate, or polycaprolactone composites (23). As these biomaterials have the opposite charge of growth factors, they form ionic complexes with the

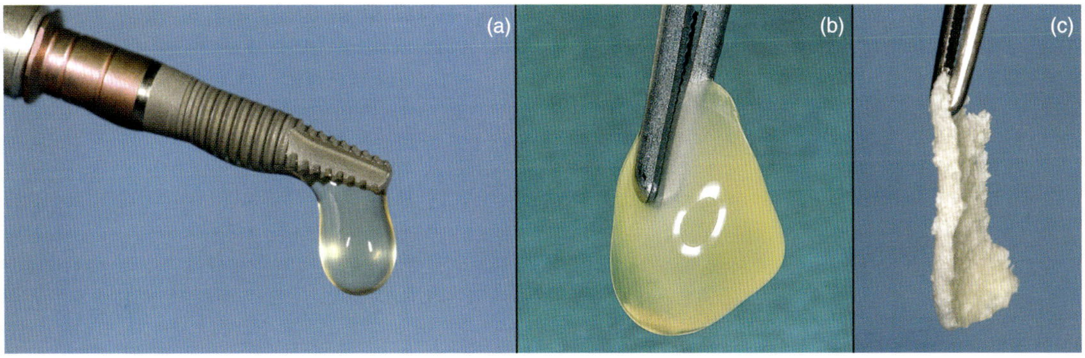

Figure 3.1 The technology of PRGF enables the production of different formulations with therapeutic potential from the same patient's blood depending on the coagulation and activation degree of the samples: (a) a BTI Tiny dental implant humidified with PRGF; (b) scaffold-like PRGF; and (c) a graft consisting of a mixture of anorganic bone and PRGF.

growth factors, controlling growth factor release through the strength of the ionic interactions.

These scaffold-like preparations only act as carriers for growth factors and proteins, and allow cellular infiltration and subsequent integration of the newly formed tissue within the native tissue. Since these fibrin scaffolds are biocompatible, noncytotoxic, and nonimmunogenic to prevent any adverse effects on recruited cells and neighboring tissue, their combination with isolated cells and growth factors has opened the door to several tissue engineering approaches for bone regeneration, and cartilage and periodontal tissue engineering (24). PRGF technology can also be used to produce elastic, dense, and hemostatic fibrin, which is an excellent tool to seal postextraction sockets and to promote epithelialization of soft tissues.

Protocol for PRGF Elaboration

To obtain a reproducible PRGF product, it is necessary to follow specific elaboration protocols, and to use the PRGF kit. The PRGF kit includes citrated tubes, the PRGF activator, and all material necessary for successful PRGF elaboration (Figure 3.2a).

Peripheral blood (10–72 mL, as required) is drawn by venipuncture just before surgery and is placed into BTI blood collecting tubes® that contain 3.8% (wt/vol) sodium citrate as an anticoagulant. Using a single-step centrifugation at 460*g* for 8 min (PRGF System®, Vitoria, Spain), blood is separated at room temperature into its three basic components: plasma containing mostly platelets, the white blood cell layer (known as the buffy coat), and red blood cells (Figure 3.2b). Usually,

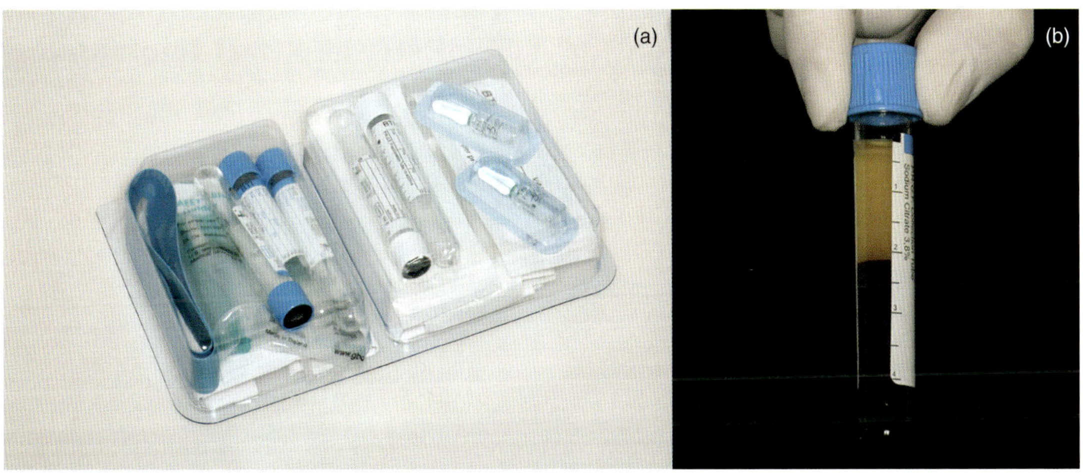

Figure 3.2 (a) The PRGF kit includes all the necessary material for a successful PRGF elaboration. (b) After centrifugation, the separation of the different fractions is clearly observable.

the plasma fraction located at the top of the tubes is used to create an autologous fibrin membrane. The latter is prepared by transferring the plasma to a glass bowl and adding PRGF activator®. It is incubated at 37°C for 20–25 min, allowing formation of a biocompatible fibrin membrane with excellent elastic and homeostatic properties.

The scaffold-like PRGF is prepared by collecting and disposing, in a fractionating tube, the contiguous plasma fraction which is located above the red blood cells. Care should be taken to avoid taking the buffy coat. In order to initiate clotting, PRGF activator® (calcium chloride) is added to the liquid preparation (50 μL PRGF activator® per mL of preparation).

Initial Research Evidence of PRGF Efficacy

The initial basic research involving PRGF was focused on the biological effects induced by growth factors and proteins released from the autologous preparation in different cells and tissues. It was demonstrated that PDGFs can stimulate the proliferation of different type of cells including myocites, chondrocites, fibroblasts, human mesenchymal stem cells, tenocytes, and osteoblasts. The culture potential of PRGF supernatants for the expansion of human tenocytes has been evaluated (14, 25). PRGF significantly stimulated the proliferation of tenocytes and induced the paracrine secretion of both VEGF and HGF. The latter is particularly important as these agents play an active role in angiogenesis and as an antifibrotic molecule. Another important consideration is that cells return to their normal fate of proliferation once the PDGFs are withdrawn, which is an obligatory biosafety requirement, if the cells are to be transplanted into humans. Furthermore, a potent angiogenic effect and a cell proliferation stimulation were observed in vivo (14).

The potential of the scaffold-like PRGF and liquid PRGF to accelerate and promote bone regeneration and faster osseointegration of dental implants has also been shown. Histological analysis at 8 weeks revealed mature bone trabeculae when PRGF was used to fill artificial defects, whereas the control samples showed mainly connective tissue with incipient signs of bone formation. In a second set of experiments, 26 BTI implants (13 humidified with liquid PRGF) were placed in the tibiae of goats. Histological and histomorphometrical results demonstrated that application of liquid PRGF increased the percentage of bone-implant contact in 84.7% of the sites treated. The complete surfaces of the PRGF-treated implants were covered by newly formed bone, whereas only the upper half of the surfaces was surrounded by bone in the control implants. Thus, the use of PRGF scaffold might have implications for the treatment of postextraction defects, especially when complete regeneration of the alveolar bone and surrounding soft tissues are necessary to ensure the future success of the implant. Dental implants should be humidified with liquid PRGF before their insertion, as such treatment accelerates osseointegration. This phenomenon can be explained in part because the growth factors derived from platelets stimulate proliferation of different cells including human trabecular bone cells, human osteoblast-like cells, human stromal stem cells, and human mesenchymal stem cells (20, 26–29). Because of the polarity of the titanium surface, the negatively charged proteins present in the liquid PRGF, such as vitronectin and fibronectin, may be adsorbed on the implant's surface. These proteins may provide specific sites for cell adhesion. Fibronectin is a well-known adhesive protein (30) which will enhance the formation of focal adhesions by osteoblasts (31) and improve the adhesion and spreading of gingival fibroblasts on the implant surface (32).

Therapeutic Applications of PRGF in Dentistry and Oral Implantology

The first report describing the therapeutic potential of PRGF involved 20 patients who underwent tooth extraction because of periodontal disease or vertical root fractures (7). In most of the patients receiving PRGF, soft tissue epithelialization was complete; bone regeneration was extensive; and the bone tissue was compact with well-organized trabeculae. In the control group connective tissue and little mature bone were found in the extraction sockets. In addition to the growth factors released from the scaffold-like PRGF, this technology also enables the production of an elastic, biocompatible, and hemostatic fibrin, which is an excellent biomaterial for the sealing of the defects (Figure 3.3).

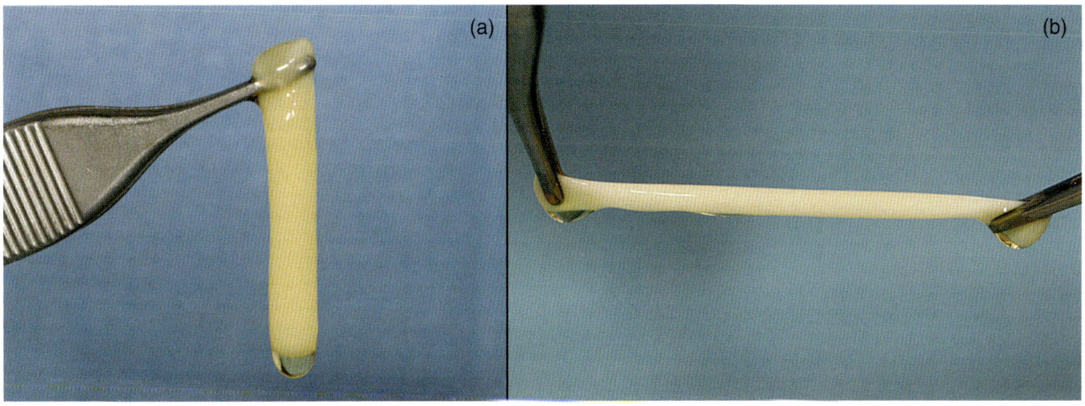

Figure 3.3 The biocompatible fibrin obtained from the patient's blood is hemostatic and very elastic.

The therapeutic opportunities derived from PRGF technology are increasing. PRGF can be used to facilitate the aggregation, manipulation, and administration of different biomaterials used in dentistry, including autologous bone. Liquid PRGF is an excellent culture medium for autologous bone, as it provides an environment rich in growth factors and proteins, which help maintain the viability and functionality of the bone particles (33). Liquid PRGF is also an aid in sinus elevation surgeries, as it provides an increased volume to fill the sinus.

As demonstrated in animal studies, the PRGF scaffold is an excellent tool by which to fill postextraction defects, with the aim of inducing rapid regeneration of the bone and adjacent soft tissues. When bone densitometry was measured using the Hounsfield scale, it was observed that bone densities in the sockets filled with PRGF were significantly higher than that in control sockets, which received no PRGF. Filling the defects with PRGF scaffold increased bone densitometry within the defects over 180%.

Clinical demonstration of efficacy and biosafety of humidifying dental implants with PRGF represents a potential breakthrough in the field of oral implantology (22). Recent reports confirm the predictability, biosafety, and efficacy of bioactivated dental implants. In a report evaluating the survival of more than 5,700 implants in 1,060 patients, the overall survival rate of BTI implants was 99.2% for the implant-based analysis. Twenty-eight out of 5,787 implants (0.48%) were lost during the observation period. Although smoking habits, implant position, implant staging (two-stage implants), and the implementation of special techniques were statistically correlated with lower implant survival rates, only implant staging and the use of special techniques were considered as risk factors associated with implant failure. In a report of the survival of more than 530 short BTI implants humidified with liquid PRGF, an overall survival rate of 99.2% was observed for the implant-based analysis. Two implants were lost during the observation period (34).

The technology of PRGF can be successfully applied to the immediate loading of implants. When evaluating over 1,130 immediately loaded bioactivated implants, a survival rate of 99.3% was observed for the implant-based analysis. Five implants were lost. Apart from the use of PRGF and fibrin, a detailed surgical and prosthetic protocol for immediately loading of implants was reported upon, which included the necessity of bone densitometries $\geq$500 Hounsfields and insertion torque values, measured by a dynamometric ratchet wrench, in the range of 45–70 Nw.

PRGF is also used as an aid in sinus elevation surgeries (35). Once the osseous window is separated, it is placed in a solution of liquid PRGF until it is replaced in its native anatomic location.

In cases of Schneiderian membrane perforation, the biocompatible fibrin may be used as autologous sealant biomaterial. The graft material used to fill the cavity is a mixture of Bio-Oss and liquid PRGF. This combination allows the formation of a clot in which the bovine bone is incorporated, facilitating the manipulation and administration of the latter, and increasing the biosafety of the approach.

This protocol for sinus elevation, which includes the use of PRGF and autologous fibrin, has

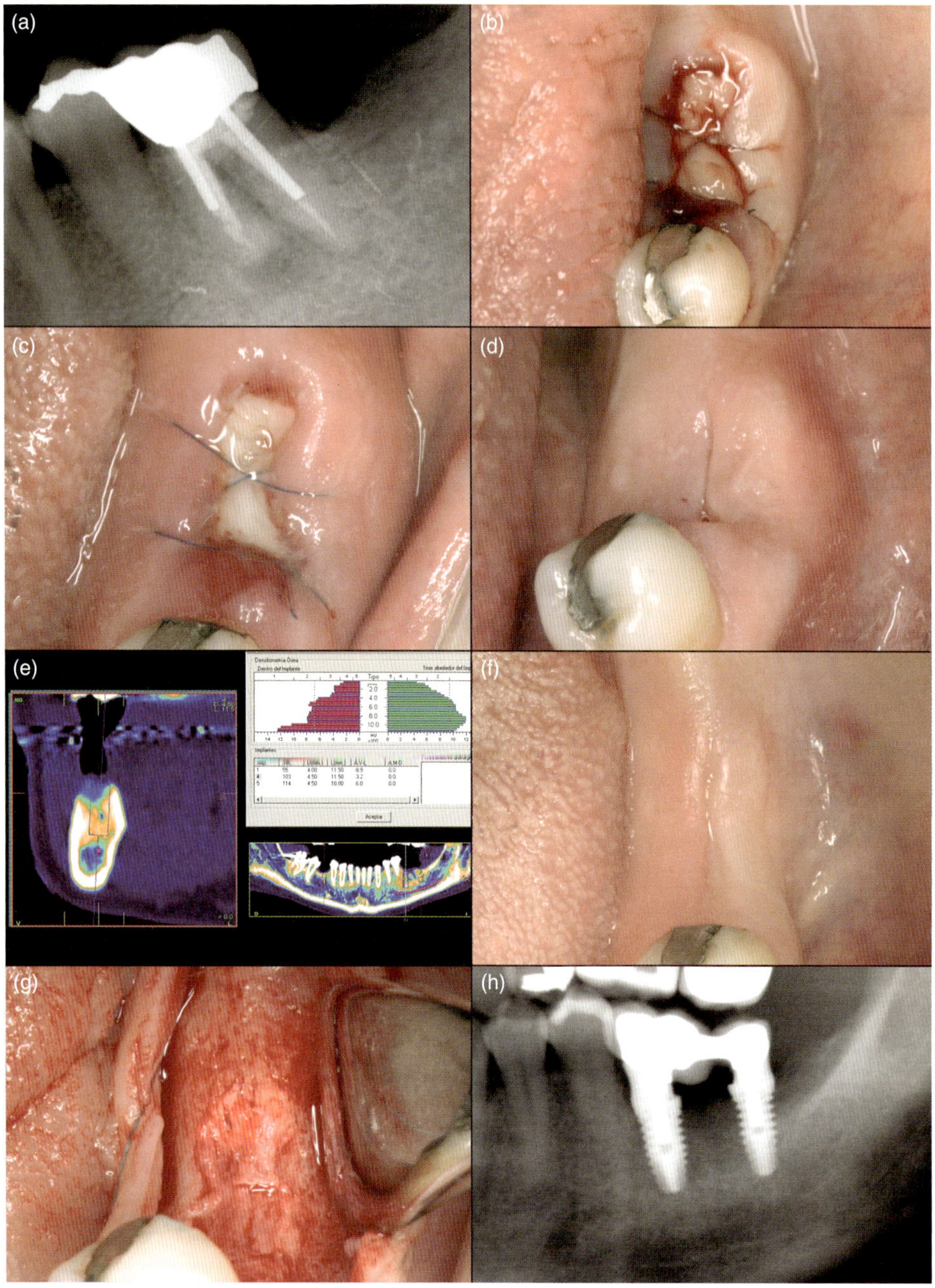

Figure 3.4 (a) A vertical fracture is noted in a 45-year-old woman. (b) Tooth extraction is carried out and the defect is filled with scaffold-like PRGF. (c) A view of the postextraction defect, 24-h posttreatment. (d) Epithelialization has occurred 10 days posttreatment. (e) Eleven weeks posttreatment, a scan is performed to visualize tissue regeneration within the defect. (f) The thickness of the keratinized tissue is evident. (g) Extensive bone regeneration is evident. (h) Dental implants were installed 11 weeks posttreatment. The final prosthesis was inserted 3 months later.

been demonstrated to be effective, safe, and predictable. A recent report documented 18 patients who received 43 dental implants after sinus floor elevation according to the protocol described above. The implants were followed for a meantime of 33 ± 7 months, ranging from 24 to 44 months. The survival rate of the implants was 100% during the observational period. Figures 3.4 and 3.5 demonstrate

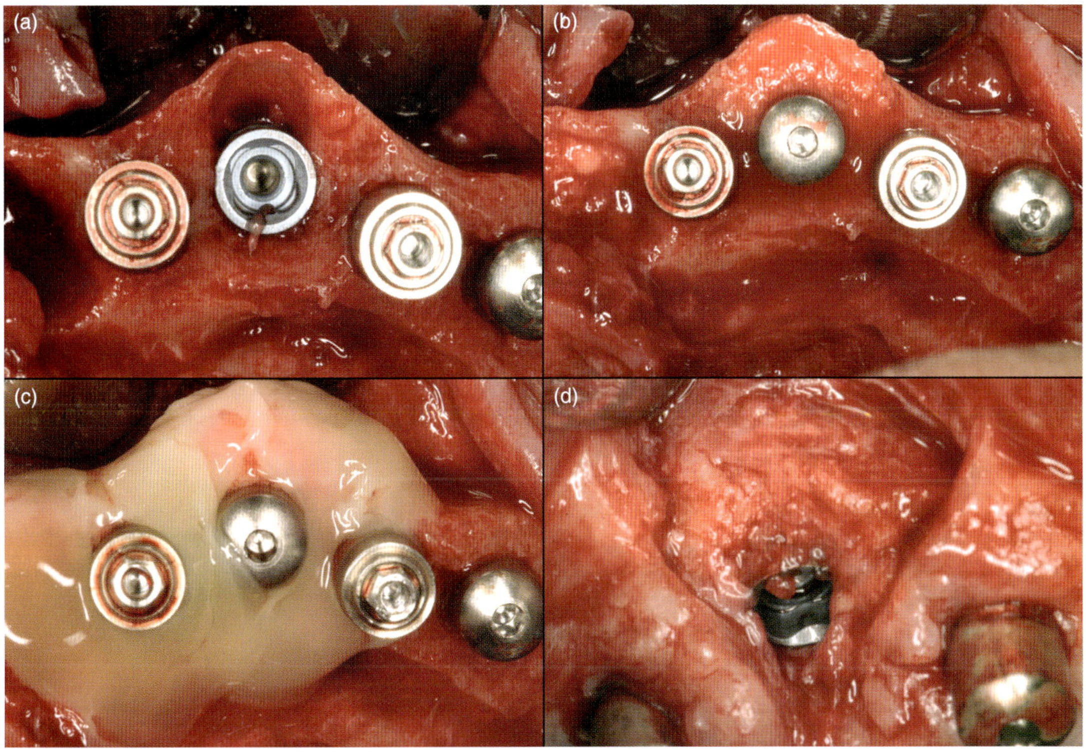

Figure 3.5 (a) Implants are immediately installed after tooth extraction in a 54-year-old man. (b) The gap is filled with autologous bone obtained from the drilling procedure. (c) The area is covered with a fibrin membrane obtained with the PRGF protocol. (d) Three months after the treatment, regeneration is clearly observed in the area.

the therapeutic potential of PRGF technology as an aid in surgery, both for dentistry and oral implantology.

PRGF in Other Medical Fields

The ability to properly formulate platelets and growth factors in novel formulations has stimulated the research and use of this type of preparation in other medical fields including orthopedics, ulcer treatment, eye disorders, and tissue engineering. Of particular note is the use of PRGF in surgery with the aim of accelerating the reconstruction and repair of musculoskeletal tissues. The activated PRGF can be injected among ruptured tendon fibers after the tendon is sutured. Using this surgical approach in six athletes, a significant acceleration in functional recovery was observed compared to a matched group that followed conventional surgery (36, 37). Encouraging results have been reported after using PRGF in arthroscopic surgery of the anterior cruciate ligament and avulsion of the articular cartilage (37, 38). In addition, the therapeutic potential of PRGF in the treatment of chronic ulcers has been documented. In a randomized open-label controlled pilot trial, the effectiveness of a protocol consisting of coagulating the PRGF in vivo within the bed ulcer and covering the area with a fibrin membrane prepared ex vivo in the treatment of chronic vascular ulcers was analyzed and compared with standard therapy (38). Results showed that at 8 weeks, the mean percentage of surface healed in the PRGF group was 73 ± 22%, whereas it was 21 ± 34% in the control group ($P < 0.05$).

Conclusions

PRGF is a new biotechnology for the stimulation and acceleration of soft tissue healing and bone regeneration. The above examples represent some of the interesting approaches of PRGF in dentistry, oral implantology, and other medical fields.

The promising results obtained up until now, and the new approaches under study, point to a future in which this technology may be broadly applied to current and exciting developments and applications.

References

1. Werner S and Grose R. 2003. Regulation of wound healing by growth factors and cytokines. *Physiol Rev* 83:835–870.
2. Street J, Bao M, deGuzman L, et al. 2002. Vascular endothelial growth factor stimulates bone repair by promoting angiogenesis and bone turnover. *Proc Natl Acad Sci USA* 99:9656–9661.
3. Saltzman WM and Olbricht WL. 2002. Building drug delivery into tissue engineering. *Nat Rev Drug Discov* 1:177–186.
4. Anitua E, Sanchez M, Orive G, and Andia I. 2008. Delivering growth factors for therapeutics. *Trends Pharmacol Sci* 29:37–41.
5. Orive G, Gascón AR, Hernández RM, Domínguez-Gil A, and Pedraz JL 2004. Techniques: New approaches in the delivery of pharmaceuticals. *Trends Pharmacol Sci* 25:382–387.
6. Marx RE, Carlson ER, Eichstaedt RM, Schimmele SR, Strauss JE, and Geuseffe KR. 1998. Platelet-rich plasma: Growth factor enhancement for bone grafts. *Oral Surg Oral Med Oral Pathol Oral Radiol Endodon* 85:638–646.
7. Anitua E, Andia I, Ardanza B, Nurden P, and Nurden AT. 1999. Plasma rich in growth factors: Preliminary results of use in the preparation of sites for implants. *Int J Oral Maxillofac Implants* 14:529–535.
8. Anitua E, Andia I, Ardanza B, Nurden P, and Nurden AT. 2004. Autologous platelets as a source of proteins and for healing and tissue regeneration. *Thromb Haemost* 91:4–15.
9. Nurden AT, Nurden P, Sanchez M, Andia I, and Anitua E. 2008. Platelets and wound healing. *Frontiers Biosci.* 13:3532–3548.
10. Thorwarth M, Rupprecht S, Falk S, Felszeghy E, Wiltfong J, and Schlegel KA. 2005. Expression of bone matrix proteins during de novo bone formation using a bovine collagen and platelet rich plasma (prp)—an immunohistochemical analysis. *Biomaterials* 26:2575–2584.
11. Sammartinno G, Tia M, Marenzi G, di Lauro AE, D'Agostino E, and Claudio PP. 2005. Use of autologous platelet rich plasma (PRP) in periodontal defect treatment after extraction of impacted mandibular third molars. *J Oral Maxillofac Surgeons* 14:529–535.
12. Froum SJ, Wallace SS, Tarnow DP, and Cho SC. 2002. Effect of platelet rich plasma on bone growth and osseointegration in human maxillary sinus grafts: Three bilateral case reports. *Int J Periodontics Restorative Dent* 22:45–53.
13. Aghaloo TL, Moy PK, and Freymiller EG. 2002. Investigation of platelet rich plasma in rabbit cranial defects: A pilot study. *J Oral Maxillofac Surg* 60:1176–1181.
14. Anitua E, Sanchez M, Nurden AT, et al. 2006. Autologous fibrin matrices: A potential source of biological mediators that modulate tendon cell activities. *J Biomed Mat Res* 77:285–293.
15. Sánchez AR, Sheridan PJ, and Kupp LI. 2003. Is platelet rich plasma the perfect enhancement factor? *Int J Oral Maxillofac Implants* 18:93–103.
16. Landesberg R, Moses S, and Karpatkin M. 1998. Risk of using platelet-rich plasma gel. *J Oral Maxillofac Surg* 56:1117–1117.
17. Weibrich G, Hansen T, Kleis W, Buch R, and Hitzler WE. 2004. Effect of platelet concentration in platelet-rich plasma on peri-implant bone regeneration. *Bone* 34:665–671.
18. Scott A, Khan KM, Roberts CR, Cook JL, and Duronio V. 2004. What do we mean by the term "inflammation"? A contemporary basic science update for sports medicine. *Br J Sports Med* 38:372–380.
19. Anitua E, Sanchez M, Orive G, and Andia I. 2007. The potential impact of the preparation rich in growth factors (PRGF) in different medical fields. *Biomaterials* 28:4551–4560.
20. Doucet C, Ernou I, Zhang Y, et al. 2005. Platelet lysates promote mesenchymal stem cell expansion: A safety substitute for animal serum in cell based therapy applications. *J Cell Physiol* 9999:1–9.
21. Lucarelli E, Beccheroni A, Donati D, et al. 2003. Platelet-derived growth factors enhance proliferation of human stromal stem cells. *Biomaterials* 24:3095–3100.
22. Anitua E. 2006. Enhancement of osseointegration by generating a dynamic implant surface. *J Oral Implantol* 32:72–76.
23. Rai B, Teoh SH, and Ho KH. 2005. An in vitro evaluation of PCL-TCP composites as delivery systems for platelet rich plasma. *J Control Rel* 107:330–342.
24. Yamada Y, Ueda M, Hibi H, and Baba S. 2006. A novel approach to periodontal tissue regeneration with mesenchymal stem cells and platelet-rich plasma using tissue engineering technology: A clinical case report. *Int J Periodontics Restorative Dent* 26:363–369.
25. Anitua E, Andia I, Sanchez M, et al. 2004. I. Autologous preparations rich in growth factors promote proliferation and induce VEGF and HGF production by human tendon cells in culture. *J Orthop Res* 23:281–286.
26. Gruber R, Varga F, Fischer MB, and Watzek G. 2002. Platelets stimulate proliferation of bone cells: Involvement of platelet-derived growth factor, microparticles and membranes. *Clin Oral Implants Res* 13:529–535.
27. Weibrich G, Gnoth Sh, Otto M, Reichert TE, and Wagner W. 2002. Stimulation of the proliferation rate of human osteoblast like cells by platelet concentrates in vitro. *Mund Kiefer Gesichtschir* 6:168–174.

28. Celotti F, Colciago A, Negri-Cesi P, Pravettoni A, Zaninetti R, and Sacchi K. 2006. Effect of platelet-rich plasma on migration and proliferation of SaOS-2 osteoblasts: Role of platelet-derived growth factor and transforming growth factor-beta. *Wound Rep Reg* 14:195–202.
29. Ye L, Peng L, Tan H, and Zhou X. 2006. HGF enhanced proliferation and differentiation of dental pulp cells. *J Endod* 32:736–741.
30. Dean JW 3rd, Culbertson KC, and D'Angelo AM. 1995. Fibronectin and laminin enhance gingival cell attachment to dental implant surfaces in vitro. *Int J Maxillofac Implants* 10:721–728.
31. Schneider G and Burridge K. 1994. Formation of focal adhesions by osteoblasts adhering to different substrata. *Exp Cell Res* 214:264–269.
32. Scheideler L, Geis-Gerstorfer J, Kern D, et al. 2003. Investigation of cell reactions to microstructured implant surfaces. *Mater Sci Eng C* 23:455–459.
33. Anitua E, Carda C, and Andia I. 2007. A novel drilling procedure and subsequent bone autograft preparation: A technical note. *Int J Oral Maxillofac Implants* 22:138–145.
34. Anitua E, Orive G, Aguirre JJ, and Andia I. 2008. 5 year clinical evaluation of short dental implants placed in posterior areas: A retrospective study. *J. Periodontol* 79:42–48.
35. Torrella F, Pitarch J, Cabanes G, and Anitua E. 1998. Ultrasonic osteotomy for the surgical approach of the maxillary sinus: A technical note. *Int J Oral Maxillofac Implants* 13:697–700.
36. Sanchez M, Anitua E, Azofra J, Andia I, Padilla S, and Mujika I. 2007. Comparison of surgically repaired Achilles tendon tears using PRGF. *Am J Sports Med* 35:245–251.
37. Sánchez M, Azofra J, Anitua E, et al. 2003. Plasma rich in growth factors to treat an articular cartilage avulsion: A case report. *Med Sci Sports Exerc* 35:1648–1652.
38. Anitua, E, Aguirre JJ, Algorta J, et al. 2008. Effectiveness of autologous preparation rich in growth factors for the treatment of chronic cutaneous ulcers. *J Biomed Mater Res B* 84:415–421.

Chapter 4
Patient Evaluation and Planning Considerations

Will Martin, DMD, MS, FACP

Outline

Introduction

The twenty-first century has introduced several advances in dental technology that benefit both the patient and clinician. The incorporation of digital technology, ranging from radiographic techniques (cone-beam computed tomography [CBCT]) to CAD/CAM restoration, fabrication, has streamlined dental rehabilitation and rendered such rehabilitation more predictable and successful. Practitioners are now armed with numerous diagnostic tools to assist in patient evaluation and planning for dental implant therapy. Utilization of these tools, in conjunction with five key diagnostic parameters, will help team members improve treatment efficacy and reduce treatment time for patients.

Historically, implant therapy took many months to years to complete. Bone augmentation procedures were unpredictable and implant surfaces were machined or coated, necessitating extended healing times which often led patients to decline therapy due to the time commitment required. Advances in implant surface design (roughened and chemically active) and simultaneous grafting procedures (where indicated) have significantly reduced these healing periods, making implant procedures more attractive to patients (1–15). Today's dental patient is often educated through internet research and propaganda, making it vital that the clinicians understand patient treatment desires from the beginning. A clear understanding of what the patient wants often may not correlate with what the patient needs. Keys to success are finding the point where "wants" meet "needs," describing the value of therapy in terms of the patient's desires, and providing therapy which satisfies both.

This chapter will highlight the key diagnostic parameters needed to evaluate and plan for implant rehabilitation.

Patient Evaluation

The patient is first evaluated regarding his or her candidacy for dental implant rehabilitation at the consultation visit. During this session, a medical risk assessment and past dental history must be reviewed, highlighting any risks that may be contraindications to implant surgery (Table 4.1). Time should be invested in educating the patient regarding the options for tooth replacement, and the benefits or drawbacks of each approach. Four major treatment options are often available:

- fixed (tooth or implant supported)
- removable (conventional or implant assisted/supported)
- a combination of fixed and removable
- no treatment

It is crucial to inform patients of the potential intraoral side effects of tooth loss, which include (Table 4.2):

- decrease in soft and/or hard tissue volume
- tooth crowding

Table 4.1 General risk factors for implant therapy.

Risk factor	Remarks
Medical	Severe bone disease causing impaired bone healing Immunologic disease Steroid use Uncontrolled diabetes mellitus Irradiated bone Others
Periodontal	Active periodontal disease History of refractory periodontitis Genetic disposition
Smoking habits	Light smoking (<10 cigarettes per day) Heavy smoking (>10 cigarettes per day)
Oral hygiene/ compliance	Home care measured by gingival indices
Occlusion	Personality Intellectual aspects Bruxism

Buser et al. (16).

- supereruption of the opposing dentition
- anatomical issues
- loss of vertical dimension
- malocclusion

These problems can usually be prevented when implants are placed simultaneously with tooth removal. However, when patients present with edentulous spans, the above-listed deficiencies should be addressed in conjunction with the tooth replacement. This discussion will help prepare the patient for the procedures necessary, in addition to the implant surgery, to render the implant rehabilitation successful. Table 4.2 lists several scenarios and the treatment options necessary to address them appropriately.

Visualization of tissue deficiencies by the patient can be enhanced with patient mirrors, intraoral cameras, dental photography, and dental radiography. CBCT is a recent addition to the dentist's armamentarium which offers the ability to view hard and soft tissue defects, and anatomical limitations, in a quick and accurate digital rendition (Figure 4.1). These views capture a volume of data that is processed and converted into slices, ranging from 0.4- to 1-mm thick, which can be viewed in several formats. Sectional views allow visualization of the hard tissue volume and its relation to anatomical structures such as nerves, sinuses, roots, etc. (Figure 4.2). Several hardware options (CBCT machines) and software programs are available which allow utilization of this technology in the dental office.

Patients who seek restoration of lost or failing teeth in the anterior maxilla, often referred to as the "esthetic zone," introduce an added level of difficulty to planning and treatment with dental implants. Utilization of an esthetic risk assessment (ERA) analysis allows the clinician to chart relevant clinical parameters and inform the patient of the potential for esthetic success or compromise in the final treatment result (Table 4.3). Successful integration of the ERA analysis is dependent upon the clinician understanding the parameters for an esthetic implant restoration (16).

Table 4.2 Side effects from tooth loss, and treatment options.

Defect	Treatment options
Soft tissue	Guided tissue regeneration (GTR), orthodontic extrusion
Hard tissue	Guided bone regeneration (GBR), ridge splitting technique, osteotome expansion, combinations
Crowding	Orthodontics, restorative therapy
Supereruption	Orthodontic, restorative, periodontic, and/or endodontic therapies
Anatomical	GBR, orthodontics, maxillofacial surgical therapy
Loss of vertical dimension	Restorative, periodontic, endodontic, orthodontic, and/or maxillofacial surgery therapies
Malocclusion	Orthodontic, restorative, and/or maxillofacial surgical therapies

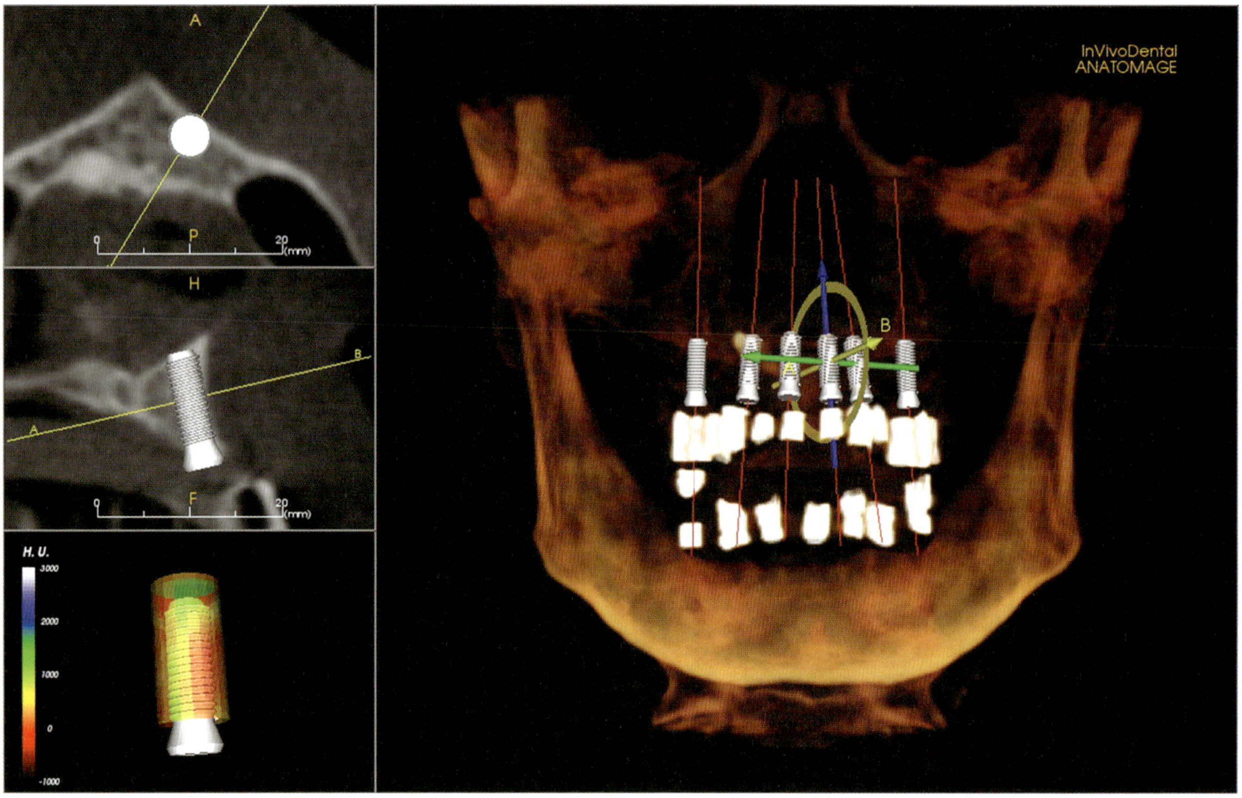

Figure 4.1 Three-dimensional rendering of DICOM data allows for sectional views of the hard and soft tissues.

STANDARDS FOR AN ESTHETIC FIXED IMPLANT RESTORATION

An esthetic implant prosthesis is defined as one that is in harmony with the perioral facial structures of the patient. The esthetic peri-implant tissues, including health, height, volume, color, and contours, must be in harmony with a healthy surrounding dentition. The restoration should imitate the natural appearance of the missing dental unit(s) in color, form, texture, size, and optical properties.

The ERA analysis establishes low-, medium-, and high-risk levels, which are based upon achieving a result as previously outlined. For example, a patient who has several high-risk levels in the ERA analysis may still elect to proceed with care, understanding that an esthetic compromise may follow. The ERA does not refer to overall implant survival.

At the conclusion of the consultation visit, the patient should have been provided with enough information to determine if he or she is a candidate for dental implant therapy. Prior to committing to treatment, a comprehensive examination must be performed. This examination includes:

- extra- and intraoral examination
- hard and soft tissue charting
- periodontal charting
- occlusal analysis
- diagnostic impressions
- radiographs
- photography

This information is utilized by the treatment team to generate viable therapeutic options, which will be presented to the patient. The appropriate treatment plan is then selected and initiated.

Treatment Planning

Patients seek out the dentist to replace what was lost, whether it be a tooth or teeth. With this fact in mind, dental implants should be thought of as root replacements for missing dental units. Successful implant therapy is grounded in a restoration-driven approach to the planning and placement of the dental implants (17, 18). Planning for implant rehabilitation becomes a "crown-down" approach to site

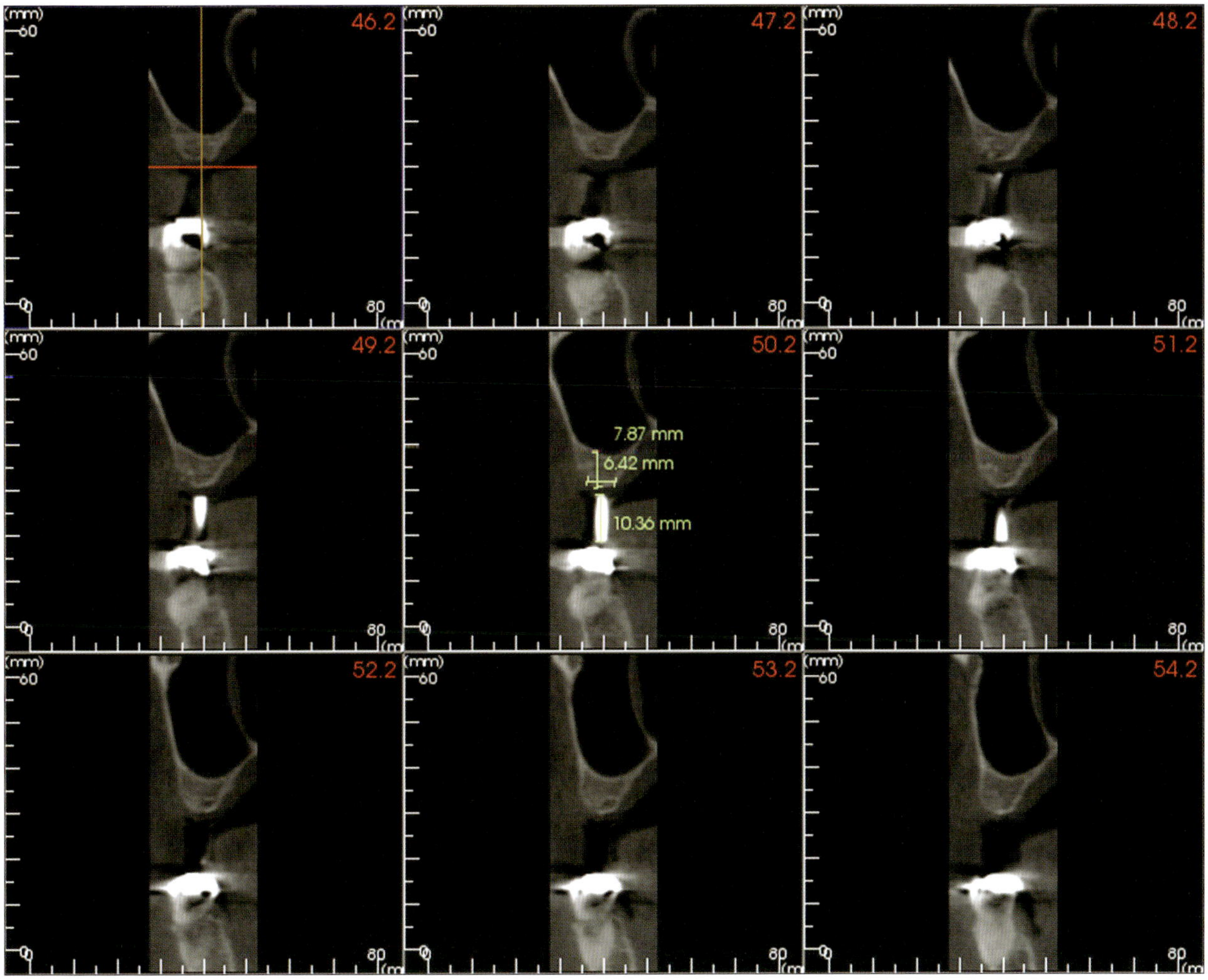

Figure 4.2 Sectional views afford visualization of alveolar dimensions to help in planning appropriate implant angulation (In Vivo Dental, Anatomage).

enhancement and implant positioning. The treatment team must adopt this concept in order to ensure predictable, efficient, and streamlined delivery of care. When planning for implants, five key parameters dictate this restoration-driven process:

- restorability
- soft tissue evaluation
- hard tissue evaluation
- anatomical considerations
- revisit restorability

Upon completion of data collection, the patient's charting, casts, photos, and radiographs are utilized by the team to determine the most advantageous options for the patient.

RESTORABILITY

Prior to performing a diagnostic wax-up, planned restoration(s) should be visualized, to analyze the therapeutic steps necessary to ensure successful implant rehabilitation. The edentulous space is examined in three dimensions. Components examined include:

- the inter-arch space
- the intradental space
- the occlusal plane
- the position of the gingival margins of the surrounding teeth

The next step is to determine if the dimensions of the planned restoration(s) are appropriate in size to the contralateral teeth (when applicable). When

Table 4.3 Esthetic risk assessment for edentulous sites.

Esthetic risk factors	Low	Medium	High
Medical status	Healthy patient and intact immune system		Reduced immune system
Smoking habit	Nonsmoker	Light smoker ($<$10 cigarettes per day)	Heavy smoker ($>$10 cigarettes per day)
Patient's esthetic demands	Low	Medium	High
Lip line	Low	Medium	High
Gingival biotype	Low scalloped, thick	Medium scalloped, medium thick	High scalloped, thin
Shape of tooth crowns	Regular		Triangular
Bone level at adjacent teeth	$<$5 mm to contact point	$=$ 5 mm to contact point	$>$5 mm to contact point
Periodontal health status	Healthy	Moderately compromised	Severely compromised
Restorative status of neighboring teeth	Virgin		Restored
Width of edentulous span	1 tooth ($\geq$7 mm) 1 tooth ($\geq$5.5 mm)	1 tooth ($<$ 7 mm) 1 tooth ($<$5.5 mm)	2 teeth or more
Soft tissue anatomy	Intact soft tissue		Soft tissue defects
Bone anatomy of alveolar crest	Alveolar crest without bone deficiency	Horizontal bone deficiency	Vertical bone deficiency

Martin et al. (18).

deficits or excesses exist in any of the previous dimensions, measures must be taken and therapeutic strategies devised, prior to proceeding with treatment. For example, a lack of adequate intra-arch space may require orthodontics to create sufficient space for the planned restoration(s); or reduction of the adjacent teeth may be incorporated into the treatment plan (Figures 4.3a–d). A diagnostic wax-up is often performed to confirm implant restorability. Prior to initiating this procedure, it is necessary to build up or reduce the edentulous space to create an ideal ridge form (Figure 4.4). This exercise ensures placement of the teeth in ideal positions related to the arch, thus creating ideal emergence profiles. Once the planned restoration is developed, a soft-tissue evaluation may be performed. Fabricating a vacuform template over a duplication of the diagnostic wax-up will allow visualization of the planned restoration on the diagnostic cast, or directly in the patient's mouth (Figure 4.5). The vacuform template serves as a means to ensure a restoration-driven process for the planning for augmentation procedures and dental implant positioning (Figure 4.6).

SOFT TISSUE EVALUATION

Evaluation of the soft tissues is based upon the clinical situation at the proposed implant site. Two scenarios max exist:

- the tooth is present
- the site is edentulous

When the tooth is present and adequate in restorative dimensions, it will function as the planned implant restoration. The soft tissue evaluation is then based upon the existing clinical crown related to the planned implant restoration's mucosal margin. Assessment of soft tissue defects around these teeth can be aided through reference to Miller's classification of gingival recessions (Table 4.4). Sites exhibiting Miller Class I defects can often be

(a) (b)

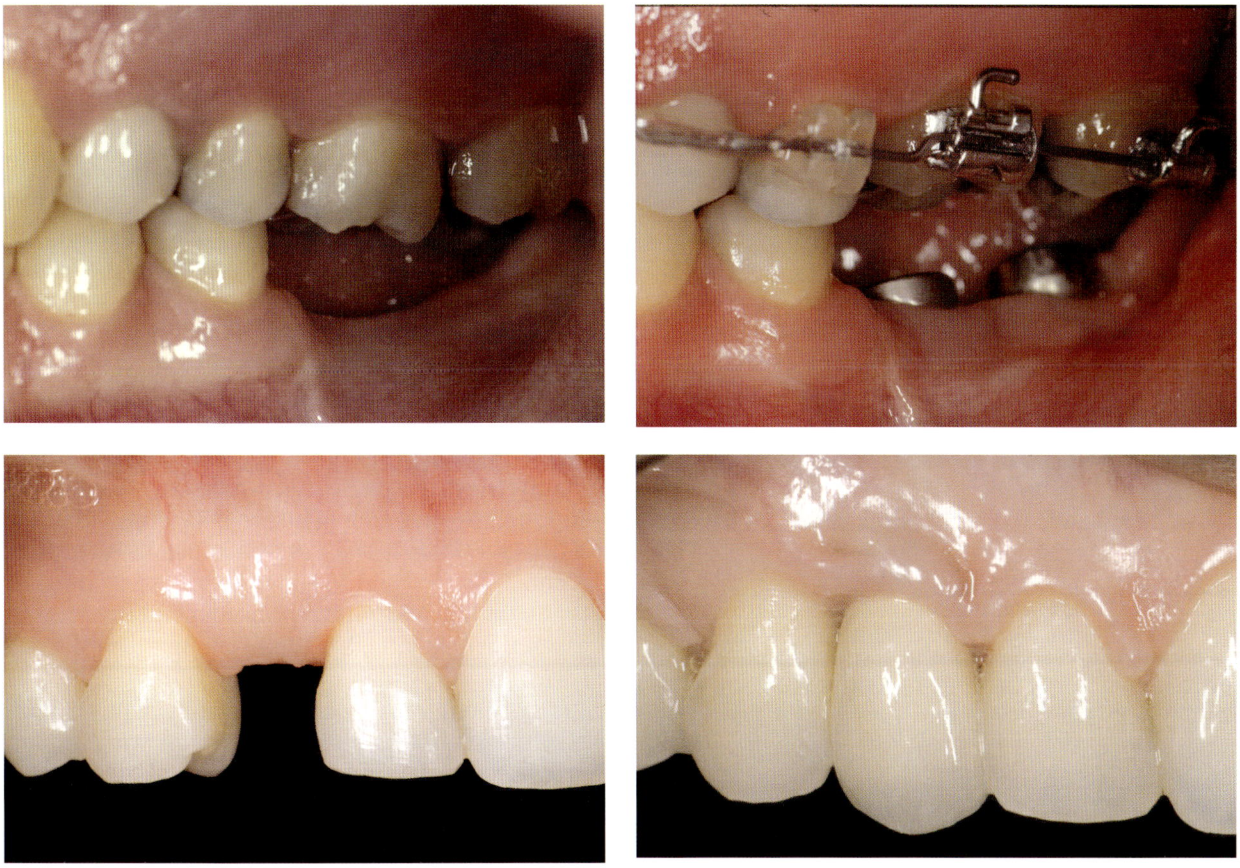

(c) (d)

Figure 4.3 (a) A lack of adequate interocclusal space in edentulous site numbers 18 and 19 is evident. (b) Orthodontic therapy is utilized to create ideal interocclusal space for restoration of implants in the positions of numbers 18 and 19. (c) There is limited interdental space for the proposed implant in site number 6. (d) Enameloplasty was performed on teeth numbers 5 and 7 to create adequate space for restoration of the implant in the position of tooth number 6.

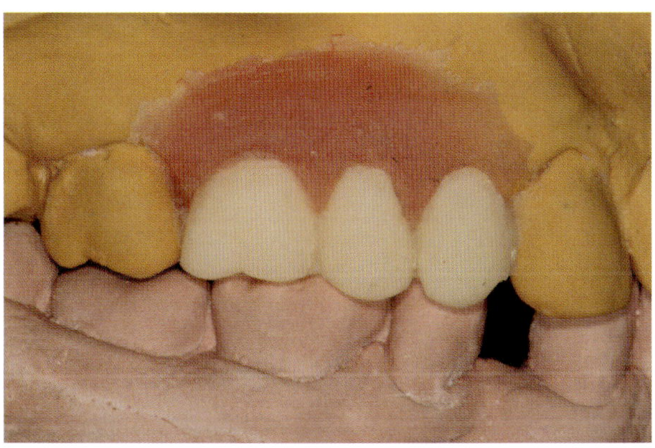

Figure 4.4 A diagnostic wax-up, highlighting alveolar deficiencies in addition to replacement of missing teeth, has been carried out.

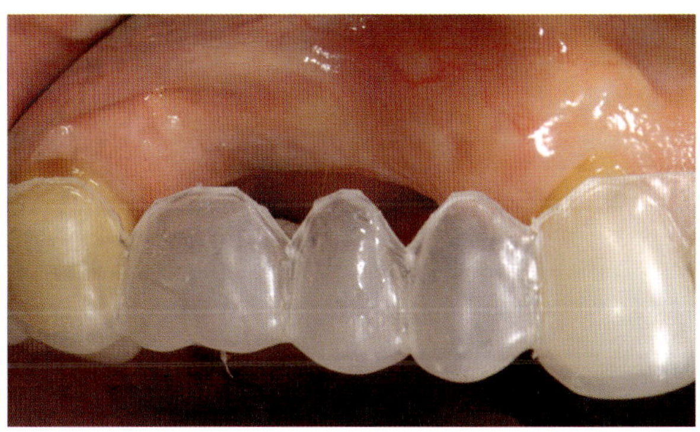

Figure 4.5 A vacuform template has been created from the diagnostic wax-up.

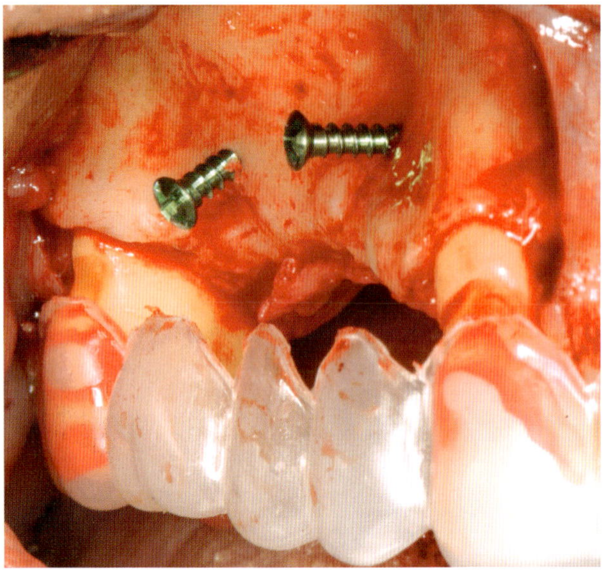

Figure 4.6 The vacuform template is utilized to assist in the hard tissue augmentation procedure.

addressed either at the time of tooth extraction or at implant placement through the use of connective tissue grafts. Miller Class II defects, where recession extends past the mucogingival junction (MGJ) but does not involve interproximal tissues, often require soft and hard tissue grafting prior to implant placement. Defects treated in this manner will yield favorable esthetic outcomes (Figures 4.7a, b). Miller Class III and IV defects require soft and hard tissue grafting procedures prior to implant placement. The esthetic result in such a situation is often compromised. Restorative measures to address potential "black triangles" are usually necessary. Long clinical crowns, broad contact points, and restoration of adjacent teeth may be required. When teeth adjacent to the proposed implant site exhibit interproximal bone loss, surgical efforts to reattain tissue attachment to the teeth are unpredictable at best.

When the proposed implant site is edentulous, the vacuform template of the diagnostic wax-up serves as a means by which to evaluate soft tissue support for the planned implant restoration. The width and height of the soft tissue volume in the edentulous space are assessed intraorally or on the diagnostic casts, using the template. Periodontal disease should be addressed prior to initiation of implant therapy, as active periodontal disease can increase the potential for complications associated with long-term survival of the dental implant(s) and result in loss of peri-implant tissue support. In sites free of active periodontal disease, a deficit of soft tissue volume is usually related to a deficiency in hard tissue volume. An example of this situation is the site of a congenitally missing tooth (Figures 4.8a, b). When adequate hard tissue is available for ideal implant positioning, soft tissue augmentation procedures can be planned (connective tissue grafts) in conjunction with implant placement. Such soft tissue grafting is important for esthetic success, as this added tissue volume creates a root form which will aid in establishing the appropriate emergence profile of the implant restoration.

HARD TISSUE EVALUATION

Upon completion of the restorability and soft tissue assessment, appropriate evaluation of the volume of hard tissue at the proposed implant site must

Table 4.4 Miller's classification of gingival recessions.

Recession defect	Expected treatment outcome
Class 1: Recession does not extend to MGJ, no loss in interdental area, tooth is well aligned in the arch	100% root coverage
Class 2: Recession extends to or beyond the MGJ, with no loss in interdental areas, tooth is well aligned in the arch	100% root coverage
Class 3: Recession extends to or beyond the MGJ, tissue loss in the interdental area, or malpositioning of the teeth	Partial root coverage
Class 4: Recession extends to or beyond the MGJ, loss in the interdental area and/or malpositioning of teeth is severe	Root coverage should not be attempted

(a) (b)

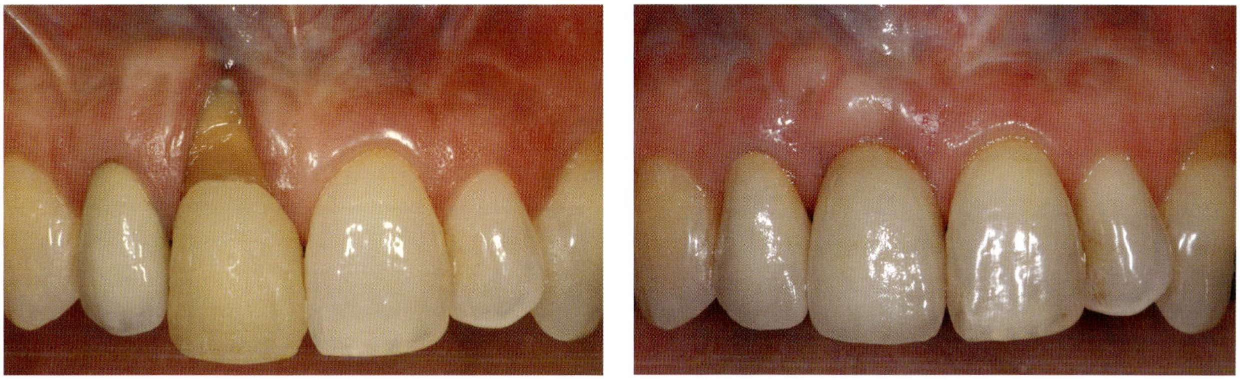

Figure 4.7 (a) A Class II Miller defect is present on the buccal aspect of tooth number 8. (b) A view postextraction, grafting and implant placement, and restoration in site number 8.

be carried out. Utilizing the vacuform template, hard tissue width and height are evaluated. When a deficit in hard tissue width exists and adequate attached soft tissue is present, onlay grafting may be considered. The degree of ridge atrophy will determine whether the site is augmented in conjunction with or prior to implant placement (16, 19). One determining factor for the appropriateness of simultaneous implant placement and grafting is whether primary stability of the implant, in a perfect position, can be achieved at the time of surgery. An advantage to this approach is a reduction in overall healing and treatment time (Figures 4.9a, b). Rough surface dental implants placed with simultaneous hard tissue augmentation are afforded three months of healing prior to commencing with implant restoration. When onlay grafts are necessary prior to implant placement, numerous grafting material options are available, including autograft, allograft, and xenografts (20, 21; Table 4.5). Autografts require up to four months of healing prior to implant placement, while allografts and xenografts require up to six months of healing. Horizontal augmentation of an atrophic site is a routine procedure. Interim restoration options are important when addressing extended healing times, as patients desire teeth during this phase of treatment. A key factor in selection of an interim restoration is that it does not place pressure on the graft site, as such pressure will lead to resorption of the graft material. Several removable and fixed temporization options exist.

When evaluating hard tissue support in a vertical dimension, the mucosal margin of the planned

(a) (b)

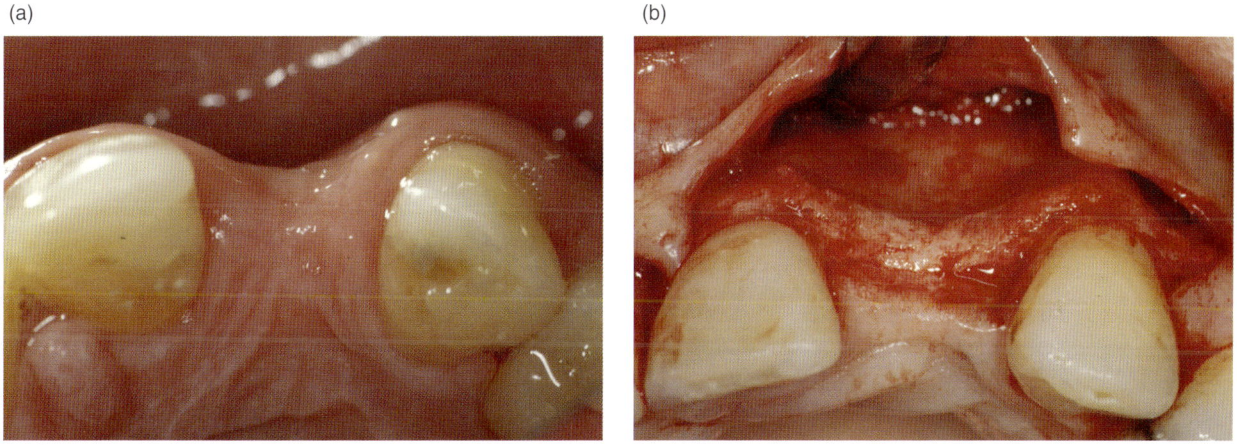

Figure 4.8 (a) An occlusal view of a congenitally missing tooth number 7. (b) A deficient ridge width is noted in site number 7.

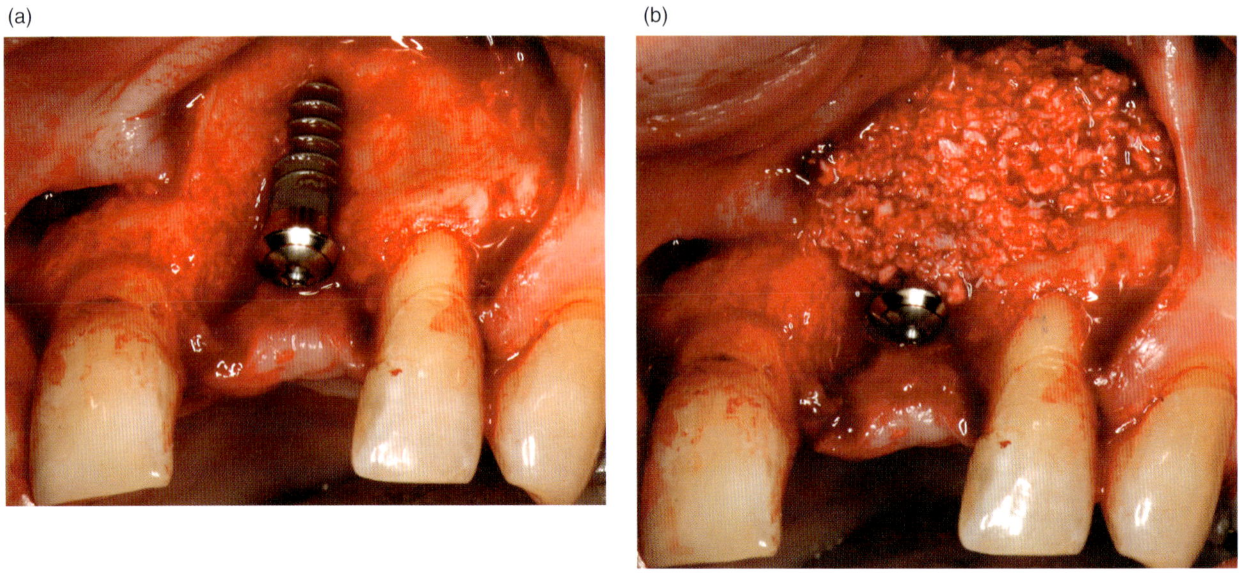

Figure 4.9 (a) Primary stability of an implant in position number 9, with a full facial dehiscence, has been attained. (b) Hard tissue augmentation is performed over the exposed implant surface with a xenograft, prior to placement of a covering resorbable membrane.

restoration, as determined by the vacuform template, is used as a reference point. When an excess of hard tissue exists, as is often seen in sites of congenitally missing teeth, it is imperative that the alveolar crest is contoured at the time of surgery to allow for proper vertical positioning of the implant (Figures 4.10a, b). Dental implants placed too shallow may result in several restorative complications, including an exposed implant collar, a compromised emergence profile, the need for ridge-lap restorations and limited restorative space. When deficiency of ridge height is present, several clinical situations may influence the treatment to be provided. Consideration should be given to the predictability of vertical augmentation, as this is a procedure that carries a higher failure rate than seen with horizontal augmentation. In the anterior maxilla, vertical deficits adjacent to teeth with adequate periodontal support are more amenable to vertical augmentation than sites bounded by teeth exhibiting attachment loss. The level of augmentation attained will usually be no more coronal than the height of the bone crests on the teeth bounding the edentulous span. In such situations, consideration must be given to addressing the potential esthetic compromise through restoration of the adjacent teeth, allowing the clinician to control the contact points and embrasure forms (Figures 4.11a–d).

ANATOMICAL CONSIDERATIONS

Addressing anatomical limitations to implant placement is the most critical step in the overall evaluation process. Such limitations can be categorized as dental, alveolar, nerve, vessel, and sinus. Dental

Table 4.5 Hard tissue grafting options.

Graft type	Description
Autograft	Tissue from same individual (i.e., ramus, chin, hip)
Allograft	Tissue from a different individual (i.e., demineralized freeze-dried bone (DFDBA) from bone bank)
Xenograft	Tissue from one species to another (i.e., pig or cow)
Synthetic	Graft made from natural occurring minerals (i.e., hydroxylapatite or surface reactive glass-ceramics)

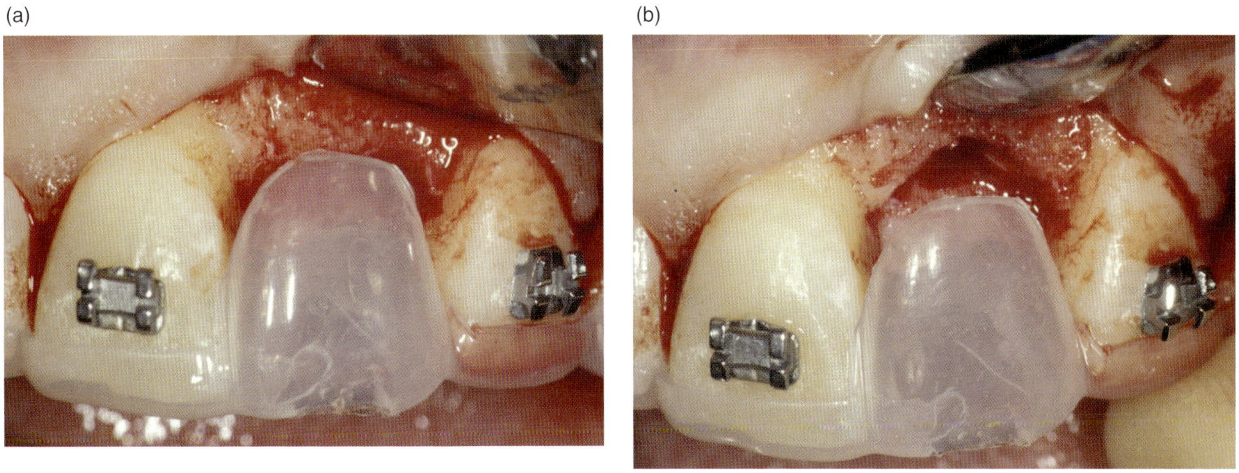

Figure 4.10 (a) A vacuform template in place highlights a vertical excess of alveolar crest height in relation to the planned implant restoration. (b) The alveolar crest has been contoured prior to placement of a dental implant.

limitations become evident during the restorability evaluation. Upon completing a diagnostic wax-up, inter-arch and intra-arch dimensions are assessed. Root positions of the teeth adjacent to the implant site are assessed during a radiographic evaluation. Orthodontic therapy may be the treatment of choice to address such limitations. However, the introduction of reduced diameter implants (i.e., −2.8 to 3.5 mm) has facilitated implant placement in areas of limited inter-root space without the need for root expansion. When planning for implants in limited areas of inter-root space, the implant should not be placed within 1.4 mm of the adjacent root surface. Alveolar considerations are addressed during the soft and hard tissue assessment. There are anatomical limitations that are present in all patients that must be addressed. In the posterior mandible, the lingual concavity should be visualized during planning, or manually during surgery. This concavity will become more important as mandibular resorption progresses. Another area of consideration is the anterior mandible. Perforation of the lingual cortical plate could lead to trauma to the lingual artery, a serious complication. Nerves and vessels are most often found in close proximity to each other, and are thus evaluated together. The inferior alveolar nerve should be evaluated through the use of a calibrated radiograph or a cross-sectional study. The introduction of guided implantology allows practitioners to place implants within 1 mm of the inferior alveolar canal. Other areas of significance are the nasopalatine nerve and anterior branch of the inferior alveolar nerve, which is anterior to the mental foramen. These anatomical areas should be isolated and avoided during implant surgery. Pneumatized maxillary sinuses are addressed with a variety of surgical procedures, as will be discussed in Chapter 6.

REVISIT RESTORABILITY

Upon completion of the evaluation process, a tentative plan for implant therapy should be evident. When adjunctive therapies such as orthodontics or soft or hard tissue grafting have been carried out, the restorability of the site must be revisited prior to proceeding with implant placement. For example, when vertical augmentation procedures are planned in the posterior mandible to address ridge atrophy and inferior alveolar nerve position, the inter-arch space would decrease postgrafting. A restorable situation pregraft could become unrestorable postgraft. It may thus become necessary to address the opposing arch in order to make the patient an implant candidate.

Another example is when orthodontic therapy is planned to align the roots of the teeth adjacent to an implant site. Incremental follow-up care by the restorative dentist is important to maintain the interdental space. In situations where orthodontics is to be utilized to create the necessary restorative space or to align roots, placement of a denture tooth on the arch wire assists in visualizing ideal tooth size, in addition to providing the patient with an esthetic interim prosthesis (Figure 4.12).

(a)

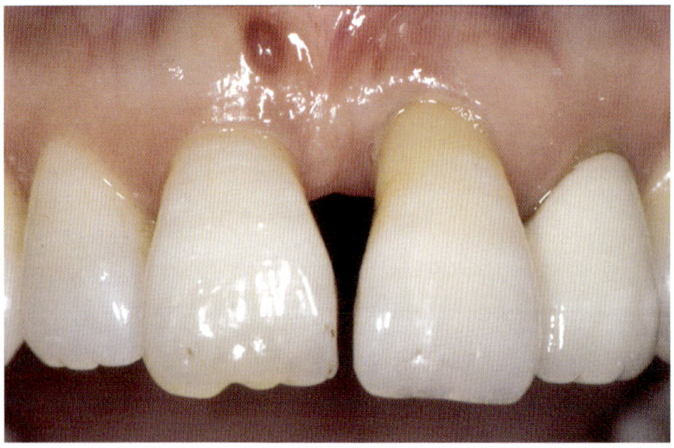

(b)

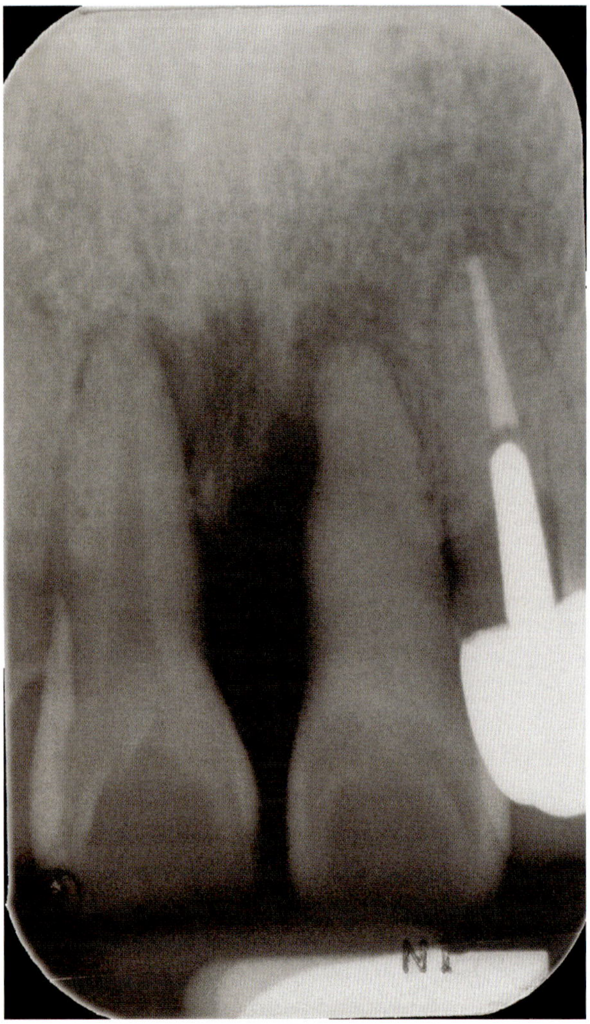

4.11

(c)

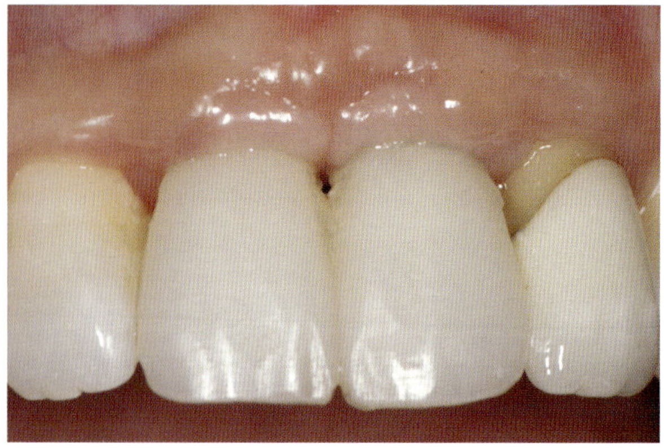

(d)

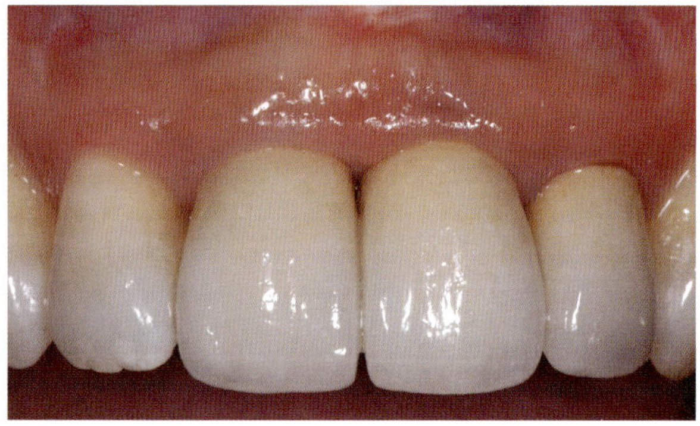

Figure 4.11 (a) A pretreatment view of failing teeth numbers 8 and 9. (b) A radiograph highlights the degree of bone loss on teeth numbers 8 and 9. (c) Provisional implant restorations have been placed on numbers 8 and 9, highlighting the posttreatment attachment loss on number 10. (d) Restoration of the implants in the positions of numbers 8 and 9, and natural tooth number 10, have been carried out.

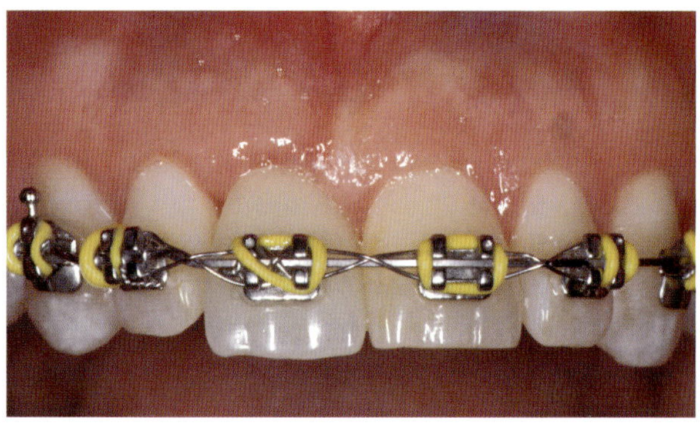

Figure 4.12 A denture tooth (number 8) has been attached to the orthodontic archwire to assist in creating an ideal restorative space for the planned implant.

Conclusions

It remains imperative to evaluate and plan treatment in an appropriate and concise manner, to ensure predictable and consistent therapeutic results. The five parameters discussed afford a systematic approach for site evaluation. Utilizing a restoration-driven approach to evaluation and planning is indispensable to providing the best care for the patient. Utilizing a restorative-driven approach for implant placement will create efficient restorative procedures and consistent esthetic and functional results. The patient visits the dentist to replace a missing tooth, not to receive a dental implant. The dental implant serves as the foundation for restorative success.

References

1. Cochran DL. 1999. A comparison of endosseous dental implant surfaces. *J Periodontol* 70:1523–1539.
2. Cochran DL, Buser D, ten Bruggenkate CM, et al. 2002. The use of reduced healing times on ITI implants with a sandblasted and acid-etched (SLA) surface: Early results from clinical trials on ITI SLA implants. *Clin Oral Implants Res* 13:144–153.
3. Oates TW, Valderrama P, Bischof M, et al. 2007. Enhanced implant stability with a chemically modified SLA surface: A randomized pilot study. *Int J Oral Maxillofac Implants*. 22:755–760.
4. Li D, Ferguson SJ, Beutler T, et al. 2002. Biomechanical comparison of the sandblasted and acid-etched and the machined and acid-etched titanium surface for dental implants. *J Biomed Mater Res* 60:325–332.
5. Buser D, Broggini N, Wieland M, et al. 2004. Enhanced bone apposition to a chemically modified SLA titanium surface. *J Dent Res* 83:529–533.
6. Attard NJ and Zarb GA. 2005. Immediate and early implant loading protocols: A literature review of clinical studies. *J Prosthet Dent* 94:242–258.
7. Barone A, Rispoli L, Vozza I, Quaranta A, and Covani U. 2006. Immediate restoration of single implants placed immediately after tooth extraction. *J Periodontol* 77:1914–1920.
8. Wismeijer D, Buser D, Belser UC. (eds) 2007. *ITI Treatment Guide. Vol. II: Loading Protocols in Implant Dentistry: Partially Dentate Patients*. Chicago: Quintessence.
9. Cochran DL, Morton D, and Weber HP. 2004. Consensus statements and recommended clinical procedures regarding loading protocols for endosseous dental implants. *Int J Oral Maxillofac Implants* 19(Suppl):109–113.
10. Cooper L, Felton DA, Kugelberg CF, et al. 2001. A multicenter 12-month evaluation of single-tooth implants restored 3 weeks after 1-stage surgery. *Int J Oral Maxillofac Implants* 16:182–192.
11. Degidi M and Piattelli A. 2003. Immediate functional and non-functional loading of dental implants: A 2- to 60-month follow-up study of 646 titanium implants. *J Periodontol* 74:225–241.
12. Ganeles J and Wismeijer D. 2004. Early and immediately restored and loaded dental implants for single-tooth and partial-arch applications. *Int J Oral Maxillofac Implants* 19(Suppl):92–102.
13. Kan JY, Rungcharassaeng K, and Lozada J. 2003. Immediate placement and provisionalization of maxillary anterior single implants: 1-year prospective study. *Int J Oral Maxillofac Implants* 18:31–39.
14. Morton D, Jaffin R, and Weber HP. 2004. Immediate restoration and loading of dental implants: Clinical considerations and protocols. *Int J Oral Maxillofac Implants* 19(Suppl):103–108.
15. Roccuzzo M, Bunino M, Prioglio F, and Bianchi SD. 2001. Early loading of sandblasted and acid-etched (SLA) implants: A prospective split-mouth comparative study. *Clin Oral Implants Res* 12:572–578.
16. Buser D, Martin W, and Belser UC. 2004. Optimizing esthetics for implant restorations in the anterior maxilla: Anatomical and surgical considerations. *Int J Oral Maxillofac Implants* 19(Suppl):43–61.
17. Buser D, Belser UC, and Wismeijer D. (eds) 2006. *ITI Treatment Guide. Vol. I: Implant Therapy in the Esthetic Zone for Single-Tooth Replacements*. Chicago: Quintessence.
18. Martin W, Morton D, and Buser D. 2006. *Diagnostic Factors for Esthetic Risk Assessment. ITI Treatment Guide*, Vol. 1. Chicago: Quintessence, pp. 11–24.
19. Grunder U, Gracis S, and Capelli M. 2005. Influence of the 3-D bone-to-implant relationship on esthetics. *Int J Periodontics Restorative Dent* 25:113–119.
20. Conner KA, Sabatini R, Mealey BL, Takacs VJ, Mills MP, and Cochran DL. 2003. Guided bone regeneration around titanium plasma-sprayed, acid-etched, and hydroxyapatite-coated implants in the canine model. *J Periodontol* 74:658–668.
21. von Arx T, Cochran DL, Hermann JS, Schenk RK, Higginbottom FL, and Buser D. 2001. Lateral ridge augmentation and implant placement: An experimental study evaluating implant osseointegration in different augmentation materials in the canine mandible. *Int J Oral Maxillofac Implants* 16:343–354.

Chapter 5

Planning and Surgical Options for Implant-Based Esthetic Treatment: The Partially Dentate Patient

Jamil Alayan, BS, BDS, MDSc, FRACDS and Dean Morton, BDS, MS, FACP

Outline

Introduction

Predictable implant-based treatment in the esthetic zone is reliant upon accurate and comprehensive patient assessment by the treatment team. The development of an esthetic and functional treatment plan, which is accepted and clearly understood by the patient, is critical to the outcome. This is of particular significance when treatment is planned in the esthetic zone, which has been objectively defined as any dentoalveolar segment visible upon a full smile. Subjectively, the esthetic zone has been considered any dentoalveolar area of esthetic importance to the patient (1).

Optimal treatment outcomes for many patients rely on the surgical augmentation of existing hard and soft tissue deficiencies (Figures 5.1 and 5.2). Restoratively, clinicians must also be cognizant of the limitations introduced by spatial and occlusal disharmonies, and their influence upon esthetic and functional outcomes (Figures 5.3a–c). Understanding the interdependence between prosthodontics, periodontics, maxillofacial surgery and orthodontics is, therefore, central to treatment success. A simple and repeatable method for the identification of esthetic and functional considerations should be routine as part of the treatment planning process. Obtaining an optimal esthetic outcome requires not only the replacement of missing teeth, but also the replacement of missing hard and soft tissues and the management of the dentition from a three-dimensional perspective (2).

Failure to adhere to these principles in the esthetic zone increases the risk of outcome complications. A comprehensive pretreatment esthetic risk analysis (3) is central to recognizing patients with a higher probability for a negative outcome. Adherence to proven treatment modalities, in conjunction with risk analysis, will improve the prospects of treatment success.

Pretreatment Considerations: Esthetic Risk Analysis

Significant factors in pretreatment assessment of patients requiring implant-based treatment in the esthetic zone have been previously described (3). Pretreatment consideration must be given to the following factors:

(a) the patient's pretreatment expectations
(b) the patient's smoking habits

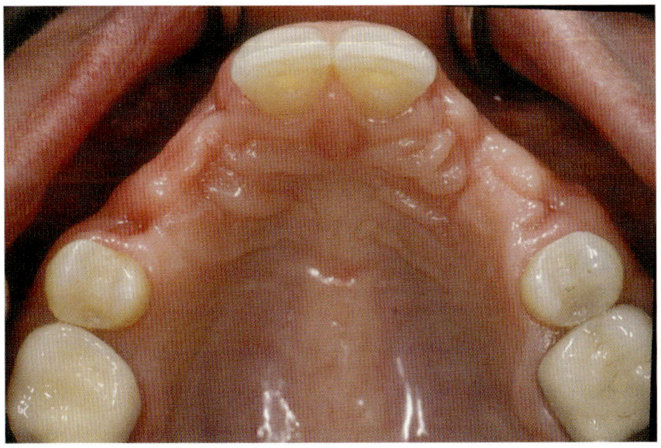

Figure 5.1 An occlusal view of a maxillary arch illustrates large bilateral horizontal tissue defects in the proposed implant sites.

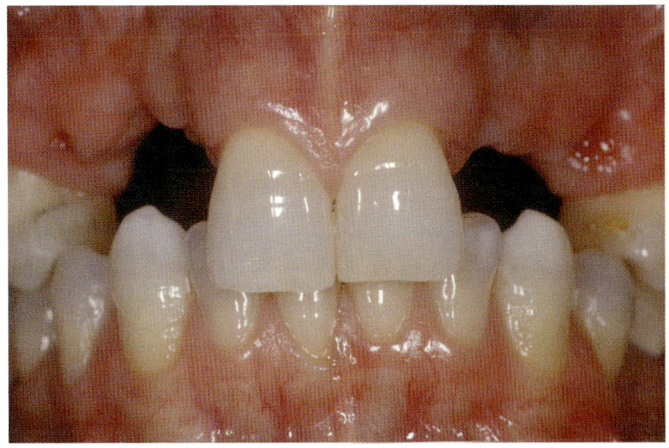

Figure 5.2 An anterior view of the maxillary arch demonstrates the bilateral vertical tissue deficiencies in the proposed implant sites.

(a)

(b)

(c)

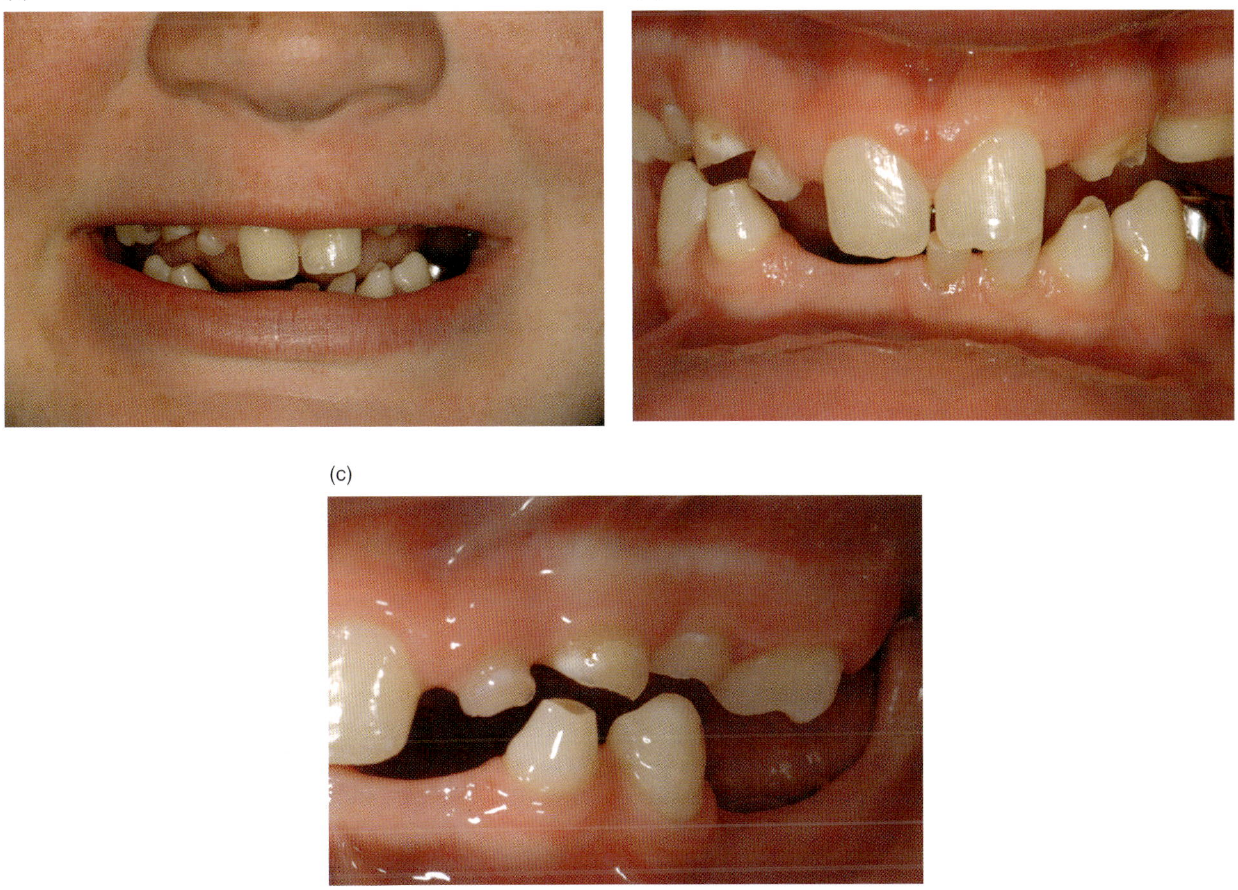

Figure 5.3 (a) An anterior profile underscores the disrupted occlusal and incisal planes, and their influence on appearance. (b) An anterior retracted view illustrates the disrupted incisal and anterior occlusal plane. (c) A lateral view demonstrates the disrupted occlusal plane and restricted interocclusal distance.

(c) the height of the lip line on smiling
(d) the gingival biotype in the treatment area
(e) the shape of the missing and surrounding teeth
(f) the presence of infection at the implant site
(g) the bone levels at the adjacent teeth
(h) the restorative status of teeth adjacent to the edentulous space
(i) the character of the edentulous space
(j) the width of the hard and soft tissues in the edentulous space
(k) the height of the hard and soft tissues in the edentulous space

Patient Concerns, Motivation, and Attitudes

Psychological and behavioral factors have significant implications when treating patients with elevated esthetic demands. Because the esthetic zone is dependent upon the individual patient's perception, and is not limited to the visibility of the smile, it is imperative that the clinician ascertains the patient's motivations and expectations prior to initiation of treatment. Attempts should be made to identify noncompliant patients with particular reference to treatment commitment, hygiene, and smoking (Figure 5.4). Where indicated, behavioral modification should be attempted. Patient's with complex medical histories and/or physical disabilities are often less capable of satisfactory dental maintenance.

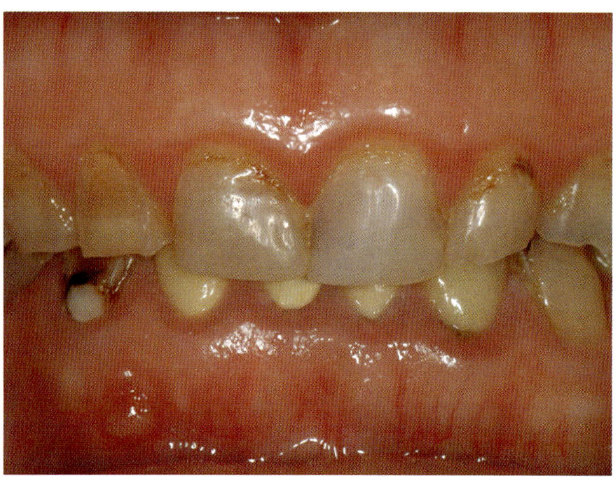

Figure 5.4 Pretreatment oral hygiene and maintenance limitations are evident.

Caution should be observed with patients for whom multiple treatment plans and procedures have been undertaken with limited patient satisfaction. Care should also be exercised when treatment is considered for patients for whom a tangible esthetic complaint is difficult to identify. As implant therapy is often elective in nature, a risk benefit analysis from the perspective of the patient must be carried out prior to the initiation of advanced, complex, or esthetic treatment.

Pretreatment evaluation of patients requiring tooth replacement in the esthetic zone should be comprehensive and holistic in nature. The importance of esthetic factors has historically been linked to the patients' sex, age, and personality. Success relies upon the timely and appropriate implementation of each stage in the treatment process. A strong relationship exists between the quality of treatment outcome and the skill and experience of the clinician. Working as a team consisting of clinicians with advanced skill sets and experiences, should be considered mandatory for patients, in this treatment category.

Basic Treatment Principles in the Esthetic Zone

The incorporation of a "restorative-based," "restoration-driven," or "crown-down" approach is fundamental to planning implant-based rehabilitation in the esthetic zone. For patient's with esthetic demands, diagnostic wax-ups aid in identifying the planned tooth form and position, and the shape and position of the planned gingival margin (Figure 5.5). Augmentation and surgical templates, based on the diagnostic wax-up, can then be fabricated and used to indicate tissue deficiencies and communicate the desired three-dimensional implant position (Figures 5.6–5.8a–c).

Optimal esthetic outcomes can only be achieved within a solid foundation of bone and soft tissue (i.e., "pink" esthetics). Bone and soft tissue architectures should be clearly developed in response to the planned restoration and the patient's restorative demands. Site development procedures, including socket preservation and provisional restorations, should be undertaken when indicated, subsequent to extraction and prior to implant placement. These measures enhance the prospects of optimal implant placement and can

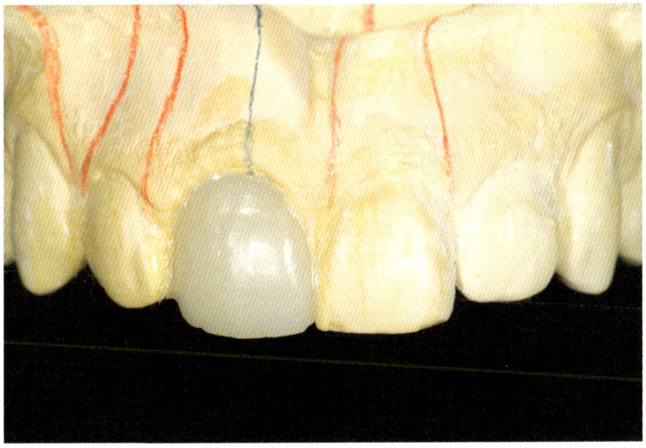

Figure 5.5 A diagnostic wax-up helps determine the desired shape of the proposed tooth and planned position of the free gingival margin.

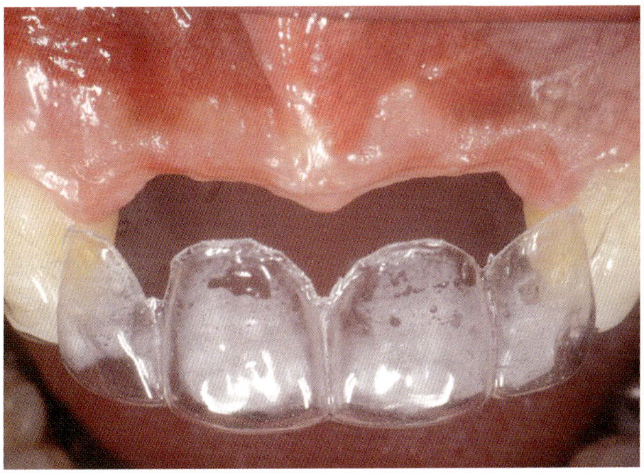

Figure 5.6 An augmentation template illustrates the three-dimensional form of the hard and soft tissue deficits.

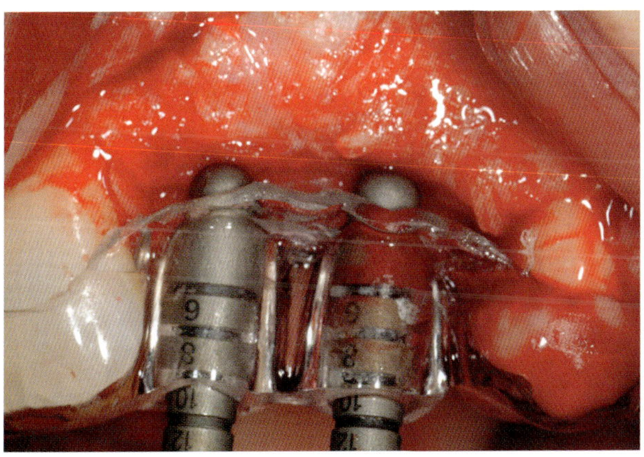

Figure 5.7 A sleeve template communicates the desired orofacial and mesiodistal positions and long-axis inclinations of the implants.

often reduce the need for more complicated enhancement procedures (Figures 5.9 and 5.10).

Site enhancement, prior to or in conjunction with implant placement, can include hard and soft tissue augmentation. Adjunctive procedures, including root coverage, crown elongation surgery and orthodontics may also be indicated (Figure 5.11). Such treatments should be planned, sequenced, and provided in a controlled manner. The least benefit is derived when these procedures are undertaken subsequent to implant placement in response to esthetic and functional complications.

Implant therapy in the esthetic zone is considered to be an advanced or complex procedure (4). As such, planning and treatment procedures should routinely address and adhere to the following concerns and principles:

1. Address the patient's concerns.
2. Identify patients with elevated risk through site analysis and a general patient assessment.
3. Employ comprehensive, interdisciplinary treatment planning.
4. Consider all treatment options.
5. Formulate a treatment chronology that will maximize benefits to the patient and minimize discomfort or inconvenience.
6. Augment deficient soft and hard tissue regions prior to or concurrent with implant placement.
7. Incorporate a restoration-based philosophy for implant placement.
8. Utilize provisional restorations for tissue development and maturation, and as templates for the definitive restoration.
9. Carry out adjunctive procedures on adjacent teeth when necessary.
10. Utilize a team approach.

Surgery associated with dental implants in the esthetic zone cannot be limited to the placement of the implant. Surgical goals during implant placement procedures should include improvement of esthetic and functional outcomes through the reestablishment of optimal bone and soft tissue profiles (Figures 5.12a–e). Deficiencies in either tissue type will compromise the esthetic outcome by positioning the implant and/or the restoration in a displeasing three-dimensional esthetic environment.

Various treatments are available to address deficiencies and esthetic anomalies. These fall into two broad categories—those that directly influence

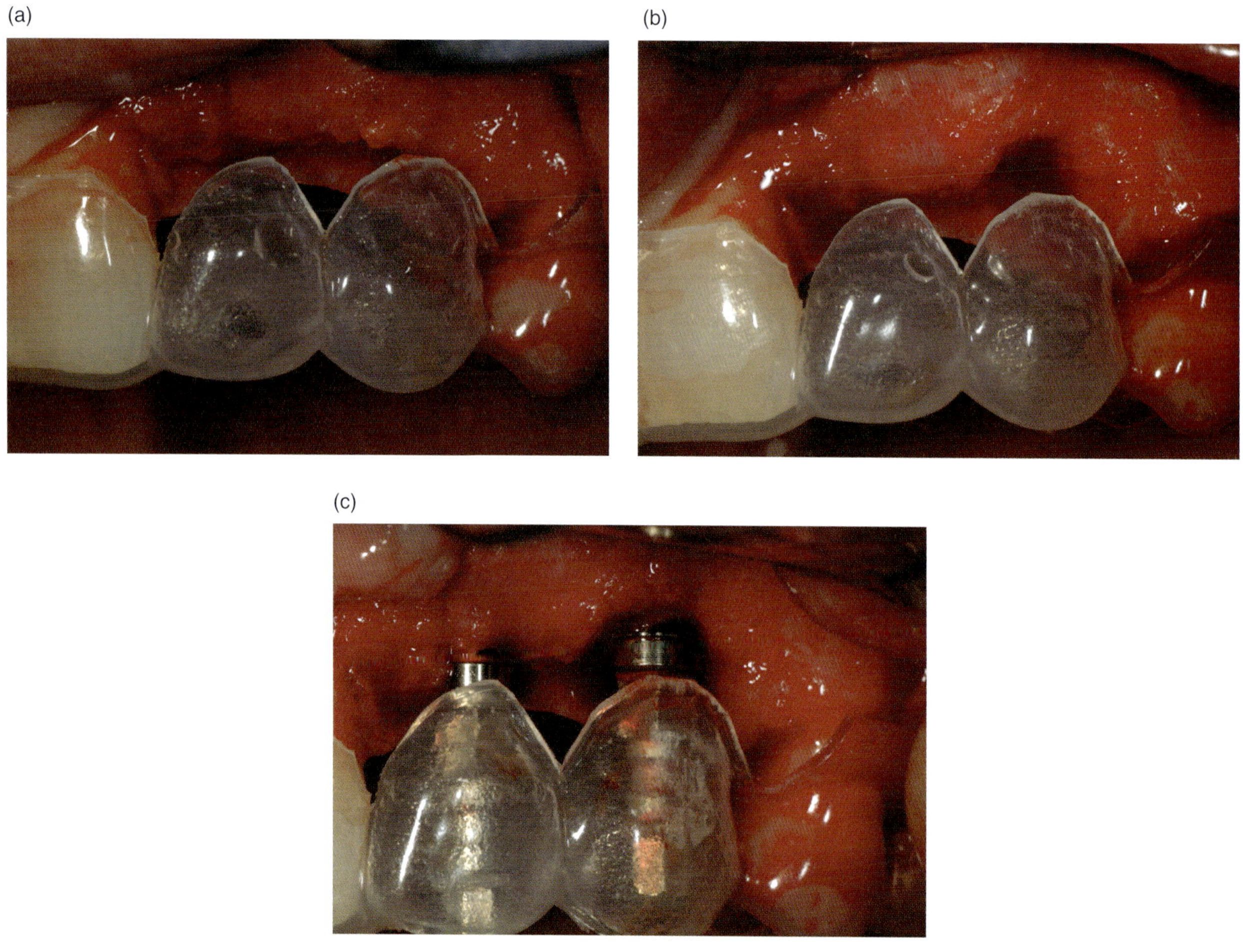

Figure 5.8 (a–c) A depth template communicates the proposed positions of the free gingival margins and desired positions of the implant restorative margins.

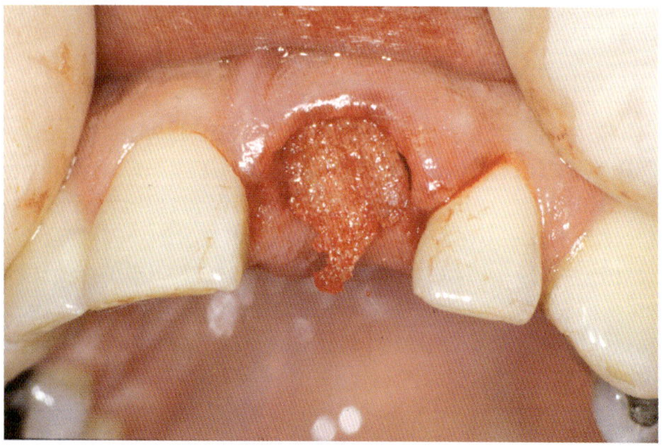

Figure 5.9 Socket preservation or osseous grafting may be carried out subsequent to tooth extraction and prior to implant placement.

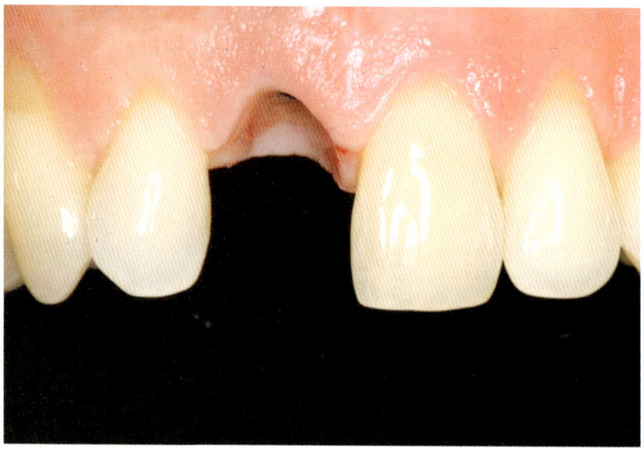

Figure 5.10 Tissue form is developed by the ovate form of the bonded provisional restoration.

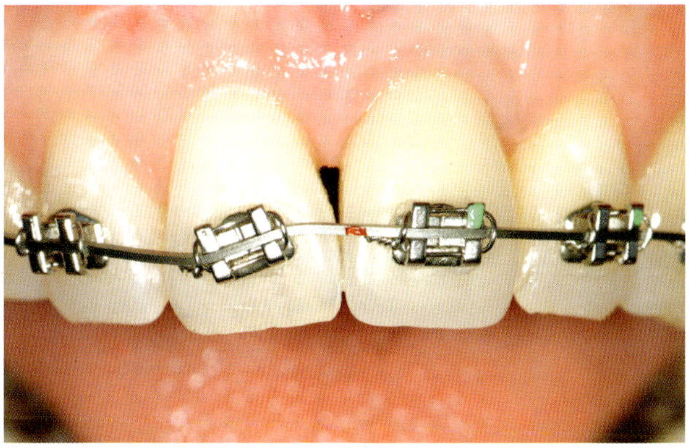

Figure 5.11 A facial view of a patient undergoing orthodontics to optimize tooth position and inclination.

the implant site and those that influence the adjacent teeth and surrounding environment.

Procedures designed to enhance the implant site include:

1. socket preservation
2. immediate and early implant placement with and without concurrent augmentation of hard and soft tissue defects
3. orthodontic tooth extrusion and
4. hard and/or soft tissue ridge augmentation as a stand-alone procedure prior to implant placement

Procedures designed to enhance the three-dimensional esthetic condition of the adjacent teeth and oral environment include:

1. orthodontics, with the establishment of appropriate tooth positioning to meet the esthetic and functional needs of the patient
2. crown-lengthening (or elongation) surgery to establish esthetic gingival contours and tooth proportions and
3. root coverage surgery

Implant Site

Clinicians have several treatment options at the time of, and subsequent to, tooth extraction. With normal healing, the internal and external socket dimensions undergo significant resorption after tooth removal. The facial bony wall is often thin to begin with in the anterior maxilla, and the healing process reduces it further with time (5). Therefore, emphasis has been placed on the preservation of bone and soft tissues through the removal of teeth with a minimum of trauma (Figure 5.13).

Dental implants predictably integrate when placed immediately into extraction wounds (Figure 5.14). Unfortunately, successful integration of the implant alone is insufficient to ensure a favorable outcome in the esthetic zone (4, 6, 7). The tissue response to immediate implant placement in the esthetic zone can be unpredictable and may result in apical migration of the free gingival margin. In an effort to further improve predictability, techniques such as orthodontic extrusion have been advocated as an alternative to extraction and augmentation.

Hard and soft tissue ridge augmentation can successfully recapture tissue contours in implant sites in the esthetic zone. A variety of clinical techniques have been advocated. Successful hard tissue augmentation has been achieved with autogenous grafts, mostly in conjunction with membranes (8, 9). Allografts and xenografts have also been successfully utilized for hard tissue augmentation, in conjunction with membranes and, where indicated, concurrent with implant placement (10–12). Soft tissue procedures designed to increase tissue bulk, improve resistance to recession, and enhance color and contour may also be utilized (13).

Adjacent Teeth and the Oral Environment

Obtaining the desired esthetic outcome often involves the surrounding teeth and oral environment. Success requires adherence to general esthetic principles, such as the establishment of favorable gingival margin contours and tooth proportion. Crown-lengthening surgery is often required as an adjunct to implant and tooth replacement. This procedure helps ensure pleasing tooth contours and proportions, in addition to establishing desired gingival symmetry and form. Crown-lengthening surgery in the esthetic zone should only be undertaken subsequent to the determination of the future incisal edge position, tooth length, and gingival form.

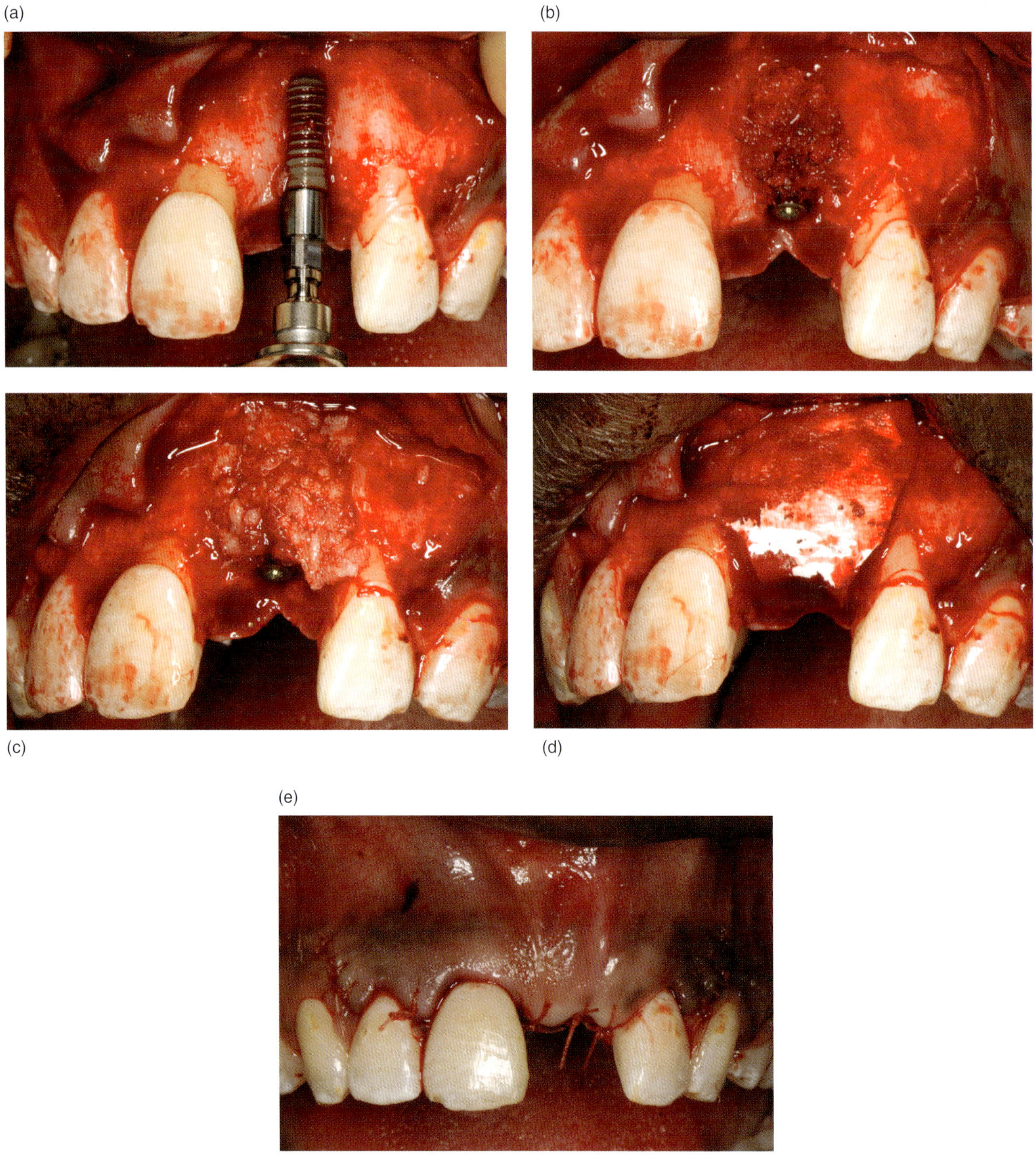

Figure 5.12 (a) Following placement of a stable implant, a total facial surface dehiscence is noted. (b) The exposed facial surface of the implant is covered with autogenous bone collected during preparation of the implant osteotomy site, or harvested intraorally. (c) The autogenous bone is covered with an allograft to establish facial ridge contours. (d) A resorbable membrane is placed to protect the graft. (e) A view of wound closure.

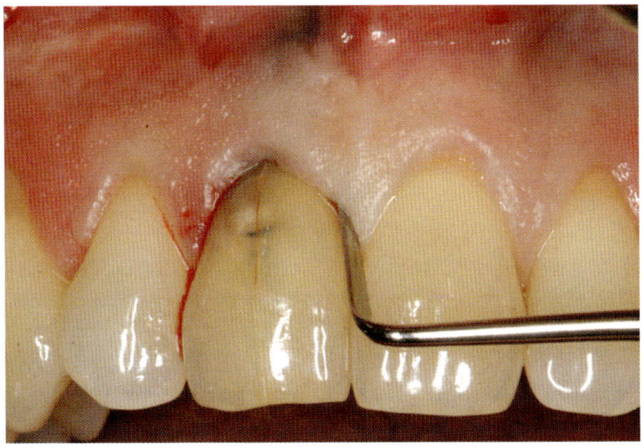

Figure 5.13 Minimally traumatic tooth extraction is carried out utilizing periotomes.

Treatment Chronology for Modification of Adjacent Teeth and the Oral Environment

1. Comprehensive patient assessment and diagnosis
2. Elimination of predisposing factors, oral disease, and inflammation
3. Development of a functional and esthetic diagnostic waxup with reference to incisal edge position, crown proportions, and gingival margin contours and position
4. Fabrication of a surgical template illustrating the desired gingival contours
5. Accurate measurement and recording of the biologic width for the treatment segment
6. Surgical removal of the indicated amount of bone

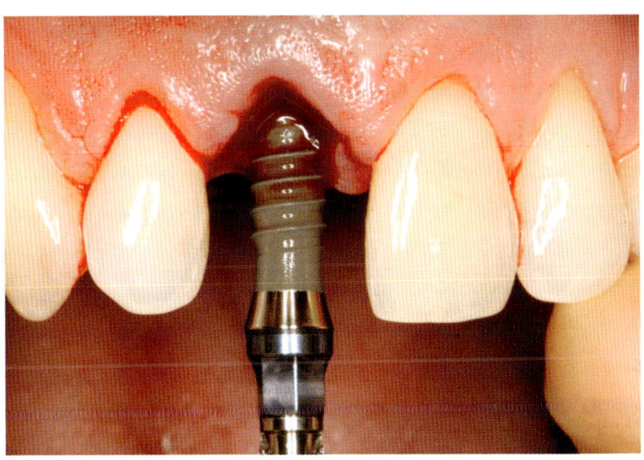

Figure 5.14 Immediate implant placement is accomplished.

7. Implant placement can be performed simultaneously if soft tissue contours subsequent to healing are considered predictable, or
8. Implant placement can be deferred until healing is complete, if any concern is evident with regard to tissue contours and healing

Radicular Coverage

Exposed root surfaces on teeth adjacent to proposed implant sites can represent considerable esthetic challenges, and influence both gingival architecture and tooth proportions. Surgical procedures designed to coronally reposition the soft tissues can significantly improve the esthetic outcome. Careful preoperative planning is critical to integrating root coverage procedures into comprehensive treatment involving implants in the esthetic zone. Root coverage procedures should be undertaken prior to implant placement. Once the surgical site has healed, and the gingival margin is stable, vertical implant position can be more accurately determined. The extent of root coverage obtained may set the reference for the entire esthetic zone, with respect to the locations and contours of the free gingival margins.

It is imperative to identify and correct the etiological factors in each instance of recession. Controlling inflammation is central to successful root coverage and long-term soft tissue stability (14). Optimizing mechanical plaque control capabilities through patient education and removal of predisposing factors (e.g., overhangs and open margins) is mandatory. Orthodontic therapy may be indicated to improve tooth alignment, and to optimize tooth position within the alveolus. In cases of thin tissue biotypes, root coverage procedures should be chosen which provide increased tissue thickness. The choice of technique should be based upon the reproducibility of success associated with the technique, and the practice environment and individual skills of the clinician.

Treatment Procedures and Chronology for Radicular Coverage Procedures in Implant Patients

- Record patient history and expectations
- Perform thorough oral, periodontal, and esthetic evaluation and examination

- Identify etiologies and classify the defect or defects
- Address etiological factors
- Ensure appropriate oral hygiene education and modify techniques when indicated
- Perform a thorough prophylaxis and debridement to establish and maintain a stable periodontal condition
- Restoratively address any predisposing conditions
- Orthodontically optimize the three-dimensional positions of teeth
- Select and execute root coverage procedures

Conclusions

Pretreatment risk analysis, along with careful assessment of treatment difficulty, will often identify patients for whom esthetic treatment may be compromised. A team approach to assessment and planning is therefore critical to avoiding compromises. Excellent esthetic restorations supported by dental implants are in demand by dentists and patients. Predictable implant-based esthetic treatment requires meticulous attention to detail in all phases of care. Clinicians should continue to seek education, experience, and skills as techniques and materials continue to improve.

Acknowledgments

We would like to thank Dr James Ruskin, Dr Emma Lewis, and Dr Dawn Martin for their clinical skills as well as Mr Todd Fridrich and Mr Mitchell Jim for their technical skills.

References

1. Higginbottom F, Belser U, Jones J, and Keith S. 2004. Prosthetic management of implants in the esthetic zone. *IJOMI* 19(Suppl):62–72.
2. Zetu L and Wang H-L. 2005. Management of the interdental/inter-implant papilla. *J Clin Periodontol* 32:831–839.
3. Buser D, Martin WC, and Belser UC. 2007. Surgical considerations for single tooth replacements in the esthetic zone: Standard procedure in sites without bone deficiencies. In: *ITI Treatment Guide*, Vol. 1. Chicago: Quintessence.
4. Botticelli D, Berglundh T, and Lindhe J. 2004. Hard tissue alterations following immediate implant placement in extraction sites. *J Clin Periodontol* 31:820–828.
5. Araujo MG, Sukekava F, Wennstrom JL, and Lindhe J. 2005. Ridge alterations following implant placement in fresh extraction sockets: An experimental study in the dog. *Clin Oral Implants Res* 14:35–42.
6. Covani U, Bortolaila C, Barone A, and Sbordone L. 2004. Bucco-lingual crestal bone jaw. Changes after immediate and delayed implant placement. *J Periodontol* 75:1605–1612.
7. Cardaropoli G, Lekhlm U, and Wennstrom JL. 2006. Tissue alterations at implant supported single tooth replacements. A 1 year prospective clinical study. *Clin Oral Implants Res* 17:165–171.
8. Fiorellini J and Nevins M. 2003. Localised ridge augmentation/preservation. A systematic review. *Ann Periodontol* 8:321–327.
9. Hammerle CH, Jung RE, and Feloutzis A. 2002. A systematic review of the survival of implants in bone sites augmented with barrier membranes (guided bone regeneration) in partially edentulous patients. *J Periodontol* 29(Suppl 3):226–231.
10. Becker W and Becker BE. 1990. Guided tissue regeneration or implants placed into extraction sockets and for implant dehiscences: Surgical techniques and case reports. *Int J Periodontics Restorative Dent* 10:376–391.
11. Nyman S, Lang NP, Buser D, and Bragger U. 1990. Bone regeneration adjacent to titanium dental implants using guided bone regeneration: A report of two cases. *Int J Oral Maxillofac Implants* 5:9–14.
12. Hammerle CH and Jung RE. 2000. Bone augmentation by means of barrier membranes. *Periodontology* 33(2003):36–53.
13. Bouchard P, Malet J, and Borghetti A. 2000. Decision making in esthetics: Root coverage revisited. *Periodontology* 27(2001):97–120.
14. Freedman AL, Green K, Salkin LM, Stein MD, and Mellado JR. 1990. An 18 year longitudinal study of untreated mucogingival defects. *J Periodontol* 70:1174–1176.

Chapter 6
Augmentation of the Posterior Maxilla

Paul A. Fugazzotto, DDS

Outline

The posterior maxilla poses a significant challenge when planning implant reconstructive therapy. The multifactorial nature of the problems which must be appropriately addressed include the buccolingual and/or apicocrestal ridge resorption which occurs following tooth removal, pneumatization of the sinus following loss of the molar teeth, and the poorer quality (type IV) bone which is often encountered in the posterior maxilla. However, it is imperative that the posterior maxilla is not visualized as a distinct entity during the diagnosis and treatment planning phase of therapy. A common sequella to the loss of posterior occlusion and the need to function exclusively in the anterior segments of the dentition is the extensive wear of the remaining anterior teeth and/or anterior protheses. Such excessive function and resultant wear may lead to acceleration of periodontal breakdown around the remaining teeth, a loss of appropriate inter-arch space for reconstructive therapy, and the development of eccentric patterns of occlusion guided by the aforementioned wear facets which develop.

As a result of these concerns, a thorough diagnosis and formulation of a multidisciplinary treatment plan, aimed at reconstructing the posterior maxilla in concert with the necessary oral rehabilitation, must be carried out prior to the initiation of therapy (1). The posterior maxilla must be seen as one component in a patient-specific overall treatment plan. Failure to consider all appropriate factors when developing such a treatment plan will undoubtedly result in a compromised final treatment outcome.

The need for an increased volume of bone in the edentulous posterior maxilla to appropriately effect implant placement and reconstruction has given rise to the sinus augmentation procedure. A variety of grafting materials and surgical approaches have been utilized to effect sinus augmentation. The report of the 1996 Sinus Consensus

Conference by the Academy of Osseointegration cited successful sinus augmentation results utilizing autografts, allografts, xenografts, and combinations of the three in various forms (2). As stated in the conclusions of the conference report, "The Conference was unanimous in agreement that the sinus graft is an efficacious procedure to be used for implant supported restoration of the posterior maxilla." These findings were confirmed by a later consensus conference on sinus grafting from the Academy of Osseointegration (3). However, as Tong et al. (4) reported in a review of literature documenting survival rates of implants placed in grafted maxillary sinuses, "Data examining short-term and long-term outcomes have been scarce and have been reported following a limited number of patients."

The utilization of osteotome techniques to effect localized sinus floor elevation and augmentation, either in anticipation of implant placement or in conjunction with implant placement, has been advocated by many practitioners. Initially proposed by Summers (5), this technique offers the advantages of a more conservative surgical entry, more localized augmentation of the sinus, a lesser degree of postoperative morbidity, and an ability to load the implants in a shorter time period than that necessary when employing a conventional LeForte osteotomy approach to sinus augmentation. While the osteotome technique has undergone a number of modifications, a paucity of papers exist that document short- and long-term success rates in a significant number of cases. In addition, disagreements abound as to the indications and contraindications for the osteotome technique in various clinical situations.

The challenge facing today's clinician is not the ability to utilize either conventional sinus augmentation therapy or the osteotome approach to sinus augmentation successfully. Rather, it is the development of a diagnostic system that allows the utilization of each therapeutic modality to its maximum advantage.

Contraindications to Sinus Augmentation Therapy

Specific contraindications to sinus augmentation therapy exist, in addition to the general systemic and psychological contraindications to any type of surgical care. These concerns specific to sinus augmentation therapy include acute or chronic sinus infections, and the presence of various sinus pathologies such as extensive polyps and unidentified masses. In addition, patients who smoke demonstrate a higher incidence of complications and a lesser degree of regeneration in augmented sinus areas than nonsmoking patients treated by similar means. A smoking habit in excess of 10 cigarettes per day should be considered a relative contraindication to sinus augmentation therapy. A smoking habit of any type, if it leads to continued tissue inflammation or a significantly suppressed healing response following surgical therapy, is a contraindication to any augmentation therapy.

Definitions of Success

The success of sinus augmentation therapy should not be viewed as a radiographic occurrence. The ability to effect bone augmentation in the sinus area with the resultant radiopacity is not a treatment end point in and of itself. Rather, successful sinus augmentation therapy must meet three specific criteria:

- The ability to place implants of ideal diameter, and overall dimension, to withstand functional forces over time in a given clinical situation, in prosthetically driven positions.
- The ability to afford adequate bone for placement of an implant of the desired dimensions, and subsequent restoration in a manner which fulfills the esthetic demands of the patient.
- Stability of regenerated bone in the augmented sinus area around implants, under function over time.

Prior to initiating augmentation of the posterior maxilla through sinus and/or ridge augmentation therapy, a number of diagnostic and treatment planning steps must be carried out. These necessary steps and their importance, if comprehensive care is to be appropriately delivered, have been discussed in Chapter 2.

Formatted CAT scan studies also afford unparalleled visualization of the precise morphology of the sinus, and the presence or absence of pathologies and/or septa, and are a significant aid to the clinician as he or she performs the planned augmentation therapy.

Buccolingual/Palatal Augmentation

As discussed in Chapter 2 (6–10), the ability to predictably effect buccopalatal or apicocrestal augmentation of an atrophic alveolar ridge through the use of a variety of appropriately employed autogenous or nonautogenous materials under fixated titanium-reinforced membranes, if soft tissue primary closure is maintained throughout the course of regeneration, is well established. Maximization of regenerative results when performing buccal and palatal ridge augmentation procedures is dependent upon adequate flap design and reflection; defect debridement; defect decortication where applicable; fixation of a titanium-reinforced space maintaining membrane; placement of materials beneath the membrane to effect clot stabilization; control of overlying forces during regeneration; and maintenance of primary closure throughout the course of regeneration. Such augmentation, in conjunction with sinus augmentations, is often critical to maximization of treatment outcomes.

Sinus Augmentation

Augmentation of the remaining alveolar bone crestal to the floor of the sinus may be accomplished through a variety of approaches including:

(a) Lateral window sinus augmentation therapy.
(b) Crestal window sinus augmentation therapy.
(c) Lateral window sinus augmentation therapy with concomitant implant placement.
(d) The Summers bone-added osteotome technique.
(e) The Summers bone-added osteotome technique with simultaneous implant placement.
(f) The trephine and osteotome technique.
(g) The trephine and osteotome technique with simultaneous implant placement.

When choosing a specific treatment modality in a given situation, it is imperative that the clinician recognizes the indications, contraindications, limitations, and predictability of the technique in question.

LATERAL WINDOW SINUS AUGMENTATION THERAPY

A horizontal incision is made approximately 1–2 mm palatal to the palatal line angle of the residual alveolar ridge (Figure 6.1). Care must be taken to extend this incision mesially and distally at least 8–10 mm beyond the area of planned augmentation therapy. Buccal vertical releasing incisions are placed at the mesial and distal extents of the horizontal incision. Horizontal releasing incisions are placed at the most apical extents of the vertical releasing incisions. A mucoperiosteal flap is reflected toward the buccal in a full-thickness manner (Figure 6.2). Full-thickness flap reflection is carried out through the area of the horizontal releasing incisions. No periosteal fenestrations are utilized. The mucoperiosteal flap must be reflected apically at least 8–10 mm beyond the area of the planned osteotomy.

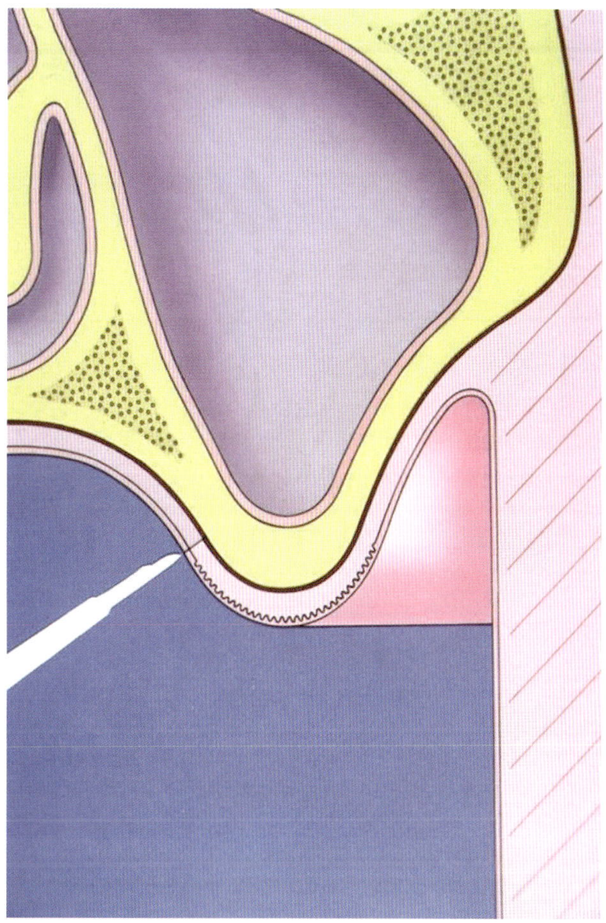

Figure 6.1 A horizontal incision is made palatal to the palatal line angle of the edentulous ridge.

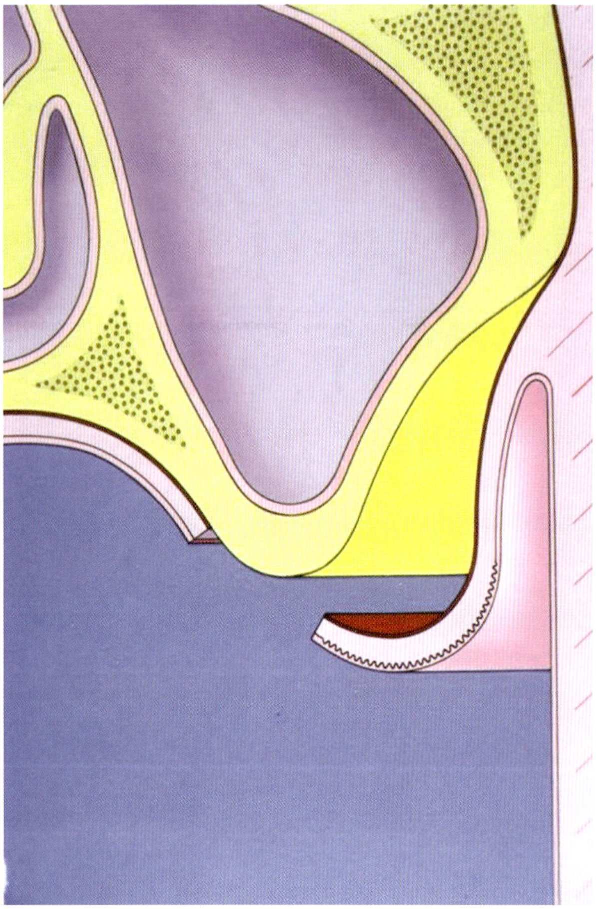

Figure 6.2 A full-thickness buccal mucoperiosteal flap is reflected.

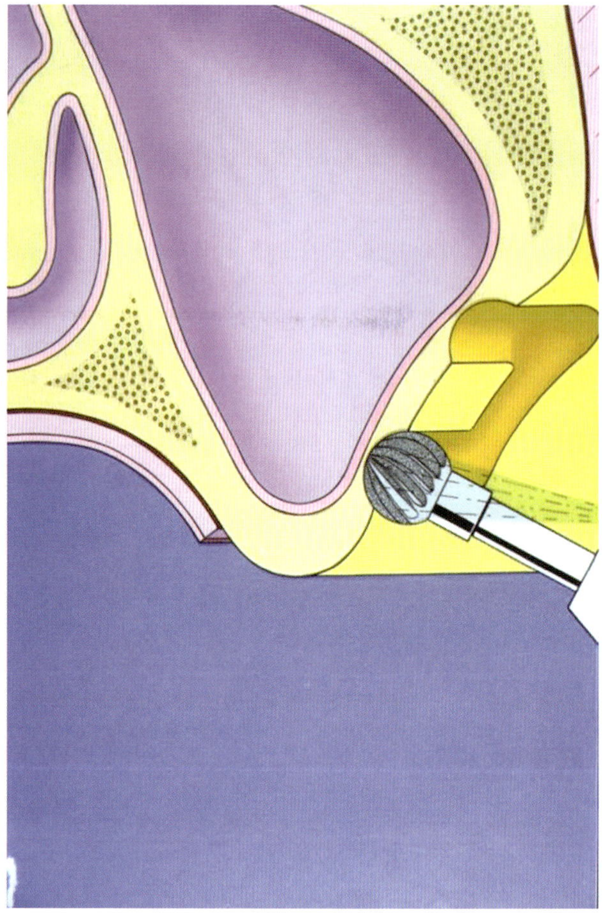

Figure 6.3 A number 8 or 10 round diamond bur on a straight handpiece is utilized to outline the osteotomy window. A carbide bur is only employed in instances in exceptionally dense bone. The complete window is outlined with the number 8 or 10 round bur until the gray membrane may be seen beneath the prepared osteotomy.

An osteotomy is prepared in the lateral aspect of the buccal alveolus in one of two ways:

Handpiece and bur utilization: A straight handpiece is employed, at a speed of 25,000–50,000 RPM, depending upon the quality and thickness of the residual buccal alveolar ridge. A number 8 or 10 round diamond bur is utilized to outline the complete extent of the osteotomy (Figure 6.3). The diameter of the bur is such that an "island" of bone will remain after the osteotomy has been completed. A carbide bur is only utilized in the presence of denser buccal alveolar bone. The osteotomy is deepened with the number 10 round bur in smooth, sweeping motions. Care must be taken not to utilize a sawing or pushing motion with the bur. These sweeping motions should extend along the complete border of the osteotomy. When connecting the apical and crestal borders of the osteotomy with the mesial and distal borders of the osteotomy, a fluid motion must be employed as the bur comes around the "corner" from one side of the osteotomy to the other. Failure to do so will result in a jagged osteotomy edge and increase the incidence of membrane perforation during osteotomy preparation and subsequent membrane reflection. The osteotomy is deepened with the number 8 or 10 round bur until the bone is thin and translucent enough to visualize the gray membrane beneath it on all aspects of the osteotomy, including its corners.

A number 4 round diamond bur is inserted into the handpiece and utilized to complete the osteotomy (Figures 6.4 and 6.5). The utilization

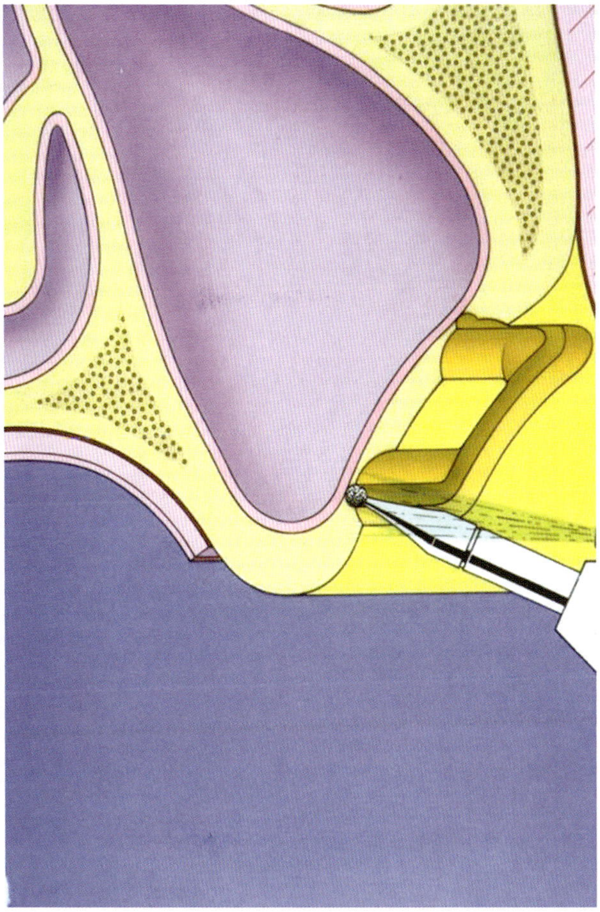

Figure 6.4 A number 4 round diamond bur on a straight handpiece is utilized to complete the osteotomy.

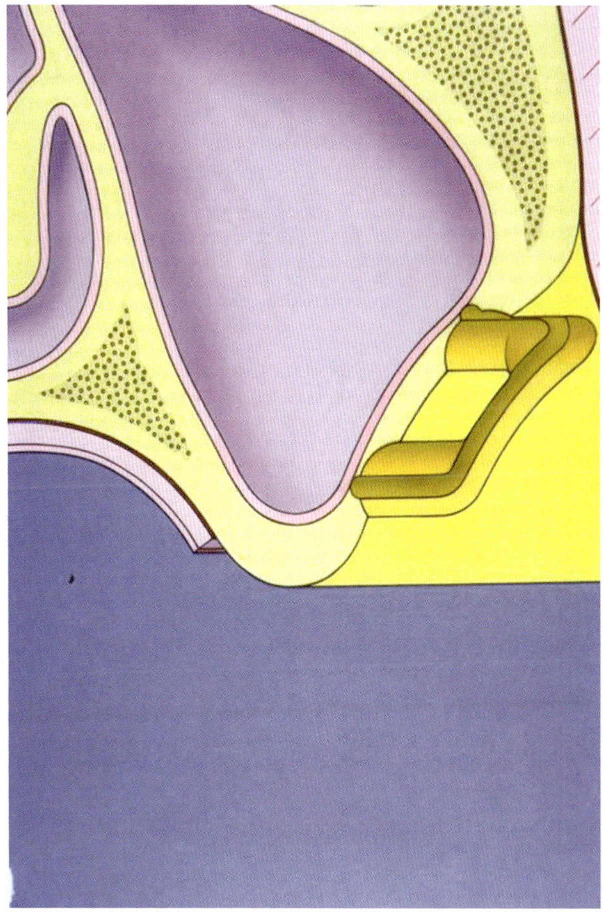

Figure 6.5 A view of both the initial osteotomy prepared with the number 8 or 10 round diamond bur and the secondary osteotomy prepared with the number 4 round diamond bur.

of this smaller bur as the sinus membrane is approached offers a number of advantages. Visualization is vastly improved through the creation of a broader channel, especially in situations where a thicker buccal alveolar wall is present. This channel also allows easy egress of the irrigating solution while the handpiece is running, once again significantly improving visualization and lessening the chance of sinus perforation during window preparation.

The island of detached bone is used to facilitate initial membrane reflection. Initial blunt dissection and constant awareness of the need for three-dimensional membrane reflection significantly decrease the incidence of membrane tears during reflection.

While it is tempting to immediately insert a curette between the detached bony window created by the osteotomy and the alveolus to begin sinus reflection, such an approach is ill advised. Forcing a sharp curette into this space will increase the incidence of membrane perforation. The following steps are taken to help minimize such a complication.

An amalgam plugger is utilized with gentle pressure to implode the detached bony window approximately 2 mm. Such movement detaches approximately 1 mm of the sinus membrane from the overlying alveolar bone. A flat, dull plastic instrument is now inserted into this created small space. The backside of the plastic instrument rests against the slightly detached osteotomy window, lifting the bony island and opening the space which has been created by the initial window implosion. The plastic instrument is carried approximately

2–3 mm mesially, distally, and medially, effecting detachment of a portion of the sinus membrane from the alveolar bone. The amalgam plugger is once again utilized to implode the bony window approximately 3–4 mm, causing further detachment of the sinus membrane from the overlying alveolar bone. The plastic instrument is reinserted in the manner previously described, approximately 3–4 mm medially. The plastic instrument is brought mesially and distally until it reaches the "line angles" of the osteotomy.

The sinus membrane is now sufficiently detached to allow the passive insertion of a curette into the created space (Figure 6.6). As the backside of the curette contacts the detached bony window, the resultant displacement of the bony window lifts the already detached portion of the sinus membrane, creating a space for the safe, passive insertion of the sinus curette. The curette is now carried mesially, distally, and medially, to effect further detachment of the sinus membrane from the alveolar bone. Care must be taken to perform a three-dimensional membrane reflection. All movements mesially and/or distally must correspond to a medial movement. Failure to perform a three-dimensional sinus membrane reflection will result in an increased incidence of sinus membrane perforation.

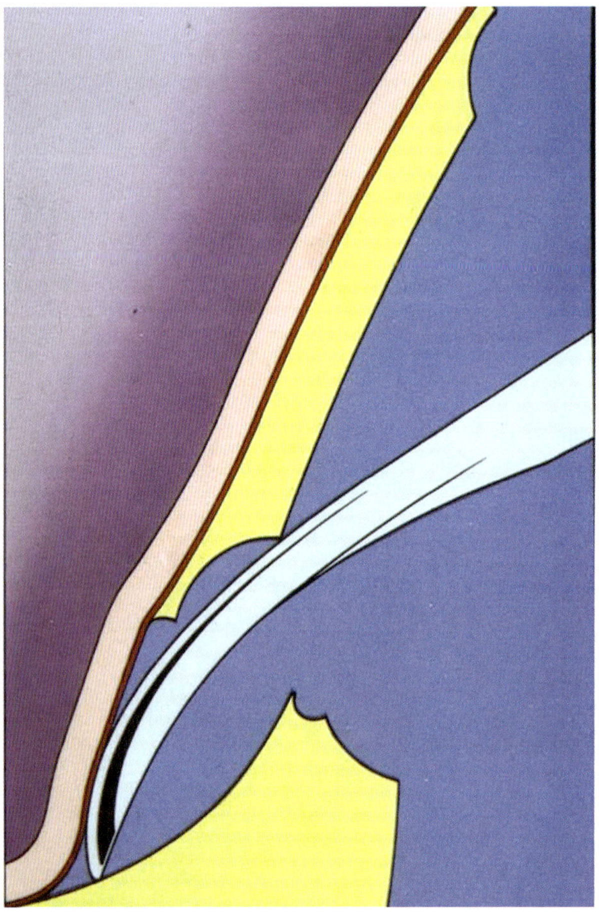

Figure 6.6 As a sinus curette is inserted into the already created space, the backside of the curette lifts the detached osteotomy window and the attached membrane, allowing passive insertion of the curette between the membrane and the residual lateral wall of the alveolus. The detached osteotomy window and membrane are elevated to the desired position.

The bony window is always wholly detached from the buccal alveolar bone. Such an approach offers a number of advantages over other techniques, including detachment of three sides of the bony window, perforation of the most apical aspect of the bony window, and reflection of the bony window in a "trap door" manner. This trap door approach is never utilized.

Detachment of the bony window offers three distinct advantages over other approaches:

- The less easily controlled technique of green stick fracturing of the window inward, and thus increasing the chances of sinus perforation, is avoided.
- The bony window offers a purchase from which to initiate minimally traumatic sinus membrane reflection.
- Failure to detach the bony window from the buccal alveolar wall limits the extent of sinus reflection which may be performed apically. By detaching the bony window, the sinus membrane and the attached window may be positioned as far apically as needed in a given situation.

Sinus membrane perforations during sinus augmentation therapy most commonly occur due to one or more of four technical errors:

- Inappropriate initial osteotomy preparation: Movement of the bur in a sawing, jagged motion, pressure on the bur resulting in penetration of the alveolus through the sinus membrane at a given point, or failure to change to a smaller bur as the sinus membrane is approached will all increase the risk of membrane perforation.

- Overly aggressive initial implosion of the sinus window to ensure its detachment from the buccal alveolar bone increases the chances of membrane perforation at the crestal aspect of the osteotomy.
- Overly aggressive insertion of a sinus curette in the initial phases of membrane reflection will lead to membrane tears at the point of insertion.
- Failure to perform a three-dimensional sinus membrane reflection in the mid to later stages of sinus membrane displacement often results in membrane tears at the most mesial and crestal aspects of the osteotomy.

When performed appropriately, the net effect of the aforementioned therapy is safe, predictable reflection of the detached bony window and sinus membrane in a contiguous unit, thus affording access for placement of the appropriate regenerative materials (Figures 6.7 and 6.8).

Piezosurgery Utilization: While many practitioners still employ handpieces and burs as described above to prepare the initial osteotomy in the lateral wall of the alveolus, the use of piezosurgery in place of burs offers a number of advantages. These advantages include:

- Greater tactile feedback as opposed to utilizing a handpiece with burs.
- Greater control of bone preparation than with burs.
- The lesser chance of soft tissue perforation utilizing piezosurgery as compared to a bur technique (11).
- A more superior osseous response, including a lesser degree of necrosis and decreased morbidity, than when a bur is employed (12).

The piezosurgery tip is not utilized to denude the membrane in the area of planned reflection, as has been proposed by other authors (11). Rather, piezosurgery is employed to prepare an osteotomy of the same shape as that prepared when utilizing rotary burs. An OP3 tip is first utilized to outline the osteotomy window and begin to thin the bone, much as the large diameter diamond bur was previously employed. Once the graying membrane is visible along the complete course of the outlined osteotomy, an OT1 tip is employed to complete the osteotomy window. Its use is analogous to that of the smaller diameter diamond bur. The initial reflection, achieved by applying some pressure to the

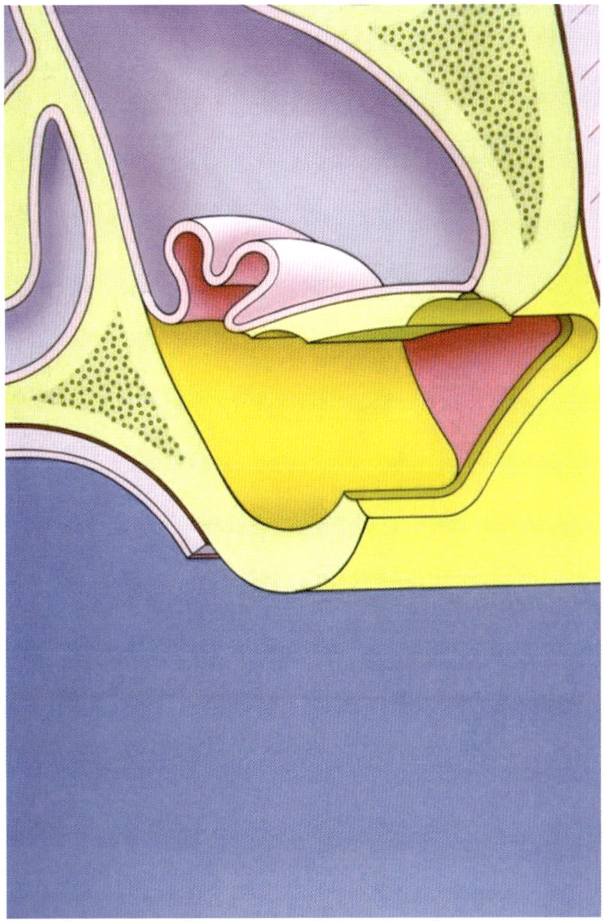

Figure 6.7 A lateral view of the elevated membrane and attached osteotomy window.

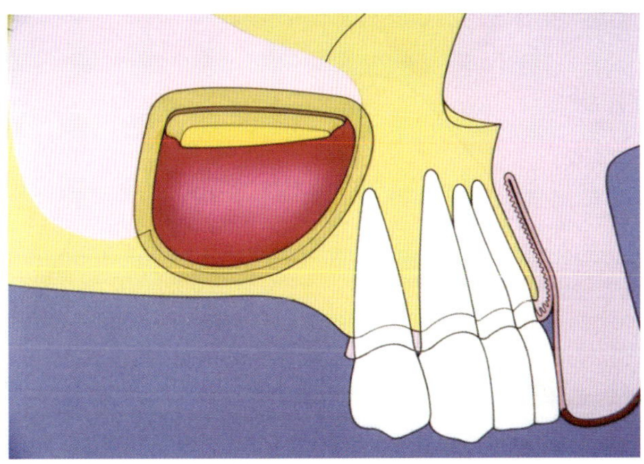

Figure 6.8 A buccal view of the elevated membrane and attached osteotomy window.

osteotomy window, is carried out utilizing the EL1 insert. In this way, the aforementioned advantages of a detached bony window are preserved.

The created subantral space is filled with the appropriate graft materials (Figure 6.9). If a particular graft material is utilized, care must be taken to fill the anterior portion of the subantral space first. If this is not done, and the medial, mesial, and distal aspects of the subantral space are filled with graft material prior to ensuring complete fill of the anterior portion of the subantral space, the clinician will find access to the anterior portion of the subantral space impeded. The net result will be insufficient augmentation of the anterior portion of the created subantral space.

When a bone paste is to be utilized in conjunction with bone putty, the paste is first injected into the created subantral space, ensuring that it reaches the anterior, medial, and posterior portions of the created subantral space. The bone putty is then inserted into the subantral space. The bone paste flows around the bone putty, and extrudes through the prepared osteotomy window. The question of whether or not to place a membrane over the osteotomy window will be discussed subsequently.

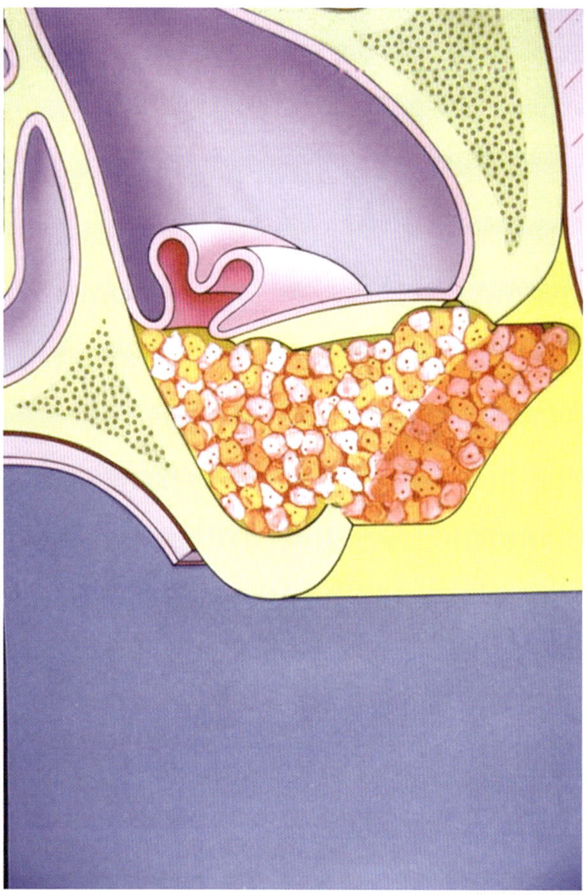

Figure 6.9 The created subantral space is filled with graft material.

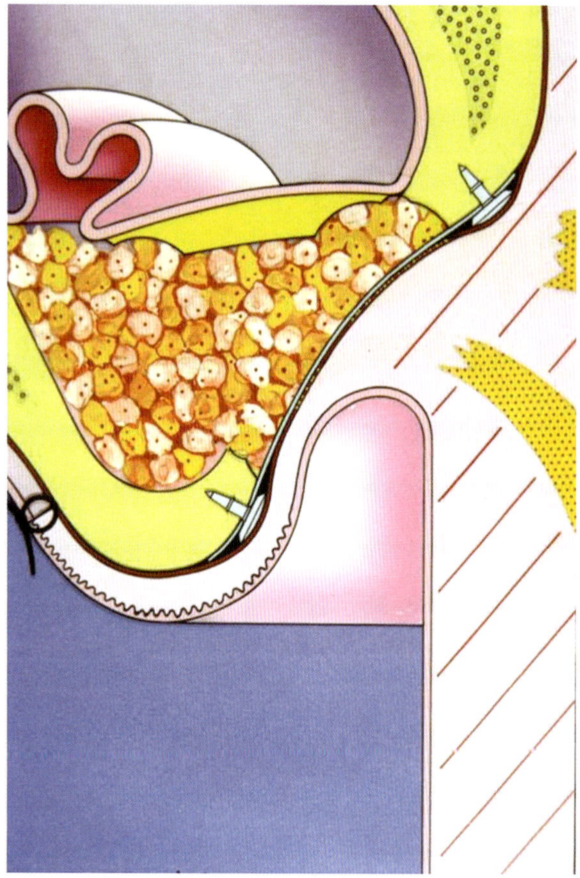

Figure 6.10 A membrane can be placed over the osteotomy window and secured with fixation tacks. The buccal mucoperiosteal flap is replaced and sutured with interrupted sutures. The need or lack of need for a covering membrane over the osteotomy window is discussed in detail in this chapter.

If concomitant ridge augmentation therapy is not to be carried out, the mucoperiosteal flap is replaced and sutured with interrupted 4-0 plain gut sutures (Figure 6.10).

CRESTAL WINDOW SINUS AUGMENTATION THERAPY

Originally employed when the floor of the sinus approached within 2 mm of the crest of the ridge, the primary advantage to crestal sinus augmentation therapy is the relative ease of window preparation and reflection when compared to lateral sinus augmentation therapy. A horizontal incision is made approximately 5 mm apical to the palatal line angle of the alveolar crest. Vertical releasing incisions with horizontal extensions and full-thickness flap reflection are carried out as previously described. Osteotomy preparation and membrane reflection are identical to the techniques employed when performing a lateral window sinus augmentation approach.

Although crestal approach sinus augmentation therapy offers the advantage of a greater ease of technical manipulation, there are potentially significant compromises which result from utilization of such a treatment modality. Unless the residual alveolar ridge demonstrates sufficient thickness buccopalatally to allow window preparation to occur wholly within the crest of the ridge and not approach closer than 2 mm from the buccal line angle of the alveolar ridge, utilization of a crestal window approach will compromise the buccal line angle of the ridge, and thus negatively impact both the buccal positioning of the planned implants, and the final esthetic treatment outcome. As a result, crestal window sinus augmentation therapy is rarely utilized.

LATERAL WINDOW SINUS AUGMENTATION THERAPY WITH CONCOMITANT IMPLANT PLACEMENT

Incision design, flap reflection, and membrane reflection are identical to those previously described for lateral window sinus augmentation therapy. Figure 6.11 demonstrates the initial stages of osteotomy preparation. The gray color of the underlying sinus membrane may be visualized through the thinned buccal alveolar wall. A 4-mm-wide round diamond bur is now utilized to complete osteotomy preparation. Following appropriate membrane reflection, the osteotomy site for the planned implant is prepared. Whether the clinician chooses to prepare this site utilizing a bur or an osteotome, a sinus curette must always be inserted into the prepared subantral space (Figure 6.12), in order that the bur or osteotome penetrating the residual alveolar bone crestal to the floor of the sinus encounters the sinus curette, rather than impacting and possibly tearing the reflected sinus membrane. In the view shown, two implants have been placed anterior to the sinus region, and an osteotomy has been prepared for placement of an implant in conjunction with sinus augmentation therapy.

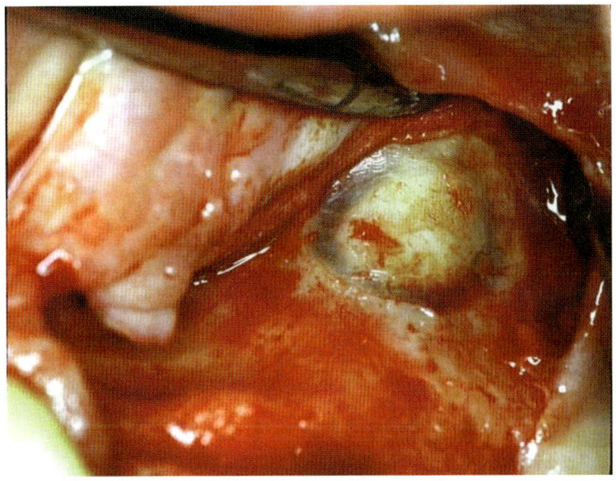

Figure 6.11 A view of an osteotomy window prepared with a number 8 round diamond bur to a depth sufficient for visualization of the gray membrane beneath the remaining alveolar bone.

When an implant is to be placed at the time of sinus augmentation therapy, an undersized osteotomy is always prepared. For example, if a wide-bodied Straumann implant is to be placed, a conventional osteotomy site would be prepared to a 4.2-mm diameter, after sequential use of 2.0-, 2.2-, 3.5-, and 4.2-mm-wide osteotomes. Such a site would only be prepared to a diameter of 3.5 mm

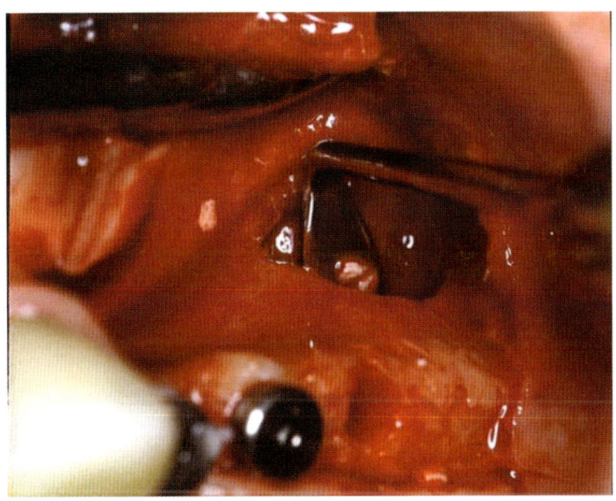

Figure 6.12 Following membrane reflection and partial filling of the subantral space with graft material, a curette is inserted into the created subantral space to protect the reflected membrane and window as an osteotomy site is prepared in anticipation of implant placement.

if an implant is to be placed at the time of sinus augmentation therapy. Precise techniques utilized for such preparation and implant insertion will be subsequently detailed. Whenever possible, the osteotomy site is prepared utilizing osteotomes rather than burs. This approach offers the advantages of both greater control during site preparation, and the compacting of bone lateral to the osteotomy site and thus to the inserted implant.

If an implant is to be placed at the time of sinus augmentation therapy, the sequencing of placement of particulate graft material is as follows:

- The anterior (mesial) aspect of the created subantral space is filled with graft material.
- The medial and distal aspects of the created subantral space are filled with graft material.
- The implant is inserted utilizing a handpiece held insertion device at 30 RPMs. Implants are never inserted with manual torque devices. It is impossible to control the lateral forces generated with the use of a torque wrench to insert implants as precisely as when a handpiece is utilized for implant insertion.
- The residual subantral space is "back filled" with graft material.

If a combination of bone paste and bone putty is to be employed to effect sinus augmentation therapy, the bone paste is inserted into the created subantral space, ensuring that it reaches the mesial, medial, and distal aspects of the created subantral space. An adequate amount of bone putty is then inserted to fill the subantral space in all of the areas except where the implant or implants will reside. The implant or implants are inserted. The subantral space is "back filled" with bone putty until the residual subantral space is completely filled.

The decision as to whether or not to place an implant at the time of sinus augmentation therapy has traditionally rested on the radiographic evidence of "available bone," defined as the height of the alveolar bone crestal to the sinus floor. Unfortunately, an assessment of the available bone is usually carried out through examination of periapical and panoramic radiographs. Such a diagnostic tool is inadequate, as it does not take into account the buccopalatal slope of the residual alveolar crest, or the morphology of the "underside" of the alveolar crest.

The implant supporting capabilities of a severely sloped alveolar ridge which presents with 5 mm of bone crestal to the sinus floor at the mid-crestal point is significantly less than that of an alveolar crest with a mid-crestal height of 5 mm of bone crestal to the sinus floor, which does not slope as it proceeds buccally or palatally. While a truer picture of residual ridge morphology is attainable with various three-dimensional scans, assessment at the time of clinical entry is indispensable to the decision-making process. The ramifications of this consideration will become obvious during development of a treatment decision tree for reconstruction of this region.

Assessment of the radiograph in Figure 6.13, taken at the time of treatment in 1989, led to the decision to perform sinus augmentation therapy in the maxillary right posterior region, and place a single implant at the time of augmentation therapy. This decision was based upon the perceived alveolar bone crestal to the floor of the sinus in the first bicuspid region. As will be discussed, such a diagnostic system is inadequate with regard to formulating an appropriate treatment plan.

Subsequent to healing (Figure 6.14), significant bone regeneration is noted both around the 19-mm-long titanium plasma-sprayed IMZ implant which had been placed, and in the area of planned implant placement in the region of the first molar. A 19-mm-long implant was placed due to crown implant ratio concerns. The need or lack of need for implants of such dimension will be discussed in Chapter 7.

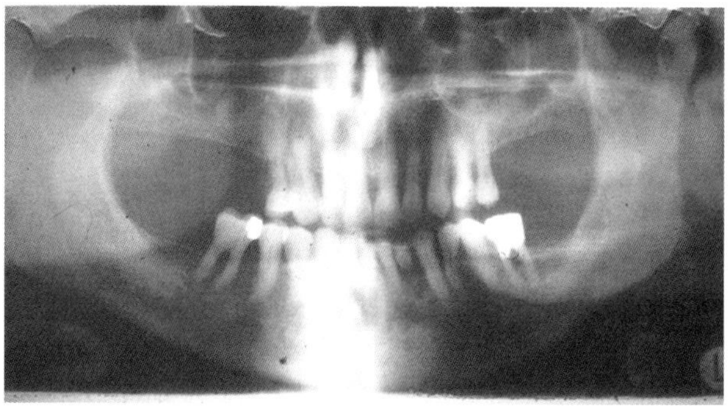

Figure 6.13 The patient presents with significant sinus pneumatization in his maxillary right posterior region. Sinus augmentation will be performed with simultaneous implant placement in the position of tooth number 4. The criteria utilized to determine the ability to simultaneously place an implant when performing sinus augmentation therapy have been modified and further developed since the time the patient was treated.

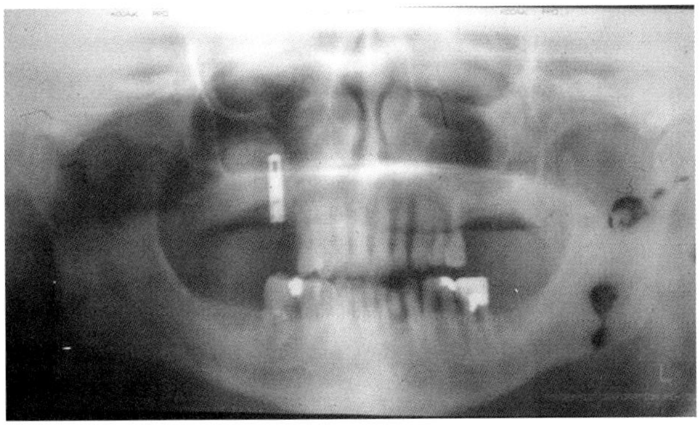

Figure 6.14 A radiograph taken eight months after sinus augmentation therapy and placement of a 19-mm-long implant demonstrates significant bone regeneration in the created subantral space.

When a patient presents with minimal residual bone crestal to the floor of the sinus (Figure 6.15), sinus augmentation therapy should be performed without simultaneous implant placement. The results are highly predictable, leading to generation of more than adequate bone for the placement of implants of sufficient dimensions to withstand functional forces over time (Figure 6.16).

It is not necessary to completely obliterate the sinus to effect implant placement. Before and after CAT scans (Figures 6.17 and 6.18) demonstrate regeneration of more than adequate bone to effect implant placement in the augmented sinus areas of a 36-year-old woman treated in 1990. Sixteen years postregenerative therapy and implant insertion, the implants are stable under function and there is no evidence of peri-implant bone loss.

Numerous authors have demonstrated the efficacy of sinus augmentation therapy, utilizing a variety of autogenous and nonautogenous graft

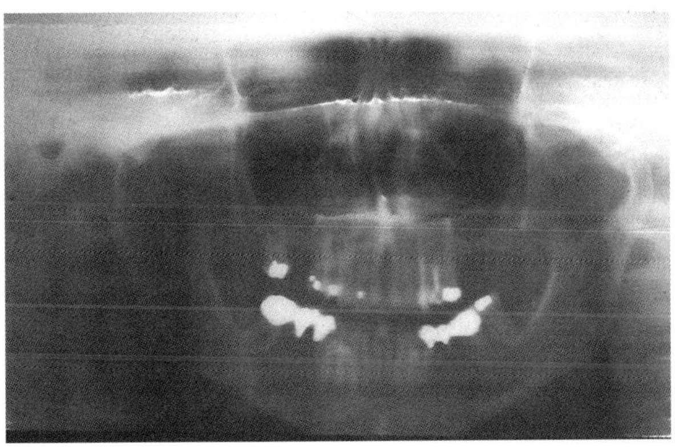

Figure 6.15 The patient presents with severe sinus pneumatization in the maxillary left posterior region.

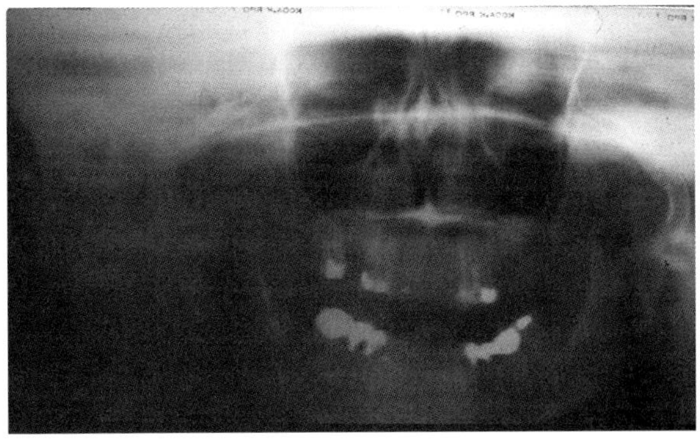

Figure 6.16 Eight months after sinus augmentation therapy utilizing Bio-Oss graft material, radiographic evidence of significant bone regeneration is noted in the created subantral space.

materials, with and without simultaneous implant placement. A recent paper documents the results of 1,633 implants placed in 814 augmented sinuses in two private practices, in function for up to 180 months (13). A variety of allografts and xenografts were employed as graft materials. The definition of

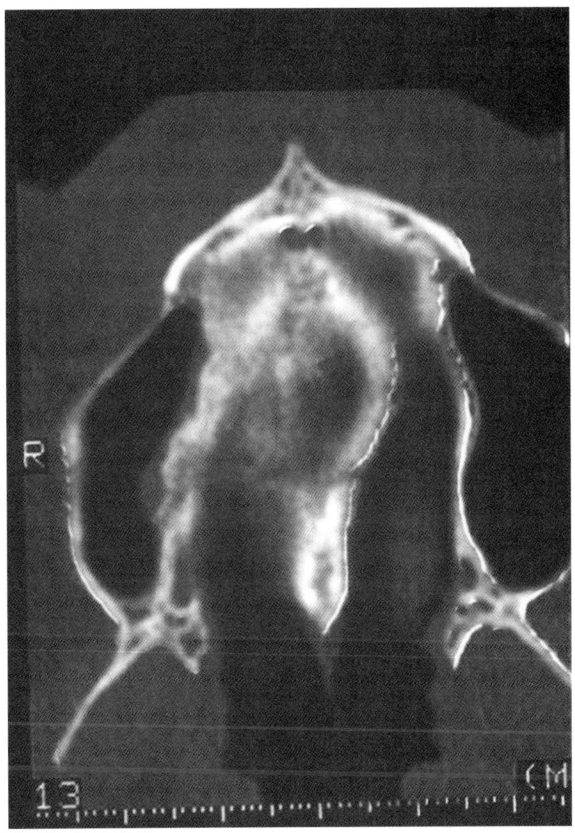

Figure 6.17 A CAT scan was taken prior to bilateral sinus augmentation therapy.

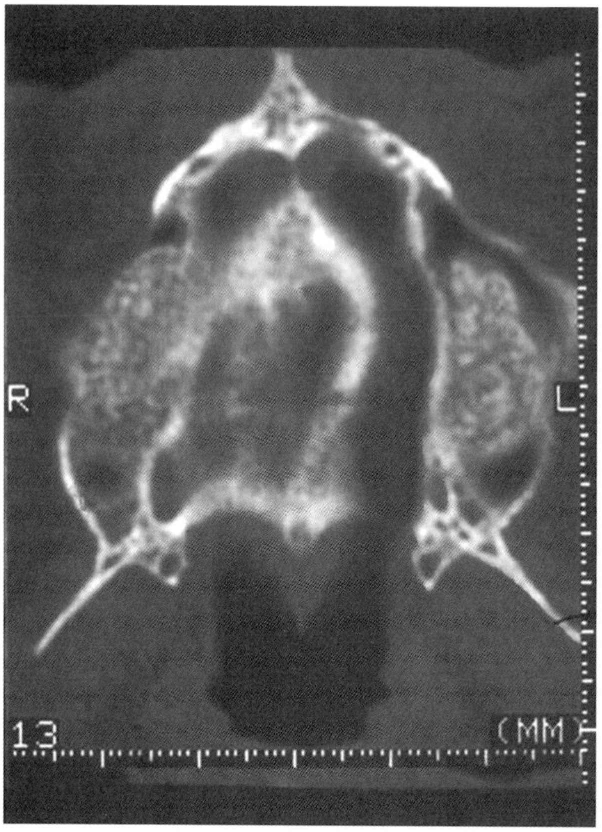

Figure 6.18 A CAT scan was taken eight months after sinus augmentation therapy was carried out utilizing Augmen (tri-calcium phosphate). Note the failure to fill the most anterior portions of the maxillary sinuses.

success was the ability to insert implants of at least 10 mm in length, which were wholly ensconced in native and regenerated bone in the augmented sinus areas. Utilizing this criterion, 608 or 614 sinus augmentation procedures were deemed successful, yielding a success rate of 99.0%.

Of greater importance is the success of the 1,633 implants placed in these augmented sinuses, in function over time. The mean time in function was 69.1 months. The success of the implants was judged via the criteria of Albrektsson et al., including sequential radiographs. The overall cumulative success rate of implants in function for up to 180 months was 98.1%. The breakdown of the augmentation procedures by approach and by materials may be seen in Tables 6.1 and 6.2.

Ridge augmentation therapy may be performed in conjunction with a sinus augmentation procedure.

Table 6.1 Sinus augmentation procedures performed by technical approach.

Clinical approach	Number of procedures	Number of procedures successful	Percent successful
Lateral	393	357	98.5
Crestal	28	28	100
Lateral approach with simultaneous implant placement	393	378	99.5
Total	814	808	99.0

In the aforementioned study, 64 cases were treated with simultaneous sinus and buccolingual ridge augmentation procedures. One hundred and twenty-seven implants were placed in these 64 augmented areas. All implants were functioning successfully at the time of data compilation for publication.

Figures 6.19–6.21 demonstrate such an approach. A 41-year-old female had been missing teeth in her maxillary right posterior sextant for approximately 20 years. Both the atrophic nature of the ridge and the pneumatized sinus are evident radiographically.

Flap reflection revealed a ridge of inadequate dimension for implant placement in the appropriate

Table 6.2 Procedures performed by augmentation materials utilized.

Material utilized	Number of procedures	Number of procedures successful	Percent successful
DFDBA/TCP	105	102	97.1
FDBA/TCP	13	13	100
DFDBA/FDBA	11	10	90.9
OGN/FDBA	40	39	97.5
Bio-Oss	370	368	99.5
Bio-Oss/DFDBA	208	208	100
Regenaform/ Regenafill	69	68	98.6

Bio-Oss, bovine bone matrix; DFDBA, demineralized freeze-dried bone allograft; OGN, osteogen; TCP, tri-calcium phosphate; Regenaform, DFDBA putty with cortical chips; Regenafill, DFDBA paste.

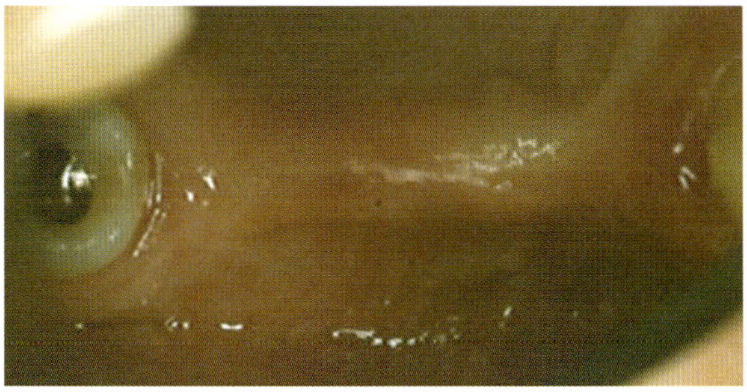

Figure 6.19 A clinical view of the atrophic residual edentulous ridge in the maxillary right posterior region.

positions. Particulate tri-calcium phosphate (Augmen) graft material was placed and covered with a laminar bone sheet. Neither titanium-reinforced Gore-Tex membranes nor fixation tacks were commercially available at the time the patient was treated.

The eight-month clinical reentry demonstrated marked buccal bone regeneration. Sinus augmentation had been effected, affording more than adequate bone for implant placement in ideal positions.

Membrane Placement

Disagreement exists in the literature regarding the need to place a membrane over the prepared osteotomy window following sinus augmentation therapy. While many authors have demonstrated successful treatment outcomes without the use of membrane over the prepared osteotomy (2, 3, 13, 14), Wallace et al. (15) have reported superior histologic and clinical results when a membrane was placed over the osteotomy window, as compared to sites where no membranes were employed.

In the study under discussion (14), 66 sites were treated with simultaneous sinus and buccal ridge augmentation. All of these sites required

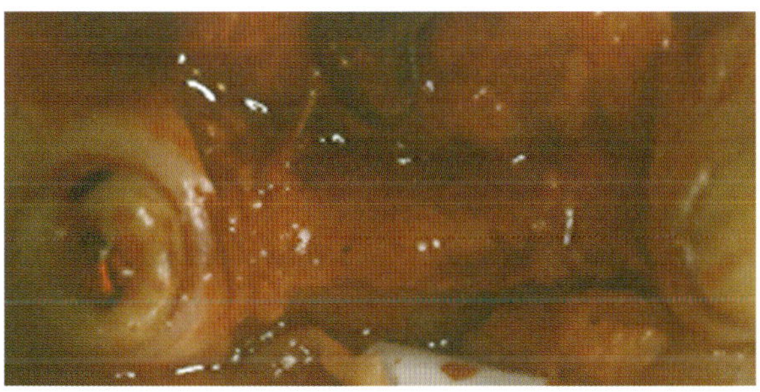

Figure 6.20 Flap reflection demonstrates inadequate buccolingual dimension of residual alveolar ridge for appropriate implant placement.

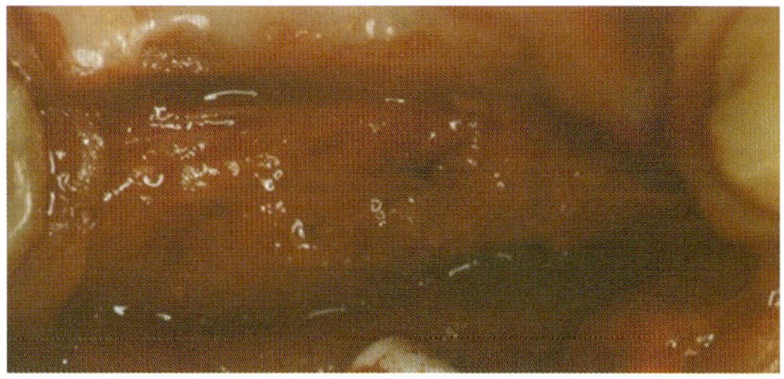

Figure 6.21 Nine months following simultaneous sinus augmentation with Augmen and guided bone regenerative therapy utilizing Augmen beneath a laminar bone sheet, marked buccal augmentation of the atrophic ridge is noted.

titanium-reinforced membrane placement to effect such regeneration. Exclusion of these sites from the data leaves 748 augmented sinus areas. Of these sites, 363 had resorbable membranes placed over the osteotomy windows at the time of sinus augmentation therapy. Five of these sinus augmentation procedures were classified as failures by the previously described criteria (1.4%). Three hundred and eighty-five sinuses were augmented without membranes being placed over the osteotomy windows. Three of these sites were classified as failures according to previously described criteria (0.78%). The difference between the two groups is not statistically significant.

The contention that a greater volume and quality of bone is regenerated in augmented sinuses, when membranes are placed over the windows, would also seem to have no clinical relevance in this study. Assessment of implant success rates over time, as defined by the criteria of Albrektsson et al. (16), demonstrates a cumulative implant success rate of 98.08% in the sites where membranes were placed over the sinus windows, and 98.11% where membranes where not placed over the sinus windows. It was necessary to compute the data to the second decimal point to see any difference between the two groups. This difference is not statistically significant.

There does not seem to be any advantage to membrane placement over prepared osteotomy windows at the time of sinus augmentation therapy unless concomitant ridge augmentation is performed, with regard to long-term implant success under function.

This data, obtained from two private practices, offers no support for the concept that membrane placement over the osteotomy window enhances sinus augmentation treatment outcomes. While there are no clinical disadvantages to placement of a membrane, it is difficult to justify the added expense to the patient of such membrane placement if no tangible clinical benefits result.

Graft Material Selection

Any graft material chosen for use in sinus augmentation therapy must meet certain criteria. The graft material must elicit no unfavorable host responses, must be easy to utilize, and must resorb predictably. Ideally, the graft material would also demonstrate a consistent level of osteoinductive capability.

There is no doubt that autogenous bone meets all of these criteria. As previously discussed in Chapter 2, the only disadvantage to autogenous bone is the need to procure graft material from a second surgical site, thus increasing the length of the surgical procedure, and resulting in a significant increase in postoperative morbidity.

The aforementioned paper documented the use of particulate demineralized freeze-dried bone allograft with tri-calcium phosphate; freeze-dried bone allograft mixed with tri-calcium phosphate; demineralized freeze-dried bone allograft mixed with freeze-dried bone allograft; osteogen mixed with freeze-dried bone allograft; Bio-Oss (bovine bone matrix); Bio-Oss mixed with demineralized freeze-dried bone allograft; and Regenaform (demineralized bone matrix block with cortical chips) mixed with Regenafill (demineralized bone matrix paste). The advantages and disadvantages of each are summarized in Table 6.3.

Table 6.3 Advantages and disadvantages of various graft materials.

Graft material	Advantages	Disadvantages
Autogenous bone	• Osteoinductive capabilities • Speed of regeneration	• Need to prepare the graft from a second surgical site
Tri-calcium phosphate	• Ease of use	• Unpredictable resorptive pattern • No predictable osteoinductive capability
FDBA/tri-calcium phosphate	• Ease of use	• Unpredictable resorptive pattern • No predictable osteoinductive capability • Greater cost than tri-calcium phosphate alone
DFDBA/FDBA	• Ease of use • Theoretical osteoinductive capability	• No predictable osteoinductive capability • Regenerated bone at eight months was softer than that following use of other graft materials
DFDBA/Osteogen	• Denser regenerated bone at the eight-month surgical reentry than DFDBA/FDBA mix	• No predictable osteoinductive capability • Unpredictable resorptive patterns
Bio-Oss	• Ease of use • Predictable resorptive patterns	• No osteoinductive capability • May take longer than 12 months to resorb if inserted inappropriately
FDBA/Bio-Oss	• None over Bio-Oss use alone	• Softer regenerated bone at eight-month reentry as compared to Bio-Oss alone
Regenaform/Regenafill	• Ease of use • Superior handling characteristics in the presence of a sinus membrane tear • Predictable osteoinductive capability	• More expensive than some other graft materials

DFDBA, demineralized freeze-dried bone allograft; Bio-Oss, BioGuide.

Tri-calcium phosphate use was discontinued due to the unpredictability of its resorptive patterns. Two patients had sinus augmentation therapy performed and moved out of the area for two and five years, respectively. When each patient returned and underwent implant placement in the augmented sinus areas, residual particles of tri-calcium phosphate were still evident.

In each of the few cases treated with a mixture of particulate demineralized freeze-dried bone allograft and particulate freeze-dried bone allograft, surgical reentry eight months post-augmentation therapy demonstrated regenerated bone of a soft, pliable consistency which was deemed inferior to that obtained with other graft materials, with regard to implant stabilization.

Particulate freeze-dried bone allograft mixed with Osteogen, while resulting in adequate regenerated hard tissue for appropriate implant stabilization eight months post-sinus augmentation therapy, often demonstrated residual Osteogen particles at that time.

Bio-Oss was employed in the greatest number of augmented sinuses. Treatment consistently resulted in generation of more than adequate hard tissue for implant placement and stabilization at the six-month surgical reentry visit.

Utilization of Bio-Oss grafts in over 3,000 guided bone regeneration and sinus augmentation sites has resulted in less than 20 sites demonstrated significant residual bone particles eight months postregenerative therapy, as was discussed in Chapter 2.

Published data document histologic results following the use of Bio-Oss grafts to effect sinus augmentation therapy, or the need for resorbable or nonresorbable membranes in fresh extraction sockets (17, 18). Both the augmented sinus areas (31 sites) and the augmented extraction socket defects (59 sites) utilized Bio-Oss alone as the graft material. While resorbable or nonresorbable membranes were placed over the extraction socket defects following graft insertion, no membranes were placed over the prepared osteotomies at the time of sinus augmentation therapy. Core biopsies were taken at various intervals between 3 and 12 months in the 90 grafted sites. The distribution and timing of the biopsies are listed in Table 6.4.

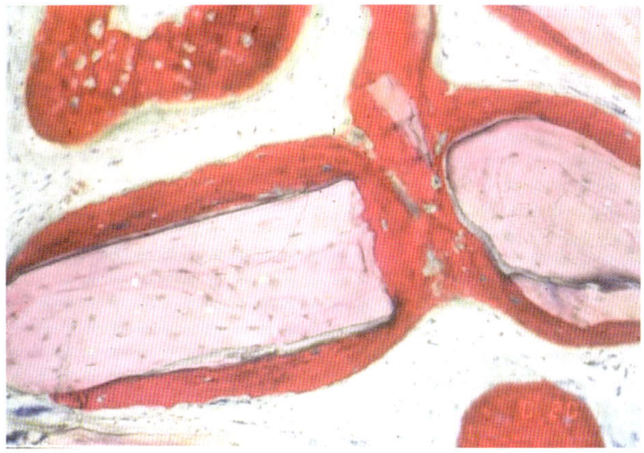

Figure 6.22 A histologic specimen taken four months following sinus augmentation therapy with Bio-Oss. Note the retained Bio-Oss particles and the viable regenerating bone surrounding the particles.

As expected, biopsies taken at 3–4 months and 5–6 months demonstrated a preponderance of Bio-Oss particles with viable regenerated bone surrounding them (Figure 6.22).

Biopsies taken at the 8- to 9-month interval demonstrated extensive regenerated bone and some residual Bio-Oss particles (Figure 6.23).

The 12- to 13-month biopsies demonstrated almost complete resorption of Bio-Oss graft material and extensive bone regeneration. The average compositions of the biopsies at the various time intervals may be seen in Table 6.5 (Figures 6.24 and 6.25).

Table 6.4 Biopsy timing following Bio-Oss use.

Therapy	3- to 4-month biopsy	5- to 6-month biopsy	8- to 9-month biopsy	12- to 13-month biopsy	Total
Sinus augmentation	3	9	14	5	31
Extraction socket/ ridge augmentation	6	40	6	7	59
Total	9	49	20	12	90

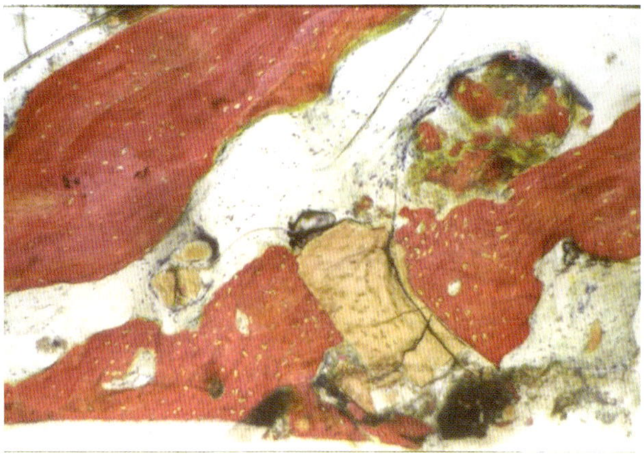

Figure 6.23 A histologic specimen taken eight months following sinus augmentation therapy with Bio-Oss. Note the extensive bone regeneration and the isolated residual Bio-Oss particle.

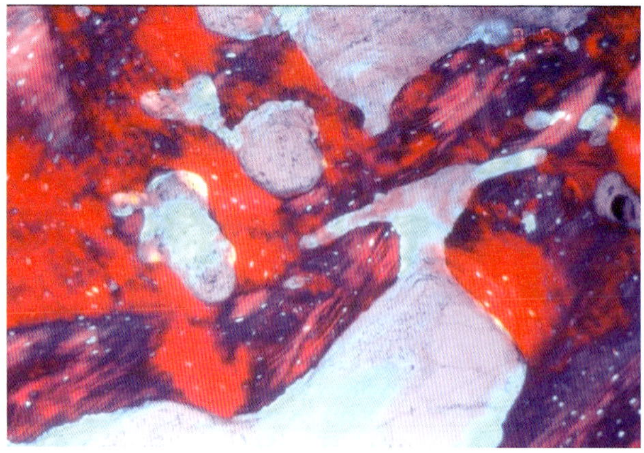

Figure 6.24 A 12-month specimen of a sinus augmented with only Bio-Oss. Note the extensive bone regeneration which has occurred.

Bio-Oss graft material has proven highly predictable in the treatment of various alveolar ridge defects and to effect sinus augmentation therapy. However, the need to wait 8–9 months to place implants in regenerating Bio-Oss grafts in larger areas, and the relative difficulty utilizing Bio-Oss when faced with a significant sinus membrane perforation, lead to the exploration of other materials.

The addition of demineralized freeze-dried bone allograft to the Bio-Oss offered no discernable advantages, and frequently resulted in generation of material of a less firm consistency at the eight-month reentry time than that attained through the use of Bio-Oss alone.

Employment of a demineralized bone matrix paste (Regenafill) in combination with a demineralized bone block impregnated with cortical chips (Regenaform) resulted in consistent regeneration of bone of adequate dimension and solidity to stabilize implants six months post-augmentation therapy. This is the only nonautogenous material utilized in this paper which predictably afforded the ability to place implants six months after augmentation therapy, as compared to the 8- to 9-month

Table 6.5 Core biopsy composition (%).

Time postoperative	Bio-Oss	Bone	Other
3–4 months			
Sinus augmentation	59.7	18.8	21.5
Extraction socket	59.1	19.4	21.5
Total	59.3	19.2	21.5
5–6 months			
Sinus augmentation	21.4	40.0	38.6
Extraction socket	18.7	34.5	46.8
Total	19.1	35.5	45.4
8–9 months			
Sinus augmentation	11.1	68.4	20.5
Extraction socket	11.3	69.1	19.6
Total	11.2	68.6	20.2
12–13 months			
Sinus augmentation	0.14	68.8	31.0
Extraction socket	0.13	68.8	31.1
Total	0.13	68.8	31.1

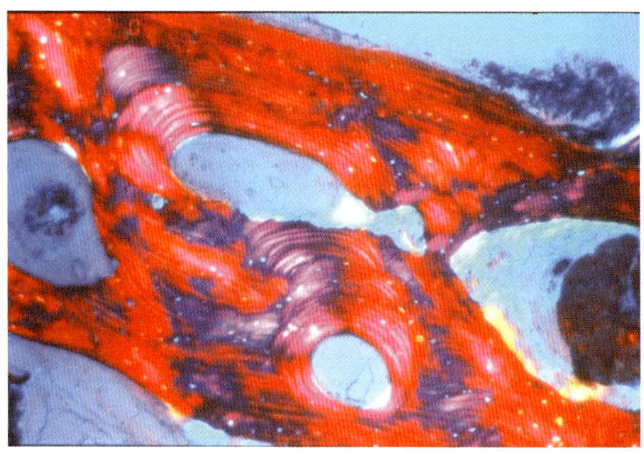

Figure 6.25 Another 12-month specimen of a sinus augmented with only Bio-Oss also demonstrates extensive bone regeneration.

time period for implant placement with all other graft materials utilized.

Regenaform and Regenafill differ from other mineralized or demineralized freeze-dried bone allografts in a number of ways. These bone allograft materials are always tested following sterilization for osteoinductive capability, utilizing the Urist model. If a certain level of osteoinductive capability is not met, the specimen is discarded. On average, 21–23% of all post-sterilization specimens are rejected in this manner. As a result, the clinician is theoretically assured of a minimum level of osteoinductive capability in each graft specimen utilized. No other commercially available allograft material undergoes such stringent testing. Six-month post-sinus augmentation histologic specimens of sites treated with a combination of Regenaform and Regenafill have consistently demonstrated new bone growth. A paper documenting the use of these materials in 87 sinus augmentation cases yielded a success rate of 98.9% (86 out of 87), with success being defined as adequate bone for placement of implants of at least 10 mm in length (19). These materials have also proven highly predictable beneath the appropriate covering membranes in effecting vertical and crestal ridge augmentation. Assessment of 334 sites treated with Regenaform, Regenafill, or a combination of both beneath resorbable and nonresorbable membranes, has yielded success rates at least comparable to those attained utilizing autogenous or other nonautogenous graft materials beneath membranes in similar situations. As explained in Chapter 2, the precise results attained following guided bone regeneration therapy are highly flap design and membrane selection dependent. However, the utilization of Regenaform and/or Regenafill beneath the appropriately selected covering membranes offers the advantage of osteoinductive capability of the graft and the ability to reenter large augmented sites six months postoperatively to effect implant placement.

This treatment approach is documented below.

Clinical Example One

A 47-year-old male presented missing his maxillary right molars. Radiographically, significant sinus pneumatization and ridge atrophy were evident (Figure 6.26). Six months following sinus augmentation therapy utilizing a combination of Regenafill and Regenaform, radiographic evidence of marked bone regeneration in the augmented sinus area is present (Figure 6.27). Regenaform and Regenafill are not radiopaque. As a result, any radiopacities noted in the augmented sinus areas are not merely a radiographic view of the bone graft materials which had been placed, but rather are indicative of regenerated bone. A six-month histologic specimen demonstrated healthy, viable bone in the augmented sinus region (Figure 6.28).

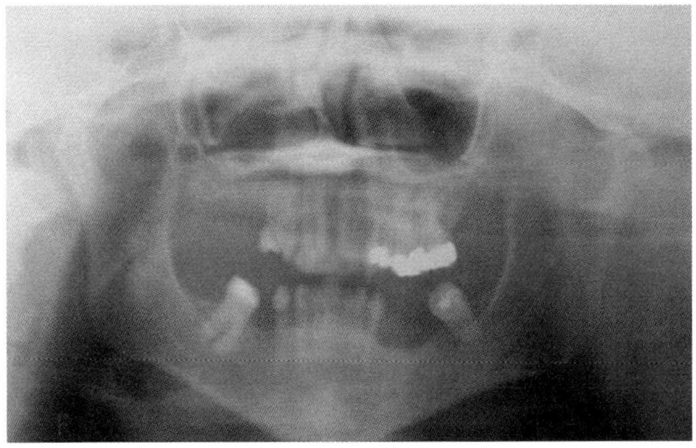

Figure 6.26 The patient presents with significant sinus pneumatization in the maxillary right posterior region and inadequate bone for implant placement.

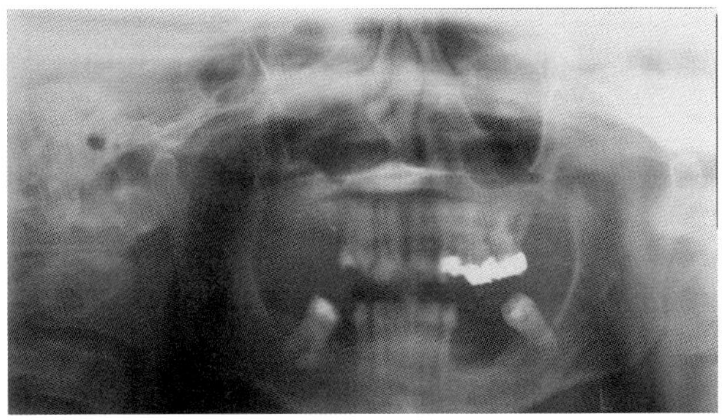

Figure 6.27 Six months following sinus augmentation therapy utilizing a combination of Regenaform and Regenafill, there is evidence of significant bone regeneration in the created subantral space.

Clinical Example Two

A 51-year-old female had been missing posterior teeth in both maxillary sextants for 19 years.

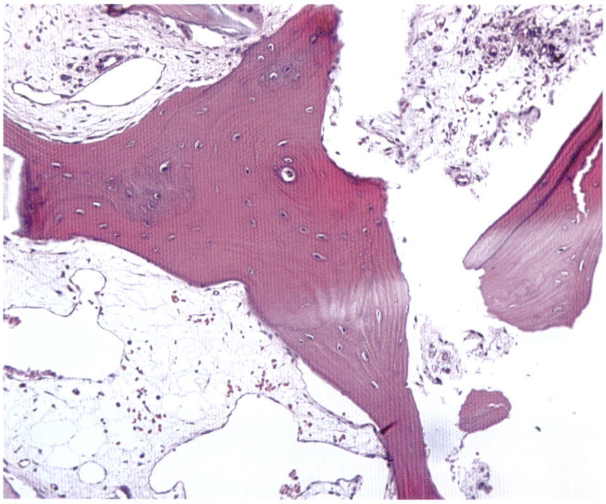

Figure 6.28 A histologic specimen taken six months after sinus augmentation with Regenaform and Regenafill. Note the healthy, viable regenerated bone.

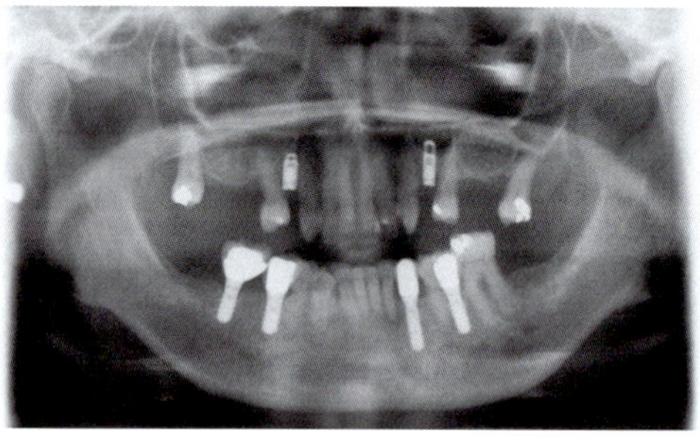

Figure 6.30 Six months following bilateral sinus augmentation therapy with a combination of Regenaform and Regenafill, marked bone regeneration is noted radiographically.

Bilateral sinus pneumatization was evident (Figure 6.29). Following sinus augmentation with a combination of Regenaform and Regenafill, extensive bone regeneration was evident radiographically (Figure 6.30). Periapical radiographs taken six months post-sinus augmentation therapy (Figures 6.31 and 6.32) demonstrated the degree of bone regeneration which had occurred in the augmented sinus areas. Histologically (Figures 6.33 through 6.37), healthy, viable bone was present in the augmented sinus regions. The delivery of this graft material in a resorbable matrix significantly enhanced its handling characteristics and decreased the length of the surgical procedure.

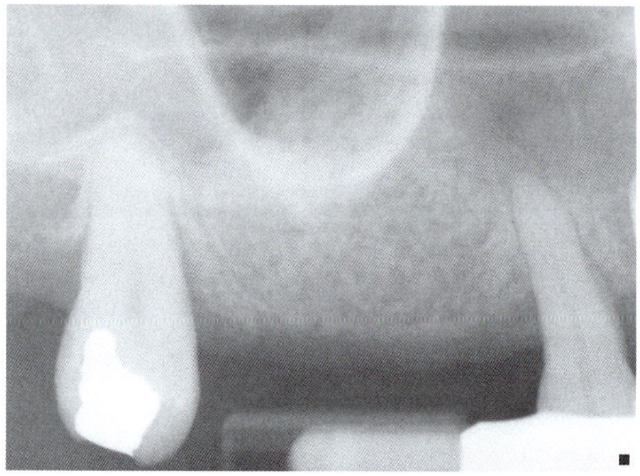

Figure 6.31 A periapical radiograph taken six months following sinus augmentation therapy with Regenaform and Regenafill in the maxillary right posterior region demonstrates extensive bone regeneration.

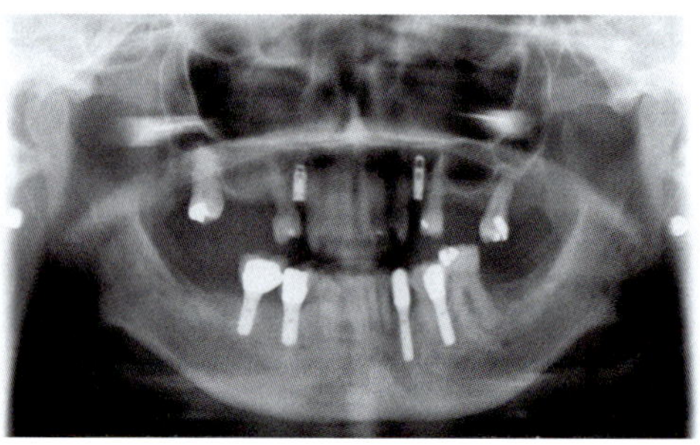

Figure 6.29 The patient presents with marked bilateral sinus pneumatization.

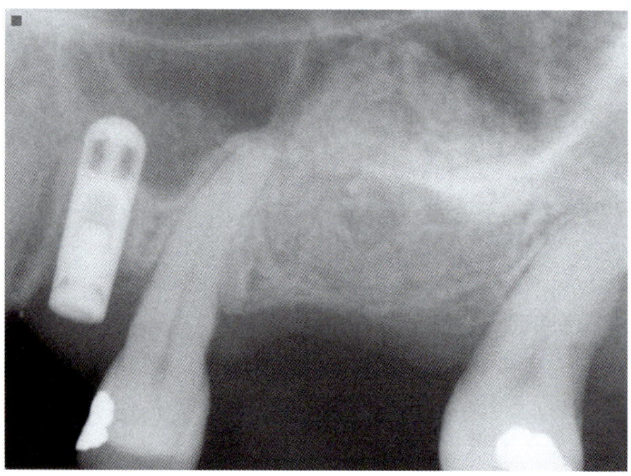

Figure 6.32 Extensive bone regeneration was also noted on a periapical radiograph of the maxillary left posterior region taken six months post sinus augmentation therapy.

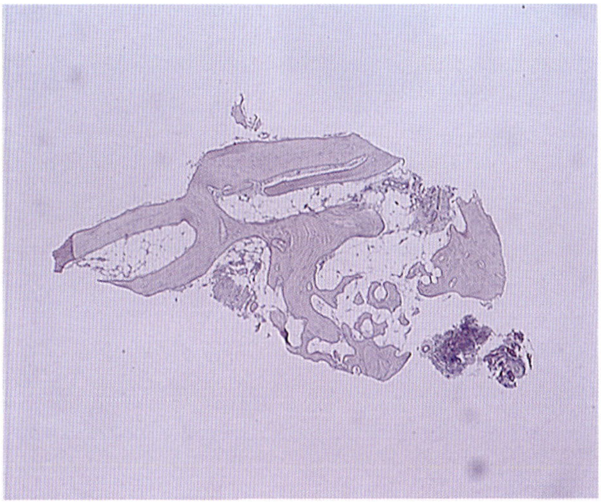

Figure 6.33 A histologic specimen of the augmented maxillary right sinus region taken six months post-sinus augmentation therapy demonstrates healthy, viable bone.

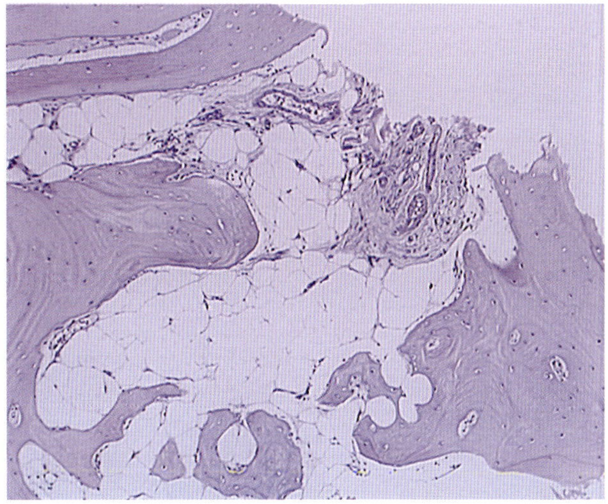

Figure 6.35 A closeup of the histologic specimen in Figure 6.37. Note the osteocytes in lacunae and the lack of retained graft particles.

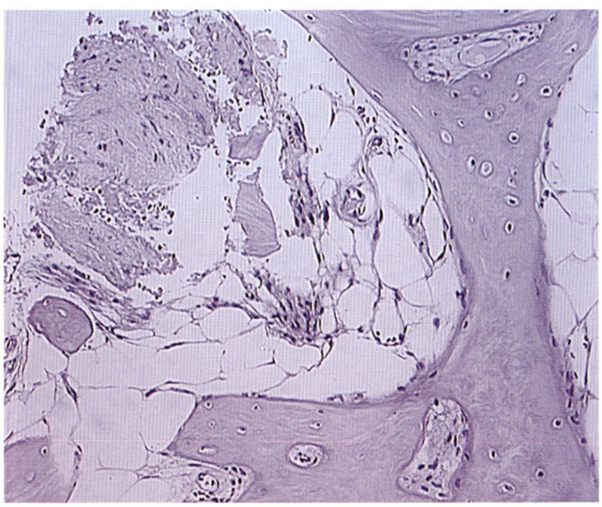

Figure 6.34 Another high magnification view of the histologic specimen in Figure 6.37 demonstrates osteocytes in lacunae and the lack of retained graft particles.

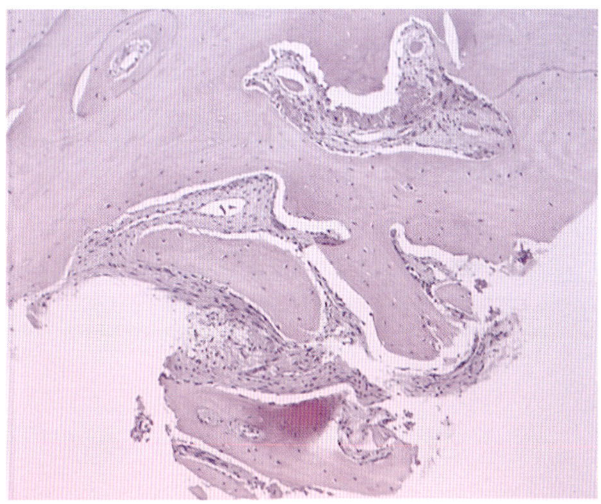

Figure 6.36 A six-month histologic specimen of the regenerated maxillary left sinus area. Note the healthy, viable bone which is present.

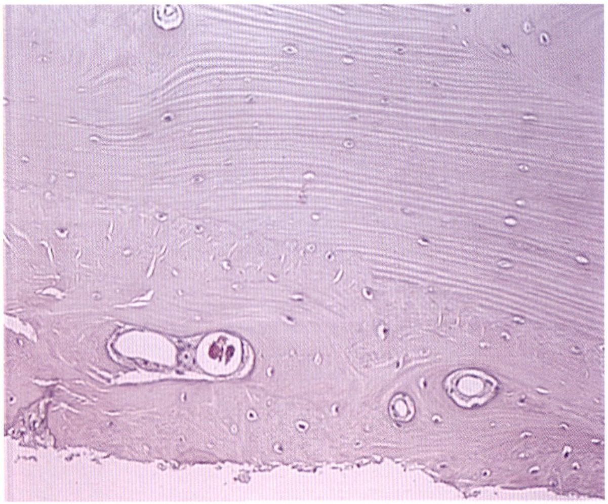

Figure 6.37 A closeup of Figure 6.40. Healthy bone and continued bone regeneration are evident.

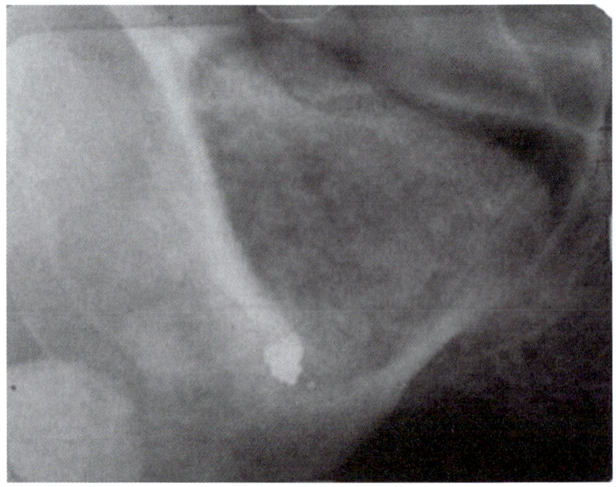

Figure 6.39 Following extraction of the maxillary first molar and sinus augmentation therapy with Regenaform and Regenafill, radiographic evidence of significant bone regeneration is noted six months postoperatively.

Clinical Example Three

A 46-year-old female presented with a fractured maxillary right first molar, which was a terminal abutment for a three-unit fixed splint (Figure 6.38). Following sectioning of the existing fixed splint on the distal aspect of the first bicuspid, both the first molar and the pontic in the position of the second bicuspid were removed. The defect was debrided, and sinus augmentation therapy was performed utilizing a mixture of Regenaform and Regenafill. Six months post-sinus augmentation therapy, radiographic evidence of extensive bone regeneration was present (Figure 6.39). Two osseointegrating implants were placed in the area of bone regeneration six-month postoperative (Figure 6.40). Histologically, healthy, viable bone was evident in the augmented sinus area (Figures 6.41 and 6.42).

As previously mentioned, the ability to successfully effect sinus augmentation with a variety of materials is highly predictable. However, such treatment outcomes must be considered merely

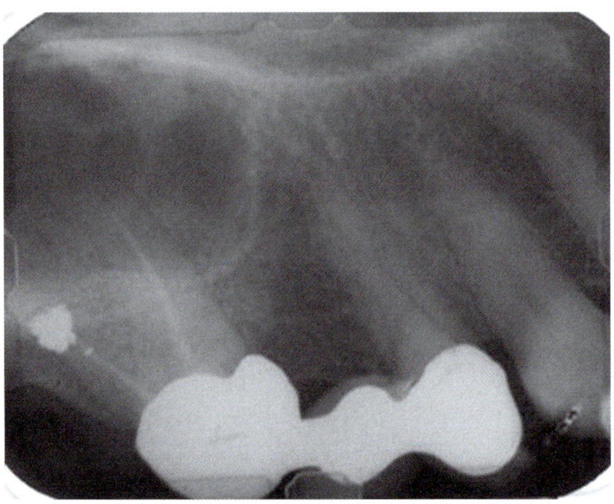

Figure 6.38 The patient presents with a hopeless prognosis for a maxillary right first molar.

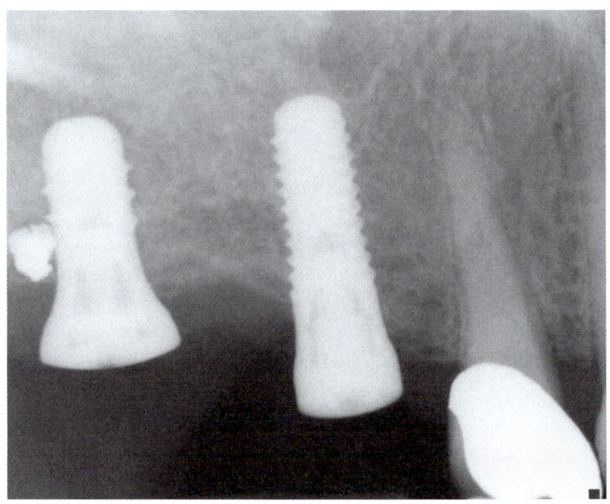

Figure 6.40 Two implants have been placed in the regenerated bone in the maxillary right sinus area.

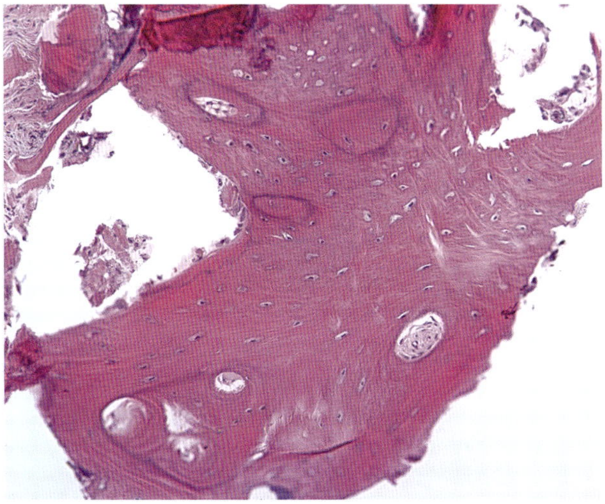

Figure 6.41 Note the healthy, viable bone which is present in a histologic specimen taken at the time of implant placement, six months after sinus augmentation therapy with Regenaform and Regenafill.

the **first-generation definition of success** when augmenting the posterior maxilla. Augmentation in an apicocrestal dimension alone, while providing function to the patient, often results in a less than satisfactory esthetic treatment outcome. In addition, in high stress situations, placement of implants in a more palatal position due to buccal alveolar ridge atrophy mandates a prosthetic design with significant buccal cantilevers, generating unfavorable forces under function. Such unfavorable force generation, coupled with the fact that narrower implants must be placed in more atrophic ridges, may lead to a compromised implant prognosis over time.

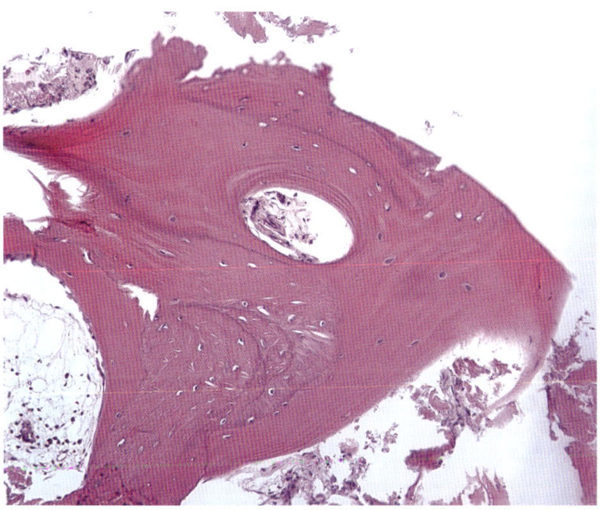

Figure 6.42 Another view also demonstrates healthy, viable bone six months after sinus augmentation therapy with Regenaform and Regenafill.

Clinical Example Four

A 41-year-old female patient presented having already undergone various levels of implant therapy. Hydroxyapatite-coated Micro-vent implants and titanium plasma-sprayed IMZ implants of different diameters had been placed in the maxillary and mandibular arches. Inadequate bone was present to allow placement of implants in the maxillary left posterior region (Figure 6.43). Examination of the patient demonstrated the presence of a severe parafunctional habit.

Utilizing techniques available in the late 1980s, sinus augmentation therapy was effected in the maxillary left posterior region. Four IMZ implants were placed eight months post-augmentation therapy. The maxillary and mandibular arches were reconstructed with fixed prostheses. The implant which had been placed in the position of the mandibular right bicuspid was not engaged due to its poor positioning (Figure 6.44). Intramobile elements were utilized with the IMZ implants in the maxillary left quadrant of the fixed prosthesis, both to allow retrievability and to help dampen parafunctional force transmission to

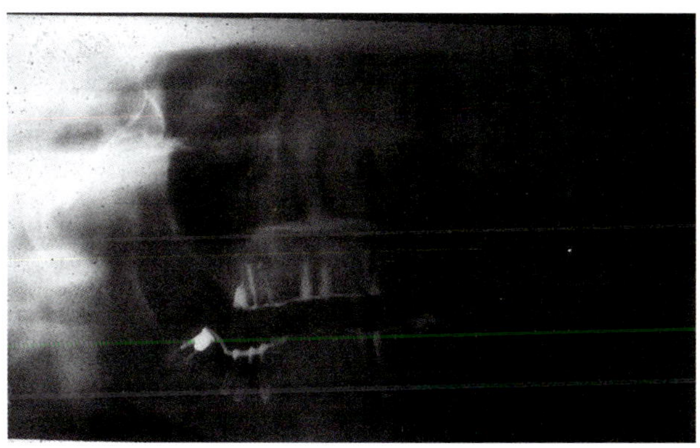

Figure 6.43 A patient presents with inadequate bone for implant placement in the maxillary left posterior region.

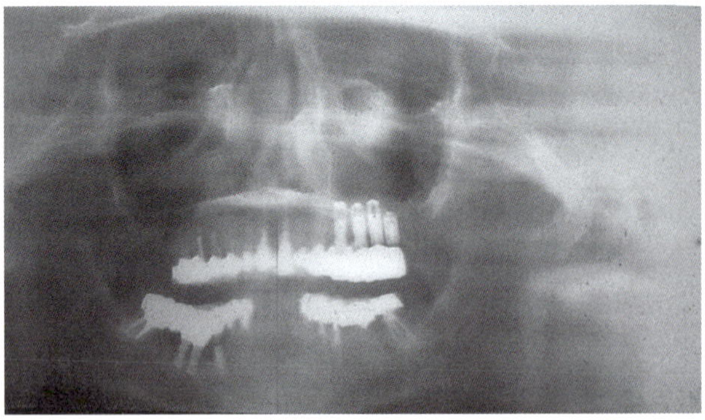

Figure 6.44 Following sinus augmentation therapy, subsequent placement of four IMZ implants and restoration of the patient's maxilla and mandible, appropriate function has been reattained.

the regenerated bone. Gold occlusal surfaces were fabricated with porcelain facings in an effort to further diminish load transmission to the implants and natural teeth, and eventually the supporting bone (Figure 6.45). A full frontal view demonstrates the compromises inherent in performing augmentation therapy in an apicocrestal direction without concomitant buccal ridge augmentation. In addition to the nonesthetic ridge lapped prosthesis which had to be fabricated in the maxillary left quadrant (Figure 6.46), narrower implants had to be utilized due to the limited buccopalatal dimension of the alveolar ridge. Fortunately, the combination of the aforementioned prosthetic design, intramobile element use, and bite appliance fabrication has yielded this patient a reasonable long-term prognosis.

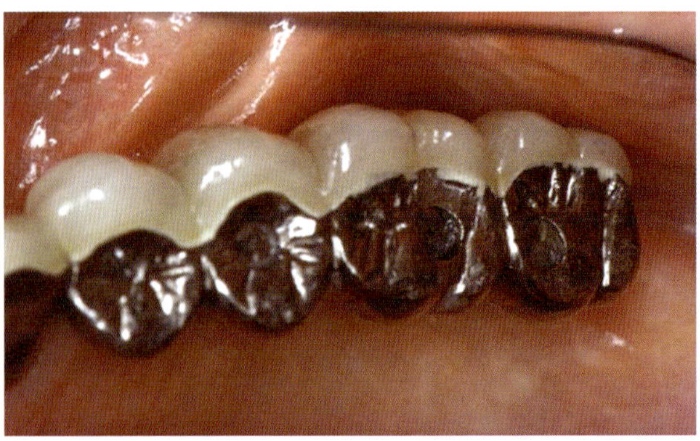

Figure 6.45 Gold occlusal surfaces were fabricated due to the patient's heavy parafunctional habit. IMZ implants were utilized with intramobile elements to help dampen the magnitude of parafunctional forces transmitted to the supporting alveolar bone. As a result, the prosthesis is screw retained.

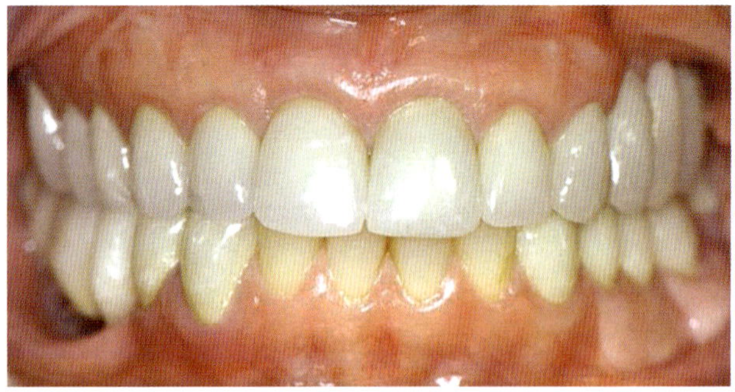

Figure 6.46 A frontal view demonstrates the compromises inherent in performing sinus augmentation therapy without concomitant buccal ridge augmentation, when significant ridge atrophy has occurred. Note the ridge-lapped implant supported crowns in the maxillary left posterior region.

LATERAL APPROACH SINUS AUGMENTATION THERAPY

The efficacy of sinus augmentation therapy, following use of a variety of graft materials, has been well established.

Blomqvist et al. (20) treated severe cases of maxillary resorption through the placement of autogenous grafts to augment both the anterior and posterior maxilla. Three hundred fourteen implants were placed in 50 patients six months after grafting. Two hundred two of these implants were placed in augmented sinuses, and demonstrated an 84% success rate in function, for a mean time of 28 months after the implant placement (approximately 20 months after loading). Seventy-five percent of the 112 implants placed in the grafted anterior maxilla demonstrated success under function during the same time period.

Cordioli et al. (21) performed simultaneous sinus augmentation and implant placement in 12 patients, placing a total of 27 implants. Three to 5 mm of bone remained crestal to the floor of the sinus prior to grafting. A 4:1 ration of bioactive glass to autogenous bone was utilized as a grafting material. Sinus augmentation resulted in an average hard tissue increase of 7.1 mm $\pm$ 1.6 mm. Twenty-six of the 27 implants were functioning successfully 12 months after loading, yielding a cumulative success rate of 96.3% at 12 months.

Daelemans et al. (22) treated 44 sinuses in 33 patients. One hundred twenty-one implants were placed, 113 of which were functioning successfully 3–80 months after loading (a mean postloading time of 40.2 months), yielding a cumulative success rate of 93.2%.

Khoury (23) placed 467 implants in 216 augmented sinuses in 216 patients. All implants were placed at the time of sinus augmentation utilizing autogenous bone blocks. Fifty-one membrane perforations were noted during sinus augmentation therapy and implant placement. Twenty-eight of the 267 implants failed. Nineteen implants failed at 0–12 months in function, and 9 implants were failing at the time of statistical compilation, yielding a 94% cumulative success rate for the period of 24 months to 6 years in function. The average time in function was 49 months. Fourteen of the failed implants were associated with sinus perforations notes during the surgical phase of therapy.

Mazor et al. (24) performed sinus augmentation therapy with concomitant placement of single implants in 10 sinuses in 10 patients. Five to 7 mm of residual bone remained crestal to the floor of the sinus prior to the augmentation surgery. Implants 13–15 mm in length were placed in all cases. At 36 months in function, all 10 implants were functioning successfully.

Olson et al. (25) placed 120 implants in 45 augmented sinuses. Eighty-eight of the implants were placed at the time of sinus augmentation. Thirty-two of the implants were placed 3–12 months after augmentation had been performed. Autogenous bone was utilized to effect sinus augmentation in all cases. Eight implants 10 or 10.5 mm in length, 74 implants 12 mm in length, and 38 implants 16 mm in length were placed. The quantity of bone present prior to augmentation therapy was not reported. After 5–71 months in function (a mean time of 38.2 months in function), the authors reported a cumulative success rate of 97.5%.

Peleg et al. (26) placed 160 implants in 63 augmented sinuses in 63 patients. Three to 5 mm of bone was present coronal to the floor of the sinus at the time of implant placement. Implant uncovery occurred nine months after placement. Sixty-four 15-mm-long implants were placed in 23 sinuses that presented with 3 mm of bone crestal to the floor of the sinus preoperatively. Thirty-nine 15-mm implants and two 13-mm-long implants were placed in 17 sinuses that presented with 4 mm of preoperative bone crestal to the floor of the sinus. Forty-two 15-mm-long implants and fifteen 13-mm-long implants were placed in 23 sinuses that demonstrated 5 mm of bone crestal to the floor of the sinus preoperatively. All implants were functioning successfully 2–4 years after loading.

Peleg et al. (27) reported the results of 20 sinuses treated in 20 patients with autogenous bone and simultaneous implant placement. All patients presented with 1–2 mm of bone crestal to the floor of the sinus prior to augmentation therapy. Implants were uncovered nine months after insertion. All 55 implants were functioning successfully 26.4 months after loading.

Valentini et al. (28) augmented 20 sinuses in 15 patients, utilizing bovine matrix. Fifty-seven implants were placed in the sinuses six months after augmentation had been performed. All patients presented with less than 5 mm of bone crestal to the sinus prior to augmentation therapy. Implants placed were 13- or 15-mm long and 4-mm wide. Fifty-six implants were functioning successfully, a mean time of four years in function, yielding a cumulative success rate of 98.2%.

van den Bergh et al. (29) augmented 62 sinuses in 42 patients utilizing iliac crest grafts. One hundred sixty-one implants were placed four months after grafting. All implants were functioning successfully 1–6 years after grafting. No mean time in function was reported.

Raghoebar et al. (30) placed 93 implants in 47 grafted maxillary sinuses. The sinus grafting material utilized was either iliac crest (86 implants), symphyseal bone (6 implants), or a maxillary tuberosity bone graft (1 implant). If less than 5 mm of residual alveolar bone was present preoperatively crestal to the floor of the sinus, sinus grafting was first performed and the implants were inserted three months later. If at least 5 mm of bone remained crestal to the floor of the sinus, the implants were placed at the time of sinus grafting. Five implants were mobile at implant uncovery (three placed at the time of sinus grafting and two placed three months subsequent to sinus grafting). All other implants were functioning successfully according to the criteria of Albrektsson et al. at a mean time of 16 months in function (ranging from 6 to 36 months in function), yielding a cumulative success rate of 94.6%.

Block and Kent (31) followed 170 implants placed in 53 autogenous bone grafted sinuses for 3–10 years. Twenty implants were lost in four patients during this time. Cumulative success rates were not reported.

Tong et al. (4) performed a retrospective analysis of 10 studies examining the efficacy of sinus augmentation therapy utilizing either autogenous bone, autogenous bone and hydroxyapatite, or hydroxyapatite alone. Four hundred eighty-four implants inserted in 130 patients following autogenous bone sinus augmentation were in function for 6–60 months and demonstrated a 90% cumulative success rate. Three hundred sixty-three implants placed in 104 patients treated with autogenous bone and hydroxyapatite to effect sinus augmentation were in function for 18 months and demonstrated a cumulative success rate of 94%. Two hundred fifteen implants placed in 50 patients whose sinuses were augmented with DFDBA and hydroxyapatite were in function for 7–60 months and demonstrated a 98% cumulative success rate. Thirty implants placed in augmented sinuses of 11 patients were in function for 18 months and demonstrated a cumulative success rate of 87%. When combined, the data from these studies yielded a 92.8% cumulative success rate of implants in function in augmented sinuses.

It should be noted that, while various authors have suggested criteria for determining the minimal amount of residual bone crestal to the floor of the sinus which is necessary for simultaneous implant placement and Caldwell-Luc approach sinus augmentation therapy, Peleg et al. carried out simultaneous implant placement with autogenous bone sinus grafting in 20 patients with only 1–2 mm of residual bone crestal to the floor of the sinus. It is also difficult to compare studies suggesting various residual bone requirements for simultaneous implant placement, when many of the studies employed autogenous bone grafts to help secure the implants while others utilized wholly particulate materials. For a list of the studies included, and a summary of their results, see Table 6.6.

Table 6.6 Sinus augmentation articles reviewed.

Reference	Number of sinuses treated/ Number of implants placed	Augmentation material	Simultaneous implant placement (Y/N)	Implant mean time in function (months)	Cumulative implant success rate
Blomqvist et al. (20)	100/202	Autogenous bone	N	20	84%
Cordioli et al. (21)	12/27	4/l bioactive glass/ autogenous bone	Y	12	96.3%
Daelemans et al. (22)	44/121	Variety		40.2	93.2%
Fugazzotto and Vlassis (14)	222/510	Autogenous bone	Y/N	12–73*	97.0%
Khoury (23)	216/467	Autogenous bone and DFDBA	Y	49	94.0%
Mazor et al. (24)	10/10	Autogenous bone	Y	36	100.0%
Olson et al. (25)	45/120	Autogenous bone	Y/N	38.2	97.5%
Peleg et al. (26)	63/160	Autogenous bone	N	31	100.0%
Peleg et al. (27)	20/55	Autogenous bone	Y	25.4	100.0%
Valentini et al. (28)	20/57	Bovine bone matrix	N	48	98.2%
van den Bergh et al. (29)	30/69	DFDBA	N	12–72*	100.0%
van den Bergh et al. (29)	62/161	Autogenous bone	N	12–72*	100%
Raghoebar et al. (30)	47/93	Autogenous bone	Y/N	16	100%
Block and Kent (31)	53/170	Autogenous bone	Y/N	36–20*	Unknown
Tong et al. (4)†	130–484	Various materials	Y/N	6–60*	Varied

Time in function reflects status at time of this publication.
*Mean time in function not reported.
†Retrospective analysis of numerous papers.
DFDBA, demineralized freeze-dried bone allograft.

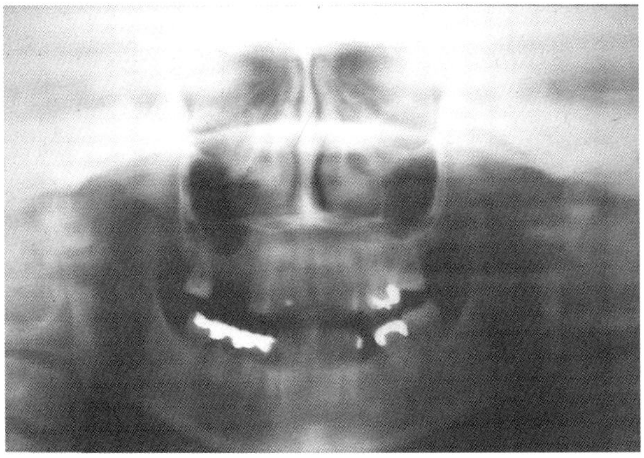

Figure 6.47 The patient presents with 6–7 mm of bone crestal to the floor of the sinus.

One of the potential complications of sinus augmentation therapy listed in various publications is the inadvertent devitalization of adjacent teeth. In the performance of over 750 Caldwell-Luc sinus augmentation procedures by the author, no adjacent teeth have been devitalized as a result of the augmentation procedures.

Clinical Example Five

Figure 6.47 illustrates a patient who presented with approximately 5–6 mm of residual bone crestal to the floor of the sinus, and a flat, buccopalatally broad alveolar ridge crest. Due to the quantity and morphology of the available bone crestal to the floor of the sinus, lateral sinus augmentation therapy with simultaneous implant placement was performed (Figure 6.48). Significant bone regeneration was evident on a radiograph taken eight months after augmentation therapy had been carried out

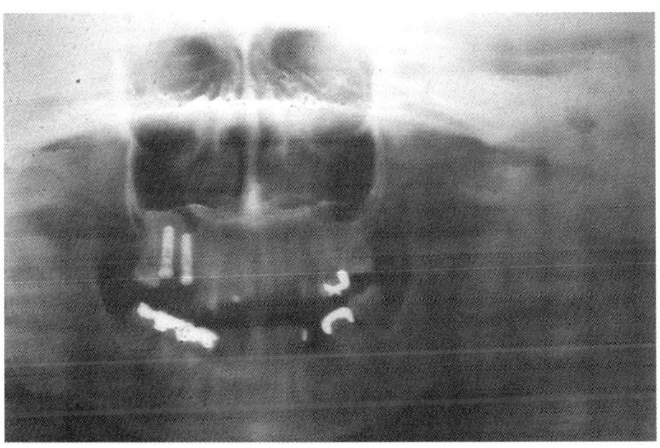

Figure 6.48 Following sinus augmentation therapy and implant placement, marked bone regeneration is noted.

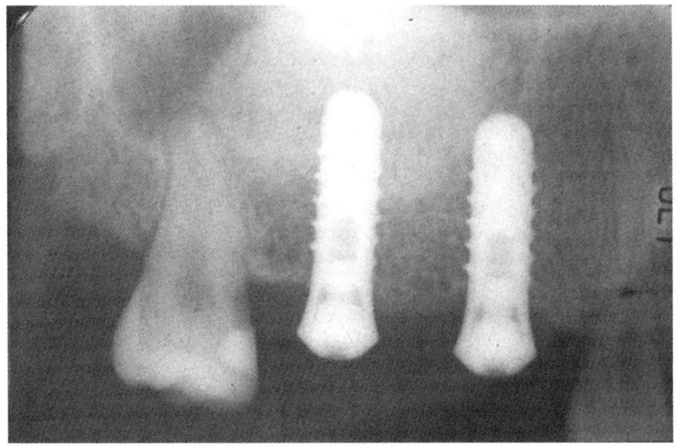

Figure 6.49 A periapical film of the augmented sinus area eight months after therapy has been performed. The second molar tests are vital.

(Figure 6.49). Despite the fact that the augmentation material was placed in close proximity to the root apices of the adjacent molar, this molar remains vital and demonstrates no symptoms of pulpal pathology.

The above outlined treatment underscored the need to develop a more demanding definition of success for augmentation of the posterior maxilla, beyond generation of adequate bone for implant placement (**the first-generation definition of success**) and simultaneous buccopalatal ridge augmentation therapy when needed to maximize esthetic treatment outcomes (**the second-generation definition of success**). It is evident from Figure 6.47 that the extent and morphology of the residual alveolar bone crestal to the floor of the sinus offered additional treatment options beside a Caldwell-Luc lateral sinus augmentation approach with simultaneous implant placement.

OSTEOTOME SINUS AUGMENTATION THERAPY

Summers (5) proposed the osteotome technique, in an attempt to augment the atrophic maxillary sinus in anticipation of implant placement in a simpler, less invasion manner. This approach eliminates the need for preparation of a bony window in the lateral aspect of the alveolus, and its subsequent rotation to displace the maxillary sinus. An "internal sinus lift" is performed through the utilization of sequentially sized osteotomes and particulate graft material. This technique may be utilized in conjunction with simultaneous implant placement, or to prepare a site for future implant placement.

Summers placed 143 implants in 55 patients at the time of performance of an osteotome sinus lift, and reported a cumulative success rate of 96% for these implants in function for 0–5 years. Implant success and failure rates were not examined relative to preoperative residual alveolar bone height crestal to the floor of the sinus.

Horowitz (32) placed 34 implants at the time of an osteotome sinus lift in 18 patients, and reported a 97% cumulative success rate for the implants, in function for 10–15 months. An average gain in alveolar bone height of 3 mm following osteotome sinus lift therapy and implant placement was noted by the author.

Coatoam and Krieger (33) placed 89 implants in osteotome-lifted sinuses of 77 implants, and reported a 92% cumulative success rate of implants in function for 6–42 months. The length of the implant placed and implant success were not evaluated in relation to the amount of residual alveolar bone crestal to the floor of the sinus preoperatively. In addition, no effort was made to document the gain in apical alveolar bone height.

Komarnyckyj and London (34) placed 16 implants in 16 patients following osteotome sinus lifts, and reported a 94% cumulative success rate of the implants in function for 3–38 months. The height of the residual alveolar bone preoperatively was 5.31 mm on the buccal and 5 mm on the palatal. The authors reported a 3.25-mm gain in alveolar bone height of 3.38 mm on the buccal aspect and 3.13 mm on the palatal aspect, following the performance of the osteotome sinus lift procedure.

Zitzmann and Scharer (35) placed 59 implants in osteotome-lifted sinuses of 20 patients, and reported a 95% cumulative success rate for the implants, in function for 30 months. An apical alveolar bone height gain of 3.5 mm after utilization of an osteotome procedure was reported. The authors stated that a minimum of 6 mm of residual bone crestal to the floor of the sinus must be present to employ an osteotome approach with simultaneous implant placement.

Deporter et al. (36) placed 26 implants in 16 patients following osteotome sinus lifts. These implants were in function for 6–36 months with a mean functional time of 11.1 months. All implants were functioning successfully at the time of statistical compilation. Greater than 3 mm of residual alveolar bone was present crestal to the floor of the sinus at the time of therapy, and the average implant length was 6.9 mm. Twenty-two of the 26 implants placed were 7 mm in length.

Cavicchia et al. (37) placed 97 implants in 86 sinuses augmented utilizing an osteotome approach. Eight implants were mobile at uncovery and three were lost in function, yielding a cumulative success rate of 88.6% after 6–90 months in function. Patients were treated utilizing this approach only if at least 5 mm of residual bone was present crestal to the floor of the sinus preoperatively. Cavicchia reported sinus displacement of 1–6 mm utilizing the osteotome approach, with a mean sinus displacement of 2.9 mm apically. Six 8-mm-long implants; twenty-eight 10- or 11-mm-long implants; forty-seven 13-mm-long implants; and sixteen 15-mm-long implants were placed. Of the eight implants mobile at uncovery, six were placed in patients in whom the amount of preoperative residual alveolar bone was less than 50% of the implant length. One patient demonstrated 5–6 mm of preoperative residual bone and had a 10-mm implant placed. Implants 13 mm in length were placed in two patients who exhibited 9–10 mm of preoperative alveolar bone, and a 13-mm-long implant was placed in a patient who exhibited 8 mm of preoperative alveolar bone.

Bruschi et al. (38) reported the results of 499 implants placed in 303 patients following utilization of a localized management sinus floor (LMSF) technique. While not identical, this technique is similar to Summers osteotome technique, but does not advocate placement of bone graft material. The 499 implants placed demonstrated a cumulative success rate of 97% in function for 2–5 years. All patients treated presented with 5–7 mm of residual alveolar bone crestal to the floor of the sinus preoperatively.

Winter et al. (39) reported the results of 58 implants placed in 34 patients following utilization of an LMSF technique. The cumulative success rate after 22 months of function was 91.4%. Winter et al. treated patients who presented with 4 mm of residual bone or less crestal to the floor of the sinus preoperatively, and reported that the sinus was "raised" an average of 9.12 mm. Four implants, or 6.9% of the implants placed, were mobile at uncovery.

Emmerich et al. (40) performed a meta-analysis of sinus floor elevation utilizing osteotomes in 2005. They concluded that "short term clinical success/survival of implants placed with an osteotome sinus floor elevation technique seems to

Table 6.7 Osteotome articles reviewed.

Reference	Sinus/ implants	Preoperative alveolar bone	Gain in bone height (mm)	Implant mean time in function (months)	Cumulative implant success rate
Summers (5)	55/143	NR	NR	0–60*	96.0%
Horowitz (32)	18/34	NR	3.0	10–15*	97.0%
Coatoam and Kreiger (33)	77/89	NR	NR	6–42*	92.0%
Komarnyckyj and London (34)	16/16	5.0–5.31	3.13–3.25	3–38*	94.0%
Zitzman and Scharer (35)	20/59	≥6.0	3.5	30.0	95.0%
Rosen et al. (41)	101/174	≥5.0, <5.0	NR	20.2	96.0%, 85.7%
Deporter et al. (36)	16/26	>3.0	NR	11.1	100.0%
Cavicchia et al. (37)	86/97	≥5.0	1–6	6–90*	88.6%
Bruschi et al. (38)	303/499	5.0–7.0	NR	24–60*	97.0%
Winter et al. (39)	34/58	≤4.0	9.12	22.0	91.4%
Fugazzotto (42)	103/116	NR	NR	32.7†	98.3%

NR, not reported.
*Mean time in function not reported.
†Time in function reflects implant status at the time of publication of current paper.

be similar to that of implants conventionally placed in the partially edentulous maxilla."

For a list of the articles reviewed, and a summary of their results, see Table 6.7.

Osteotomes are always utilized in conjunction with trephines of varying diameters when augmenting the edentulous posterior maxilla. The type of osteotome utilized is immaterial, as long as it meets the following criteria:

- The osteotome has parallel lateral walls.
- The osteotome has a concave end.
- The osteotome is offset to allow attainment of an appropriate angle for utilization.
- The osteotomes correspond to the bur diameters specific to the implant system being utilized, if implants are to be placed at the time of osteotome therapy.
- Applicable depth markings are easily visible on the osteotome bodies.

Trephines of internal diameters ranging from 2.0 to 12.0 mm are utilized, depending upon the planned treatment approach. The trephines have a 0.4-mm wall thickness. Therefore, a trephine with a 2.0-mm internal diameter has an outer diameter of 2.8 mm.

Osteotomes and trephines are utilized in one of the following manners to effect "external" sinus augmentation therapy in the edentulous posterior maxilla:

"External" sinus augmentation therapy utilizing trephines and osteotomes without simultaneous implant placement: A trephine is chosen of the largest diameter possible for utilization, without compromising the buccal and/or palatal line angles of the residual alveolar ridge. An osteotomy is prepared to within 1 mm of the sinus membrane, at 500 RPMs under copious sterile irrigation. If the floor of the sinus is not flat, the osteotomy is prepared to within 1 mm of the most shallow aspect of the floor of the sinus. A flat-ended osteotome is utilized to implode the prepared alveolar core to a depth 1 mm less than the depth of the initial trephine osteotomy. Should the core fail to move under gentle malleting of the osteotome, the osteotomy is prepared 0.5 mm deeper than the original cut, and malleting with an osteotome is repeated. The created alveolar defect is filled with particulate graft material and the flaps are sutured with interrupted plain gut sutures. The end result of treatment will be generation of alveolar bone both in the osteotomy site, and beneath the sinus membrane which has been lifted by the imploded core (Figures 6.50–6.55).

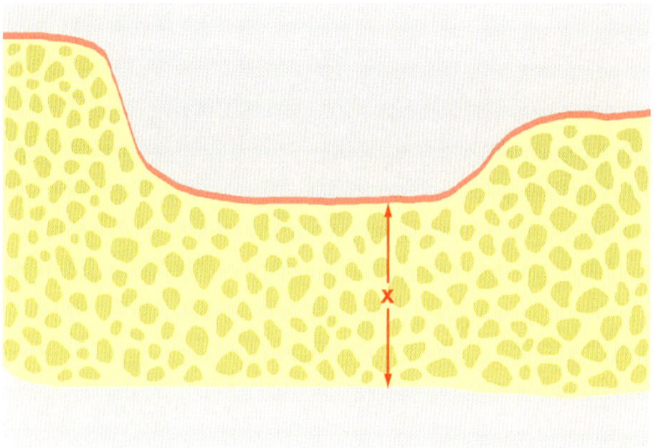

Figure 6.50 A diagrammatic representation of an edentulous maxillary posterior region. X is the residual bone crestal to the floor of the sinus.

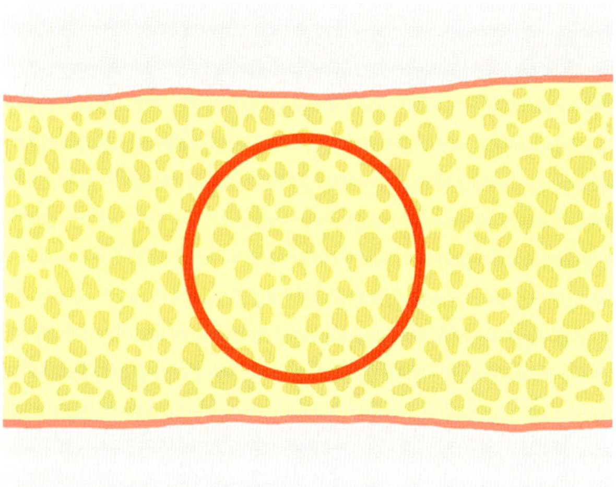

Figure 6.51 A trephine cut is made in the crest of the ridge utilizing the largest diameter trephine possible without compromising the buccal and palatal line angles of the ridge.

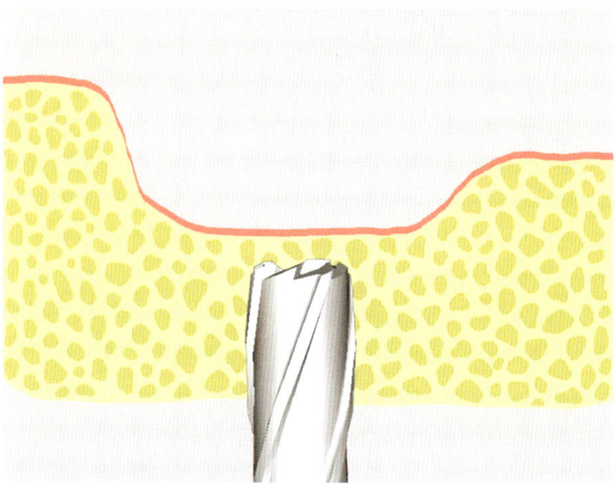

Figure 6.52 The trephine is carried to a depth 1-mm short of the sinus floor.

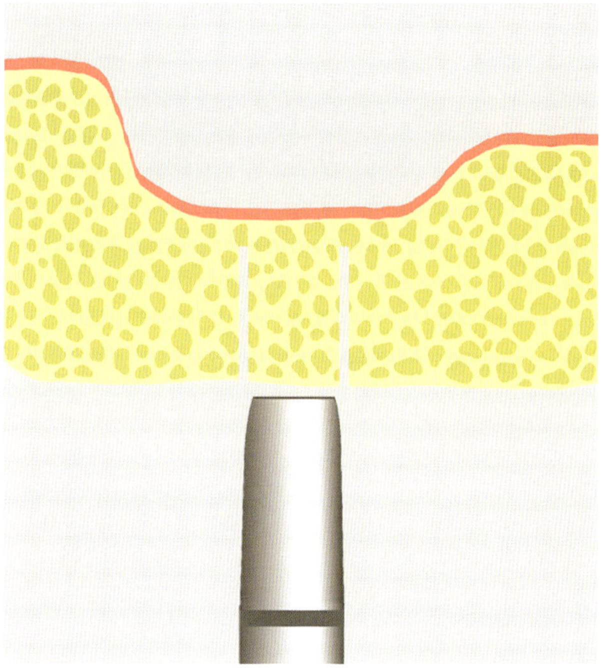

Figure 6.53 The prepared bone core is displaced with an osteotome.

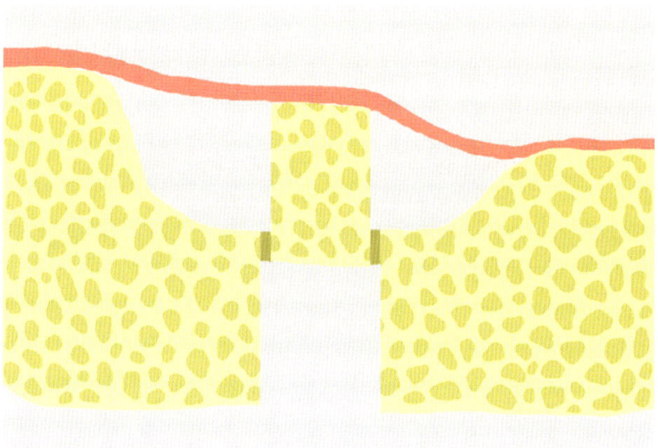

Figure 6.54 Core displacement occurs to a depth 1-mm less than that of the original osteotomy prepared with the trephine. The net result is both localized lifting of the sinus membrane and containment of the crestal aspect of the core within the residual alveolar ridge.

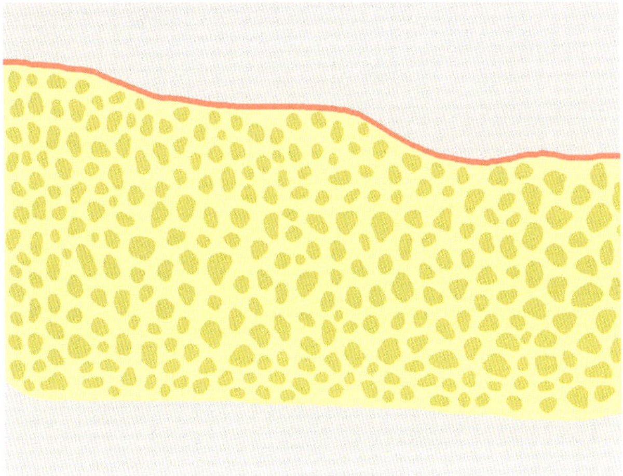

Figure 6.55 Following regeneration, more than adequate bone is present to effect implant placement.

It is imperative that the imploded core be displaced 1 mm less than the depth of the initial osteotomy. For example, if the initial osteotomy is cut to a depth of 5 mm, the core is imploded 4 mm. Considering the compressibility of the maxillary posterior alveolar bone, this means that the core will extrude beyond the most apical extent of the residual alveolus approximately 3.5 mm, lifting the sinus membrane as it does so. Such an approach is utilized to ensure maintenance of the integrity of the displaced sinus membrane, and its containing function. Displacement of the bone core from the osteotomy site beyond the most apical confines of the residual alveolar bone runs the risk of membrane perforation and displacement of both the alveolar core from the site to be augmented, and membrane containment of the core or any subsequently placed graft materials.

This technique of osteotomy preparation and implosion of an alveolar bone core is always chosen over that of the conventional Summers technique, which involves use of a tapered osteotome through the residual alveolar bone crestal to the floor of the sinus until the sinus membrane is reached, followed by incremental placement of particulate graft material which is displaced apically by osteotome use, thus displacing the sinus membrane. Use of the alveolar bone core technique offers a number of advantages over the conventional Summers technique, including:

- The ability to effect membrane displacement without risking contact of a tapered osteotome with the membrane itself, either during the initial penetration of the residual alveolar bone crestal to the floor of the sinus, or following placement of particulate graft material. Such contact between a tapered osteotome and the sinus membrane increases the chance of sinus membrane perforation and loss of particulate graft material from the site.
- Better support of the displaced sinus membrane through the use of an imploded core rather than compacted particulate material.
- A means by which to "plug" any sinus tears which occur with an autogenous bone core.
- Delivery of autogenous bone to the site of desired regeneration, thus hastening bone regeneration when compared to use of nonautogenous particulate grafts.

It is certainly possible that, even taking care to displace the core 1 mm less than the depth of the initial osteotomy cut, a membrane tear could occur at the most apical extent of the displaced core. However, such a tear will not result in displacement of the core through the sinus membrane as it is gently malleted to place. In addition, the core would serve as an autogenous bone plug at the site of membrane perforation, certainly improving bone regeneration in this region and helping to hasten membrane repair.

It is unrealistic to expect the displaced membrane to behave in precisely the manner diagrammed. Rather, it should be expected that the membrane will begin to "droop" as one proceeds further away from the supporting core. Nevertheless, such a technique will result in creation of more than adequate space for bone regeneration and eventual implant placement.

A 48-year-old female presented having lost her maxillary right first molar approximately 20 years previously. Radiographically, extensive sinus pneumatization and limited residual alveolar bone crestal to the floor of the sinus were evident (Figure 6.56). Following implosion of a bone core as previous described graft material was placed within the osteotomy space. Radiographic evidence of significant bone regeneration is present on the six-month postoperative radiograph (Figure 6.57).

There are two potential complications to this therapeutic approach.

When the trephine is removed after osteotomy preparation, the alveolar bone core may be within the trephine. In such a situation, the core is

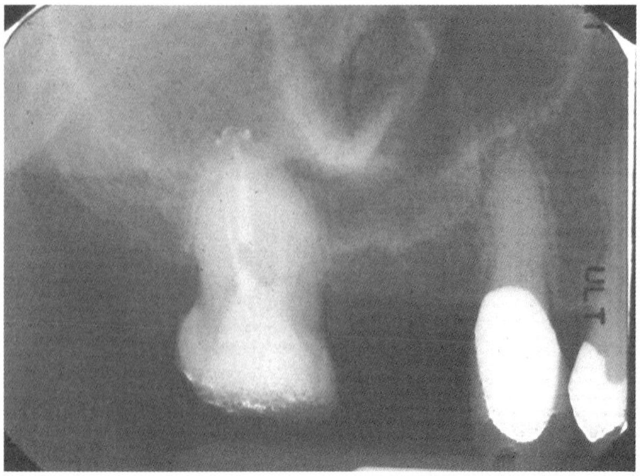

Figure 6.56 The patient presents with inadequate bone for implant placement in the maxillary first molar position.

carefully removed from the trephine and replaced in the osteotomy site. It is then gently malleted to the desired position.

The second potential complication is the presence of the bone core from the osteotomy site in the trephine upon its removal, compounded by evidence of a perforation through the sinus membrane. In such a situation, the alveolar bone core is once again carefully removed from the trephine, replaced in the osteotomy, and gently malleted to the desired position. The tear in the sinus membrane will be of no consequence, as an alveolar bone "plug" is now in place to help aid regeneration and repair.

When a membrane tear occurs utilizing a more "conventional" technique, repair is more difficult to achieve, as no autogenous bone plug is available to help effect such repair.

While it is tempting to utilize this technique and extend well beyond the guidelines presented, it is imperative to differentiate between anecdotal case reports and predictable treatment outcomes.

Clinical Example Six

A 61-year-old male presented with a failing fixed prosthesis in his maxillary left quadrant. A radiograph of the area demonstrated significant sinus pneumatization and limited bone crestal to the floor of the sinus (Figure 6.58).

The patient was treated through the implosion of two bone cores, in the positions of the second bicuspid and first molar. The cores were imploded well beyond the apical border of the residual alveolar bone. Demineralized bone paste was injected into the osteotomy sites, and demineralized bone putty imbedded with cortical chips was placed into the osteotomy sites following paste injection. A six-month postoperative radiograph demonstrated

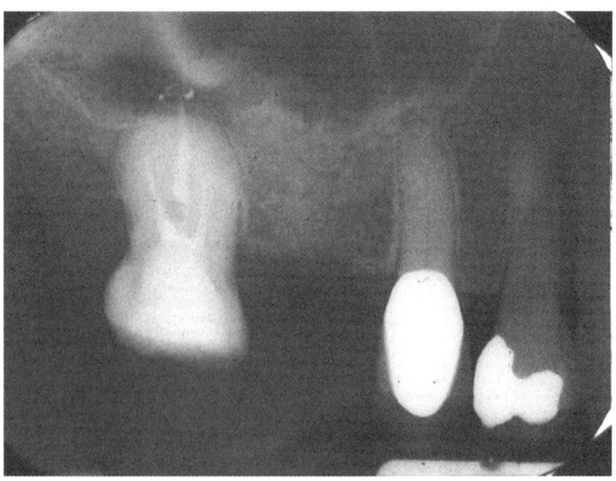

Figure 6.57 Five months after performance of a trephine and osteotome sinus lift as described, marked bone regeneration and sinus augmentation are evident. An implant of sufficient dimension to withstand functional forces may now be safely placed.

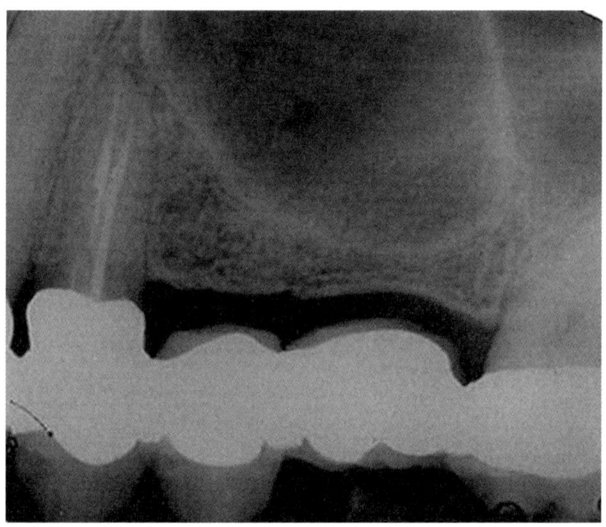

Figure 6.58 A patient presents with severe sinus pneumatization and inadequate bone for implant placement in the positions of the maxillary left second bicuspid and first molar.

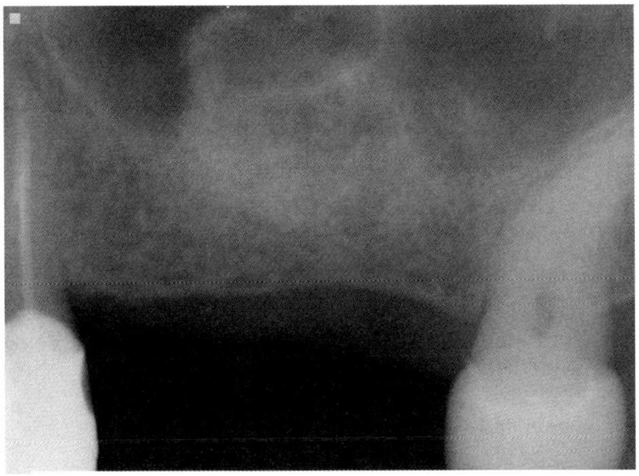

Figure 6.59 Following a dual trephine and osteotome technique and placement of particulate graft material, marked sinus augmentation is noted. However, imploding trephine bone cores apical to the residual alveolar crest should not be considered a predictable procedure.

marked bone regeneration in the augmented sinus area (Figure 6.59).

Despite the dramatic regenerative result of the case described above, such a treatment approach is not predictable. There is a danger inherent in examining the results of one or two cases and forming a treatment protocol from this assessment. Of the eight cases of similar severity treated in the manner outlined above, only the case shown demonstrated a satisfactory regenerative result. In contrast, all of the cases treated with the aforementioned approach in which the guideline of displacing the alveolar bone core 1 mm less than the depth of the prepared osteotomy was followed, resulted in more than adequate bone regeneration for appropriate implant placement.

A publication by Rosen et al. (41) documented the use of the Summers bone-added osteotome technique for simultaneous implant placement in the treatment of 174 sites. Following tapered osteotome use to penetrate the residual bone crestal to the floor of the sinus and lift the sinus membrane, particulate graft material was placed. Osteotome use was continued, to apply pressure to the sinus membrane through the graft material, furthering its displacement. Particulate graft materials were added incrementally followed by osteotome use, until the desired degree of membrane displacement was achieved. The implant was then inserted according to conventional manufacturer protocols.

A dichotomy was found between the sites of two subsets in this report. Of the 160 implants placed in sites which demonstrated at least 5 mm of residual bone crestal to the floor of the sinus preoperatively, the inserted implants demonstrated a success rate of 96.3% in early function.

In contrast, when implants were placed following use of the Summers osteotome technique in sites which presented with less than 5 mm of residual bone crestal to the floor of the sinus preoperatively, implant success in early function was 85.7%.

Extraction of this author's data from the paper yields the following findings. When implants were placed in 61 sites, which demonstrated at least 5 mm of residual alveolar bone crestal to the floor of the sinus preoperatively, all implants demonstrated success in early function. Of the two implants which had been placed in sites which demonstrated less than 5 mm of residual bone crestal to the floor of the sinus preoperatively, one implant was functioning successfully and one had failed, yielding an implant success rate in early function of 50%. Of course, a data pool of two implants is insufficient for meaningful analysis.

It is evident from these findings that the amount of residual bone crestal to the floor of the sinus available for implant stabilization is of significance. However, there is another piece of information which is necessary if we are to formulate an appropriate therapeutic decision tree. The length of the implant to be placed at the time of osteotome augmentation therapy must be considered. Placement of an implant which protrudes further beyond the apical border of the residual alveolar bone will require a greater degree of membrane displacement, and thus increase the chances of membrane perforation. Such perforation is especially important if particulate graft materials are being utilized, rather than a displaced bone core against the membrane.

Sinus augmentation, with or without simultaneous implant placement, is attainable through the utilization of the Summers osteotome technique or modified osteotome techniques as described by Bruschi et al. (38), Winter et al. (39), and Fugazzotto (40). However, Rosen et al. (41) reported a decrease in predictability when implant placement is performed at the time of osteotome sinus lift therapy, if less than 5 mm of preoperative alveolar bone is present crestal to the floor of the sinus.

Bruschi et al. (38) report a significantly higher success rate following localized management sinus floor augmentation with simultaneous implant placement in the presence of 5–7 mm of alveolar bone coronal to the sinus floor preoperatively, than Winter et al. (39) reported when employing this technique with simultaneous implant placement when 4 mm or less of residual alveolar bone was present coronal to the floor of the sinus. The papers by Bruschi et al. and Winters et al. seem to indicate a relationship between the ratio of implant length to residual alveolar bone and success rate both at the time of implant uncovery and under function. This fact is underscored by the findings of Cavicchia et al. (37), who reported that six out of eight implant failures (75%) at the time of osteotome sinus augmentation and simultaneous implant placement occurred when the height of residual alveolar bone crestal to the floor of the sinus was less than half that of the implant placed following osteotome therapy.

The performance of Caldwell-Luc or osteotome sinus augmentation therapy with simultaneous implant placement in the presence of minimal preoperative residual alveolar bone crestal to the floor of the sinus poses a number of challenges. Because minimal bone remains to help afford primary stability for the inserted implant following augmentation therapy, any inadvertent surgical trauma or widening of the osteotomy site will have a much greater effect than would be expected when implants were placed in a greater volume of bone. This fact may account for Winter et al. having reported that 6.9% of the implants placed in 4 mm or less of preoperative residual bone crestal to the floor of the sinus were mobile at implant uncovery.

The relationship between preoperative residual alveolar bone crestal to the floor of the sinus and the length of the implant placed at the time of osteotome sinus augmentation therapy appears to be significant. With the exception of Winter et al., who stated that they raised the sinus membrane an average of 9.1 mm, all authors reporting average height gain through raising the sinus membrane following osteotome therapy were all in the range of 3–3.25 mm. When taken in conjunction with the reported residual alveolar bone crestal to the floor of the sinus preoperatively by the same authors, it is obvious that the extent of the bone available following osteotome therapy for implant placement is limited by the amount of preoperative bone the clinician is working with. If the imploded alveolar bone is lifted well beyond the floor of the sinus, the clinician runs the risk of losing control of the position of the imploded alveolar bone, as well as tearing the sinus membrane and forfeiting its graft-containing characteristics. While there is no doubt that long implants can be placed after implosion of relatively minimal amount of preoperative alveolar bone, Rosen et al. demonstrated a significant difference in success rates when less than 5 mm of preoperative alveolar bone was present crestal to the floor of the sinus.

"External" sinus augmentation therapy utilizing trephines and osteotomes, with simultaneous implant placement: As a result of an analysis of cases previously treated with osteotome therapy and simultaneous implant placement over a number of years, and available literature as described above, the following formula is now utilized whenever contemplating implant placement at the time of trephine and osteotome augmentation in the posterior maxilla:

If X is the quantity of bone crestal to the floor of the sinus, the longest implant which will be placed following core displacement through trephine and osteotome use is an implant of length 2X-2 (42). It is important to realize that the implant length derived from this formula is the length of the implant in bone. For example, if a Straumann implant is utilized with a 1.8- or 2.8-mm collar and an 8-mm roughened surface body, the implant is classified as an 8-mm-long implant. Such an implant would be appropriate for use if 5 mm of residual alveolar bone remained crestal to the floor of the sinus ($(2 \times 5) - 2 = 8$).

The success and failure rates of 116 implants placed following osteotomy preparation with a trephine and displacement of the alveolar core with an osteotome as previously described, in function for up to four years, has been documented. All implants were placed following the guidelines of 2X-2, with X being the height of the residual bone crestal to the floor of the sinus. Two implants were mobile at abutment connection. No implants were lost in function, yielding a cumulative success rate of 98.3% (43).

Implants are mobile at uncovery in systemically healthy patients due to one of two causes: The first is failure to control forces generated on the healing site by an overlying removable prosthesis. The second cause of an implants failure to achieve osseointegration is technical in nature. If the osteotomy preparation results in excessive heat generation, undue mechanical trauma to the receptor site bone, or over widening of the site in situations where minimal bone height is present for initial stabilization of the implant, implant failure may result. While a cumulative success rate of 98.3% is comparable to the 98.4% cumulative success rate of implants in function obtained following "conventional" Caldwell-Luc sinus augmentation therapy, the two implants mobile at abutment connection mandated the development of a less traumatic surgical approach.

To avoid such a problem, the following protocol is employed when placing implants at the time of trephine and osteotome use.

A trephine is utilized with a 2-mm internal diameter and a 2.8-mm external diameter to prepare an osteotomy to within 1 mm of the floor of the sinus, at 550 RPM. The prepared core of bone is imploded to a depth of 1 mm less than that of the initial trephine osteotomy. Flat-ended osteotomes are utilized to widen the osteotomy site to one bur size less than conventional preparation. For example, if a 4.8-mm-wide body Straumann implant is to be placed, osteotome widening of the site occurs to 3.5 mm. A 4.2-mm-wide bone tap is then employed to a depth of 2 threads. A 4.8-mm-wide body Straumann implant is placed at 30 RPMs. The conventional diameter osteotomy attained to the depth of 2 threads of the bone tap allows placement of the implant without any "wiggling" and undesirable overenlarging of the entry to the osteotomy. The undersized osteotomy results in compression and compaction of the bone lateral to the implant as it is inserted (Figures 6.60–6.69).

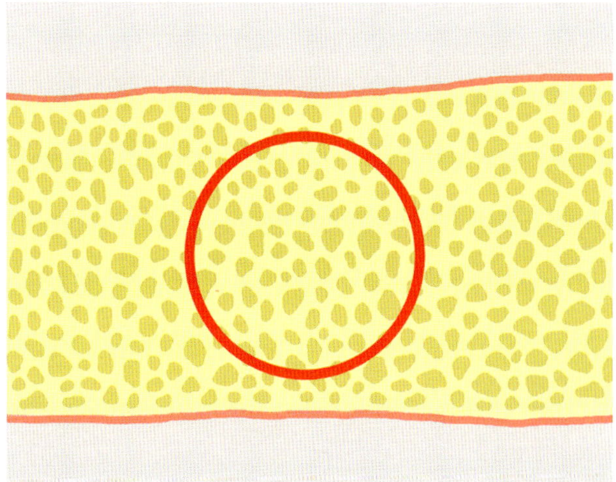

Figure 6.61 When simultaneous implant placement is to be carried out, a trephine is utilized with a 2.0-mm internal diameter, a 0.4-mm wall thickness, and a 2.8-mm external diameter.

This modified implant insertion technique has proven highly predictable. Following its utilization for placement of over 450 implants, no implants have been mobile at abutment connection. A further modification of this technique is employed when implants are placed in the posterior maxilla without concomitant internal sinus lift therapy. A 2.2-mm-wide bur at 500 RPMs is taken to the desired depth of the osteotomy. Sequentially sized osteotomes are next utilized as outlined to prepare an undersized osteotomy. A normal size bone tap is employed for two revolutions, and an appropriately

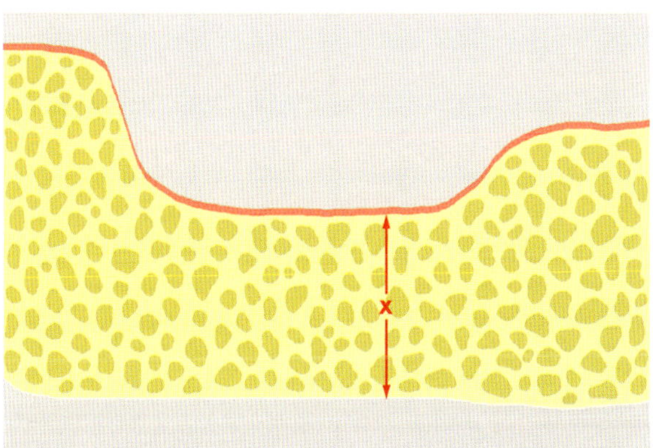

Figure 6.60 Another view of an edentulous posterior maxilla. X is the residual bone crestal to the floor of the sinus.

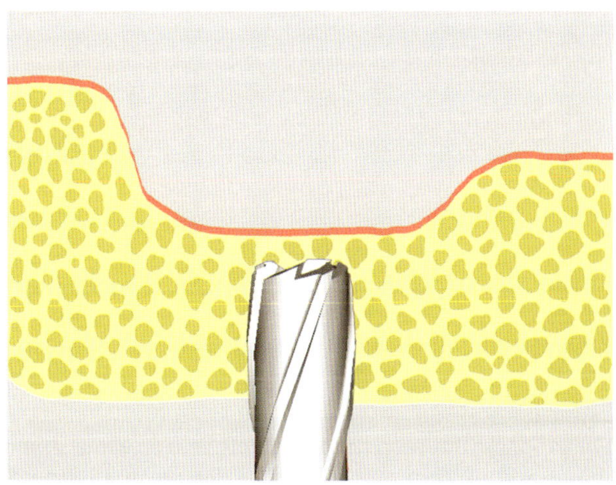

Figure 6.62 A trephine is carried to a depth of 1 mm less than the floor of the sinus.

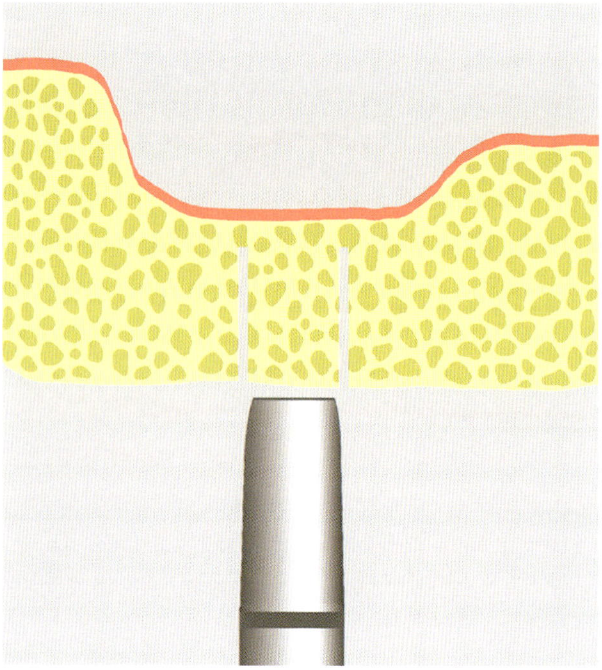

Figure 6.63 The 2.0-mm bone core is displaced utilizing an osteotome and gentle malleting.

sized implant is placed. This modified technique has been employed in the insertion of over 500 implants in the posterior maxilla. No implants have been mobile at uncovery.

The predictability of this modified implant insertion technique in conjunction with an osteotome

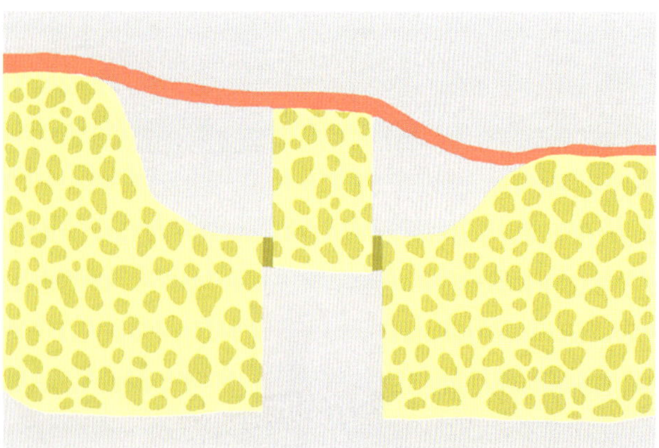

Figure 6.64 The prepared bone core is displaced 1 mm less than the depth of the original trephine cut to ensure that its most crestal aspect is contained within the confines of the residual alveolar bone.

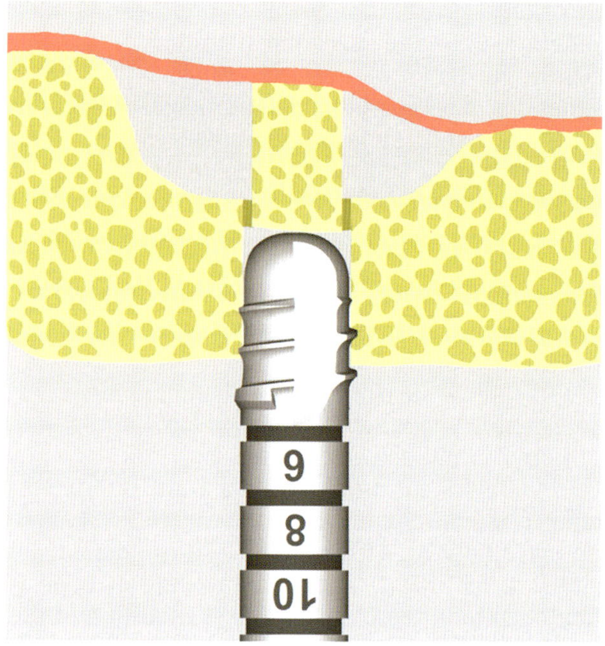

Figure 6.65 The osteotomy is enlarged to one bur size smaller than a conventional osteotomy for the implant to be placed. A conventional size bone tap is utilized to a depth of two revolutions.

and trephine sinus lift is demonstrated below. A patient presents missing all molars and the second premolar in her maxillary right posterior sextant. An implant was inserted in the first molar position following use of the modified osteotomy technique in conjunction with a trephine and osteotome sinus

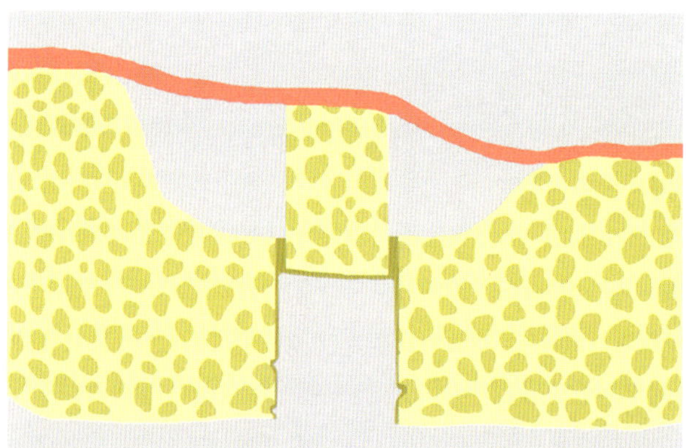

Figure 6.66 The prepared osteotomy site is now characterized by conventional size tapping at its most crestal aspect and an undersized diameter along the remaining lateral walls of the osteotomy.

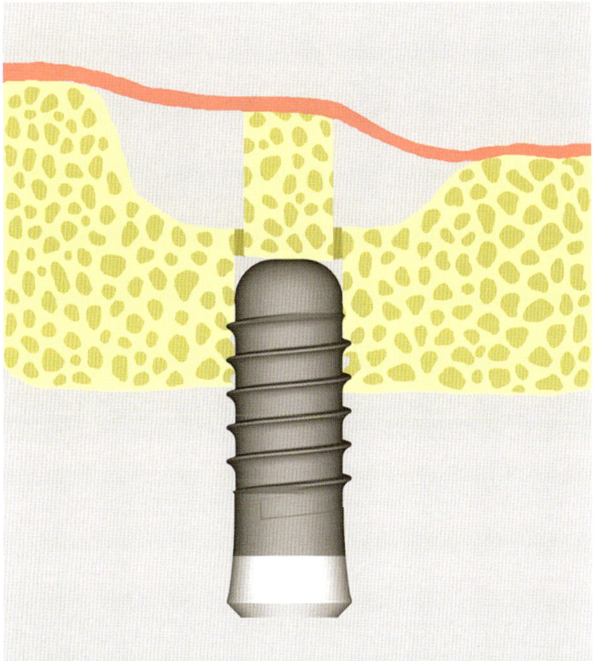

Figure 6.67 An implant is inserted utilizing a handpiece at 30 RPMs. The implant will engage the tapped area of the osteotomy without wobbling and distorting the osteotomy site. As the implant proceeds along the length of the osteotomy, the bone on the lateral walls of the implant in the undersized area is compressed.

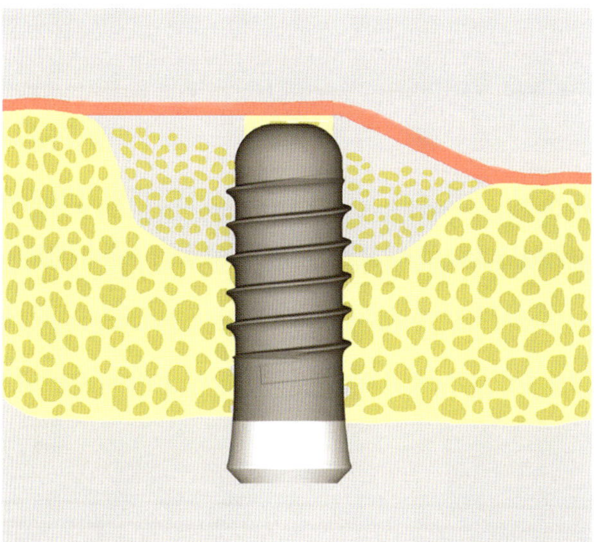

Figure 6.68 The implant encounters the displaced alveolar bone core and rotates the core; displaces the core further apically; compresses the core and crushes and displaces portions of the core laterally. An implant which is inserted at 30 RPMs under gentle pressure will not force the core through the displaced sinus membrane.

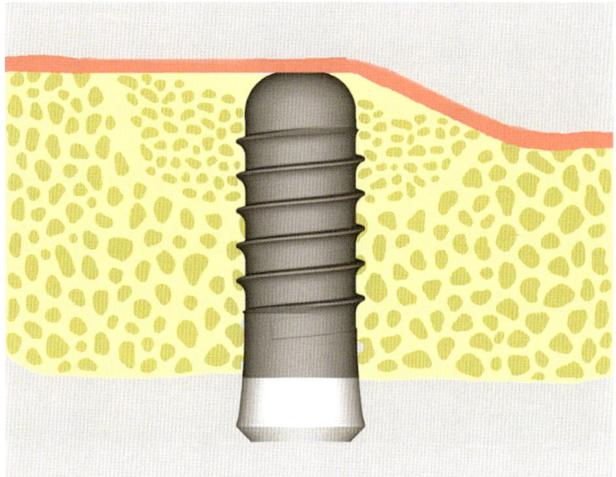

Figure 6.69 Following bone regeneration, the implant is surrounded by healthy, viable bone.

lift. An implant was placed in the second premolar position utilizing the modified osteotomy preparation technique without sinus lift therapy (Figure 6.70).

A radiographic view of the implants five-plus years in function demonstrates maintenance of both crestal bone around the implants and the bone around the "apex" of the implant placed at the time of osteotome and trephine sinus lift therapy (Figure 6.71).

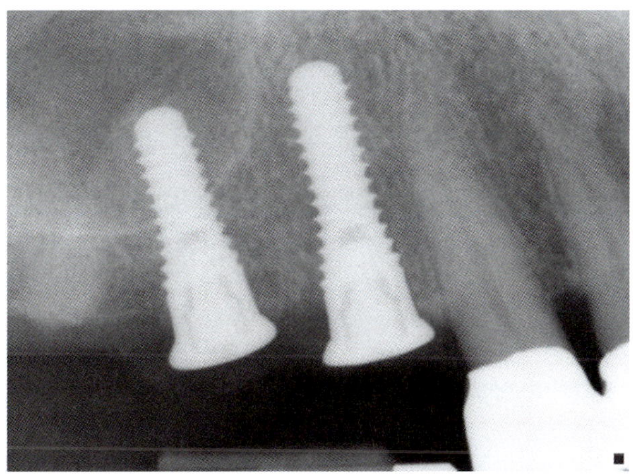

Figure 6.70 An implant has been placed in the first molar position following trephine and osteotome utilization and site preparation as previously described. No sinus augmentation was performed in the site of a second premolar.

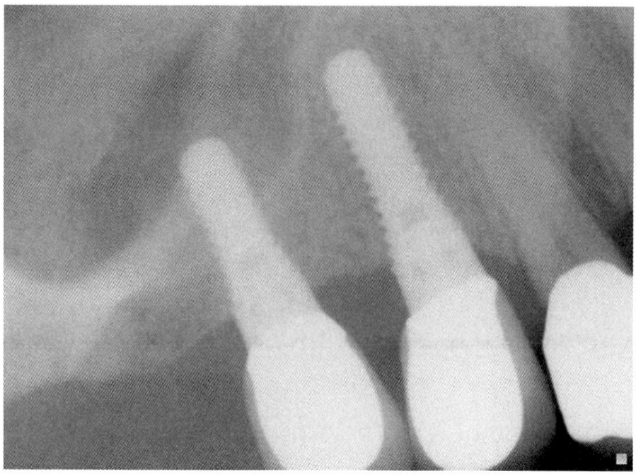

Figure 6.71 After five-plus years in function, the stability of the crestal bone and the bone surrounding the "apex" of the implant in the first molar position is evident radiographically.

Clinical Example Seven

A 53-year-old male presented having lost his maxillary right molars. Moderate sinus pneumatization had occurred. Approximately 5 mm of residual alveolar bone remained crestal to the floor of the sinus. Following osteotomy preparation with a trephine to a depth of 4 mm, and implosion of the alveolar core to a depth of 3 mm, an 8-mm-long wide platform titanium plasma-sprayed Straumann implant was placed (Figure 6.72). The imploded, compressed, and displaced alveolar bone core was well contained beneath the intact sinus membrane.

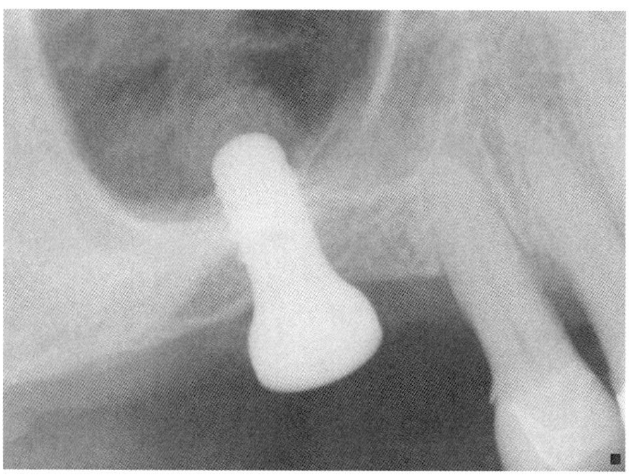

Figure 6.72 A bone core has been imploded following trephine and osteotome preparation as previously described, and an implant has been placed.

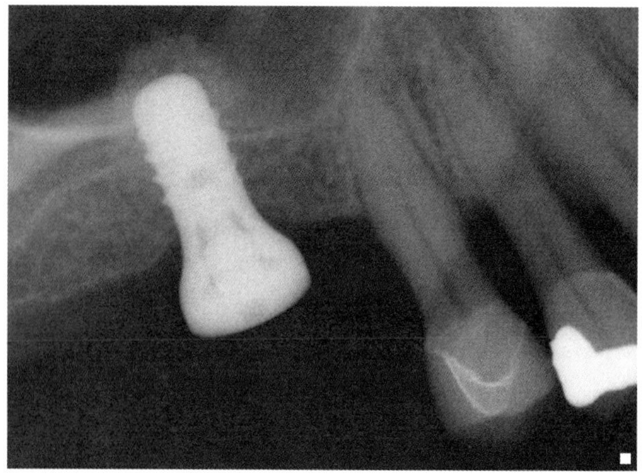

Figure 6.73 Six months posttherapy, consolidation of the imploded alveolar bone around the most apical extent of the implant is evident.

Six months post-augmentation therapy, a radiograph demonstrated containment and consolidation of the displaced alveolar bone surrounding the apex of the implant (Figure 6.73).

No loss of either crestal bone or apical bone is noted around the implant after five-plus years in function (Figure 6.74).

Such a therapeutic approach is highly predictable when utilized appropriately. Care must be taken to thoroughly assess the morphology and quantity of the available residual bone crestal to the floor of the sinus, and to realistically appraise the ability to both maintain the integrity of the

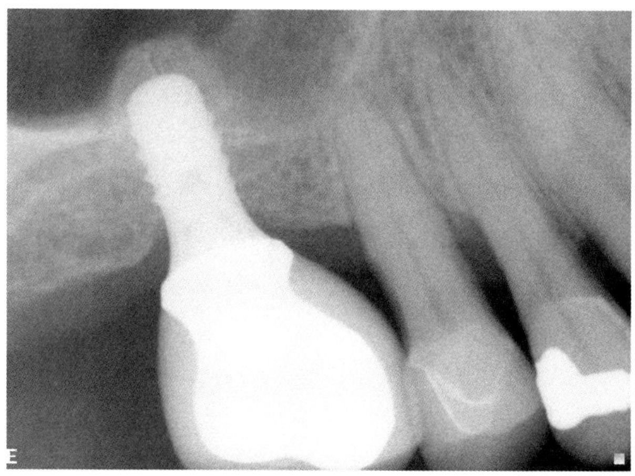

Figure 6.74 After five-plus years in function, the stability of the consolidated bone around the "apex" of the implant is evident radiographically.

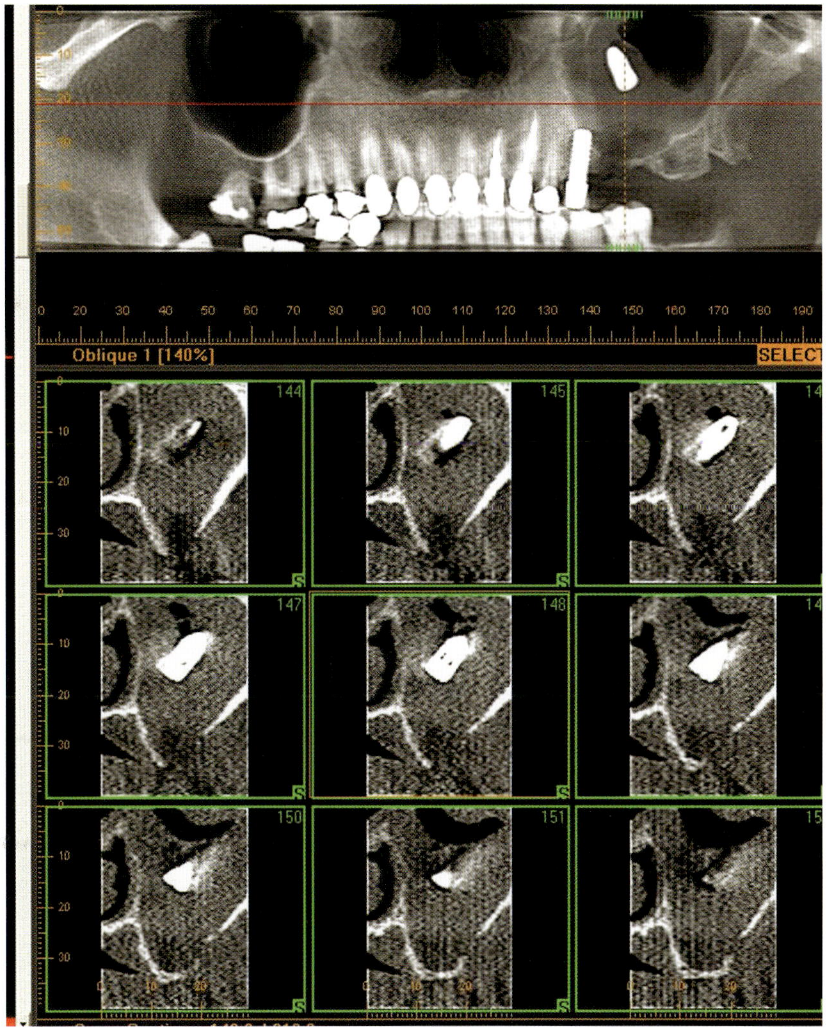

Figure 6.75 A patient was treated inappropriately utilizing a trephine and osteotome technique in the area where inadequate bone was present to support the implant at the time of placement. Note the position of the implant in the sinus and the significant inflammation surrounding the implant.

displaced sinus membrane and to attain initial stability of the implant, prior to initiating such treatment. Failure to do so will often lead to highly problematic treatment outcomes. Figure 6.75 demonstrates such a situation. A patient presented after unsuccessful treatment utilizing a trephine osteotome and immediate implant placement approach. At implant uncovery, six months after insertion, the clinician "could not find" the implant. A CAT scan revealed that the implant had been imploded into the sinus cavity. Unfortunately, the treating clinician's delay in referral for this problem resulted in development of significant inflammation and sinus congestion.

Clinical Example Eight

In contrast, a 64-year-old patient presented with extensive buccopalatal ridge atrophy in the maxillary left posterior region. Between 5 and 7 mm of residual alveolar bone height was apparent crestal to the floor of the sinus. The buccopalatal width of the residual alveolar ridge was insufficient for implant placement in the desired positions. Buccopalatal ridge augmentation therapy was carried out to improve upon the 1.5-mm buccopalatal dimension of the residual alveolar crest. Ongoing regeneration, including a titanium-reinforced membrane

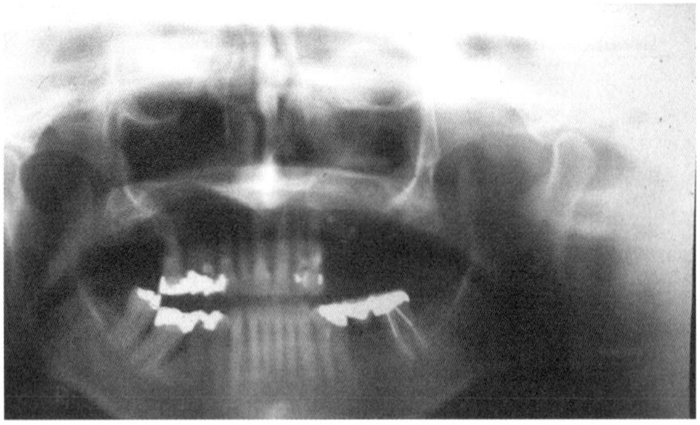

Figure 6.76 Simultaneous sinus augmentation and ridge augmentation therapy have been performed. Note the radiographic evidence of the tacks supporting the membrane to help effect appropriate ridge augmentation therapy.

secured with fixation tacks, is evident radiographically (Figure 6.76).

Following maturation of the regenerated buccal alveolar bone, three implants were placed utilizing the aforementioned trephine and osteotome technique (Figure 6.77). Six months postimplant insertion, containment and consolidation of the displaced alveolar bone around the apices of the implants was evident radiographically (Figure 6.78). A radiograph taken five-plus years in function demonstrated maintenance of the bone surrounding the implants, and no evidence of peri-implant pathology (Figure 6.79).

Utilization of an osteotome and trephine technique to effect implant placement in the posterior maxilla, and guided bone regenerative therapy at the time of tooth removal, offers the potential to significantly simplify therapy and shorten the overall course of treatment, as demonstrated below.

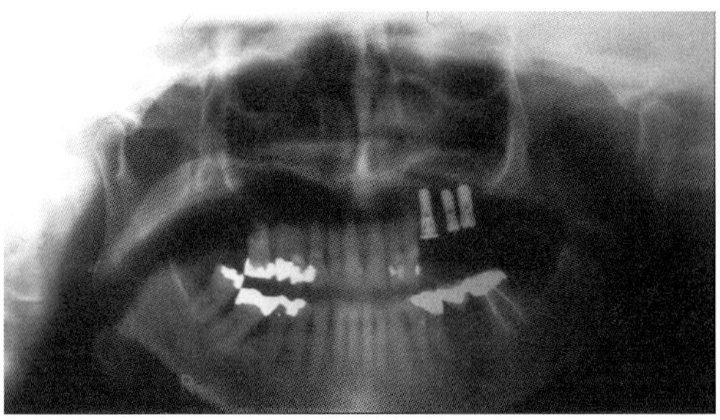

Figure 6.77 Following maturation of the regenerating hard tissues, three Straumann implants were placed.

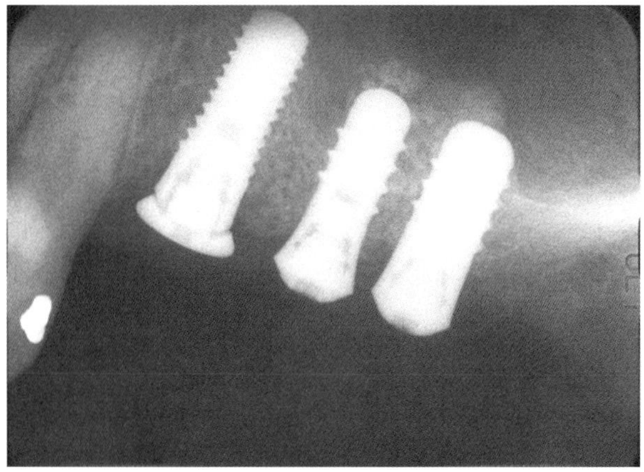

Figure 6.78 Note the regenerated bone around the implants at the time of abutment connection, six months after original augmentation therapy was performed.

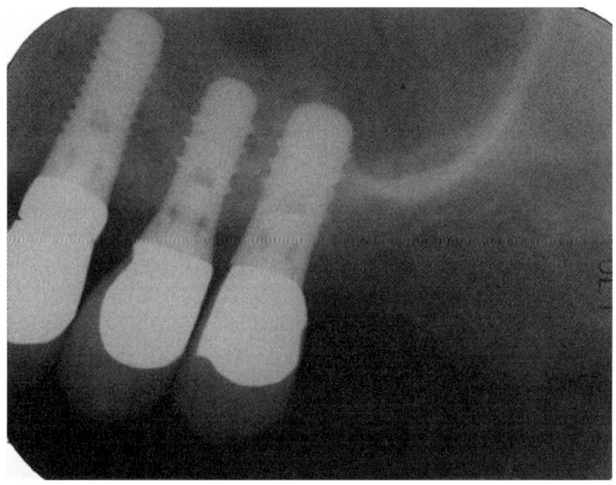

Figure 6.79 A radiograph taken after the implants have been in function for five-plus years demonstrates stability of the bone surrounding the implants.

Clinical Example Nine

A 58-year-old female presented with a hopeless prognosis for her maxillary left first and second bicuspids and second molar, which were serving as abutments for a four-unit fixed prosthesis. There was no opposing mandibular tooth in the second molar position. Following extraction of the three teeth, and debridement of the extraction socket defects, significant alveolar ridge destruction and mild to moderate sinus pneumatization were evident (Figure 6.80). An 8-mm-long, tapered end Straumann was placed in the position of the first bicuspid. Following trephine and osteotome

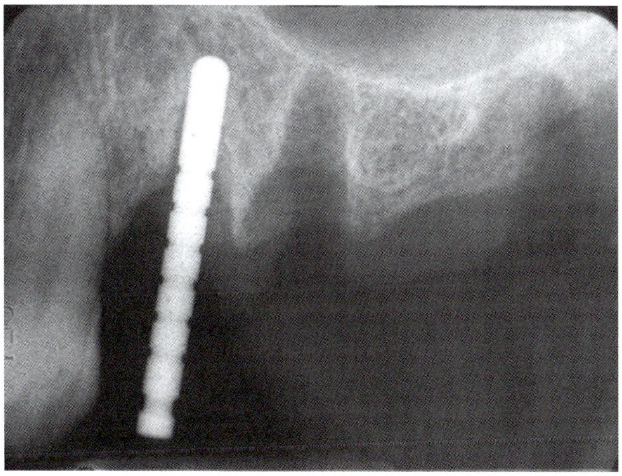

Figure 6.80 The patient presented with a hopeless prognoses for three teeth supporting a fixed bridge in the maxillary left posterior sextant. The teeth have been extracted.

utilization as previously described, an 8-mm-long, wide platform Straumann implant was placed in the first molar position. Particulate graft material was placed in the extraction socket areas of the second bicuspid and second molar, and in the residual extraction socket defect which surrounded the implant in the position of the first bicuspid. Membranes were utilized as previously described, and soft tissue primary closure was attained and maintained throughout the course of regeneration.

Six months postimplant placement and regenerative therapy, consolidation of the regenerating bone was evident (Figure 6.81). Radiographic and

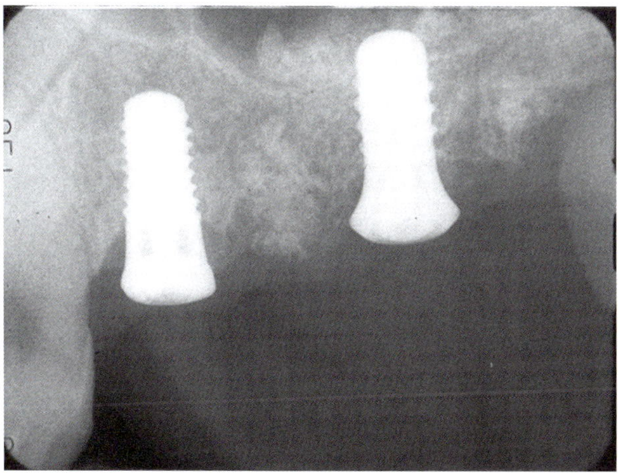

Figure 6.81 Following a trephine and osteotome approach, a wide neck Straumann implant has been placed in the first molar position. An implant was also placed in the first bicuspid position, and regenerative therapy was performed in the residual extraction socket defects.

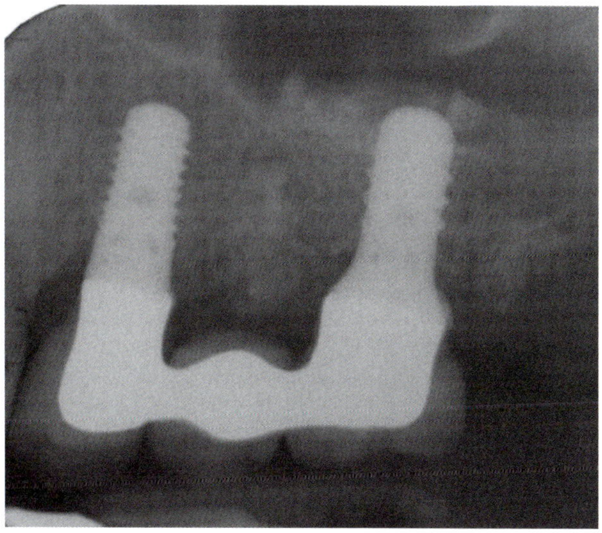

Figure 6.82 A radiograph taken after the implants have been in function for six years demonstrates the stability of the bone surrounding the implants.

clinical views of the area after six years in function demonstrated no evidence of crestal or apical bone loss around the implants, and healthy soft tissues surrounding the implant supported fixed prosthesis (Figures 6.82 and 6.83).

The ability to utilize short implants (i.e., implants of 8 mm or less in bone) for the replacement of missing teeth in maxillary posterior areas has been repeatedly called into question. An in-depth discussion of implant length and the concept of crown to implant ratio as it relates to clinical implant therapy will be carried out in Chapter 7. However, one publication is especially applicable to the discussion of reconstruction of the maxillary posterior region.

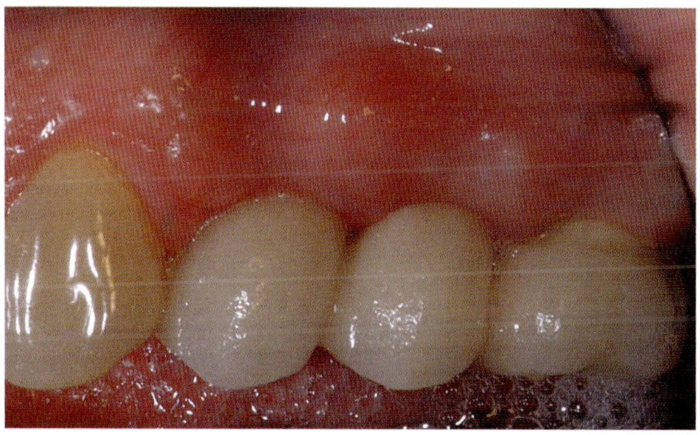

Figure 6.83 A clinical view of the restored implants.

The success and failure rates of 987 implants of 9 mm or less in length were documented in the replacement of missing maxillary molars (44). All implants were restored with single crowns. The implants were in function for up to 84 months, with a mean time in function of 29.3 months. The cumulative success rate in function was 95.1%. This success rate is comparable to success rates reported for implants of greater length, in function in the posterior maxilla.

The ability to utilize shorter implants of specific designs in replacement of missing maxillary posterior teeth offers a means by which to greatly simplify therapy for patients.

Clinical Example Ten

For example, a 75-year-old male presented missing his maxillary right second molar, and with a hopeless prognosis for his fractured maxillary right first molar (Figure 6.84). The first molar was extracted, and the residual alveolar bone in both the first and second molar positions was imploded utilizing a trephine and osteotome technique. Specific techniques for bone implosion at the time of extraction of maxillary molar teeth will be discussed in a subsequent chapter. Particulate graft material was placed in the osteotomy sites, and the residual extraction socket area of the first molar. A membrane was placed over the first molar extraction socket. Passive soft tissue primary closure was attained and maintained throughout the course of regeneration.

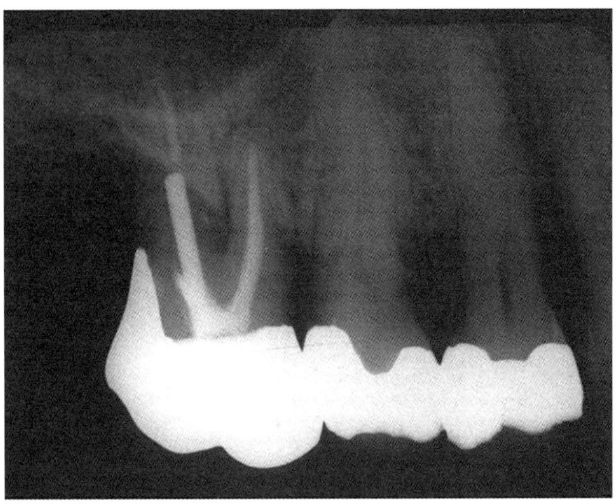

Figure 6.84 A patient presents with a hopeless prognosis for a maxillary right first molar. Following tooth extraction and implosion of bone cores with an osteotome and trephine technique, two implants were placed and restored with single crowns.

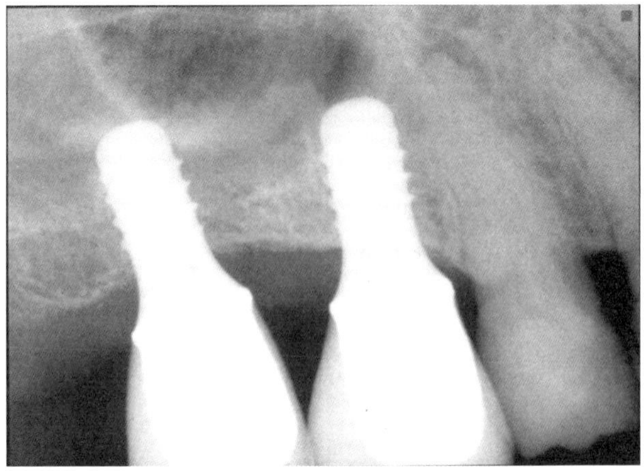

Figure 6.85 A radiograph of the implants after six-plus years in function demonstrates stability of the bone around the implants.

Following maturation of the regenerating hard tissues, two 8-mm-long, wide platform Straumann implants were placed and subsequently restored with individual crowns. These implants were in occlusion with two mandibular Straumann implants restored with porcelain fused to gold crowns. After six years in function, the stability of the bone surrounding the implants was evident radiographically (Figure 6.85).

FORMULATING A HIERARCHY OF TREATMENT SELECTION

With these facts in mind, the conscientious clinician must determine when to perform Caldwell-Luc lateral window sinus augmentation therapy; when to perform such treatment with simultaneous implant placement; when to incorporate ridge augmentation therapy into treatment of the site; and when to perform lateral window augmentation with concomitant implant placement and ridge augmentation (Flow chart 6.1).

Decisions must also be made as to when it is appropriate to utilize osteotomes and trephines to effect augmentation of the edentulous posterior maxilla, and when to incorporate simultaneous implant placement into the use of osteotomes and trephines during such augmentation therapy.

While the advantages inherent in utilizing osteotomes and trephines as opposed to Caldwell-Luc approach augmentation therapy include performance of a less invasive procedure, reduction of operating time, less postoperative morbidity, and shortening of the overall course of therapy, such a treatment approach must only be employed if there is a reasonable expectation of attaining a level of success comparable to that documented with more "conventional" sinus augmentation techniques. The following factors should be assessed before choosing a specific therapeutic approach:

I **The need for buccolingual ridge augmentation therapy to effect appropriate implant positioning and allow use of implants of desired diameters:** If buccal and/or palatal ridge augmentation therapy is necessary, osteotomes and trephines cannot be utilized to augment the edentulous posterior maxilla. Inadequate bone is present in the appropriate positions for osteotome implosion following osteotomy preparation. Therefore, a lateral approach Caldwell-Luc surgery must be utilized as follows:

A. **Caldwell-Luc sinus augmentation therapy with concomitant buccopalatal ridge augmentation, with or without simultaneous implant placement:** The need or lack of need for buccopalatal ridge augmentation does not affect the decision as to whether to place implants at the time of lateral window sinus augmentation. Such buccopalatal ridge augmentation is performed following sinus augmentation therapy, with or without implant placement, according to the same principals and techniques that would be employed when augmenting an atrophic edentulous ridge without concomitant sinus augmentation therapy.

(1) If simultaneous lateral approach sinus augmentation therapy and implant placement will result in at least 4 mm of bone supporting the implant circumferentially, implants are placed at the time of augmentation therapy. Implants are placed in such a situation utilizing the same modified osteotomy preparation that was outlined for implant placement at the time of osteotome and trephine use. No burs are employed in the osteotomy preparation. Osteotomes are utilized to widen the osteotomy to one bur size less than that usually developed for placement of an implant of a specific diameter. The conventional diameter bone tap is placed into the osteotomy, and the site is tapped two revolutions, as previously described. The implant is inserted in conjunction with the appropriate bone placement technique. 4 mm of residual alveolar bone circumferentially around the implant is adequate to ensure attainment of initial implant stability when this insertion technique is employed.

(2) If the implant or implants will not be supported by at least 4 mm of preexisting alveolar bone on all aspects following sinus augmentation therapy, a staged approach is utilized. While implants can be inserted if less than 4 mm of alveolar bone will be present circumferentially around the implant, the danger of overinstrumenting the site prior to implant placement, and compromising the initial implant stability and hence the final treatment outcome, is greatly increased in such instances. It is for this reason that implants are not be placed in areas where less than 4 mm of bone will be present circumferentially around the implant during sinus augmentation therapy.

II When buccal and/or palatal ridge augmentation is not necessary, additional treatment approaches may be possible, including osteotome and trephine use.

A. If less than 4 mm of alveolar bone are present crestal to the floor of the sinus radiographically, lateral approach sinus augmentation therapy is accomplished followed by implant placement 6–8 months postoperatively, depending upon the graft material utilized, for reasons already discussed.

B. If adequate alveolar bone is present so that 2X-2, with X representing the alveolar bone crestal to the floor of the sinus, is an implant length of sufficient dimension to withstand functional forces over time in a given situation, a trephine and osteotome approach is utilized to lift a core of bone. The implant is placed at the time of osteotome sinus augmentation, as previously described. Multiple cores may be lifted to effect placement of additional implants during the same visit.

C. If 2x-2 is an insufficient dimension for the implant length desired, but 4x-6 is a sufficient dimension for the length of the required implant in a given clinical situation, a core of bone is imploded to a depth of 1 mm less than the extent of alveolar bone coronal to the sinus floor. Graft material is placed in the osteotomy and allowed to heal. The area is re-entered approximately eight weeks postoperatively and an osteotome and trephine approach is once more utilized with simultaneous implant placement. The length of the implant does not exceed 2x-2, with x being the residual alveolar bone present crestal to the floor of the sinus, now that early healing has occurred following prior augmentation.

D. If 2x-2 and 4x-6 are both insufficient lengths for placement of the desired implant in a given clinical situation, lateral approach sinus augmentation therapy is carried out with subsequent implant placement.

Utilization of this hierarchy of treatment selection affords the clinician the means by which to assess a given situation and employ the treatment approach which both renders the course of therapy as simple and problem-free as possible for the patient, and ensures an optimal degree of predictability in the final result.

SINUS MEMBRANE PERFORATIONS

The presence of preexisting Schneiderian membrane perforations, or the creation of a membrane perforation at the time of sinus augmentation, may cause clinicians to pause and reevaluate the feasibility of performing the planned augmentation therapy and implant placement during the same visit. However, Karabuda et al. (45) reported upon 91 patients undergoing sinus augmentation therapy and concomitant implant placement. Twelve membrane perforations were detected during surgery. Implant survival rate was not effected by the presence or absence of sinus membrane perforation.

Is the presence of a sinus membrane perforation cause to either abort the planned augmentation procedure, or modify a planned augmentation with simultaneous implant procedure so that only the augmentation is performed during the first surgical visit?

These questions may be answered, and predictable treatment results obtained, through the utilization of a simple framework by which to deal with sinus membrane perforations and effect predictable sinus augmentation, with or without simultaneous implant placement.

Treatment of sinus membrane perforations involved the following steps:

- Classification of the perforation.
- Management of the perforation.
- Modification of particulate graft material, if utilized.
- Modification of the graft packing technique, when particulate graft material is utilized.

A simplified classification and repair system for sinus membrane perforations has been previously published (46). It has been successfully utilized in the treatment of 24 sinus membrane perforations (Table 6.8).

Upon discovery of a sinus membrane perforation, specific steps must be taken prior to any attempts at membrane repair. The clinician must avoid manipulation of the membrane to ascertain the size of the tear, as such manipulation only worsens the tear. The buccal mucoperiosteal flap may have to be extended through lengthening of the mesial and distal vertical releasing incisions and their horizontal extensions and further full-thickness flap reflection, in order to gain greater visualization and access to the prepared sinus window area. Following additional mucoperiosteal flap reflection as required, the membrane perforation is evaluated, classified, and treated.

Membrane perforations are first classified with respect to location (Figure 6.86). Class I perforations occur at any point along the most apical wall of the prepared sinus window. Class II perforations occur along the lateral or crestal aspects of the prepared sinus window and are further subdivided according to their relative position to the most mesial, distal, or crestal bony walls of the underlying sinus. Class III perforations occur at any location within the body of the prepared sinus window (Flow chart 6.2).

Table 6.8 Results of treated sinus perforations.

Perforation classification	Grafting material	Simultaneous implant placement (Y/N)	Implant types and sizes (mm)	Final restoration
I	BBM	Y	IMZ 4 × 15 4 × 15	Fixed splint
I	BBM	Y	ITI 4.8 × 10 4.8 × 10	2 Crowns
I	BBM	Y	ITI 4.8 ×10 wn	Crown
I	DFDBA/BBM	Y	ITI 4.8 ×10 wn 4.8 ×10 wn	2 Crowns
I	Autogenous bone, DFDBA/PRP	Y	ITI 4.1 ×10 4.1 ×10	Fixed splint
I	BBM	Y	ITI 4.8 ×12	Crown
I	Autogenous bone, BBM/PRP	Y	ITI 4.8 ×10 wn 4.8 ×10 wn	2 Crowns
I	DFDBA/BBM	Y	ITI 4.1 ×12	Crown
I	BBM	Y	ITI 4.8 ×8 wn 4.8 ×8 wn	2 Crowns
I	Regenaform	Y	ITI 4.8 ×10 wn 4.8 ×10 wn 4.8 ×10 wn	3 Crowns
IIA	BBM	Y	ITI 4.8 ×10 4.8 ×12	Fixed splint
IIA	BBM	Y	ITI 4.8 ×10 4.8 ×10	Fixed splint
IIA	BBM	Y	ITI 4.1 ×10 4.1 ×10	2 Crowns
IIA	BBM	Y	ITI 4.8 ×10 wn 4.8 ×10 wn	Fixed splint
IIA	BBM	N	ITI 4.1 ×12 4.1 ×12	Fixed splint

Table 6.8 (*Continued*)

Perforation classification	Grafting material	Simultaneous implant placement (Y/N)	Implant types and sizes (mm)	Final restoration
IIA	Regenaform/ Regenafill	Y	ITI 4.8 × 10 wn 4.8 × 10 wn	2 Crowns
IIB	BBM/DFDBA	N	ITI 4.1 × 12	Crown
IIB	BBM	N	IMZ 4 × 11 4 × 13 4 × 13	Fixed splint
IIB	DFDBA/BBM	N	ITI 4.1 × 12 4.1 × 13	Fixed splint
IIB	BBM	N	ITI 4.8 × 10 wn 4.8 × 8 wn	Fixed splint
IIB	BBM	N	ITI 4.8 × 10 wn 4.8 × 12 wn	2 Crowns
III	DFDBA/BBM	N	ITI 4.1 × 12 4.1 × 12	Fixed splint
III	BBM/PRP	N	ITI 4.1 × 10 4.1 × 10	Fixed splint
III	BBM	N	ITI 4.8 × 10 wn 4.8 × 10 wn	2 Crowns

BBM, bovine bone matrix; DFDBA, demineralized freeze-dried bone allograft; PRP, platelet-rich plasma; wn, wide neck.

CLASS I SINUS MEMBRANE PERFORATIONS

The presence of a Class I sinus membrane perforation poses no concerns with regard to either sequencing of therapy or the final treatment result, assuming appropriate perforation management. While the clinician must take care not to apply direct pressure during sinus membrane reflection in the area of the perforation, so as to avoid increasing the perforation's dimensions, sinus membrane elevation should be easily affected. The apical displacement of the sinus membrane that occurs following its reflection results in the membrane folding over itself. The Class I sinus membrane perforation is thus "sealed." To alleviate any concerns about the presence of this perforation after it has been covered over by the displaced and "folded" membrane, a piece of collagen tape may be placed over the area. If simultaneous implant placement had been planned, such implant placement may now be carried out.

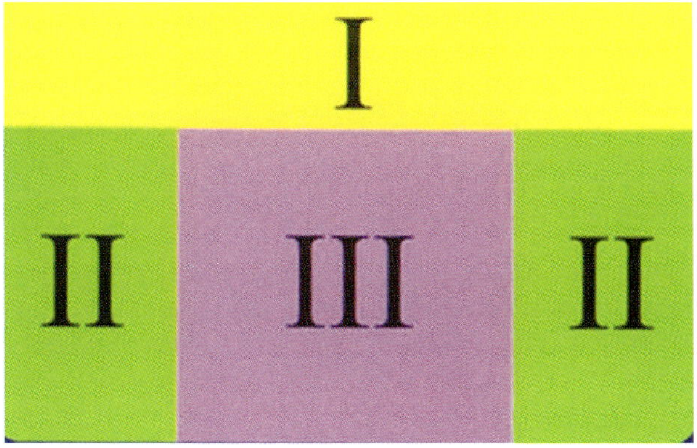

Figure 6.86 A diagrammatic representation of the locations of various sinus membrane perforations.

Clinical Example Eleven

A 53-year-old female required sinus augmentation therapy in the maxillary right posterior region due to severe sinus pneumatization following tooth loss (Figure 6.87). During sinus augmentation therapy, a Class I perforation developed in the sinus membrane (Figure 6.88). The perforation was managed as previously described. A Bio-Oss graft was placed in the subantral space. No covering membrane was utilized over the created osteotomy window. Primary soft tissue closure was attained and maintained throughout the course of regeneration.

Extensive bone regeneration in the augmented sinus area was evident eight months following therapy (Figure 6.89). Two 4.0-mm-wide, 15.0-mm-long titanium plasma-sprayed IMZ implants were placed eight months post-augmentation therapy, and restored with a fixed splint.

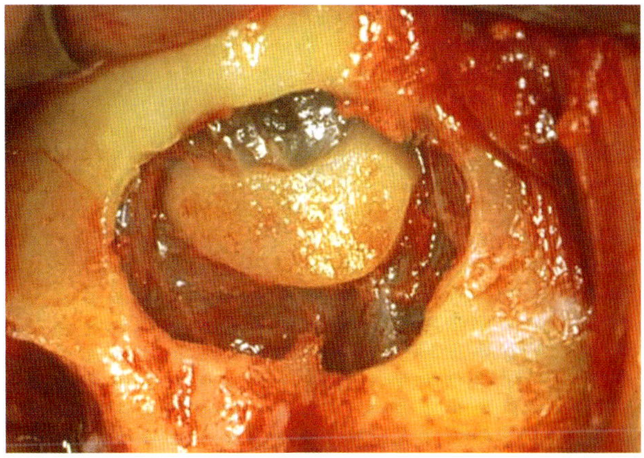

Figure 6.88 A Class I sinus membrane perforation developed during sinus augmentation therapy. Following appropriate flap reflection, the sinus augmentation procedure was continued.

CLASS II SINUS MEMBRANE PERFORATIONS

Both the repair of a Class II sinus membrane perforation, and the need or lack of need to alter the proposed course of therapy, are dependent upon the position of the membrane perforation with relation to the bordering walls of the subantral space to be augmented. If the initial sinus window was precisely prepared to approximate the bordering

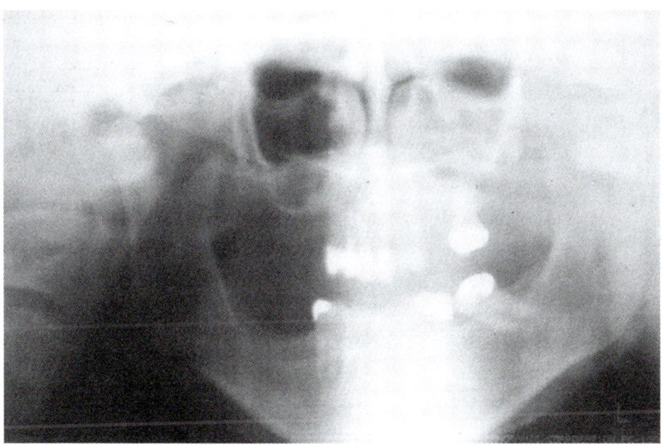

Figure 6.87 A patient presents with severe sinus pneumatization and the need for sinus augmentation therapy before contemplating implant placement in her maxillary right posterior sextant.

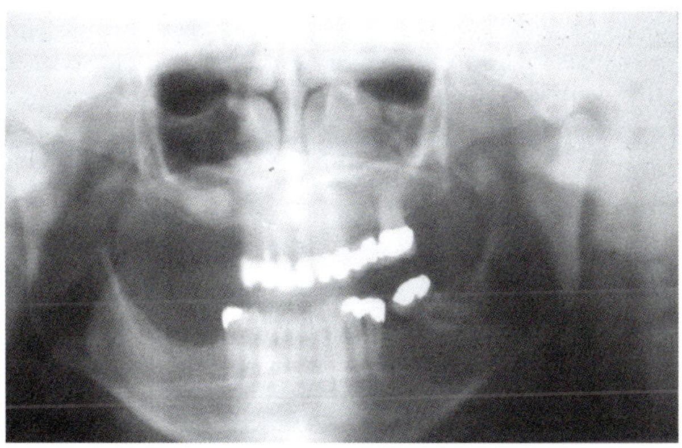

Figure 6.89 A radiograph taken eight months after sinus augmentation therapy demonstrates extensive bone regeneration in the created subantral space. Implants were placed at this time.

sinus cavity walls, repair of a Class II sinus membrane perforation is more difficult and has a greater impact upon the course of therapy than if the initial sinus window preparation was undersized and did not approximate the bordering sinus cavity walls.

CLASS IIA SINUS MEMBRANE PERFORATIONS

A Class IIA sinus membrane perforation may occur anywhere along the expanse of the lateral or coronal walls of the prepared sinus window, when the sinus cavity to be augmented extends a minimum of 4–5 mm beyond the position of the membrane perforation. For example, if the membrane perforation is on the mesial aspect of the sinus window, and the sinus extends at least 4–5 mm mesially beyond the prepared sinus window, this perforation is classified as IIA. In such a situation, care is taken following mucoperiosteal flap extension to gently extend the osteotomy further mesially utilizing a piezosurgery tip, thus exposing intact sinus membrane mesial to the perforation. A plastic instrument, followed by a curette of sufficient dimension to bridge the membrane perforation, are utilized to continue membrane reflection in the normal manner. The exception to standard protocol is that the reflecting instrument is extended over the membrane perforation to the intact sinus membrane area, thus bridging the tear and allowing gentle reflection of the intact sinus membrane and rotation of the membrane and the attached bony window medically and apically. Preparation rich in growth factors (PRGFs) is placed over the perforation area prior to placement of regenerative materials. If simultaneous implant therapy had been planned preoperatively, it can be accomplished at this time.

CLASS IIB SINUS MEMBRANE PERFORATIONS

If the prepared aspect of the sinus window approximates the extension of the sinus cavity in this area, no additional space exists for performance of a further osteotomy. For example, when the mesial wall of the prepared sinus window approximates the mesial extent of the sinus to be augmented, it is impossible to remove additional bone mesial to the prepared sinus window in an effort to uncover intact sinus membrane for use during reflection. Attempts to reflect the remnants of the sinus membrane will increase the size of membrane perforation, rendering it unmanageable. It is imperative that a new "membrane" be recreated, so as to provide the clinician with a containing element for reception of the planned regenerative materials. Insertion of collagen tape or other pliable, nonsecured materials in an attempt to form a containing element within the augmented sinus is unpredictable. A resorbable membrane is shaped and inserted into the sinus window, with its ends extruding out of the window. The extruding aspects of the membrane are secured to the surrounding alveolar bone with one or two fixation tacks. A curette is utilized to gently mold the morphology of the membrane within the sinus cavity to be augmented, ensuring the creation of adequate space to receive and contain the augmentation materials. If preoperative planning called for simultaneous implant placement at the time of sinus augmentation, this course of therapy is abandoned. When faced with an extensive membrane perforation requiring the aforementioned reconstructive therapy, only augmentation is carried out during this surgical session. Implant placement will occur at a second visit, following maturation of the regenerating hard tissues in the augmented sinus area.

Modification of Graft Material

If PRGF is to be utilized during the augmentation procedure, a PRGF membrane is laid into the created sub-antral space, to serve as a sealant over the evident perforation and any undetectable microperforations, as well as to begin the healing cascade. The need or lack of need to modify the graft material to be placed following management of a sinus membrane perforation is dependent upon the regenerative approach being utilized. When particulate graft materials are employed, in the absence of PRGF, they should be mixed with microfibrillar collagen so as to provide cohesiveness and enhance placement and compaction. If PRGF is utilized, it will gather the particulate material into a highly manageable mass. When bone matrix paste is employed in conjunction with a demineralized bone matrix putty impregnated with cortical chips, the graft is enveloped in PRGF. No microfibrillar collagen is added to the graft material.

Modification of Graft Packing Techniques

When a particulate graft is to be placed, after it has been mixed with either microfibrillar collagen or PRGF, care must be taken to gently lay the graft against the recreated "membrane" so as not to displace the membrane and the graft from the planned site of augmentation.

If bone paste and putty are employed, they are inserted as previously described, injecting the paste into the created subantral space and then inserting the demineralized bone matrix putty, whether or not PRGF is to be utilized.

Development of a sinus membrane perforation during sinus augmentation therapy should not be seen as a contraindication to carrying out treatment. Rather, it is a modifying factor which will demand specific alterations in techniques employed, and may mandate delayed implant placement.

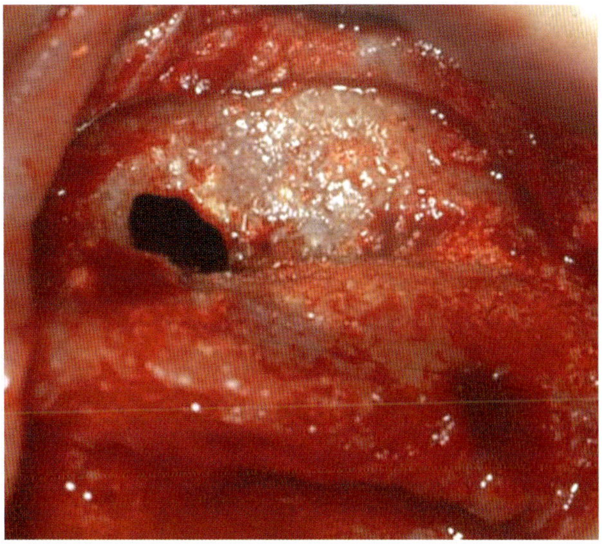

Figure 6.91 A Class IIB sinus membrane perforation developed during sinus augmentation therapy. Following membrane reflection, a subantral "pouch" was recreated with a Resolut membrane secured with fixation tacks to the outer aspect of the lateral wall of the alveolus. Sinus augmentation therapy was carried out.

Clinical Example Twelve

A 31-year-old female presented with the need for sinus augmentation therapy to effect implant placement in the maxillary first molar region (Figure 6.90). During sinus membrane reflection, a Class IIB mesial membrane perforation occurred (Figure 6.91). A small portion of the membrane remained attached to the rotated and apically displaced osseous window. A resorbable membrane was utilized to create a containing environment for the anticipated graft material. The membrane was secured with fixation tacks to the external lateral aspect of the alveolus. Bio-Oss and demineralized freeze-dried bone allograft were placed. Eight months postoperatively, significant bone regeneration in the augmented sinus area was evident radiographically (Figure 6.92). A 12-mm-long, 4.1-mm-wide Straumann implant was placed eight months

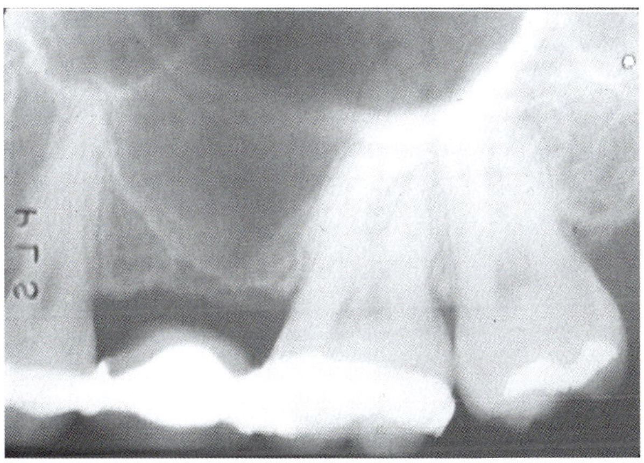

Figure 6.90 A patient presents with significant sinus pneumatization, precluding implant placement in the first molar position.

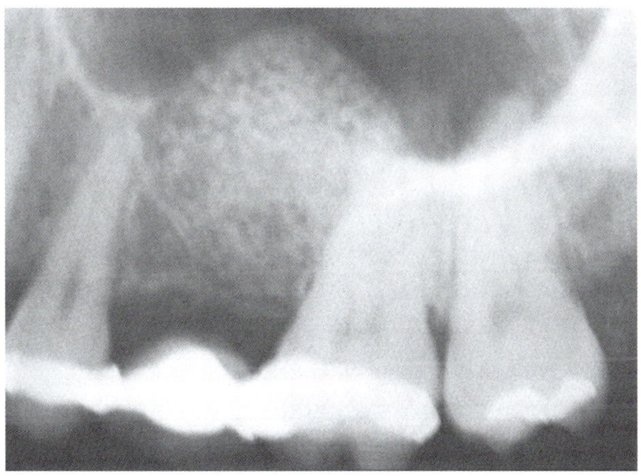

Figure 6.92 Eight months postoperatively, extensive bone regeneration is noted in the recreated subantral space.

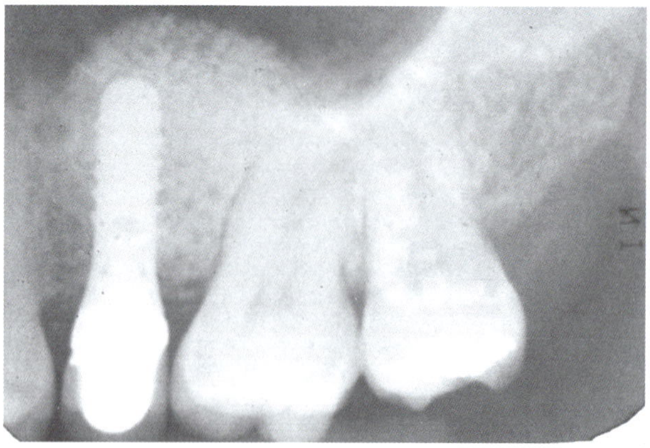

Figure 6.93 An implant has been placed in the regenerated bone and restored. Note the radiographic evidence of bone stability around the implant under function.

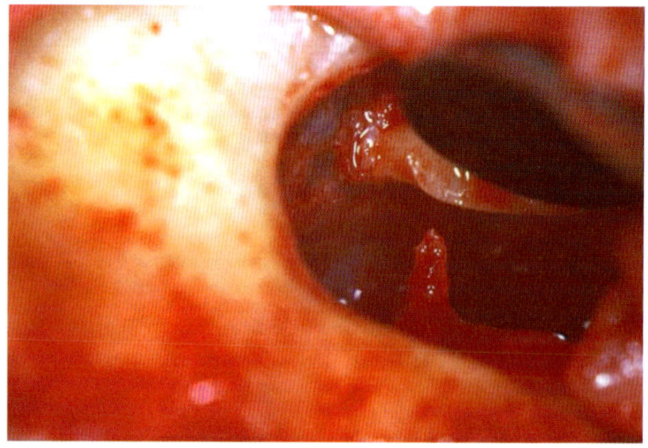

Figure 6.95 A Class III sinus membrane perforation developed during sinus augmentation therapy. The subantral space was recreated with a Resolut membrane and secured with fixation tacks to the outer aspect of the lateral wall of the alveolus. Sinus augmentation therapy was continued with a Bio-Oss graft.

after sinus augmentation therapy had been performed. This implant was uncovered three months after insertion and restored with a single cemented crown (Figure 6.93).

Clinical Example Thirteen

A 61-year-old patient presented missing multiple teeth in her maxillary left posterior sextant. Radiographically, significant sinus pneumatization was evident (Figure 6.94). During sinus augmentation therapy, a Class III sinus membrane perforation developed (Figure 6.95). A containing space was reestablished as previously described utilizing a resorbable Resolut membrane. The membrane was secured with fixation tacks on the lateral wall of the external aspect of the alveolus. Bio-Oss was mixed with microfibrillar collagen and placed into the created sinus space. Eight months postoperatively, marked regeneration of hard tissue in the augmented sinus area was evident radiographically (Figure 6.96). Three standard diameter IMZ implants were placed and restored upon their uncovery three months after insertion with a fixed splint (Figure 6.97). A radiograph of the implants after 10-plus years in function demonstrates

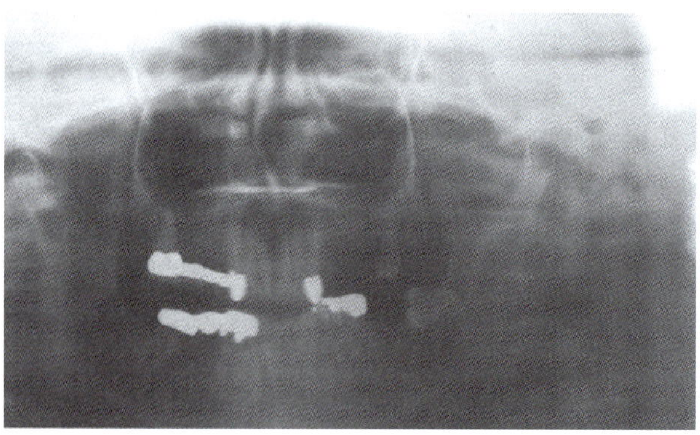

Figure 6.94 A patient presents with significant sinus pneumatization and the need for sinus augmentation therapy prior to implant placement in her maxillary left posterior sextant.

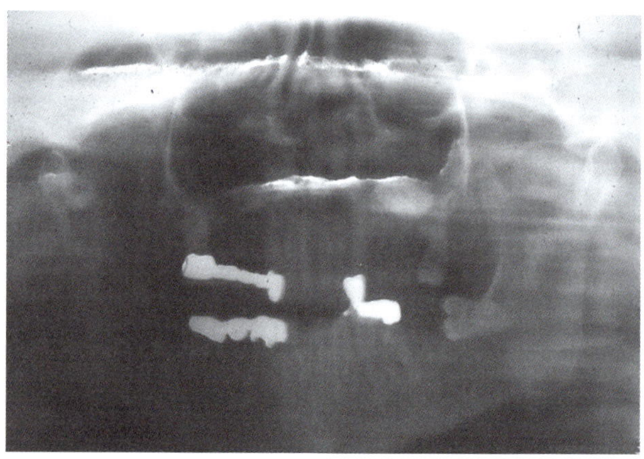

Figure 6.96 Eight months following sinus augmentation therapy, radiographic evidence of extensive bone regeneration in the created subantral space is noted.

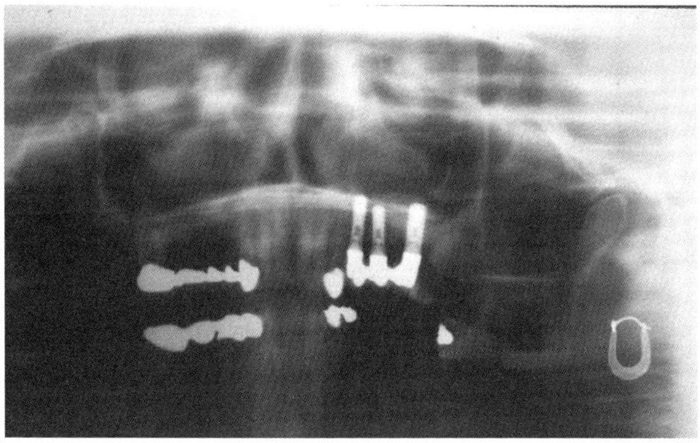

Figure 6.97 Three IMZ implants were placed and subsequently restored.

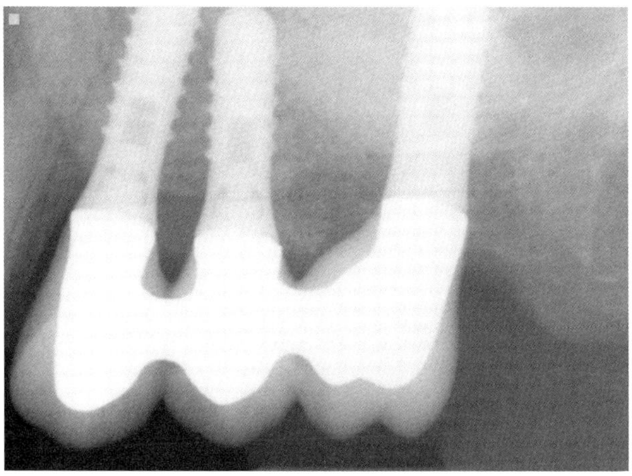

Figure 6.98 A radiograph taken after the implants have been in function for 10-plus years demonstrates the stability of the regenerated bone surrounding the implants.

stability of both the crestal peri-implant bone and the augmented bone surrounding the "apices" of the implants (Figure 6.98).

CLASS III SINUS MEMBRANE PERFORATIONS

A Class III membrane perforation is treated in an identical manner to that of a Class IIB sinus membrane perforation. It is rare to be able to utilize longer curettes to bridge a small Class III sinus membrane perforation, and thus effect regeneration, without enlarging the perforation.

PRGF UTILIZATION IN SINUS AUGMENTATION PROCEDURES

The incorporation of PRGF into sinus augmentation therapy offers a number of advantages including:

- Enhancement of the regenerative process, as described in Chapter 3.
- Ease of manipulation of particulate and putty materials through the development in the PRGF/fibrin membrane graft complex.
- Fabrication of a "biologic membrane" to place over the osteotomy window. Such "membrane" utilization entails no additional expense to the patient.
- A "biologic membrane/sealant" which is placed into the created subantral space against the reflected membrane. This PRGF/fibrin membrane complex helps to seal any microperforations which may be present.
- Utilization of the PRGF/fibrin complex over detectable, larger sinus membrane perforations to help further contain graft materials and promote regeneration and repair.

PRGF is now utilized during every sinus augmentation procedure performed by the author.

Postoperative Management

Prescribed postoperative medications following sinus augmentation therapy include Augmentin 875 mg bid for 10 days (patients allergic to Augmentin receive Clindamycin 300 mg bid for 10 days), and 500 mg bid for 10 days, unless medically contraindicated.

Patients are instructed not to blow their noses for 14 days postoperatively.

A decongestant may be utilized. However, patients are instructed not to use an antihistamine.

Conclusions

Reconstruction of the atrophic posterior maxilla through appropriate diagnosis, treatment planning and utilization of applicable techniques should be viewed as a highly predictable, straightforward treatment option which affords numerous advantages to the patient in both the short and long terms.

References

1. Bahat O, Fontanesi RV, and Preston J. 1993. Reconstruction of the hard and soft tissues for optimal placement of osseous integrated implants. *Int J Periodontics Restorative Dent* 13:255–275.
2. Jensen OT, Shulman LB, Block MS, and Iacono VJ. 1998. Report of Sinus Consensus Conference of 1996. *Int J Oral Maxillofac Implants* 13(Suppl):11–45.
3. Geurs NC, Wang IC, Shulman LB, and Jeffcoat MK. 2001. Retrospective radiographic analysis of sinus graft on implant placement procedures. Academy of Osseointegration Consensus Conference on sinus grafts. *Int J Periodontics Restorative Dent* 21:523–527.
4. Tong DC, Roux K, Drangsholt M, and Beirne OR. 1998. A review of survival rates for implants placed in grafted maxillary sinuses using META analysis. *Int J Oral Maxillofac Implants* 13:175–182.
5. Summers RB. 1994. A new concept in maxillary implant surgery: The osteotome technique. *Compend Contin Educ Dent* 15:152–160.
6. Buser D, Dula K, Belser U, Hirt H-P, and Bertholb H. 1993. Localized ridge augmentation using guided bone regeneration. I. Surgical procedure in the maxilla. *Int J Periodontics Restorative Dent* 13:29–45.
7. Fugazzotto PA, Shanaman R, Manos T, and Shectman R. 1997. Guided bone regeneration in implant therapy: Success and failure rates in 1503 sites. *Int J Periodontics Restorative Dent* 7:293–299.
8. Fugazzotto PA. 1998. Report of 302 consecutive ridge augmentation procedures: Technical considerations and clinical results. *Int J Oral Maxillofac Implants* 13:358–368.
9. Buser D, Dula K, Belser U, Hirt H-P, and Bertholb H. 1995. Localized ridge augmentation using guided bone regeneration II. Surgical procedure in the mandible. *Int J Periodontics Restorative Dent* 15:11–29.
10. Nevins M and Mellonig J. 1992. Enhancement of the damaged edentulous ridge to receive dental implants: A combination of allograft and the Gore-Tex membrane. *Int J Periodontics Restorative Dent* 12:97–111.
11. Vercellotti T, De Paoli S, and Nevins M. 2001. The Piezo electric bony window osteotomy and sinus membrane elevation: Introduction of a new technique for simplification of the sinus augmentation procedure. *Int J Periodontics Restorative Dent* 21:561–567.
12. Vercellotti T, Nevins ML, Kim DM, et al. 2005. Osseous response following resective therapy with Piezosurgery. *Int J Periodontics Restorative Dent* 25: 543–549.
13. Fugazzotto PA and Vlassis J. 2007. Success and failure rates of 1633 implants in 814 augmented sinuses in function for up to 180 months. *Implant Dent* 16:369–378.
14. Del Fabbro T, Testori T, Francetti L, and Weinstein R. 2004. Systematic review of survival rates for implants placed in the grafted maxillary sinus. *Int J Periodontics Restorative Dent* 24:513–519.
15. Wallace SS, Froum SJ, Cho SC, et al. 2005. Sinus augmentation utilizing an organic bovine bone (Bio-Oss) with absorbable and nonabsorbable membranes placed over the lateral window: Histomorphometic and clinical analyses. *Int J Periodontics Restorative Dent* 25:551–559.
16. Albrektsson T, Zarb G, Worthington P, and Eriksson HA. 1986. Long term efficacy of currently used dental implants: A review and a proposed criteria of success. *Int J Oral Maxillofac Implants* 1:11–25.
17. Fugazzoto PA. 2003. GBR using bovine bone matrix and resorbable and nonresorbable membranes. Part 1: Histologic results. *Int J Periodontics Restorative Dent* 23:361–369.
18. Fugazzotto PA. 2003. GBR using bovine bone matrix and resorbable and nonresorbable membranes. Part 2: Clinical results. *Int J Periodontics Restorative Dent* 23:599–605.
19. Fugazzotto PA, Nale J, and Ruskin J. 2009. Alveolar ridge and sinus augmentation utilizing demineralized bone matrix allograft. *J Periodontol* (submitted for publication).
20. Blomqvist JE, Alberius P, and Isaksson S. 1998. Two stage maxillary sinus reconstruction with endosseous implants: A perspective study. *Int J Oral Maxillofac Implants* 13:758–766.
21. Cordioli G, Mazzocco C, Schepers E, Brugnolo E, and Majzoub Z. 2001. Maxillary sinus floor augmentation using bioactive grafts granules and autogenous bone with simultaneous implant placement. Clinical and histological findings. *Clin Oral Implants Res* 12: 270–278.
22. Daelemans P, Hermans M, Godet F, and Malevez C. 1998. Autologous bone graft to augment the maxillary sinus in conjunction with immediate and osseous implants: A retrospective study up to five years. *Int J Oral Maxillofac Implants* 13: 52–58.
23. Khoury F. 1999. Augmentation of the sinus floor with mandibular bone block and simultaneous implantation: A six-year clinical investigation. *Int J Oral Maxillofac Implants* 14:557–564.
24. Mazor Z, Peleg M, and Gross M. 1999. Sinus augmentation for single tooth replacement in the posterior maxilla: A three-year follow-up clinical report. *Int J Oral Maxillofac Implants* 14:55–60.
25. Olson JW, Dent CD, Morris HF, and Ochi S. 2000. Long term assessment (5–71 months) of endosseous dental implants placed in the augmented maxillary sinus. *Ann Periodontol* 5:152–156.
26. Peleg M, Mazor Z, and Garg AK. 1999. Augmentation grafting of the maxillary sinus and simultaneous implant placement in patients with three to five millimeters of residual alveolar bone height. *Int J Oral Maxillofac Implants* 14:549–556.

27. Peleg M, Mazor Z, Cjaushu G, and Garg AK. 1998. Sinus floor augmentation with simultaneous implant placement in severely atrophic maxilla. *J Periodontol* 69:1397–1403.
28. Valentini P, Abensur D, Wenz B, Petz M, and Schenk R. 2000. Sinus grafting with porous bone mineral (Bio Oss) for implant placement: A five-year study on fifteen patients. *Int J Periodontics Restorative Dent* 20: 245–253.
29. van den Bergh JPA, ten Bruggenkate CM, Krekeler G, and Tuinzing DB. 1998. Sinus floor elevation and grafting with autogenous lilac crest bone. *Clin Oral Implants Res* 9:429–435
30. Raghoebar GM, Broewer TJ, Reintsema H, and van Oort RP. 1993. Augmentation of the maxillary sinus floor with autogenous bone for the placement of endosseous implants: A preliminary report. *J Oral Maxillofac Surg* 51:1198–1203.
31. Block MS and Kent JN. 1997. Sinus augmentation for dental implants: The use of autogenous bone. *J Oral Maxillofac Surg* 55:1281–1286.
32. Horowitz RA. 1997. The use of osteotomes for sinus augmentation at the time of implant placement. *Compend Contin Educ Dent* 18:441–452.
33. Coatoam GW and Krieger JT. 1997. A four-year study examining the results of indirect sinus augmentation procedures. *J Oral Implantol* 23:117–127.
34. Komarnyckyj OG and London RM. 1998. Osteotome single stage dental implant placement with and without sinus elevation: A clinical report. *Int J Oral Maxillofac Implants* 13:799–804.
35. Zitzmann NU and Scharer P. 1998. Sinus elevation procedures in the resorbed posterior maxilla. Comparison of the crestal and lateral approaches. *Oral Surg Oral Med Oral Pathol* 85:8–17.
36. Deporter D, Todescan R, and Caudry S. 2000. Simplifying management of the posterior maxilla using short, porous, surfaced dental implants and simultaneous indirect sinus elevation. *Int J Periodontics Restorative Dent* 20:477–485.
37. Cavicchia F, Brevi F, and Petrelli G. 2001. Localized augmentation of the maxillary sinus floor to a coronal approach for the placement of implants. *Int J Periodontics Restorative Dent* 21:475–485.
38. Bruschi GB, Scipioni A, Calesini G, and Bruschi E. 1998. Localized management of the sinus floor with simultaneous implant placement: A clinical report. *Int J Maxillofac Implants* 13:219–226.
39. Winter AA, Pollack AS, and Odrich RB. 2002. Placement of implants in the severely atrophic posterior maxilla using localized management of the sinus floor: A preliminary study. *Int J Oral Maxillofac Implants* 17:687–695.
40. Emmerich D, Att W, and Stappert C. 2005. Sinus floor elevation using osteotomes: A systematic review and meta-analysis. *J Periodontol* 76:1237–1251.
41. Rosen PS, Summers R, Mellado JR, et al. 1999. The bone added osteotome sinus elevation technique: Multicenter retrospective report of consecutively treated patients. *Int J Oral Maxillofac Implants* 14:853–858.
42. Fugazzotto PA. 2003. Augmentation of the posterior maxilla: A proposed hierarchy of treatment selection. *J Periodontol* 74:1682–1691.
43. Fugazzotto PA. 2002. Immediate implant placement following a modified trephine/osteotome approach: Success rates of 116 implants through four years in function. *Int J Maxillofac Implants* 17:113–120.
44. Fugazzotto PA, Beagle JR, Ganeles J, Jaffin R, Vlassis J, and Kumar A. 2004. Success and failure rates of nine millimeter or shorter implants in the replacement of missing maxillary molars when restored with individual crowns: Preliminary results 0–84 months in function. A retrospective study. *J Periodontol* 75:327–332.
45. Karabuda C, Arisan V, and Hakan O. 2006. Effects of sinus membrane perforations on the success of dental implants placed in the augmented sinus. *J Periodontol* 77:1991–1997.
46. Fugazzotto PA and Vlassis J. 2003. A simplified classification and repair system for sinus membrane perforations. *J Periodontol* 74:1534–1541.

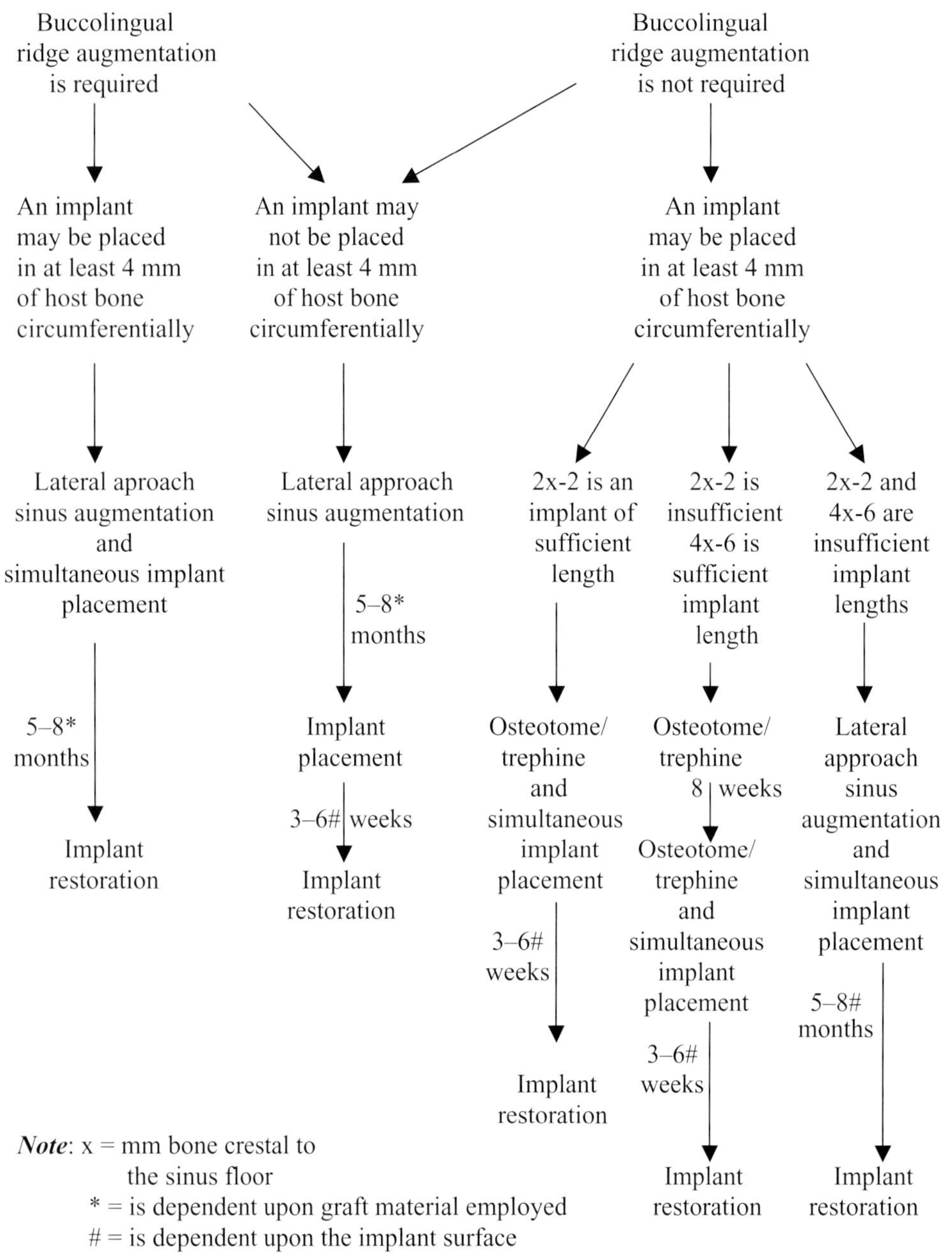

Flow chart 6.1 Selecting a treatment approach for augmentation of the edentulous posterior maxilla.

Simultaneous implant placement was planned		Simultaneous implant placement was planned
Collagen tape; Continue as planned	Class I	PRGF: Continue as planned
Collagen tape; Continue as planned	Class II A	PRGF: Continue as planned
Secured resorbable membrane; Convert to a two-stage procedure	Class II B	Secured resorbable membrane; PRGF; Continue as planned
Secured Rresorbable membrane; Convert to a two-stage procedure	Class III	Secured resorbable membrane; PRGF; Continue as planned

Flow chart 6.2 Treatment selection following sinus membrane perforation (platelet-rich plasma is always utilized).

Chapter 7

The Use of Shorter Implants in Clinical Practice

Paul A. Fugazzotto, DDS

Outline

The concept of crown to root ratio, as described by Wheeler and discussed by various clinicians with regard to treatment of the natural dentition, is well established. The positive effects of a shorter crown to root ratio on the prognoses of teeth in various clinical scenarios have been well documented, as have the potential deleterious effects of a longer crown to root ratio on the prognoses of both individual teeth and treatment outcomes as a whole.

Crown to root ratio is often seen as an indicator of the presence or absence of loss of supporting bone around tooth roots due to periodontal disease and/or other factors. Normally proportioned teeth exhibit a greater crown to root ratio as periodontal disease progresses, and the supporting bone is lost. The lever arm of functional and parafunctional forces is also increased following loss of supporting bone. These are the two primary reasons crown to root ratio is often cited as a significant influence on long-term prognosis.

Conversely, a crown to root ratio within the "normal" range of 0.60 for maxillary teeth and 0.55 for mandibular teeth is not an indicator of periodontal health, or an assurance that periodontal bone destruction has not occurred around a given tooth in the past. Should a patient exhibit a parafunctional habit, which results in excessive loss of tooth structure of the anatomical crown, in conjunction with periodontal bone loss around the root of the tooth, the crown to root ratio may fall within a "normal" range. In addition, a reduced crown to root ratio demands that the clinician examines the patient for potential parafunctional habits and excessive tooth wear.

Ante's law, stating that the surface area of the roots of the abutments of a fixed prosthesis must at least equal the surface area of the roots of the teeth to be replaced by pontics, may be seen as an offshoot of crown to root ratio considerations. Because Ante's law does not take into consideration the periodontal status of the abutment teeth, a modification of Ante's law has arisen which states that the surface area of the roots of the abutment teeth remaining within supporting bone must be at least equal to the surface area of the roots of the teeth to be replaced by pontics.

Crown to root ratio considerations and modifications of Ante's law have long been utilized as cornerstones in treatment planning a prosthetic course of therapy in both periodontally healthy patients, and those requiring periodontal prosthetic reconstruction.

When osseointegrating implants were introduced to the dental community, an assumption was made that longer implants (i.e., implants with a greater surface area for potential osseointegration) would prove more advantageous, and present with a superior long-term prognosis when compared to shorter implants, in most if not all clinical situations. Early publications documenting the extensive use of machined screw Branemark implants seemed to bear out this belief (1–4). As will become evident, it is important to note that the osseointegrating implants documented in these studies were machined screw, hex-headed implants placed in a countersunk manner. The advantages of rough surface implants, as compared to their smooth-surfaced counterparts, will be subsequently discussed.

There are many theoretical advantages to being able to utilize shorter implants, if success rates are attainable which are comparable to those of their longer counterparts. Shorter implant use will help the clinician avoid vital structures, including the sinus floor and the inferior alveolar canal. The use of shorter implants will often eliminate the need to perform augmentation therapy. Even when augmentation therapy is still necessary, the extent of augmentation required will be significantly decreased. Before advocating the utilization of shorter implants in various situations, it is important to examine the available finite element analyses and clinical data. Only if shorter implant use may be grounded in a biomechanical rationale, and reinforced by available clinical data, should the conscientious clinician consider shorter implant use as routine therapy which does not represent a compromise to the patient (Flow chart 7.1). If the finite element analyses available are not adequate to make a compelling argument for the feasibility of shorter implant use, such utilization of shorter implants should be abandoned.

However, if the available finite element analyses support and reinforce shorter implant use, the relevant clinical studies must be critically examined, through the extraction and analysis of available clinical data from published papers.

Once again, if the available clinical data does not support the predictable use of shorter implants with no statistical disadvantages over their longer counterparts, utilization of shorter implants must be abandoned. However, if the clinical data does appropriately demonstrate a predictability of shorter implant use which is equal to or greater than the predictability of use of longer implants, utilization of shorter implants should not be considered experimental. Rather, shorter implants should be integrated into the clinician's everyday treatment armamentarium in an appropriate manner.

It will then become critical to define the parameters which must be appropriately managed to ensure the successful utilization of short implants.

Finite Element Analyses

Lum (5) utilized finite element analysis to examine the distribution of occlusal forces placed on implants to the surrounding bone. He found that the occlusal forces were distributed primarily to the crestal bone, regardless of implant length. These masticatory forces were well tolerated by the crestal bone. However, parafunctional forces were not well tolerated by the crestal bone, leading Lum to state that parafunctional forces must be attenuated. Lum also suggested the use of wider implants and a greater number of implants in patients demonstrating a significant parafunctional habit.

Pierriesnard et al. (6) performed a finite element analysis on 3.75-mm-wide hex-headed screw implants of lengths of 6, 7, 8, 9, 10, 11, and 12 mm. The authors found that the magnitude and distribution of bone stress was constant, and was independent of either implant length or bicortical anchorage of the implant.

Lai et al. (7) performed finite element analysis on 3.75-mm-wide and 10-mm-long hex-headed implant cylinders. They applied 35 Ncm of vertical load to the implant cylinders, and found that the greatest stress was always concentrated at the neck of the implant. The peak stress was independent of implant length, but was inversely proportional to the extent of osseointegration. This fact will prove important in determining the prerequisites for shorter implant use.

Conversely, Petrie and Williams performed finite element analysis of implants in the premolar area. These implants ranged from diameter of 3.5 to 6 mm, and in length from 5.75 to 23.5 mm (8). The authors found a reduction in peak crestal stress with an increased implant diameter or increased implant length. Peak crestal stress increased with implant taper.

Holmgren et al. (9) performed a finite element analysis of stepped and straight press fit implants, and found that implant length had no effect on either peak stress magnitude or stress distribution. Stress was concentrated at the bone crest regardless of implant length. Holmgren et al. stated that wider implants did not offer an advantage with regard to stress distribution, and may not always be the best treatment option due to other considerations, such as bone width and the potential need for concomitant regenerative therapy.

Himmlova et al. (10) found, during a finite element analysis of implants in mandibular molar positions, that the greatest force concentration upon force application was always at the bone crest. Contrary to Holmgren et al., Himmlova et al. stated that wider diameter implant use decreased the peak stress at the bone crest.

Many more finite element analyses have been carried out to examine stress distribution following force application to implants in various areas of the mouth. The preponderance of these studies comes to a common conclusion. The greatest magnitude of stress is always found at the bone crest, at the bone implant interface. The peak stress is independent of implant length. Occlusal stresses (forces) are better tolerated than parafunctional stresses (forces).

Finite element analyses strongly support the use of shorter implants if they offer advantages over the longer counterparts in a given clinical situation. These finite element analyses suggest that such utilization represents no compromise to treatment outcomes in either the short or long term.

Shorter implant use also helps eliminate the need for cantilevered prostheses. Akca and Iplikciogou (11) demonstrated, in a finite element analysis of mandibular cantilevered prosthesis versus prosthesis with short implants placed in the areas of the cantilevers, that significantly lower peak stress values were noted with shorter implant use, as compared to the cantilevered prostheses.

Cantilevered prostheses, whether they are supported by natural teeth or implants, represent a compromise with regard to stress distribution and long-term prognosis. Figure 7.1 demonstrates a cantilevered prosthesis which has been in place for approximately four years. Note both the infrabony defect on the distal aspect of the most distal abutment (the second bicuspid) and recurrent caries on the cuspid. This patient occluded against a porcelain fused to gold mandibular prosthesis. The excessive forces placed on the second bicuspid, due in part to the presence of the distal cantilever, resulted in both significant periodontal destruction on the distal aspect of the abutment as a result of the torquing action of the cantilevered portion of the prosthesis, and eventual root fracture of the second bicuspid. This continued torquing, which was magnified following the fracture of the bicuspid, led to flexure of the prosthesis and contributed to loss of the cement seal on the cuspid and subsequent recurrent caries development. Following sectioning of the fixed prosthesis, extraction of the cuspid and second bicuspid, and implosion of the bone crestal to the floor of the sinus in the area of the first molar, 8-mm-long Straumann implants were placed and restored with individual crowns. The most anterior implant is a tapered implant with a 4.1-mm apical diameter. The middle implant is a tapered implant with a 3.3-mm apical diameter. A 4.8-mm-wide body implant with a 6.5-mm-wide restorative platform has been placed in the first molar position. These implants have been in function for over five years, with no evidence of loss of supporting bone or implant mobility (Figure 7.2).

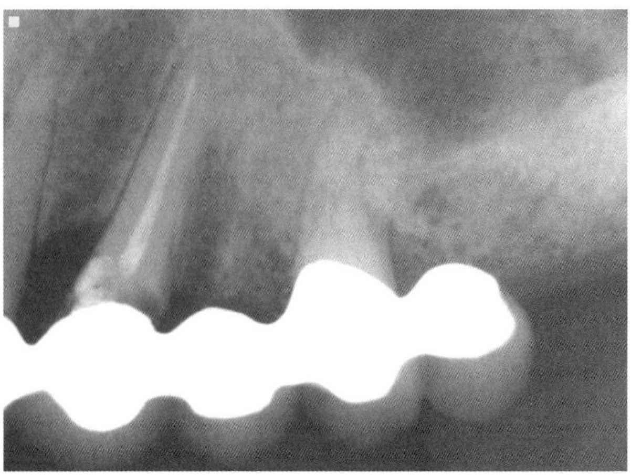

Figure 7.1 A cantilevered fixed prosthesis which has been in function for approximately four years, demonstrates both caries and periodontal breakdown.

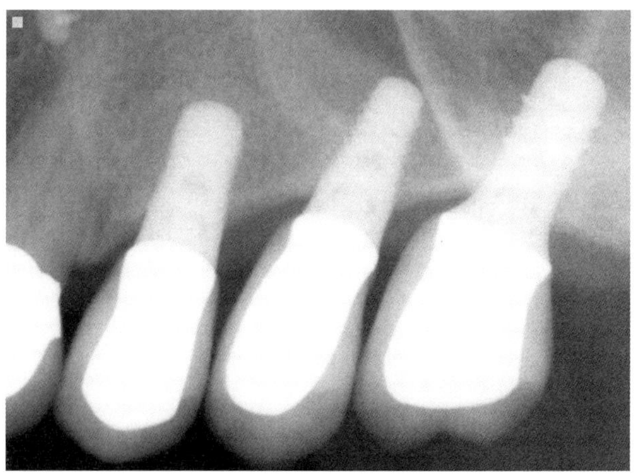

Figure 7.2 The cantilevered prosthesis has been removed, and the teeth extracted. Three 8-mm-long Straumann implants have been placed and restored with single crowns. The implants have been in function for five-plus years.

In another example, a patient presented in 1981 with an inability to tolerate a maxillary removable prosthesis. Due to esthetic considerations, he desired two cantilevers in the maxillary right quadrant and one cantilever in the maxillary left quadrant to replace missing posterior teeth, at the time of maxillary reconstruction with a fixed prosthesis. It was explained to the patient during the treatment planning phase of therapy that, if such cantilevers were placed, they could not be in occlusion with any mandibular teeth or prosthesis, as the excessive forces which would be generated would jeopardize his few remaining maxillary abutments. This was especially true as the patient demonstrated an occlusion of significant force. The patient agreed to this limitation, and the desired prosthesis was fabricated. After 10 years in function, there was no radiographic evidence of periodontal breakdown or root fracture beneath the prosthesis (Figure 7.3).

Unfortunately, the patient was subsequently seen by another practitioner who placed a mandibular fixed prosthesis, with single posterior cantilevers on each side, which were in occlusion with the maxillary prosthetic cantilevers. Within three years of the mandibular prosthesis being placed, the patient presented with root fractures of the maxillary right cuspid and the maxillary left bicuspid, due to the excessive forces now being placed upon these teeth (Figure 7.4). The patient was subsequently treated through staged selective extractions and implant placement, to ensure that adequate support was present for a temporary fixed prosthesis throughout the course of therapy. Following final implant placement and osseointegration, an implant-supported fixed prosthesis was fabricated (Figures 7.5–7.7).

Cantilevered forces may prove destructive to supporting bone around implants as well. A

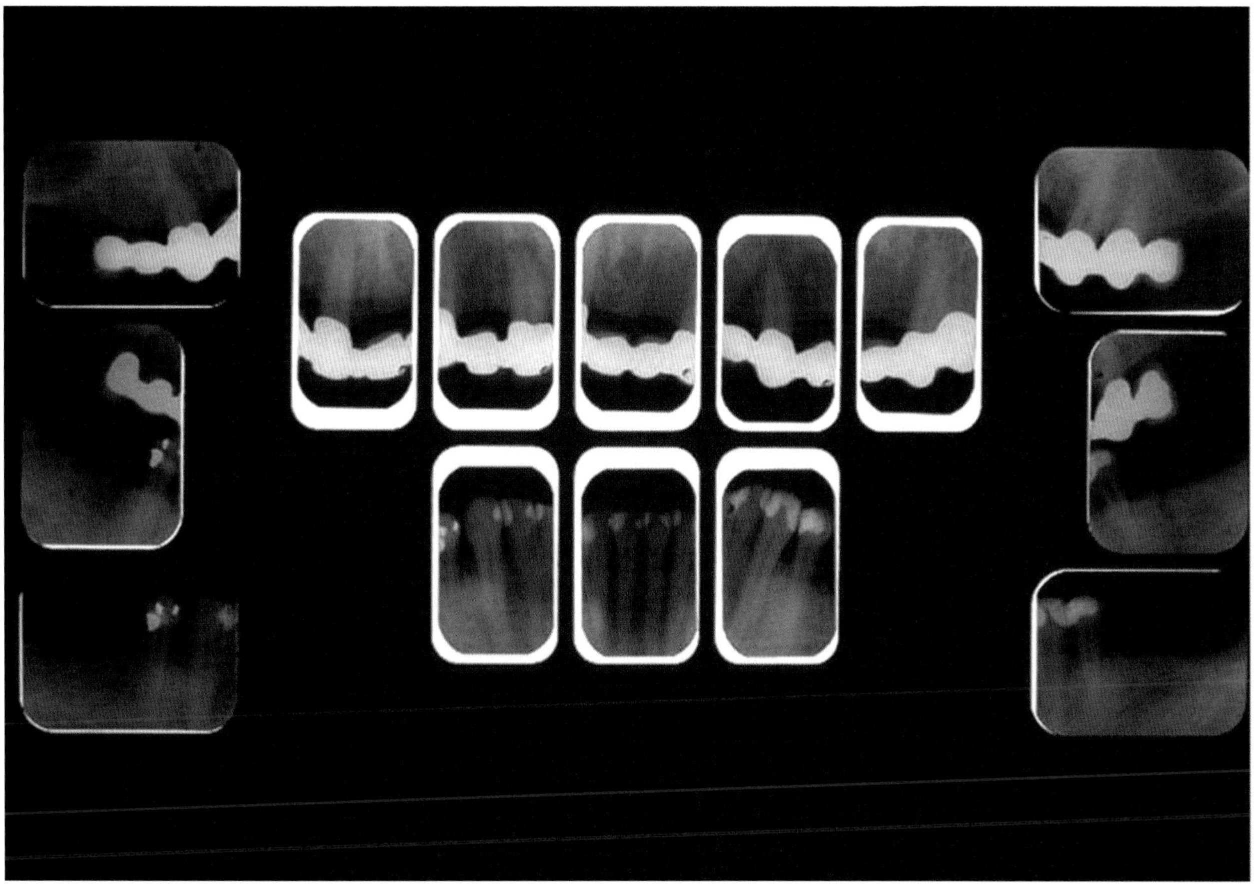

Figure 7.3 The maxillary arch has been restored with a fixed prosthesis employing three cantilevers which are not in function. After 10 years in function, both the supporting roots and the surrounding alveolar bone are stable.

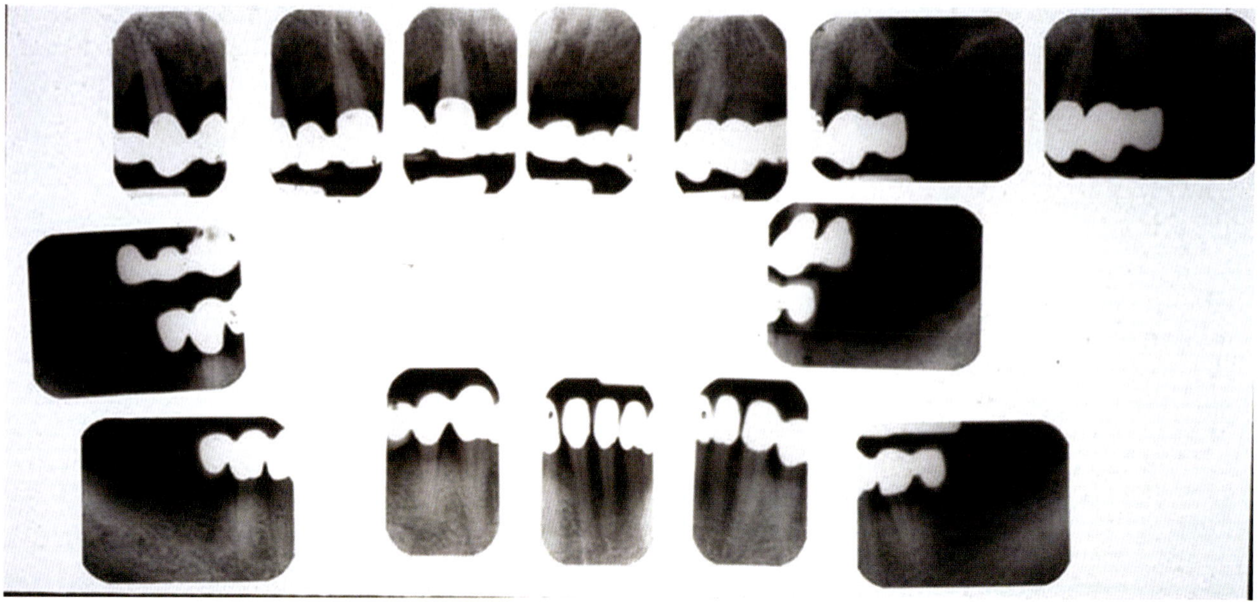

Figure 7.4 Within three years of placement of a mandibular prosthesis with cantilevers which occluded with the maxillary cantilevers, the maxillary right cuspid and left bicuspid roots fractured, undoubtedly due to the excessive forces being placed upon them.

48-year-old male had two titanium plasma-sprayed IMZ cylinder implants placed in 1986, and restored with a cantilevered fixed prosthesis. The patient demonstrated a significant parafunctional habit, for which a bite appliance was prescribed and fabricated. However, the patient was unwilling to wear the appliance during working hours, and only utilized the appliance while sleeping. Approximately 12 years after the implants had been restored, the patient presented with significant bone loss around both implants, despite immaculate home care efforts. As a result, an 8-mm-long Straumann implant was placed in the position of the cantilever. Following removal of the cantilever from the existing implant prosthesis, the implant was subsequently restored with a single crown (Figure 7.8). A radiograph taken eight years after implant restoration demonstrated the stability of the supporting bone both around the new implant which had been placed, and around the previously affected IMZ implants, albeit at a reduced level. No further loss of supporting bone has occurred around the titanium plasma-sprayed IMZ implants over the eight years since the cantilever was removed and function was provided through the use of the third implant and its subsequent restoration (Figure 7.9).

Clinical Studies

As previously noted, the studies most frequently quoted to support the need for longer implants document success and failure rates for smooth surfaced, screw type, hex-headed implants. Buser et al. demonstrated no difference in implant

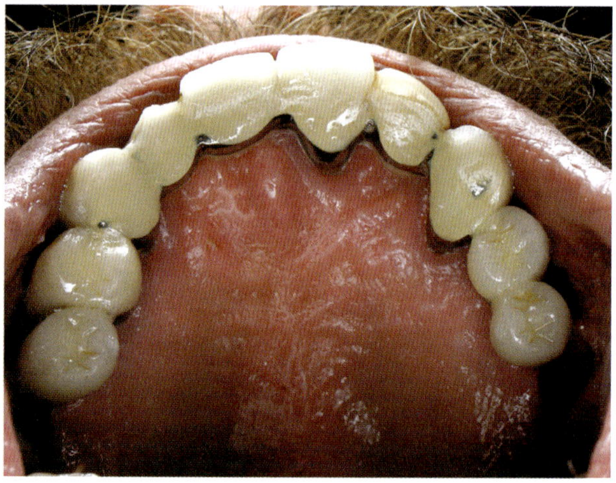

Figure 7.5 A view of the maxillary fixed prosthesis. The maxillary right cuspid and maxillary left bicuspid roots are fractured.

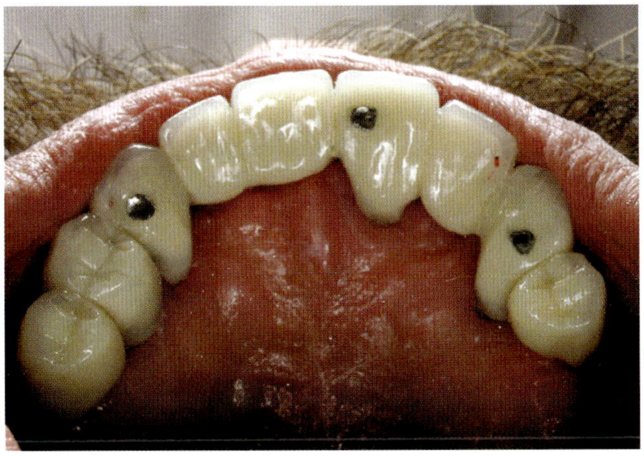

Figure 7.6 A metal frame temporary fixed splint has been placed. Note the metal occlusal stops which have been included in the prosthesis.

success rates between shorter and longer in an eight-year life table analysis of 2,359 titanium plasma-sprayed Straumann implants (12).

Feldman et al. (13) examined five-year survival rates of 2,294 rough surface Osseotite implants, and 2,597 smooth machine-surfaced implants. The difference in cumulative success rates between shorter and longer rough implants was 0.7%. However, the difference in cumulative success rates for smooth versus rough surface implants was 2.2%. Implant surface is another factor to be strongly considered in the decision to utilize shorter implants in various clinical situations.

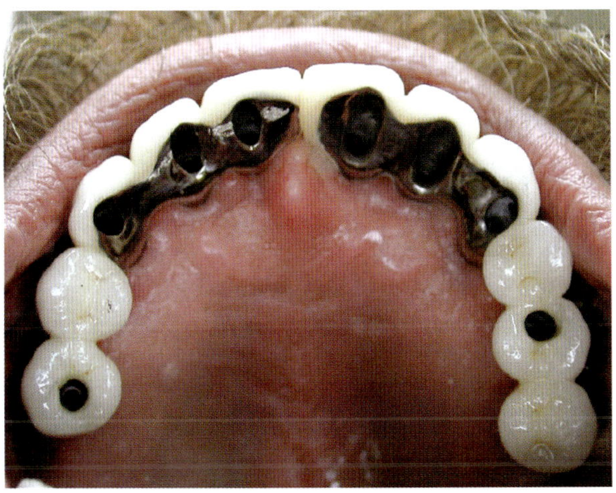

Figure 7.7 Following sequential placement of eight osseointegrated implants and fixed restoration, the patient has been afforded a stable, predictable treatment result.

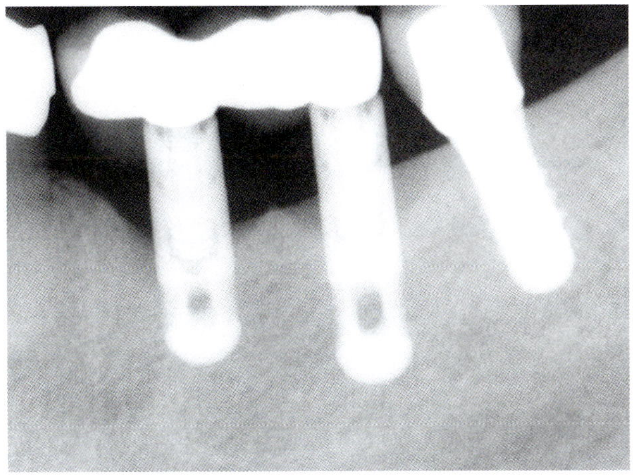

Figure 7.8 An 8-mm-long standard diameter Straumann implant has been placed in the mandibular left first molar position, beneath the cantilever of the existing implant-supported fixed prosthesis. Note the significant bone loss around the two implants supporting this prosthesis.

das Neves et al. (14) collated the results of 33 studies of 16,344 "Branemark type" implants, to assess success and failure rates over time. There were 786 failures in these studies, representing a failure rate of 4.8%. Implant length could not be correlated with implant success or failure, with one exception. 3.75-mm-wide and 7-mm-long smooth-surfaced, hex-headed, countersunk screw implants demonstrated the highest

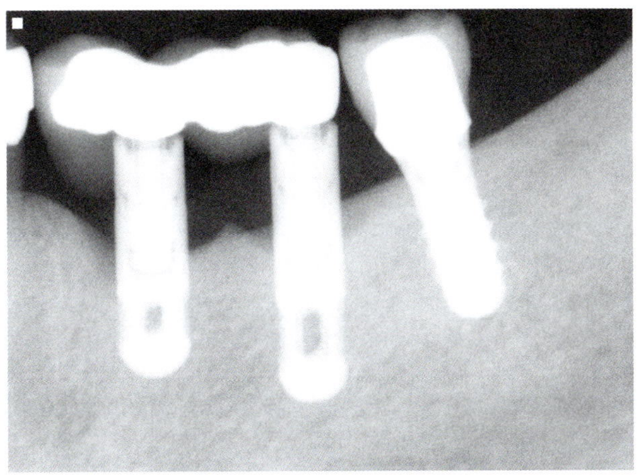

Figure 7.9 Eight years after cantilever removal and restoration of the Straumann implant with a single crown, the patient is functioning in a stable manner. No further bone loss has occurred around the IMZ implants, which initially supported the cantilevered prosthesis.

failure rate (66.7%) when placed in "poor quality" (i.e., type IV) bone. Before citing this finding as evidence that shorter implants represent a treatment compromise, a number of factors must be recognized, including:

- The 7-mm implants were countersunk. As a result, following abutment connection approximately 5.2–5.5 mm of implant was available to potentially osseointegrate with the surrounding bone.
- Smooth-surfaced implants demonstrate a higher failure rate than rough-surfaced implants, regardless of implant length.
- The failure rate of smooth-surfaced implants in type IV bone, regardless of implant length, has been documented by Jaffin and Berman (15).

With the exception of the 7-mm-long hex-headed implants, implant length could not be correlated with implant success and failure rates, even when utilizing smooth-surfaced implants.

Deporter et al. (16) documented the survival rates of 46 mandibular overdentures, each supported by three short Endopore implants. The cumulative survival rate 5–6 years posttherapy was 93.4%.

ten Bruggenkate et al. (17) demonstrated a cumulative success rate of 93.8% for 253 6-mm-long Straumann screw and hollow cylinder implants utilized to support mandibular prostheses for 1–7 years.

Nedir et al. (18) performed a 7-year life table analysis of 528 Straumann implants. The mean posterior implant length was 9.90 mm. The overall cumulative success rate was 99.4%. Cumulative success rates were not related to implant length.

Arlin (19) evaluated 630 Straumann implants of various lengths placed in 264 patients. Thirty-five implants were 6 mm long; 141 implants were 8 mm long; and 454 implants were 10–16 mm long. Two-year survival rates were 94.3, 99.3, and 97.4% for the 6, 8, and 10–16 mm implants, respectively. Arlin stated that "the results indicated that the two year outcome for 6 mm and 8 mm implants was comparable to that for longer (10–16 mm) implants in this patient population."

A publication assessing the clinical results of 5,526 Straumann implants documented the use of implants of different lengths in a variety of clinical applications (20). The implants were followed for up to 72-plus months in function. The mean time in function was 32-plus months. Implant length had no influence on the reported cumulative success rates.

Anitua et al. (21) reported a cumulative success rate of 99.2% for 532 implants of up to 7–8.5 mm in length, after a mean time in function of 31 months.

Despite the plethora of articles demonstrating success rates with shorter implants comparable to their longer counterparts, the literature quoted is not yet convincing. It is possible that, in the studies which have been documented, the patients could have been reconstructed at a reduced vertical dimension, resulting in a crown to root ratio more in line with the "ideal" numbers postulated by Wheeler in the natural dentition (i.e., 0.60 for maxillary teeth and 0.55 for mandibular teeth). It is therefore critical to assess the available literature regarding the influence of crown to implant ratio on implant success and failure rates.

Rockni et al. (22) examined 199 implant which had been restored with fixed prosthesis. Implant length ranged from 5 to 12 mm. Mean crown to implant ratio was 1.5. The implants were in function for an average four years. Neither crown to implant ratio nor implant length had any effect on the supporting bone levels around the implants.

Tawil et al. (23) assessed 262 machine-surfaced Branemark implants in function for a mean time of 53 months, and found no relationship between crown to implant ratio and either peri-implant bone loss, or implant success and failure rates.

Blanes et al. (24), in a 10-year prospective study of ITI implants in the posterior maxilla, reported a cumulative success rate of 94.1% for 192 ITI implants restored with crown to implant ratios between 2 and 3, well in excess of the "ideal" crown root rations reported by Wheeler.

In situations where significant ridge resorption has occurred, it has often been suggested to either perform extensive vertical ridge augmentation procedures, or to place long implants in an effort to better idealize the crown implant ratio. In the past, it was believed that such therapy was not only warranted but necessary. As a result, when a patient presented in 1989 with severe ridge atrophy and a desire to replace the missing teeth in his maxillary right posterior region (Figure 7.10), a 19-mm-long, 4-mm-wide titanium plasma-sprayed IMZ implant was placed at the time of sinus augmentation therapy, due to crown to implant ration concerns (Figure 7.11). An implant of similar length was

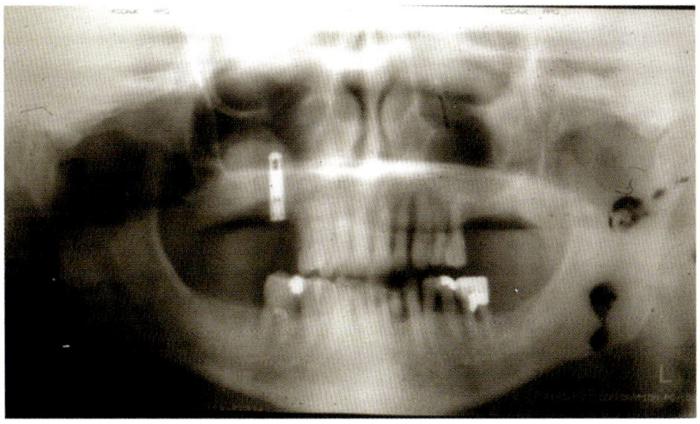

Figure 7.10 A patient presented with severe ridge atrophy and the need to replace missing teeth in his maxillary right posterior region.

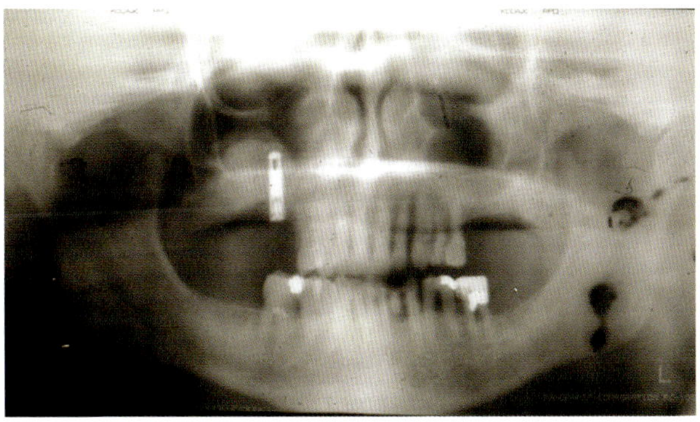

Figure 7.11 A 19-mm-long, 4-mm-wide titanium plasma-sprayed IMZ implant was placed at the time of sinus augmentation therapy. An implant of this length was utilized due to crown to implant ratio concerns. Such an approach would not be employed today.

planned for placement following maturation of the bone in the augmented sinus in conjunction with extraction of the mandibular right lower molar, and placement of two implants in this quadrant. Today, neither the treatment approach employed for the sinus augmentation therapy, nor the implant length utilized, should be deemed appropriate, as will be subsequentially explained.

Preconditions for Shorter Implant Use

A discussion of the preconditions for shorter implant use is a misguided concept. The conditions which must be present for shorter implant use are no different than those which are mandated for

Table 7.1 Global prerequisites of successful implant utilization.

- Appropriate examination, diagnosis, and case workup
- Development of a comprehensive treatment plan
- Amelioration of parafunctional forces
- Regenerative therapy, as necessary, to ensure ideal implant size and position

implant therapy in general (Table 7.1). They are as follows:

- It is critical that an appropriate diagnosis and case work up be carried out, so that a comprehensive treatment plan may be formulated. While it is possible that a patient who presents with nothing more than a fractured maxillary incisor, and an otherwise intact dentition with no periodontal or occlusal concerns, may require nothing more than clinical and radiographic examination prior to immediate implant therapy, such a situation is the exception rather than the rule.

  More often, patients demonstrate a greater degree of dental pathology, whether it be carious, periodontal, endodontic, orthodontic, or occlusal, or a combination of a number of these factors. In such situations, the patient must undergo a thorough examination and assessment, including facebow-mounted models. Periodontists, restorative dentists, laboratory technicians, and other treating dental specialists are then able to examine these models in conjunction with clinical photographs and the information gleaned from their clinical examinations, to formulate a comprehensive, unified treatment plan which addresses the patient's specific needs and desires. Failure to do so will result in less than ideal treatment outcomes (Figures 7.12–7.15).
- All parafunctional forces must be recognized and ameliorated through appropriate equilibration and/or reconstructive therapy and appliance utilization. Failure to manage parafunctional forces will lead to significant bone loss and increased implant failure, regardless of implant length.
- Regenerative therapy must be performed as necessary. Extensive ridge resorption is often encountered in areas where shorter implant

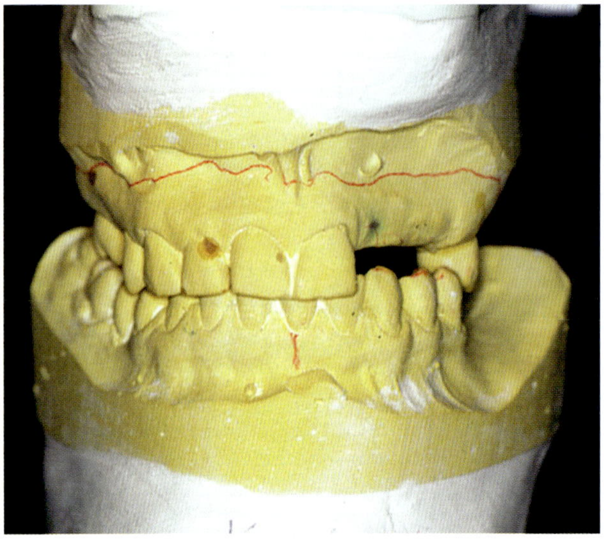

Figure 7.12 Facebow-mounted models demonstrate the maxillary hard and soft tissue deficiencies which must be managed if appropriate implant reconstructive therapy is to be carried out.

placement is contemplated. Such resorptive patterns seldom proceed in a wholly apical direction. Rather, there is almost always concomitant buccal and lingual/palatal ridge resorption, and thinning of the ridge. While it may be possible to place shorter implants in these narrowed ridges, either with generation of minor dehiscences, or with no resulting dehiscences but very thin (less than 2 mm wide) buccal and/or lingual/palatal residual bony plates, such scenarios cannot be deemed stable, regardless of implant length. There is no reason to expect thin, sometimes translucent, alveolar bone to withstand functional forces and maintain itself over time on the buccal or lingual/palatal aspects of implants. Clinicians can expect these areas of thin residual bone to resorb over time.

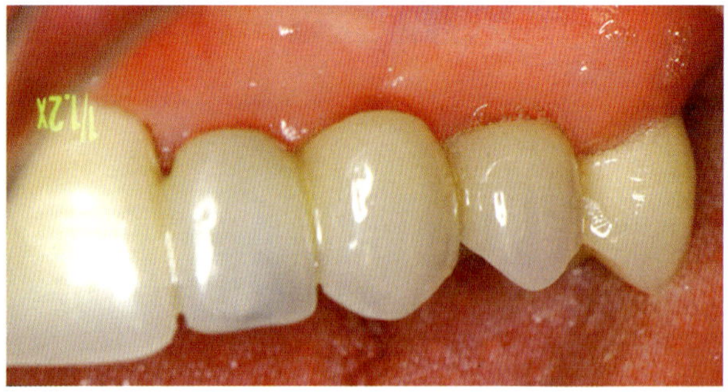

Figure 7.14 Following regenerative therapy, hard and soft tissues have been rebuilt to the desired levels in anticipation of implant placement and restoration.

It is also crucial to regenerate adequate alveolar ridge width for placement of ideal diameter implants in prosthetically driven positions. Placement of an implant narrower than one which would ideally be chosen for replacement of a given tooth in

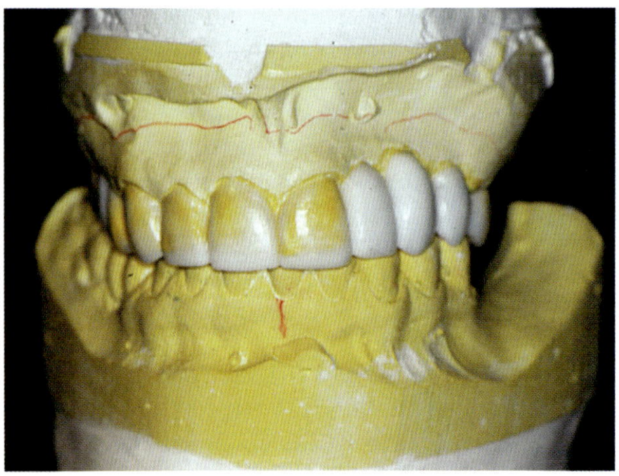

Figure 7.13 A diagnostic wax-up has been performed on the facebow-mounted models. The wax-up will now be cut back to the desired level so that a temporary prosthesis may be fabricated, which will serve as a regenerative guide.

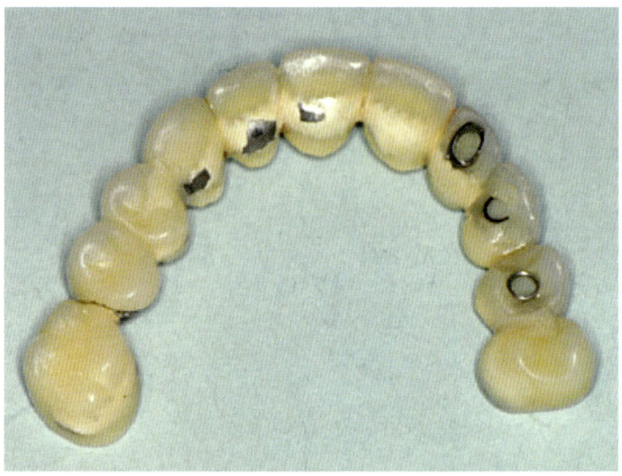

Figure 7.15 A metal frame temporary fixed prosthesis has been in place for approximately 17 months. Note that the prosthesis serves multiple functions, including stabilization of the occlusion, provision of teeth for function, and as a guide for both regenerative therapy and implant placement.

an ideal prosthetic position, due to alveolar ridge resorption, is a significant compromise with regard to long-term treatment outcomes. Because forces applied to implants are distributed primarily to the crestal bone, the implant diameter is crucial to appropriate amelioration of these forces.

A significant paradigm shift must occur in our definitions of appropriate implant placement and success. The decision process must proceed as follows:

- The ideal implant diameter for the tooth to be replaced is determined.
- The ideal position for the selected implant is determined, through use of facebow mounted models and waxups, when necessary.
- A comprehensive patient workup elucidates the clinical steps which must be taken to attain such positioning of appropriate diameter implant (ridge augmentation therapy, orthodontics, etc.).
- The necessary preimplant placement therapies are carried out.
- The appropriately sized implant is ideally positioned.
- The implant is subsequently restored.

It is only through such an approach that long-term treatment outcomes may be maximized.

Hsu et al. (25) performed finite element analyses on implants at loading angles of 0, 30 and 60°. Each 30° increase in off angle loading increased stress magnitude to the bone crest three to four times. Placement of narrower implants at off angles, and their esthetic restoration through axial surgical and restorative wizardry, represents a significant compromise for the patient.

Implant Characteristics to Maximize Prognosis

Regardless of clinicians' allegiances to various implant companies, the available data and common sense clearly demonstrate that implants should present with specific characteristics to maximize the available bone for the attainment of osseointegration, and to contribute to predictable long-term implant success. Such considerations include (Table 7.2):

Table 7.2 Implant prerequisites for successful utilization.

Roughened implant surface
Internal abutment attachment
Appropriate neck diameter for the tooth to be replaced
Specific implant body configurations

- **A roughened implant surface:** Numerous authors have documented the superior degree of osseointegration and the greater pull out and back torque strengths of rough surface implants when compared to their smooth surface counterparts. It is difficult to find a rationale for the use of smooth surface implants in today's clinical practice.
- **Internal versus external attachment implants:** Meada et al. (26) applied 30 Ncm of vertical and horizontal load to implants with internal or external hex connections. They reported increased strain at the cervical area with external hex fixtures, as compared to their internal hex counterparts. Meada et al. also found that the load was better distributed around internal hex implants than around external hex implants. These findings have been documented by a number of authors in both finite element analyses and histologic animal studies. Only internal attachment implants should be utilized if the clinician wishes to lessen peak stress levels to the crestal bone, and thus enhance implant prognosis.
- **An implant with an appropriate neck diameter should be utilized for replacement of a given tooth:** Considering the variety of implant configurations available today, there is no reason to utilize an implant with an undersized neck diameter to effect tooth replacement. Such a situation often results in a crown whose contours pose a greater challenge to a patient's home care efforts, thus compromising long-term treatment outcomes. The argument that the use of a wider implant with a wider neck diameter would result in the need for buccal ridge augmentation therapy is not valid. If augmentation therapy is required, it should be performed. Shorter implant use is not indicated only because it potentially avoids augmentation therapy. In a situation with an atrophic buccal ridge, shorter implant use will simplify augmentation therapy, allowing the clinician to perform only a buccal ridge augmentation procedure instead of buccal and vertical augmentation therapy. As already discussed, the implant body width and neck dimension should be chosen with consideration of the tooth to be replaced, not the width of available residual

bone. Once the appropriate implant dimension is selected, augmentation therapy is performed as needed to encompass this implant in bone of adequate dimensions to withstand functional forces over time.

- **Specific implant configurations:** While buccal ridge augmentation therapy should be performed wherever necessary to house the required wide-bodied implant, there is no reason to subject the patient to such augmentation therapy if it can be avoided without compromising treatment outcomes. When wider diameter implants were first introduced, they were greeted in many quarters as the solution to all of our problems regarding molar tooth replacement. Unfortunately, many clinicians failed to realize two important points. The first is that the use of a wider implant will often require buccal augmentation therapy due to the atrophic nature of the ridge, if the implant is to be placed in an ideal position rather than more lingually than ideally desired from a prosthetic point of view (Figures 7.16–7.18). The second consideration, which has already been discussed, is the fact that placement of a wider implant, even if it does not generate a fenestration or dehiscence, may result in a very thin buccal and/or lingual/palatal bone plate which will resorb relatively quickly under function. The value of specific implant configurations is easily demonstrated when considering the replacement of a mandibular molar. If an implant is placed at the time of mandibular molar extraction, two basic implant configurations may be utilized. The first is a tapered end configuration which has a narrower base, and begins to flare to final restorative platform (in the case of a Straumann implant to 6.5 mm) significantly subcrestal. The second configuration to be utilized is an implant with a paralled wall 4.8-mm-wide body, which only begins to flare to its 6.5-mm-wide restorative platform at the osseous crest. Utilization of either of these implants, with appropriate regenerative therapy to rebuild bone in the residual extraction socket defect surrounding the implant, will result in thick buccal and lingual bony plates to help withstand functional forces over time (Figures 7.19 and 7.20).

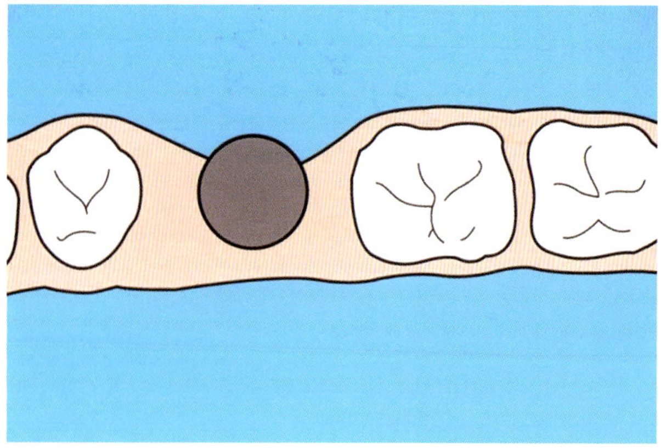

Figure 7.17 Placement of a wide-bodied implant in the appropriate position results in a significant buccal dehiscence.

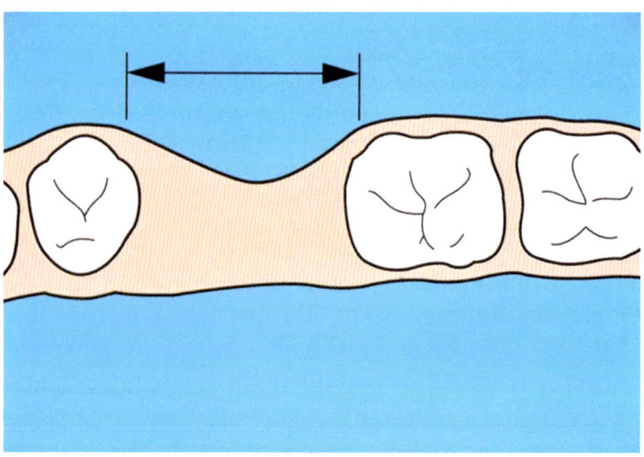

Figure 7.16 A patient presents with an atrophic mandibular ridge.

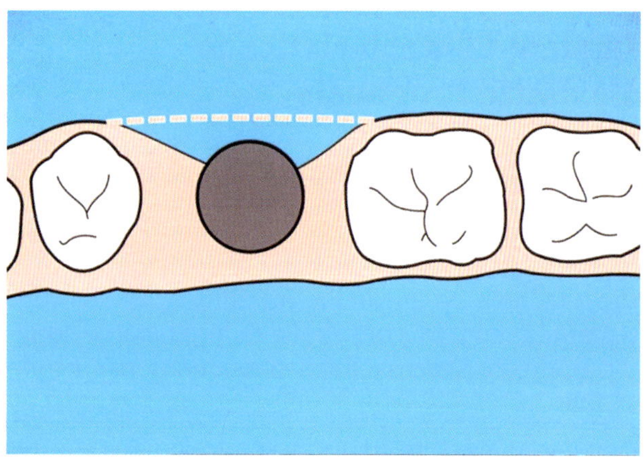

Figure 7.18 Regenenerative therapy is necessary to rebuild bone over the dehisced portion of the implant.

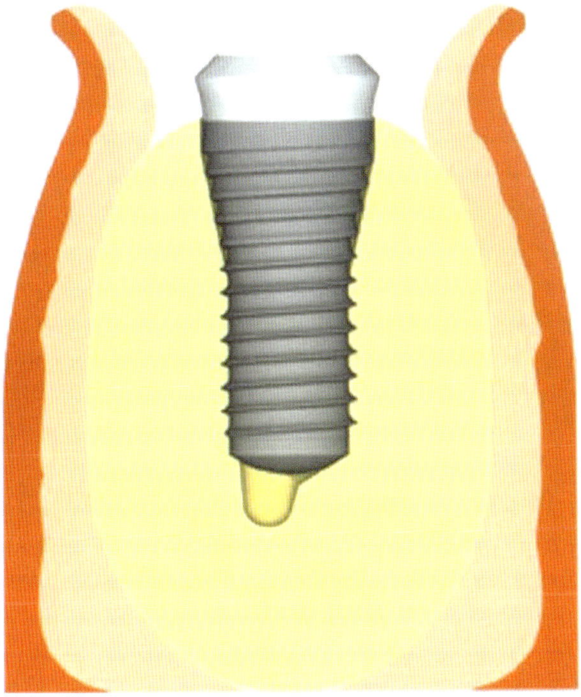

Figure 7.19 A tapered end implant which has a narrow "apex," and begins to flare to the final restorative platform of 6.5 mm subcrestally, is placed at the time of molar extraction.

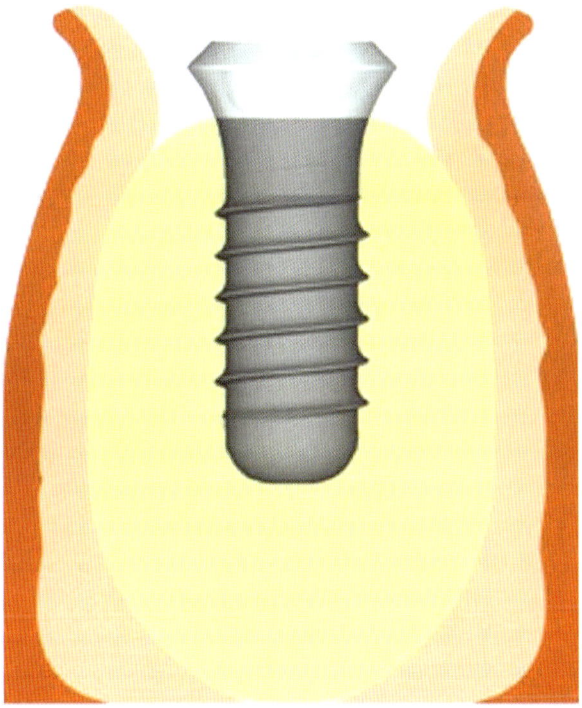

Figure 7.20 A parallel-walled 4.8-mm-diameter implant is placed at the time of mandibular molar extraction. This implant begins to flare to the final restorative platform of 6.5 mm at the osseous crest.

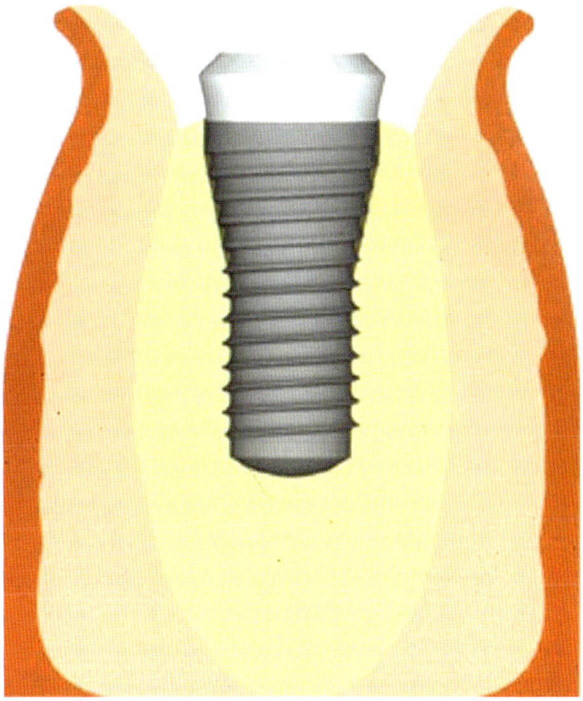

Figure 7.21 A tapered end implant which begins to flare to the final restorative diameter subcrestally has been placed in an atrophic mandibular molar region. Note the thinner buccal and lingual bone remaining around the implant.

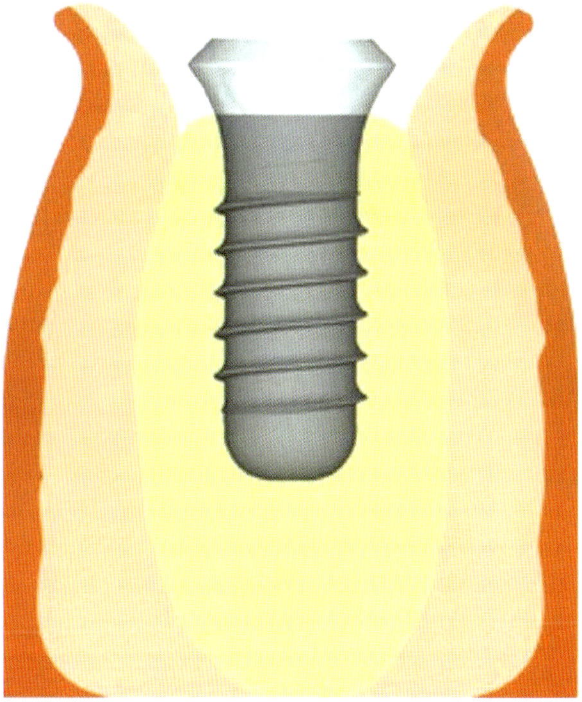

Figure 7.22 A 4.8-mm-diameter parallel-walled implant which begins to flare to the final restorative platform of 6.5 mm at the osseous crest has been placed in an atrophic mandibular molar region. Note the thicker bone buccally and palatally, as compared to when a tapered end implant, which begins its flaring subcrestally, was placed.

This is not the scenario encountered when an implant is to be placed where a mandibular molar has been missing for some time and the expected ridge atrophy has occurred. In such a situation, if a tapered implant is utilized which begins to flare to the final restorative platform dimension subcrestally, the result is often a thin buccal and/or lingual bony plate which is susceptible to resorption over time. The Straumann implant design of a 4.8-mm-wide body which has parallel walls subcrestally, and begins to flare to the 6.5-mm-wide neck at the osseous crest offers significant advantages in such areas. When utilizing this configuration in an atrophic ridge, the result is thicker buccal and lingual bony plates at the neck of the implant, the area of the greatest stress concentration under function. In these situations, this configuration is by far the most advantageous implant design to utilize (Figures 7.21 and 7.22).

CLINICAL APPLICATIONS OF SHORTER IMPLANT USE

For the purpose of discussion, Straumann type implants of 6, 7, 8, and 9 mm in length will be considered short implants. It is important to realize that these measurements represent the roughened surface of the implant. The measurements do not include the polished implant neck which, except in the instances of the need to countersink an implant due to esthetic considerations, is not countersunk. Thus, the available bone is more effectively utilized to support the implant than in a countersunk situation. For example, if an 8-mm-long Straumann implant is utilized with a 1.8-mm-long polished collar, and is not countersunk, no crestal bone cupping occurs at the time of abutment connection. All 8 mm of available bone potentially may be utilized to support the implant body.

In contrast, if a hex-headed implant is placed in a countersunk manner, approximately 1.2–1.6 mm of crestal cupping occurs following abutment connection. This means that an 8-mm countersunk hex-headed implant is at most engaging approximately 6.5 mm of bone to lend support over time under function.

Shorter Implant Use in the Posterior Mandible

Three hundred fifteen standard neck ITI implants were placed in atrophic posterior mandibular areas, and followed for up to 84 months in function, with a mean time in function of 36.2 months (27). Four implants were mobile at uncovery, and one implant was lost during the first 12 months of function, yielding a cumulative success rate of 98.4%. Implant size and duration of time in function are noted in Table 7.3.

While this cumulative implant success rate was comparable to that reported for longer implants in function in the posterior mandible, the actual cumulative success rate of the shorter implants in function over this mean time of 36.2 months was 99.7% when the four implants mobile at uncovery are excluded. Implants mobile at uncovery cast no reflection up on the ability or inability of shorter implants to withstand functional forces over time. Implants are mobile at uncovery for two reasons in a healthy patient. Either forces generated by an overlying prosthesis were not controlled during the initial stages of osseointegration, resulting in excessive micromotion of the implant; or the surgical therapy performed for a given site generated too much trauma, heat, osteotomy widening, etc.

While it is important to report implants mobile at uncovery for appropriate statistical analysis of implant success and failure, it is inappropriate to consider such implants when deciding whether or not shorter implants may be used as alternatives to their longer counterparts in a given situation. Rather, efforts should be made to develop modified surgical techniques to avoid excessive traumatization of the osteotomy site during preparation.

Shorter implants are routinely utilized to replace missing mandibular posterior teeth with abutments and single crowns. Figure 7.23 demonstrates the use of an 8-mm-long, wide body, standard neck Straumann implant to replace a missing first molar. Anterior to this implant is a standard body, standard neck 10-mm-long Straumann implant, also restored with an abutment and single crown (Figure 7.24). The implant crowns are not splinted. Implant crowns are only splinted together when there is a pontic between them.

Figure 7.25 demonstrates radiographic stability of crestal peri-implant bone around two 8-mm-long tapered end Straumann implants utilized to restore a missing mandibular second bicuspid and first molar respectively, three years after restoration.

Shorter implants may also be successfully utilized to support a fixed prosthesis, as noted in

Table 7.3 Cumulative implant success rates for standard neck short implants restored as single crowns in the posterior mandible.

Months after abutment connection	Implants beginning of interval	Failures during interval	Interval failure rate	Cumulative failure rate	Cumulative success rate
0–12	315	5	1.6	1.6	98.4
13–24	275	0	0	1.6	98.4
25–36	240	0	0	1.6	98.4
37–48	165	0	0	1.6	98.4
49–60	74	0	0	1.6	98.4
61–72	23	0	0	1.6	98.4
73–84	13	0	0	1.6	98.4

Figure 7.26. A 6-mm-long standard neck Straumann implant serves as the distal abutment for a fixed bridge, and an 8-mm-long standard neck Straumann abutment serves as the mesial abutment for the three-unit fixed prosthesis. This prosthesis has been in function for over five years, with no change in bone crest levels around either of the implants.

Two hundred twenty-nine standard diameter, standard neck Straumann implants were utilized to restore 114 fixed prostheses in the mandibular posterior regions. One hundred thirteen of these prostheses were three-unit prostheses made up of two implant crowns and a pontic. One prosthesis was a five-unit prosthesis made up of three implant crowns with two pontics between the terminal abutments and the center implant. The implants were followed for a mean time in function of 40.5 months. Three implants were mobile at abutment connection, and one implant was lost during the 25–36 months in function interval, yielding a cumulative success rate of 98.1%. If the implants mobile at abutment connection were excluded from the calculations, so as to more accurately assess the ability of shorter implants to support a fixed prosthesis and withstand functional forces over time,

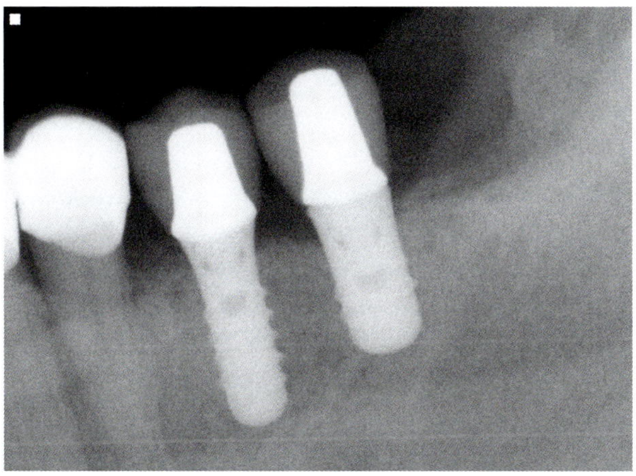

Figure 7.23 A radiograph taken four years postinsertion of 8- and 10-mm-long Straumann implants, replacing a mandibular molar and bicuspid respectively, demonstrates stable crestal peri-implant bone levels.

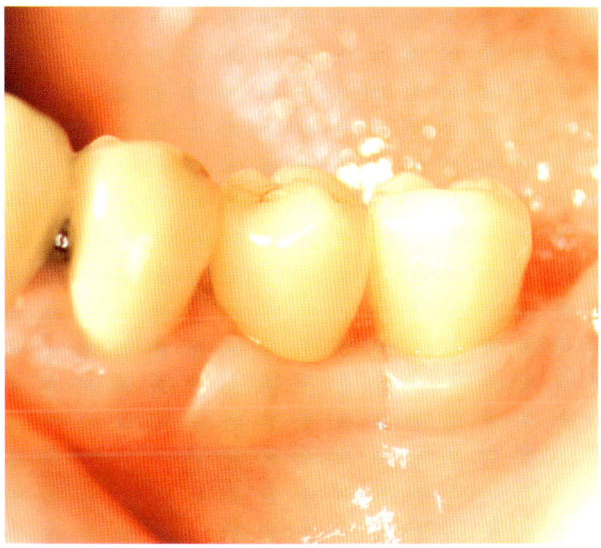

Figure 7.24 A clinical view of the implants in place.

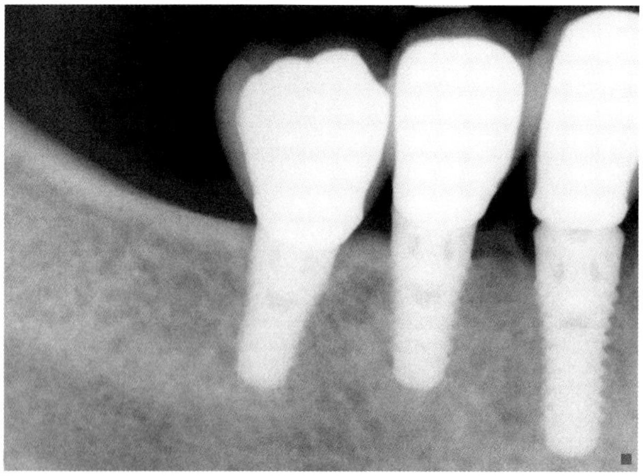

Figure 7.25 A radiograph demonstrates stability of the crestal peri-implant bone around two 8-mm-long tapered end Straumann implants utilized to restore a missing mandibular second bicuspid and first molar respectively, three years after restoration. Note the incomplete seating of the comented crown on the implant in the first bicuspid position.

the cumulative success rate of the shorter implants under function in such an application was 99.6% (Table 7.4).

Clinicians have advocated utilization of prostheses with reduced occlusal tables buccolingually, and in the case of terminal abutments mesiodistally, to lessen the magnitudes of functional and parafunctional forces, when shorter implants are restored. However, such an approach results in less reattainment of functional capabilities for the patient following therapy, and must be viewed as a compromise.

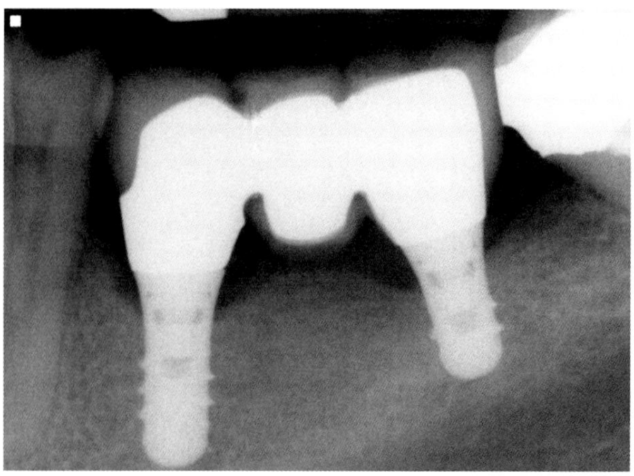

Figure 7.26 A 6-mm-long standard diameter Straumann implant has been utilized as a terminal abutment for a three-unit fixed splint in the mandibular posterior region. A radiograph taken 42 months after restoration demonstrates peri-implant crestal bone stability.

A more appropriate approach, assuming it demonstrates an acceptable level of success under function, is to utilize a shorter implant with a wider prosthetic platform, so as to incorporate a crown of appropriate dimensions to ideally replace the function which has been lost. Figures 7.27 and 7.28 demonstrate the transition to this type of concept. The initial implant was placed in the second molar position over 10 years ago. At that time, a standard diameter implant was placed, and restored with a solid abutment and a reduced occlusal table as previously described. The patient lost the first molar subsequent to this care and had it replaced 5.8 years ago with an 8-mm-long wide neck Straumann implant, which affords a 6.5-mm-wide restorative implant. The implant was restored with a solid abutment and a crown with an occlusal table of sufficient dimensions to replace all lost function for the patient.

Utilization of this approach is not limited to 8 mm or longer wide platform Straumann implants. Seven hundred twenty-two wide platform Straumann implants of 6–8 mm in length were restored with solid abutments and single crowns, and followed for a mean time of 28.5 months in function. Two implants were mobile at abutment connection. No implants were lost during function for up to 72 months, demonstrating a cumulative success rate under function of 99.9% (Table 7.5). These implants were not only utilized in "protected" situations where either a restored or natural tooth bordered each side of the implant in question. As evidenced in Figure 7.29, short, wide platform Straumann implants were also employed in terminal molar positions, and restored with abutments and single crowns.

Implant Placement at the Time of Mandibular Molar Extraction

As will be discussed in Chapter 9, wide platform and/or wide diameter implants are often placed at the time of mandibular molar extraction, in conjunction with appropriate regenerative therapy. Such an approach lessens the number of surgical

Table 7.4 Cumulative implant success rates for short implants utilized as abutments for fixed prostheses in posterior mandible.

Months after abutment connection	Implants beginning of interval	Failures during interval	Interval failure rate	Cumulative failure rate	Cumulative success rate
0–12	229	3	1.3	1.3	98.7
13–24	181	0	0	1.3	98.7
25–36	156	1	0.6	1.9	98.1
37–48	110	0	0	1.9	98.1
49–60	70	0	0	1.9	98.1
61–72	20	0	0	1.9	98.1
73–84	7	0	0	1.9	98.1

sessions for the patient, and contracts the overall time of therapy.

Two hundred eighty-three wide platform Straumann implants of various lengths were placed at the time of mandibular molar extraction, and followed for a mean time of 36.4 months in function (27). Of the 283 implants placed, 204 were 8 or 9 mm in length, and 79 were 10 or 12 mm in length. The mean time in function for the 8 or 9 mm length implants was 36.5 months. The mean time in function for the 10- or 12-mm-long implants was 34.7 months. The overall cumulative success rate of these implants in function was 98.7%.

In the 8- to 9-mm-long implant group, one implant was mobile at the time of abutment connection and one implant was lost in function during the 25- to 36-month time interval, yielding a cumulative success rate of 98.5%. The 10- to 12-mm-long implant group demonstrated one implant mobile at the time of abutment connection. No other

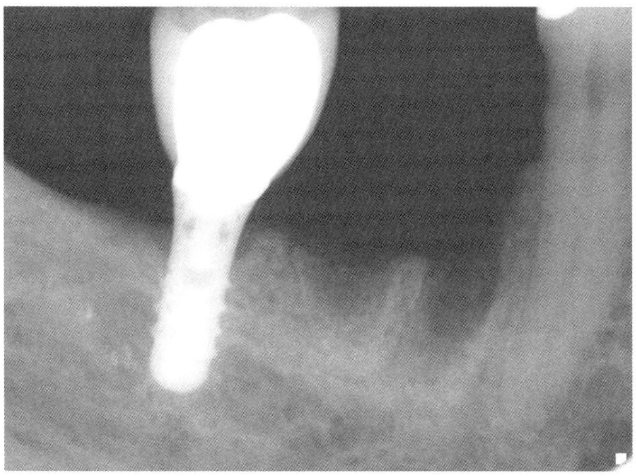

Figure 7.27 An 8-mm-long standard diameter Straumann implant has previously been replaced and restored with a single crown in the mandibular second molar position. This radiograph demonstrates both the stability of the crestal bone around the implant 84 months after restoration, and the fact that the first molar has now been lost.

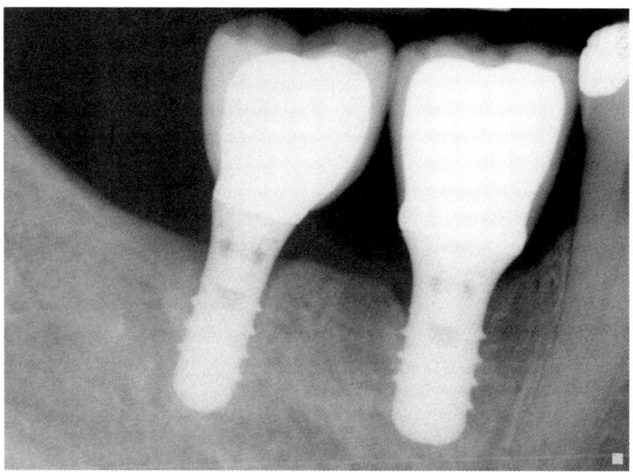

Figure 7.28 An 8-mm-long Straumann implant with a 4.8-mm-wide body and a 6.5-mm-wide restorative platform has been inserted and restored to replace the missing mandibular first molar.

Table 7.5 Cumulative implant success rates for short wide platform implants restored with single crowns in the posterior mandible.

Months after abutment connection	Implants beginning of interval	Failures during interval	Interval failure rate	Cumulative failure rate	Cumulative success rate
0–12	722	1	0.1	0.1	99.9
13–24	578	0	0	0.1	99.9
25–36	416	0	0	0.1	99.9
37–48	246	0	0	0.1	99.9
49–60	93	0	0	0.1	99.9
61–72	20	0	0	0.1	99.9

implants were lost in function, yielding a cumulative success rate of 98.7%. The difference between the cumulative success rates for the two groups was not statistically significant (Tables 7.6 and 7.7).

Shorter Implant Utilization in Maxillary Posterior Areas

The use of 9 mm or shorter noncountersunk Straumann implants in the posterior maxilla has previously been documented (28).

Nine hundred eighty-seven implants replaced missing maxillary molars and were restored with solid abutments and unsplinted single crowns. The implants were followed for up to 84 months in function with a mean time in function of 29.3 months, yielding a cumulative success rate in function of 95.1%. Followed to the present day, and including implants placed since this publication, a total of 1,757 implants have been placed and restored with solid abutments and single crowns in intact arches, in maxillary molar positions, of lengths between 6 and 12 mm. The cumulative success rate of the implants in function was 95.7%.

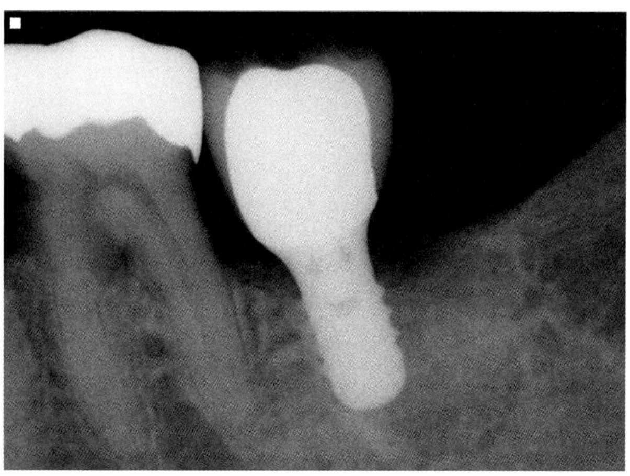

Figure 7.29 A radiograph taken 72 months after restoration of a wide platform 8-mm-long Straumann implant in the position of the mandibular second molar demonstrates stability of the peri-implant crestal bone.

Figure 7.30 demonstrates the stability of the peri-implant crestal bone around an 8-mm-long standard diameter Straumann 84 months after its placement and restoration in a maxillary first molar position.

As will be discussed in Chapter 8, implants of various lengths are often placed in conjunction with trephine and osteotome use to implode a core of the residual bone crestal to the floor of the sinus. A paper published in 2002 (29) documented the cumulative success and failure rates of 116 Straumann implants 6, 7, 8, 9, 10, or 11 mm long which were placed at the time of trephine and osteotome utilization. The implants demonstrated a cumulative success rate of 98.3% under function.

Data that examine implants placed in such situations up to the present time, as well incorporating the implants placed at the time of previous publication, demonstrate that 306 implants 6, 7, 8, or 9 mm long, placed at the time of trephine and osteotome use and restored with single crowns, have been in function for up to eight years with a meantime in function of 30.9 months. The cumulative success rate of these implants in function is

Table 7.6 Cumulative implant success rates for short, wide platform implants placed at the time of mandibular molar extraction and restored with single crowns.

Months after abutment connection	Implants beginning of interval	Failures during interval	Interval failure rate	Cumulative failure rate	Cumulative success rate
0–12	204	1	0.5	0.5	99.5
13–24	153	0	0	0.5	99.5
25–36	113	1	1.0	1.5	98
37–48	94	0	0	1.5	98.5
49–60	52	0	0	1.5	98.5
61–72	23	0	0	1.5	98.5

99.0% (27). During the same time frame, the cumulative success rate of 10- and 11-mm-long implants placed at the time of trephine and osteotome use and restored with single crowns is 98.9%. There is no statistically significant difference between the cumulative success rates of the two groups, which have been separated based upon implant length.

Ferrigno et al. (30) assessed 588 Straumann implants of 8, 10, and 12 mm lengths restored with abutments and single crowns, over a mean observation time of 60 months. The cumulative

Table 7.7 Cumulative success rates for wide platform implants placed at the time of mandibular molar extraction and restored with single crowns.

Implant length	Months after abutment connection	Implants beginning of interval	Failures during interval	Interval failure rate	Cumulative failure rate	Cumulative success rate
8–9 mm	0–12	204	1	0.5	0.5	99.5
	13–24	153	0	0	0.5	99.5
	25–36	113	1	1.0	1.5	98.5
	37–48	84	0	0	1.5	98.5
	49–60	52	0	0	1.5	98.5
	61–72	23	0	0	1.5	98.5
10–12 mm	0–12	79	1	1.3	1.3	98.7
	13–24	72	0	0	1.3	98.7
	25–36	47	0	0	1.3	98.7
	37–48	21	0	0	1.3	98.7
	49–60	8	0	0	1.3	98.7
	61–72	2	0	0	1.3	98.7
Total	0–12	283	2	0.7	0.7	99.3
	13–24	225	0	0	0.7	99.3
	25–36	160	1	0.6	1.3	98.7
	37–48	105	0	0	1.3	98.7
	49–60	60	0	0	1.3	98.7
	61–72	25	0	0	1.3	98.7

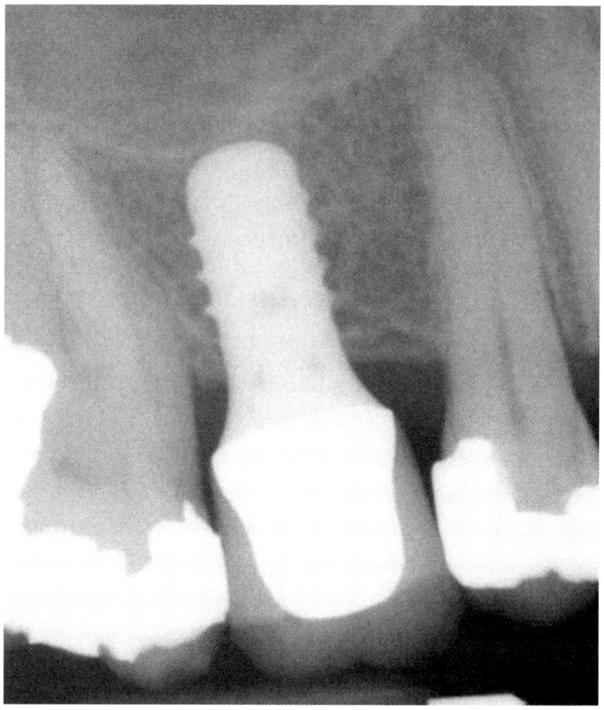

Figure 7.30 An 8-mm-long, standard diameter Straumann implant has been restored in a maxillary first molar position. A radiograph taken 84 months after restoration demonstrates the stability of the crestal peri-implant bone.

success rates noted were 88.9% for the 8-mm-long implants; 90.5% for the 10-mm-long implants; and 93.4% for the 12-mm-long implants. Although the authors stated that there was no difference in cumulative success rates between the various implant lengths, the difference between 88.9% and 93.4% could certainly give pause to the utilization of a specific treatment modality or implant length. However, as previously mentioned, such discrepancies have not been discovered following examination of the other clinical data presented.

Shorter Implant Utilization at the Time of Maxillary Molar Extraction

A previous publication documented the placement of implants in the manipulated interradicular bone at the time of maxillary molar trisection and extraction (31). The implants documented were 10, 12, and 14 mm in length, and of a specific design with a 4.1-mm-wide "apex," a tapering body, and a 6.5-mm-wide restored platform. Subsequent examination of all implants placed at the time of maxillary molar insertion documents the results of 297 implant placements (32). Two hundred nine of these implants were 10, 12, or 14 mm long and were of the aforementioned tapered design. However, 88 of these implants were 8-mm-long implants with a 4.8-mm-wide nontapered body and a 6.5-mm-wide restorative platform. The mean time in function for all implants was 18.9 months. The mean time in function for the 8-mm-long implants was 20.6 months, while the mean time in function for the implants of 10, 12, and 14 mm lengths was 18.3 months. No implants from either group were lost during function.

Conclusions

There is no doubt that both finite element analyses and available clinical data support the use of shorter implants, where it will prove advantageous to the patient with regard to simplification of therapy and lessening of the time of the overall course of treatment. However, as with any treatment modality, utilization of shorter implants must be grounded in a framework of a comprehensive treatment plan and an understanding of the specific challenges of each patient's care.

Severe osteoporosis, the presence of a nonideal maxillomandibular occlusal relationship which cannot be treated through orthodontics and/or surgical correction due to either structural or patient-imposed limitations, or the presence of a significant parafunctional habit, are all comorbidities which may mandate the use of significant regenerative therapy, longer implants, and possible splinting of implants.

The challenge is not to decide whether or not shorter implants may be successfully utilized in the majority of situations; they may. Rather, the challenge facing the conscientious clinician is to identify those situations where such utilization is appropriate, and the instances where other avenues of therapy must be explored.

References

1. Adell R, Eriksson B, Lekholm U, Branemark P-I, and Jemt T. 1990. A long term follow-up study of osseoin-

tegrated implants in the treatment of totally edentulous jaws. *Int J Oral Maxillofac Surg* 5:347–359.
2. Albrektsson T. 1988. A multi center report on osseointegrated oral implants. *J Prosthet Dent* 60: 75–84.
3. Fugazzotto PA, Gulbransen H, Wheeler S, and Lindsay J. 1993. The use of IMZ osseo integrated implants in partially and completely edentulous patients: Success and failure rates of 2023 implant cylinders up to sixty plus months in function. *Int J Oral Maxillofac Implants* 8:635–640.
4. Albrektsson T, Dahl E, Enbom L, et al. 1998. Osseointegrated oral implants: A Swedish multi center study of 8139 consecutively inserted Nobelpharma implants. *J Periodontol* 59:287–296.
5. Lum LB. 1991. A biomechanical rationale for the use of short implants. *J Oral Implantol* 17:126–131.
6. Pierriesnard L, Reinouard F, Renoult P, and Barquins M. 2003. Influence of implant length and bicortical anchorage on implant stress distribution. *Clin Implant Dent Relat Res* 5:254–262.
7. Lai H, Zhang F, Zhang B, Yang C, and Xue M. 1998. Influence of percentage of osseointegration on stress distribution around dental implants. *Chin J Dent Res* 1:7–11.
8. Petrie CS and Williams JL. 2005. Comparative evaluation of implant designs: Influence of diameter, length and taper. *Clin Oral Implants Res* 16:486–494.
9. Holmgren EP, Seckinger RJ, Kilgren LM, and Mate F. 1998. Evaluating parameters of osseointegrated dental implants using finite element analysis: A two dimensional comparative study examining the effects of implant diameter, implant shape, and load direction. *J Oral Implantol* 24:80–88.
10. Himmlova L, Dostalova T, Kacovsky A, and Konbickova S. 2004. Influence of implant length and diameter on stress distribution: A final element analysis. *J Prosthet Dent* 1:20–25.
11. Akca K and Iplikciogou H. 2002. Finite element analysis of short implant usage in place of cantilevers. *J Oral Rehabil* 29:350–356.
12. Buser D, Mericske-Stern R, Bernard J, et al. 1997. Long term evaluation of non submerged ITI implants. *Clin Oral Implants Res* 8:161–172.
13. Feldman S, Boitel N, Weng D, Kohles SS, and Stach RM. 2004. Five year survival of short machined surface/Osseotite implants. *Clin Implant Dent Relat Res* 6:16–23.
14. das Neves FD, Fones D, Bernardeds SR, do Prado CJ, and Neto AJ. 2006. Short implants—an analysis of longitudinal studies. *J Oral Maxillofac Implants* 21: 86–93.
15. Jaffin RA and Berman CL. 1991. The excessive loss of Branemark fixtures in type IV bone: A 5 year analysis. *J Periodontol* 62:2–4.
16. Deporter D, Watson P, Pharoah M, Levy D, and Todescan R. 1999. Five to six year results of prospective clinical trials using the Endopore dental implant and a mandibular overdenture. *Clin Oral Implants Res* 10: 95–102.
17. ten Bruggenkate CM, Asikainen P, Foitzik C, Krekeler G, and Sutter F. 1998. Six millimeter non-submerged dental implants: Results of multicenter clinical trial of 1 to 7 years. *J Oral Maxillofac Implants* 13: 791–798.
18. Nedir R, Bischof M, Briaux J-M, Beter S, Smukler-Moncler S, and Bernard J-P. 2004. A seven year life table analysis from a prospective study on ITI implants with special emphasis on the use of short implants. Results from a private practice. *Clin Oral Implants Res* 15:150–157.
19. Arlin ML. 2006. Short dental implants as a treatment option: Results from an observational study in a single private practice. *Int J Oral Maxillofac Implants* 21:769–776.
20. Fugazzotto PA, Vlassis J, and Butler B. 2004. ITI implant use in private practice. Clinical results with 5526 implants followed up to 72+ months in function. *Int J Oral Maxillofac Implants* 3:408–412.
21. Anitua E, Orive G, Aguirre JJ, and Andia I. 2008. Five year clinical evaluation of short dental implants placed in posterior areas: A retrospective study. *J Periodontol* 79:42–48.
22. Rockni S, Todescan R, Watson P, Pharoah M, Adegbembo AO, and Deporter D. 2005. Assessment of crown to root ratios with short sintered porous surface implants. *Int J Oral Maxillofac Implants* 20:69–76.
23. Tawil G, Aboujaoude N, and Younan R. 2006. Influence of prosthetic parameters on the survival and complication rates of short implants. *Int J Oral Maxillofac Implants* 21:275–282.
24. Blanes RJ, Bernard JP, Blanes ZM, and Belser VC. 2007. A ten year prospective study of ITI implants in the posterior maxilla: Influence of crown implant ratio. *Clin Oral Implants Res* 18:707–714.
25. Hsu M-L, Chen F-C, Kao H-C, and Cheng C-K. 2007. Influence of off access loading on an anterior maxillary implant: A three dimensional finite element analysis. *Int J Oral Maxillofac Implants* 22:301–309.
26. Meada Y, Satoh T, and Sogo M. 2006. In vitro differences of stress concentrations for internal and external hex connections. *J Oral Rehabil* 33:75–78.
27. Fugazzotto PA. 2008. Shorter implants in clinical practice: Rationale and treatment results. *Int J Maxillofac* 23:487–496.
28. Fugazzotto PA, Beagle J, Vlassis J, Ganeles J, Jaffin R, and Kumar A. 2004. Success and failure rates of 987 implants 9 millimeters or shorter replacing missing maxillary molars. *J Periodontol* 75:327–332.

29. Fugazzotto PA. 2002. Immediate implant placement following a modified trephine/osteotome approach: 116 implants up to four years in function. *Int J Oral Maxillofac Implants* 17:113–120.
30. Ferrigno N. 2006. Dental implant placement in conjunction with osteotome sinus floor elevation. *Clin Oral Implants Res* 17:194–205.
31. Fugazzotto PA. 2008. Implant placement at the time of maxillary molar extraction: Treatment protocols and report of results. *J Periodontol* 79:216–223.
32. Fugazzotto PA. 2008. Implant placement at the time of mandibular molar extraction: Description of technique and preliminary results of 341 cases. *J Periodontol* 79:737–747.

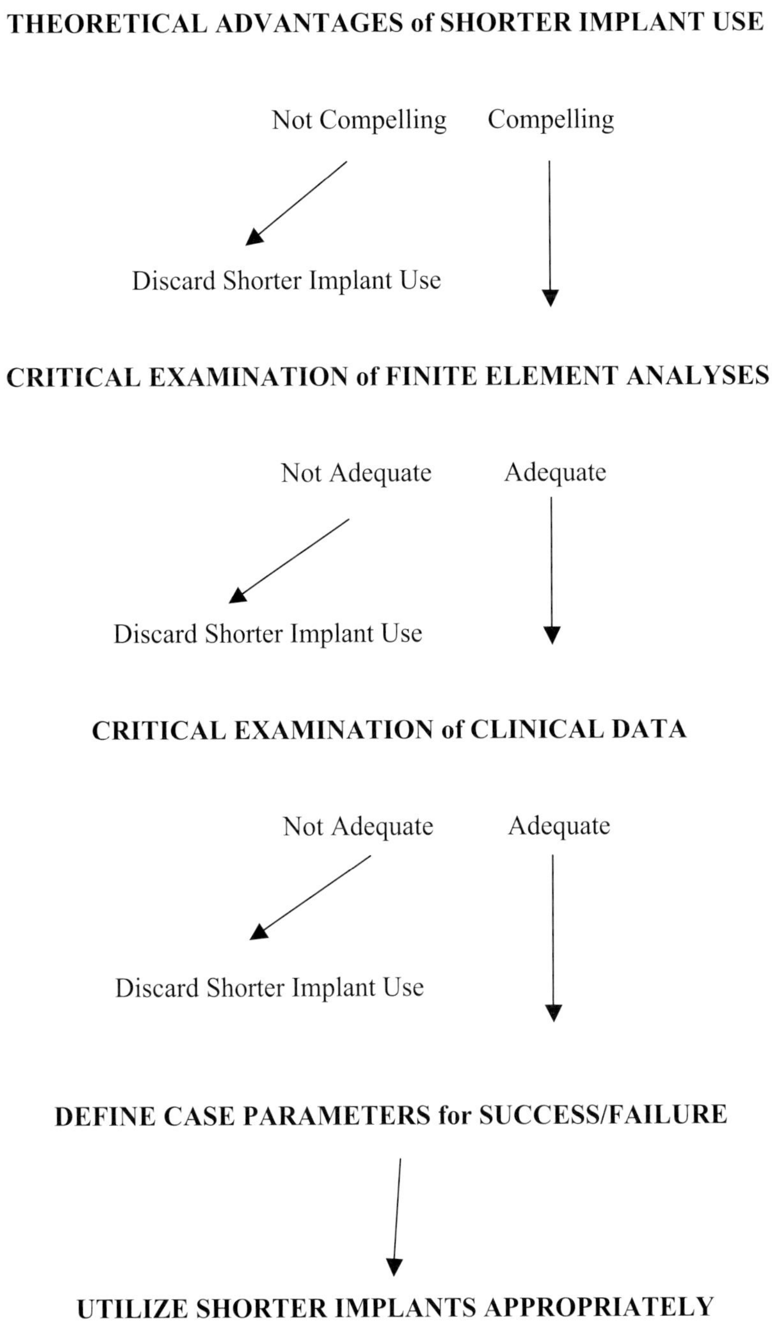

Flow chart 7.1 Assessing the feasibility of shorter implant use.

Chapter 8

Decision Making Following Extraction of Multirooted Maxillary Teeth

Paul A. Fugazzotto, DDS

Outline

Implant placement and regenerative therapy at the time of removal of maxillary multirooted teeth offers the potential to lessen both the number of surgical sessions for the patient and the overall length of treatment to be performed. However, such a treatment option should only be utilized if the final treatment outcomes are not compromised as compared to more conventional treatment approaches, which include tooth extraction with simultaneous augmentation therapy followed by implant placement 6–8 months later, and subsequent implant restoration.

As with other treatment approaches, a fundamental need in order to appropriately assess treatment outcomes is standardization of the definitions of successful therapy. Numerous authors have demonstrated the ability of implants immediately placed in single- or multirooted extraction sockets to attain predictable osseointegration in the presence or absence of various grafting materials, depending on the specific clinical situation. Lazzara (1) first documented such therapy in 1989. Included in the cases presented by Lazzara was insertion of an implant in the maxillary bicuspid site at the time of tooth extraction. Clinical reentry demonstrated osseointegration, and "fill" of the residual extraction socket defect surrounding the implant. However, while the treatment presented certainly resulted in an osseointegrated implant capable of bearing the planned restoration, it revealed a number of potential concerns, including the fact that the buccal and palatal walls of the alveolus had demonstrated some resorption despite the placement of a covering membrane. In addition, the implant had been placed subcrestally, a position now advocated by few practitioners and implant manufacturers. Nevertheless, Lazzara's paper led the way to further exploration of the possibilities of implant placement at the time of tooth removal.

Unfortunately, implant placement has all too often been dictated by the residual extraction socket morphology. Nowhere is this more evident than when discussing implant placement in extraction sockets of multirooted teeth. Schwartz-Arad et al. (2) reported on the placement of implants at the time of maxillary molar extraction, and their subsequent restoration with single crowns. While they reported that all implants were functioning successfully, this definition of success was limited to short-term implant stability (i.e., maintenance of bone levels around the implants and lack of clinical mobility). The one clinical case presented in the paper demonstrated the fact that the implants were placed in the palatal root sockets at the time of tooth removal and angled toward the buccal, so that crowns could be fabricated in acceptable restorative positions. While these implants demonstrated stability under early function, such an approach is certainly not ideal. The patient is left with a potential hindrance to plaque control efforts due to the necessary buccal cantilever of the implant restoration. In addition, the severe off-angle forces being placed upon the implant during occlusion and any possible parafunction which may be present are not desirable, if they can be avoided.

Any definition of success utilized to assess various treatment approaches for implant placement at the time of extraction of multirooted maxillary teeth must include the need to place the implants in ideal restorative positions. The implants must be placed in the exact positions they would occupy if being inserted into intact ridges rather than fresh, multirooted extraction sockets.

The challenge is not only to develop the technical means by which to effect such insertion. As important is the utilization of appropriate diagnostic techniques and acumen to recognize situations in which it is more prudent to effect regeneration at the time of tooth removal, and reenter the site once regeneration has been completed to insert the implant in the rebuilt alveolar ridge.

Finally, the conscientious clinician must recognize situations in which he or she is unable to predict the ability to immediately insert the implant until the time of tooth removal. This information must be communicated to the patient prior to initiation of care, and each possible course of therapy must be discussed and explored with the patient. Failure to do so will result in misunderstandings and a potential compromise in both treatment outcomes and patient experience.

Augmentation and Implant Placement Following Tooth Extraction in the Posterior Maxilla

A variety of treatment options present themselves at the time of tooth extraction in the posterior maxilla, including the following:

1. Augmentation of the extraction socket defect utilizing particulate material and a secured covering membrane: This option may be mandated when faced with one or more of the following:
   (a) Anticipated implant placement and restoration within the patient's esthetic zone, in the face of a severely compromised buccal alveolar ridge.
   (b) Anticipated implant placement in an extraction socket defect with inadequate residual interradicular bone for fixation of the implant in the desired restorative position, as a result of root morphology or pathologic bone destruction.
   (c) Anticipated implant placement in a residual extraction socket that is too wide to stabilize the implant in the desired restorative position.
2. Implant placement in a residual extraction socket defect, followed by utilization of appropriate particulate materials and covering membranes to facilitate regeneration of alveolar bone in the residual extraction socket defect surrounding an appropriately sized implant.
3. Implant placement in the extraction socket, following implosion of a core of autogenous bone apical to the extraction socket utilizing previously described techniques: Particulate materials and a covering membrane are placed around the implant to facilitate regeneration of alveolar bone in the residual extraction socket defect surrounding the implant.
4. Lateral sinus augmentation therapy and augmentation of the residual extraction socket defect utilizing particulate material and membranes, as described in Chapter 6.
5. Lateral sinus augmentation therapy with simultaneous implant placement and regeneration of alveolar bone in the residual extraction socket defect surrounding the implant, utilizing appropriate particulate material and covering membranes.

Although use of various materials and techniques to effect augmentation of extraction socket defects has been documented, it is nevertheless important to establish definitions of success when employing such a therapeutic approach. Regenerating alveolar bone in the extraction socket defect, while predictable with a variety of approaches, does not always comprehensively address the area to be treated. A comprehensive definition of success following augmentation of extraction socket defects must include both regeneration of bone within the body of the extraction socket and regeneration of the prepathologic alveolar ridge morphology, including the buccal and palatal and/or lingual alveolar ridge line angles. Such an approach affords the necessary alveolar ridge morphology for support of the soft tissue drape of esthetics around a restored implant. While this approach mandates specific flap designs and material utilization, it diminishes and often eliminates the need for secondary soft tissue grafting procedures, maximizes esthetics treatment outcomes, and allows placement of appropriate diameter implants in ideal positions.

The placement of implants at the time of tooth extraction in the posterior maxilla is highly patient and site-specific. The first determination that must be made is the minimum implant dimensions necessary in the context of a given treatment plan for a specific patient. Once these parameters have been established, it must be decided whether or not successful placement of an implant of the desired dimensions in a specific situation is feasible.

The second decision is site-specific and is dependent upon the tooth to be replaced and the morphology of the residual alveolar housing of the extraction socket, including the interradicular bone. This interradicular bone should be maintained whenever possible. Such maintenance is significantly enhanced by sectioning all multirooted teeth to be extracted, and removing each root individually following gentle utilization of piezosurgery, periotomes, and elevators. A further advantage of sectioning the tooth and removing each root separately is the significantly decreased chance of root tip fracture. The apical extents of the roots of most multirooted teeth demonstrate significant curvature, often in directions which are mutually exclusive from removal as one unit without significant bone resection. Sectioning the tooth into individual roots allows each root to be removed along the path most conducive to its extraction without fracture.

Augmentation Without Simultaneous Implant Placement

If adequate bone is not present in the appropriate areas to allow ideal implant positioning following tooth removal, implant placement should not be attempted. Neither the patient nor the clinician benefits from a malpositioned implant. Rather, it is better to regenerate the prepathologic alveolar ridge morphology as previously discussed, and place the implant in a reconstructed ridge at a second surgical visit.

Effecting such regenerative therapy in a maxillary bicuspid region, and ensuring the attainment and maintenance of soft tissue primary closure throughout the course of regeneration, is a highly predictable treatment approach which will result in regeneration of the prepathologic alveolar ridge morphology, and covering soft tissues of sufficient thickness to help maximize final esthetic treatment outcomes. Useful flap designs, criteria for membrane selection, and graft utilization have all been discussed in detail in Chapter 2.

Augmentation following extraction of a maxillary first bicuspid should not be viewed as merely a means to obtain fill of the extraction socket defect and rebuild the buccal and palatal line angles of the alveolar ridge. If such regeneration will result in inadequate height of bone for placement of an implant of a desired length in a specific clinical situation, apical augmentation should be performed during the same visit. This apical augmentation is easily effected through the use of trephines and osteotomes as previously described, or osteotomes alone if the most apical extent of the extraction socket approaches or is contiguous with the floor of the sinus. Following implosion of an alveolar core where appropriate, or gentle reshaping and lifting of the floor of the sinus through osteotome use alone, graft materials are placed and a covering membrane, selected according to defect morphology is secured with fixation tacks as already discussed. The net effect of this therapy will be not only complete regeneration of prepathologic ridge morphologies, but also provision of additional height of bone for placement of a longer implant.

Implant Placement at the Time of Extraction of Two-Rooted Maxillary Bicuspids

A two-rooted maxillary bicuspid presents a unique challenge to implant placement following mesiodistal hemisection and separate removal of the buccal and palatal roots. The residual interradicular bone, while too thin to provide a set point for osteotomy preparation, is usually of sufficient thickness to guide the bur into either the buccal or palatal root socket. Neither location is ideal for placement of the planned implant. An implant placed in the palatal root socket will necessitate the need to fabricate a crown with a large buccal cantilever, which represents a potential plaque control and force distribution compromise. Placement of the implant in the buccal root socket will often lead to compromise of the buccal alveolar bone, and a less than ideal final esthetic result (Flow chart 8.1).

Such problems are easily overcome as follows.

Two-rooted maxillary bicuspids are hemisected, and each root is atraumatically extracted. A Rongeur is utilized to remove the often problematic interradicular bone, providing a stable base for osteotomy preparation (3). This bone is placed in sterile saline for future utilization. Therapy now proceeds in one of four manners:

(a) If adequate bone height is present crestal to the floor of the sinus for placement of an implant of the desired size, implant placement is carried out. The osseous coagulum that was collected during osteotomy preparation and the previously removed interradicular bone are packed around the implant in the residual extraction socket defect. If the buccal and palatal extraction socket walls are not compromised, a bone swaging technique is utilized to implode the coronal 3 mm of the buccal and palatal extraction socket ridges against the implant. No covering membrane is placed (Figures 8.1–8.9). However, if a bone swaging technique cannot be

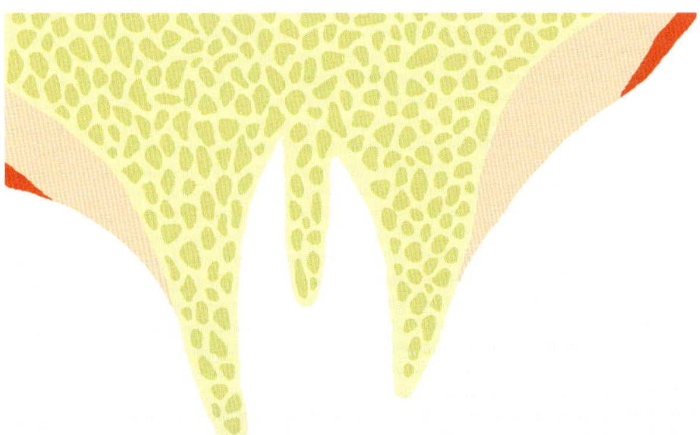

Figure 8.1 A maxillary first bicuspid has been hemisected and extracted.

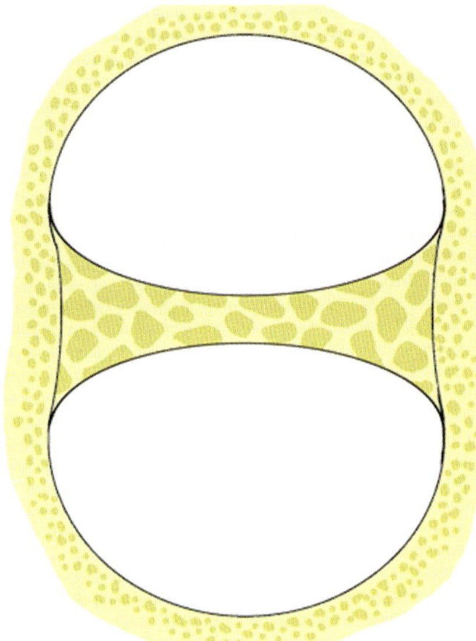

Figure 8.2 An occlusal view demonstrating the position of the interradicular bone and the buccal and palatal root extraction sockets.

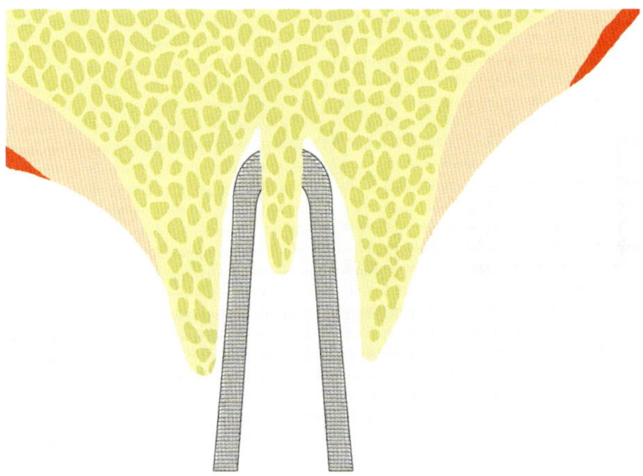

Figure 8.3 A Rongeur is utilized to remove the interradicular bone. This bone is placed in sterile saline for further use.

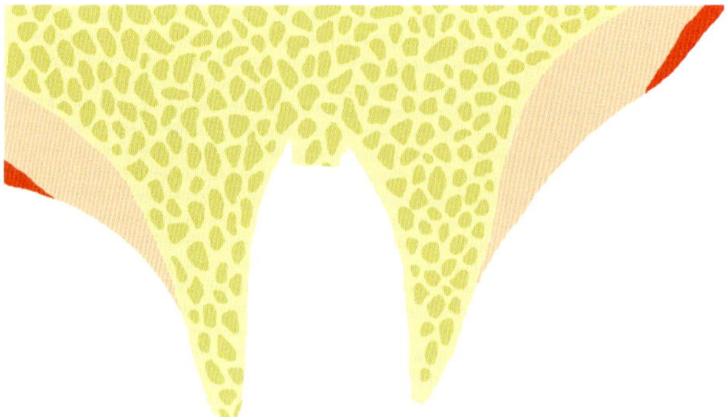

Figure 8.4 A view of the extraction socket with the interradicular bone removed. A stable base is now present for osteotomy preparation in an ideal position.

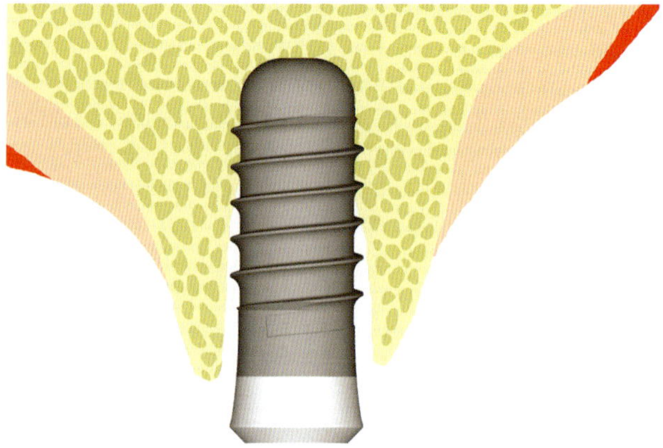

Figure 8.6 An implant is placed in an ideal position within the extraction socket. Narrow implants are not utilized in maxillary bicuspid extraction sockets.

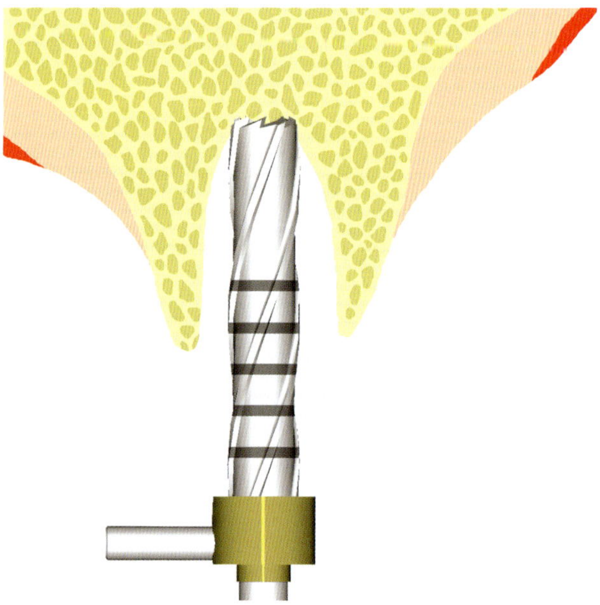

Figure 8.5 Osteotomy preparation is carried out in the conventional manner.

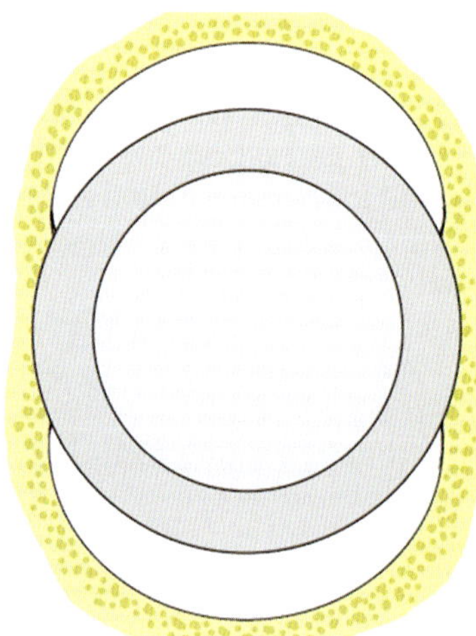

Figure 8.7 An occlusal view demonstrating the diameter of the neck of the implant in relation to the extraction socket morphology.

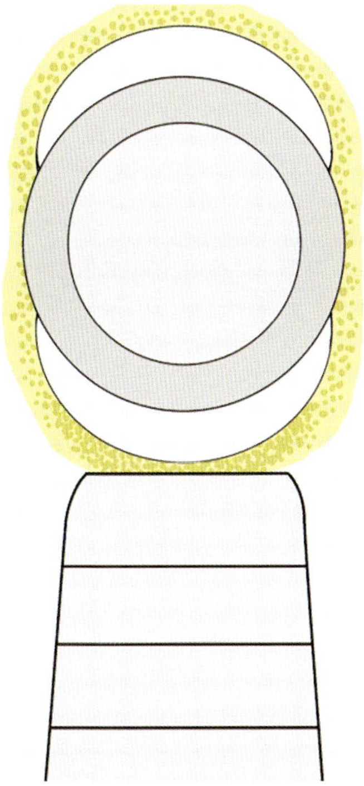

Figure 8.8 After a combination of the removed interradicular bone and osseous coagulum collected during osteotomy preparation are packed into the residual extraction socket defect, an osteotome is employed to perform a bone swage on the most crestal aspects of the buccal and palatal extraction socket walls.

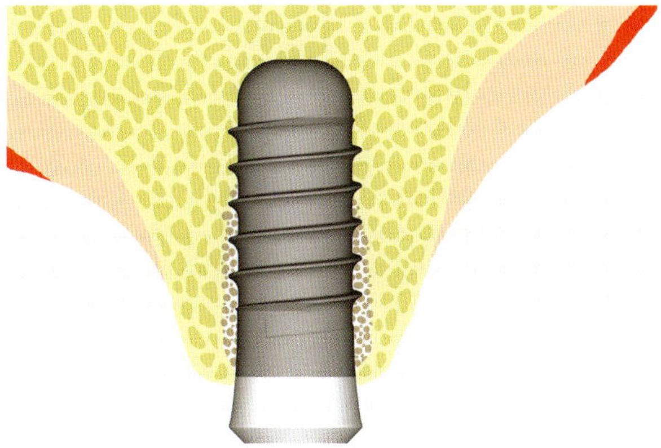

Figure 8.9 A view demonstrating the graft material in place and the swaged buccal and palatal crestal bone.

utilized due to buccal or palatal extraction wall compromise, a covering membrane is placed according to previously described criteria.

(b) If adequate bone height is not present crestal to the floor of the sinus for placement of an implant of the desired length, but 2x-2 is an adequate dimension for implant placement, with x equalling the apicocrestal dimension of the bone crestal to the floor of the sinus, the residual bone crestal to the floor of the sinus is imploded utilizing an osteotome and trephine technique, and the implant is placed. Once again, particulate material, bone swaging and/or possible membrane use are employed as already described.

(c) If 2x-2 is not an adequate dimension for the length of the implant to be placed, but 4x-6 is an adequate dimension for the implant to be placed, an osteotome and trephine technique are employed as previously described, in conjunction with augmentation of the extraction socket defect utilizing particulate material and an appropriate secured, covering membrane. The area is reentered eight weeks later and an osteotome and trephine technique is once again utilized to implode the bone crestal to the floor of the sinus. The implant is placed at this time. It is rare to utilize the "double external sinus augmentation" technique in the maxillary bicuspid region.

(d) If 4x-6 is not an adequate dimension for the desired size of the implant to be placed, a lateral approach sinus augmentation procedure is carried out with concomitant augmentation of the extraction socket defect utilizing appropriate materials. The area is reentered 4–6 months after augmentation, depending upon the extent of augmentation which was necessary, and implant placement is completed.

AUGMENTATION AND IMPLANT PLACEMENT AT THE TIME OF EXTRACTION OF MAXILLARY MOLARS

Once again, it is imperative to ensure that implant placement at the time of removal of multirooted maxillary molars is effected in an ideal prosthetic position. If the final implant position will be less than ideal due to the residual extraction socket morphology, inadequacies in the techniques utilized, or a combination of both, regeneration must first be carried out, and the implant placed in a second surgical visit. In such a situation, all diagnostic criteria and technical considerations discussed in Chapter 2 apply, and are aimed at regeneration of prepathologic alveolar ridge morphologies (Flow chart 8.2).

AUGMENTATION AT THE TIME OF MAXILLARY MOLAR EXTRACTION

If inadequate bone is present interradicularly to allow stabilization of an implant in an ideal position following sectioning and extraction of a maxillary molar, therapy proceeds as follows. The tooth to be extracted is hemisected, and each root is removed individually, taking care to preserve the interradicular bone wherever possible (Figure 8.10). Following defect debridement, a trephine is chosen of sufficient diameter to encompass the interradicular bone (Figure 8.11). This trephine is placed over the interradicular bone (Figure 8.12), and an osteotomy is prepared to within 1 mm of the sinus floor (Figure 8.13). If the clinician is unsure of a safe depth to which to prepare the osteotomy as a result of invagination of the sinus membrane between the extracted roots of the molar in question, an osteotome is applied to the interradicular bone prior to trephine utilization, and gently malleted. If implosion of the residual interradicular bone can be effected without use of a trephine in this manner,

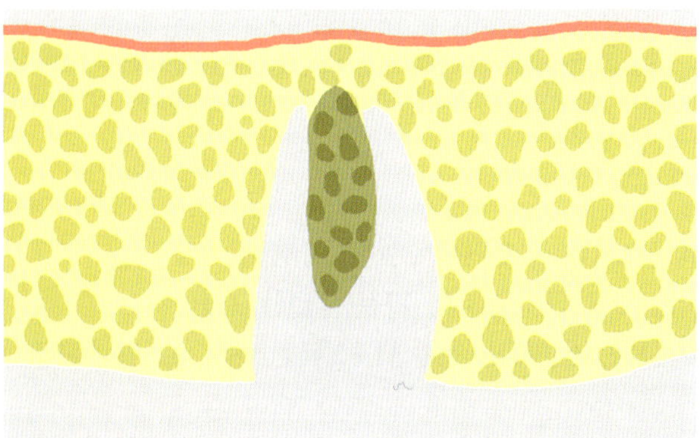

Figure 8.10 A maxillary molar has been trisected and the roots have been extracted individually, with care being taken to preserve the residual interradicular bone.

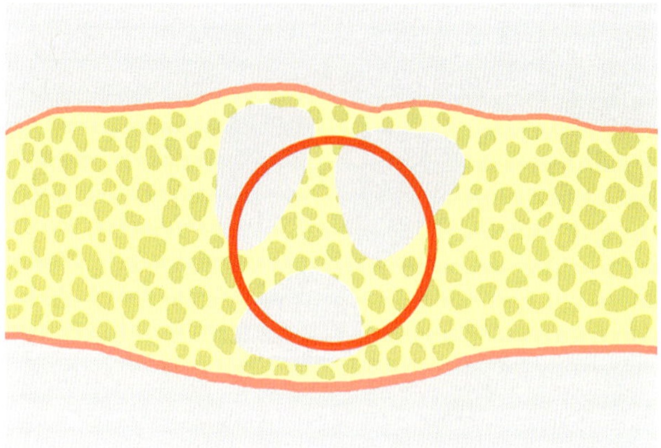

Figure 8.11 A trephine is chosen of sufficient diameter to encompass the interradicular bone.

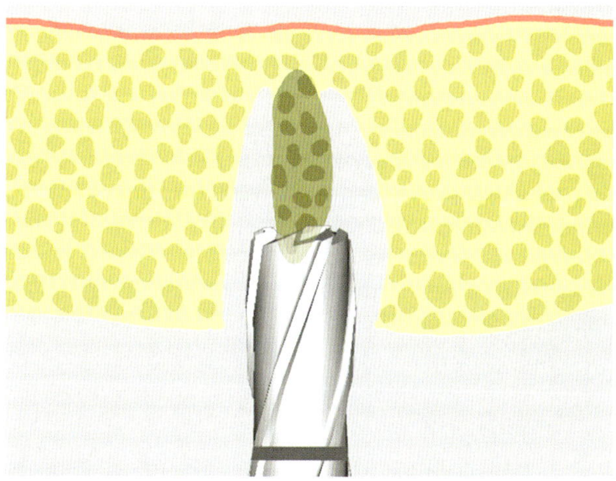

Figure 8.12 The trephine is placed over the interradicular bone.

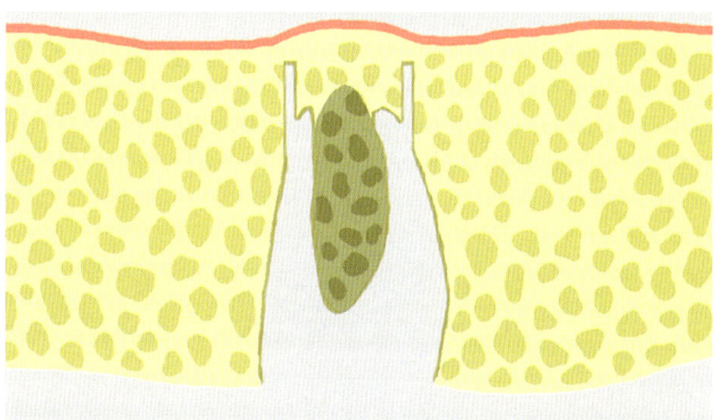

Figure 8.13 An osteotomy is prepared to within 1 mm of the sinus floor.

the interradicular bone is imploded to a depth 1 mm less than the apices of the adjacent root sockets. However, if the interradicular bone proves immobile in the face of gentle osteotome malleting without trephine utilization, a trephine is employed as described, and an osteotome is utilized to apically displace the prepared core of bone (Figure 8.14). Malleting of this core of bone will lift the sinus membrane in the area of the interradicular bone (Figure 8.15). The core is imploded to a depth 1 mm less than the depth of the osteotomy preparation (Figure 8.16). A titanium-reinforced or resorbable membrane is now chosen depending upon defect morphology as previously described, and is secured with fixation tacks. The extraction socket defect is filled with the appropriate graft material, the membrane is folded over the extraction socket (Figure 8.17), and soft tissue primary closure is attained and maintained throughout the course of regeneration.

The net result of therapy is regeneration of an ideal ridge form following complete fill of the extraction socket and the space created beneath the membrane, as well as attainment of additional bone height in the area of the interradicular bone, in anticipation of eventual implant placement (Figure 8.18). Such regeneration allows ideal implant positioning and subsequent restoration (Figure 8.19).

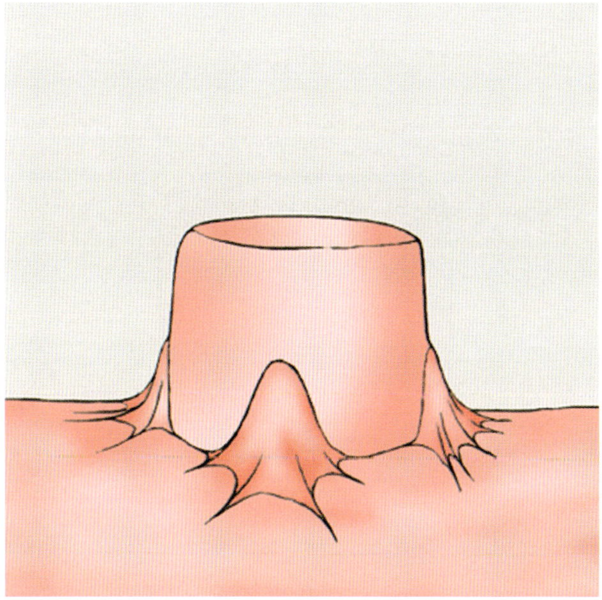

Figure 8.15 A view from within the sinus demonstrates the imploded core and lifted sinus membrane.

Clinical Example One

A 36-year-old female presented with hopeless prognoses for her maxillary right first and second molars and second bicuspid, due to a combination of periodontal destruction, caries and multiple root

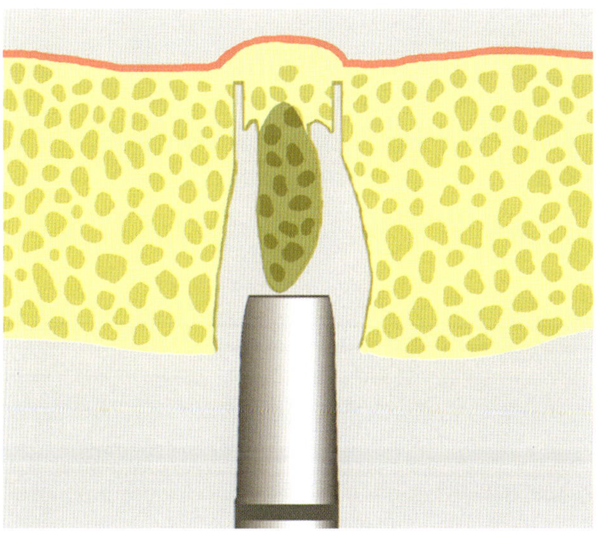

Figure 8.14 The detached bone core is imploded with an osteotome.

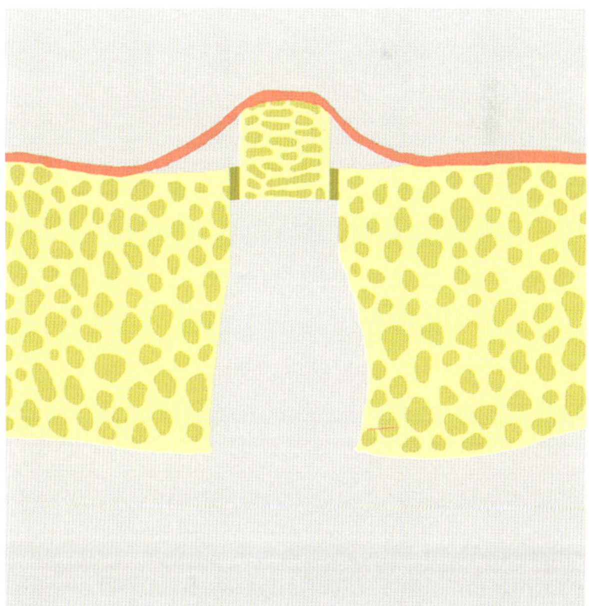

Figure 8.16 The core has been imploded and the sinus membrane has been displaced.

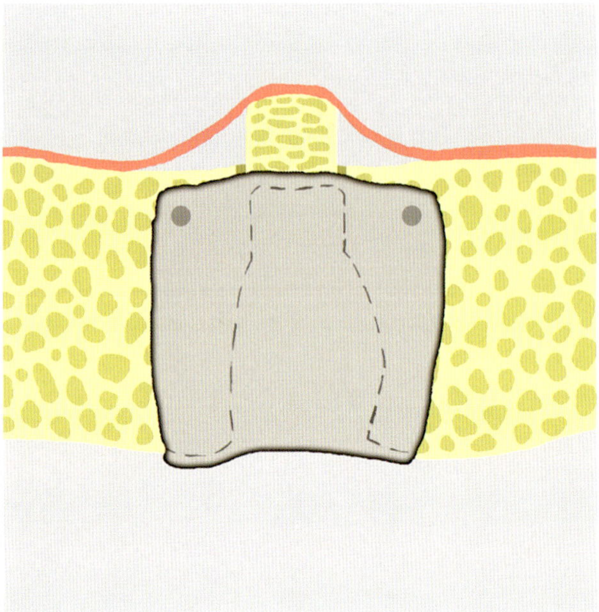

Figure 8.17 Following placement of appropriate grafting materials, a covering membrane is secured with fixation tacks. Membrane selection is a result of previously discussed criteria.

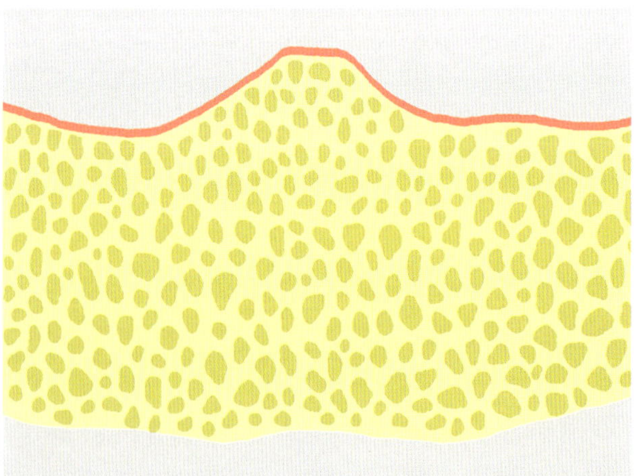

Figure 8.18 Following healing, a localized sinus augmentation procedure has been performed in the desired implant position.

fractures (Figure 8.20). The determination was made that adequate bone was not present to afford stabilization of implants in the desired restorative positions in either the molar or bicuspid extraction socket areas. Interradicular bone cores were therefore imploded in both molar areas, titanium-reinforced membranes were trimmed and secured

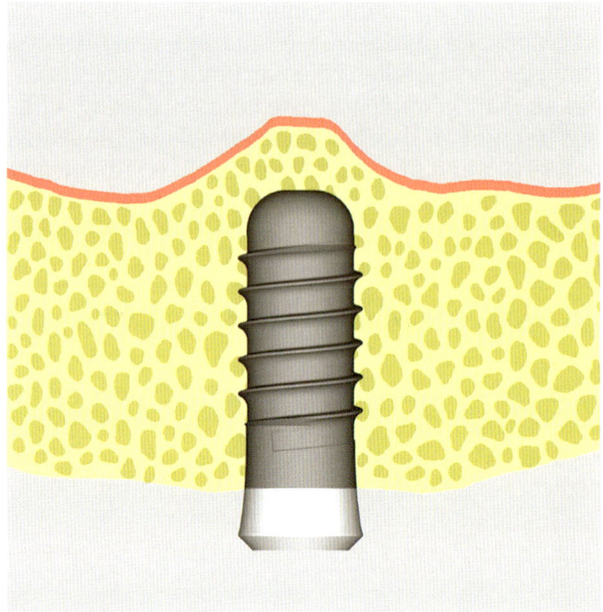

Figure 8.19 An implant may now be placed in an ideal restorative position.

with fixation tacks, and Bio-Oss grafts were placed in the socket areas. Soft tissue primary closure was attained and maintained throughout the course of regeneration.

Six months postregenerative therapy, extensive bone regeneration is evident radiographically (Figure 8.21), affording more than adequate bone for ideal implant positioning in all three sites.

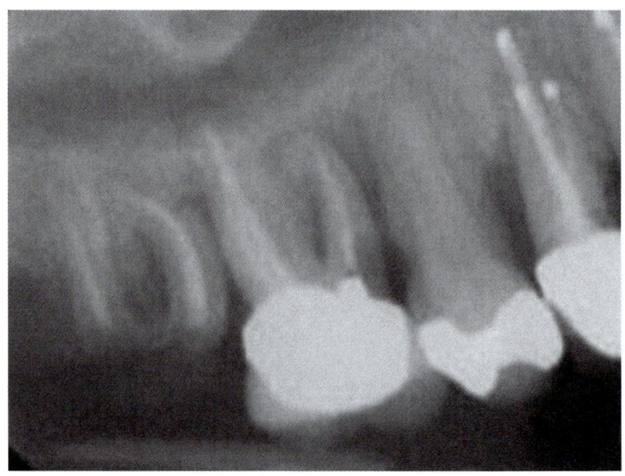

Figure 8.20 A patient presents with hopeless prognoses for both maxillary molars and the maxillary second bicuspid. Inadequate bone is present for appropriate implant stabilization in an ideal restorative position.

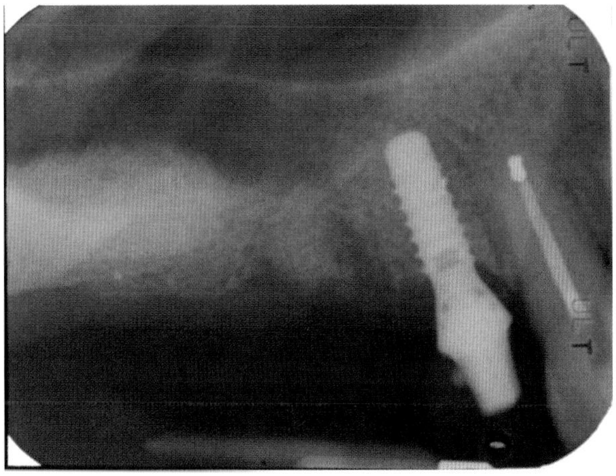

Figure 8.21 Six months after core implosion and utilization of appropriate regenerative materials extensive bone regeneration is evident radiographically, providing more than adequate bone for ideal implant placement.

TREATMENT PLANNING EXERCISE # 1

A 52-year-old male presented with a hopeless prognosis for a fractured and fistulating maxillary right second molar (Figure 8.22). No endodontic or periodontal problems were noted on either the maxillary right third molar or first molar. Opposing teeth were in occlusion through the third molar position. Treatment options include:

- Extraction of the second molar without its replacement: Such a treatment option will undoubtedly lead to loss of supporting bone on the distal aspect of the first molar, as the distobuccal root of the first molar approximates the mesiobuccal root of the second molar, leaving only a thin, cortical, highly labile septum of bone between the two roots. In addition, the net result of treatment will be a diminution of patient function.
- Extraction of the second molar with concomitant regenerative therapy using graft materials and an appropriately chosen membrane, without subsequent replacement of the second molar: While such a treatment approach would help ensure preservation of the supporting bone on the distal aspect of the first molar, the net result of treatment would be a reduction in the patient's function.
- Extraction of the second molar without concomitant regenerative therapy, followed by placement of a three-unit fixed splint from the third molar to the first molar: Such a treatment option will lead to loss of supporting bone on the distal aspect of the first molar. Two potential complications must be considered if such a treatment approach is to be employed. The first is that endodontic therapy and post and core build-up may be necessary on one or both abutment teeth due to the presence of large amalgam restorations. Such an occurrence would significantly increase the expense of therapy for the patient, as compared to other treatment options. The second potential compromise is that of depending upon the third molar as a terminal abutment for a three-unit fixed splint, considering its root form and the inherent difficulty in performing appropriate plaque control measures around it.
- Extraction of the second molar with concomitant regenerative therapy, followed by fabrication of a three-unit fixed bridge from the third molar to the first molar: While this treatment approach would help ensure preservation of the supporting bone on the distal aspect of the first molar, the other two aforementioned potential complications must once again be considered.
- Extraction of the second molar with concomitant regenerative therapy. Once bone regeneration has been completed, a single implant could be placed in the second molar position, which would be subsequently restored with an abutment and crown: This treatment option affords the multiple advantages of preservation of the supporting bone on the distal aspect

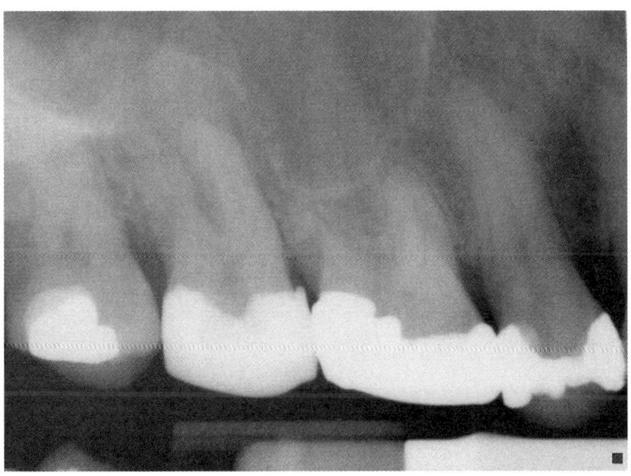

Figure 8.22 A patient presents with a hopeless prognosis for a maxillary right second molar.

of the first molar, no need to involve adjacent teeth in a fixed prosthesis with the attendant possibilities of endodontic involvement and/or plaque control problems, and a lesser financial commitment to care by the patient as compared to a three-unit fixed bridge option, should endodontic therapy be required. In addition, patient function is not compromised.

Treatment Performed

Six months following tooth extraction with concomitant regenerative therapy, marked bone regeneration in the extraction socket area and preservation of the supporting bone on the distal aspect of the first molar were evident radiographically (Figure 8.23). An implant was subsequently placed and restored with an abutment and single crown. A radiograph taken after five-plus years in function demonstrated maintenance of supporting bone around the implant (Figure 8.24).

Due to the unique configurations of maxillary molars, it is often impossible to determine the quantity and quality of the interradicular bone either clinically or radiographically prior to tooth removal. As a result, a final decision upon the precise course of therapy to be utilized must be made following tooth sectioning, minimally traumatic root removal, and defect debridement.

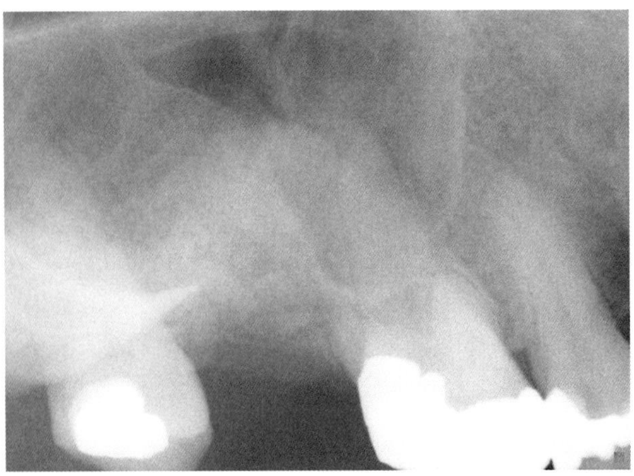

Figure 8.23 Six months following tooth extraction and appropriate core implosion and regenerative therapy, both marked bone regeneration in the extraction socket defect and preservation of the interradicular bone in the adjacent teeth are evident.

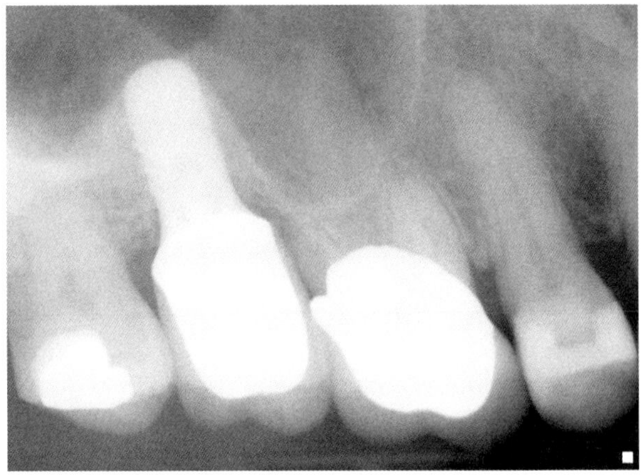

Figure 8.24 A radiograph taken five-plus years after implant restoration demonstrates stable peri-implant hard tissues.

Clinical Example Two

A 49-year-old male presented with a hopeless prognosis for his maxillary right first and second molars due to severe periodontal destruction (Figure 8.25). Following flap reflection and defect debridement, it was determined that inadequate interradicular bone was present to effect ideal implant positioning at the time of tooth removal. A titanium-reinforced membrane was trimmed and secured with fixation tacks, and placed over a demineralized bone matrix putty. Passive soft tissue primary closure was

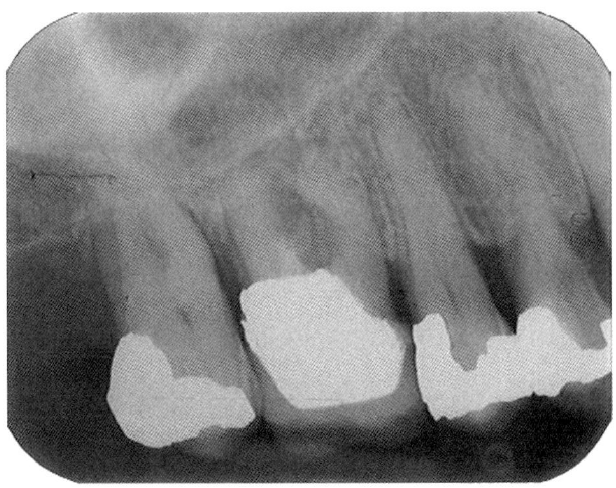

Figure 8.25 A patient presents with hopeless prognoses for his maxillary right first and second molars. Inadequate bone was present for implant stabilization in the desired restorative positions.

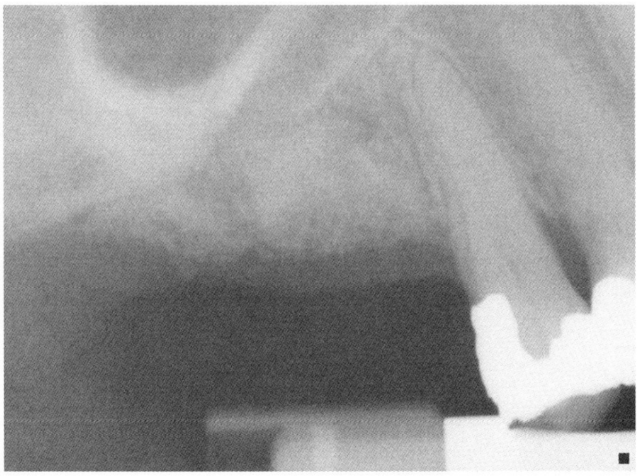

Figure 8.26 A six-month posttherapy radiograph demonstrates regeneration of more than adequate bone for implant placement.

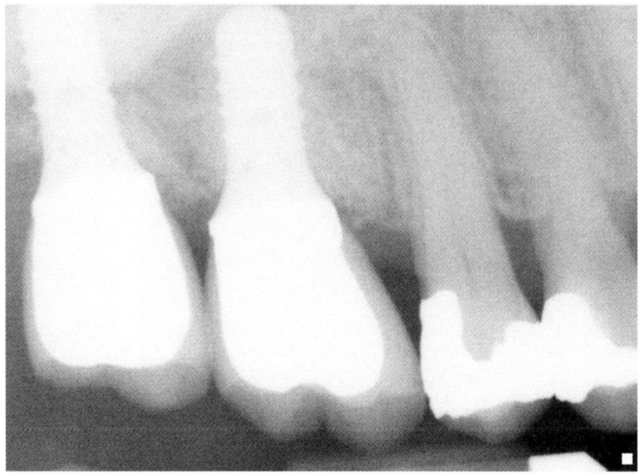

Figure 8.28 A radiograph taken after the implants have been in function for over four years demonstrates stable peri-implant bone.

attained and maintained throughout the course of regeneration.

A radiograph taken six-month posttherapy (Figure 8.26) demonstrated regeneration of more than adequate bone for placement of implants of the desired dimensions. Two 8-mm-long, wide platform Straumann implants were placed (Figure 8.27). The implants were subsequently restored with abutments and single crowns.

A radiograph taken after the implants had been in function for over four years demonstrated preservation of the supporting bone around the implants (Figure 8.28).

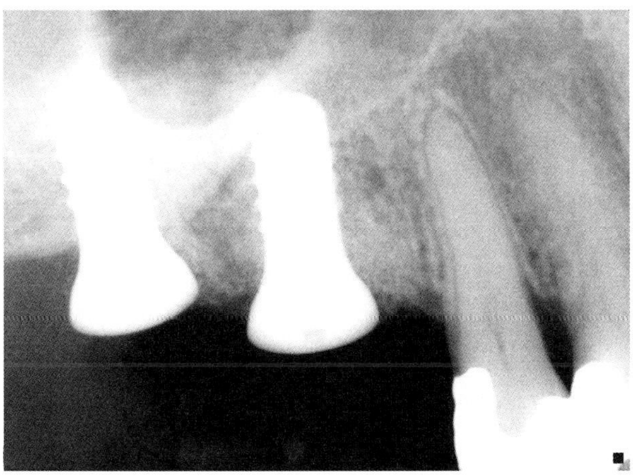

Figure 8.27 Two wide platform implants have been placed.

In situations where adequate buccal root divergence is present to visualize the interradicular bone, minimal periodontal destruction of the interradicular bone has occurred, and minimally traumatic removal of the individual roots will be possible, the clinician is able to determine that implant placement will occur at the time of tooth extraction prior to surgical entry.

TREATMENT EXERCISE PLAN # 2

A 49-year-old female presented with a hopeless prognosis for a maxillary left first molar (Figure 8.29). A buccal fistula was present, which had resulted in extensive damage to the buccal alveolar bone between the first and second molars. The compromised, tenuous nature of the interproximal bone protecting the mesial furcation of the second molar is evident.

Treatment options include:

- Extraction of the maxillary right first molar without concomitant regenerative therapy or tooth replacement: This option represents a number of significant compromises in care. If no regenerative therapy is performed, the resultant ridge resorption will lead to loss of the thin septum of bone protecting the entrance to the mesial furcation of the second molar, as well as bone in the region of the first molar. The net result of this bone loss will be significant compromise of the long-term prognosis of

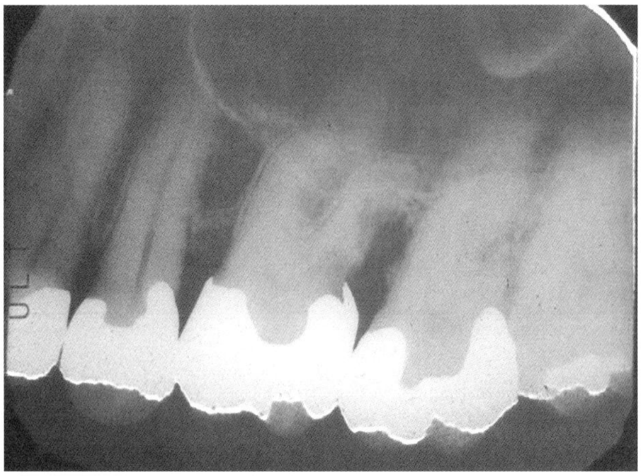

Figure 8.29 A patient presents with a buccal fistula and a hopeless prognosis for a maxillary first molar. The remaining bone protecting the mesial furcation of the second molar is at risk.

the second molar, and the inability to consider implant placement in the first molar position without sinus augmentation therapy. In addition, if the first molar is not replaced, patient function will be compromised.

- Extraction of the first molar without concomitant regenerative therapy, followed by fabrication of a three-unit fixed splint extending from the second molar to the second bicuspid: This option represents a number of significant compromises in care. Once again, if no regenerative therapy is performed, the resultant ridge resorption will lead to loss of the thin septum of bone protecting the entrance to the mesial furcation of the second molar, as well as bone in the region of the first molar, as previously described. In addition, involvement of the adjacent teeth in a three-unit fixed prosthesis will almost certainly lead to the need for endodontic therapy and post and core build-up in one or both teeth, significantly increasing both the complexity and cost of care.
- Extraction of the first molar without concomitant regenerative therapy. Once healing had occurred, a sinus augmentation procedure could be performed, followed by implant placement in an additional surgical visit, and subsequent restoration with an abutment and single crown: This option represents a number of significant compromises in care. If no regenerative therapy is performed, the resultant ridge resorption will lead to loss of the thin septum of bone protecting the entrance to the mesial furcation of the second molar, as well as bone in the region of the first molar. If such a treatment approach is employed, the patient will have to undergo a second surgical procedure to effect sinus augmentation. The overall course of therapy will be significantly protracted, and the cost of therapy will be increased.
- Extraction of the first molar with concomitant regenerative therapy. Following healing of the regenerating bone, an implant would be placed and subsequently restored with an abutment and single crown: This treatment approach offers numerous advantages. By performing regenerative therapy at the time of tooth removal, all existing bone is maintained, thus protecting the entrance to the mesial furcation of the second molar. Sufficient bone will be regenerated to obviate the need for sinus augmentation therapy. Utilization of a single implant and crown affords significant advantages over a three-unit fixed splint, as it eliminates any question of endodontic and prosthetic involvement of the adjacent teeth.

Treatment Performed

Following tooth extraction, implosion of a core of bone in the interradicular area, and placement of particulate graft material beneath a titanium-reinforced membrane, passive soft tissue primary closure was attained and maintained throughout the course of regeneration. A radiograph taken six-months postregenerative therapy (Figure 8.30) demonstrated regeneration of bone in the residual extraction socket area, marked regeneration of bone apical to the previous extraction socket area, and preservation of the bone protecting the entrance to the mesial furcation of the second molar. An 8-mm-long, wide platform Straumann implant was easily placed in an ideal position within this regenerated bone (Figure 8.31). Radiographic and clinical views of the implant and its restoration after eight-plus years in function demonstrated preservation of the supporting bone around the implant, and healthy peri-implant soft tissues (Figures 8.32 and 8.33).

There are only two reasons not to utilize this course of therapy: The first is a failure to conceptually understand the various treatment options

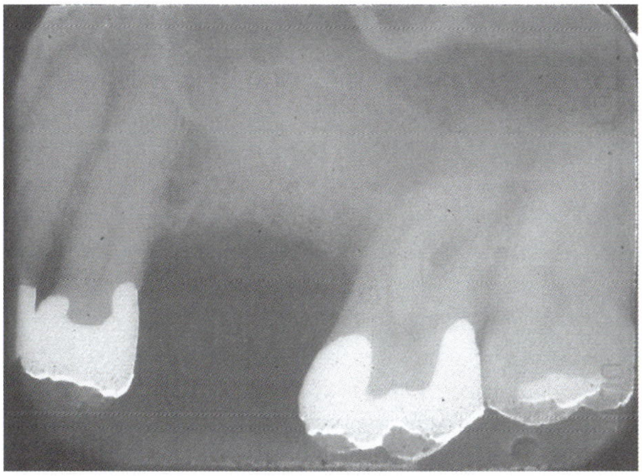

Figure 8.30 Following tooth extraction, implosion of the interradicular bone, and utilization of appropriate regenerative materials, a six-month radiograph demonstrates bone regeneration, and preservation of the bone protecting the entrance to the mesial furcation of the second molar.

and their advantages and disadvantages. The second reason is an inability to perform the technical procedures necessary to ensure attainment and maintenance of passive soft tissue primary closure throughout the course of regeneration. Either reason is unacceptable.

Appropriate diagnosis and treatment selection requires both recognition of existing problems and anticipation of host response to therapy with regard to hard and soft tissue resorptive patterns. Failure to do so will lead to dramatic compromises in therapy.

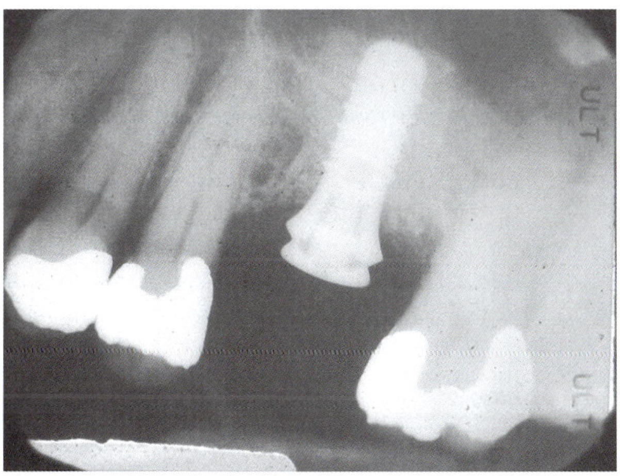

Figure 8.31 A wide platform implant is placed in the imploded and regenerated bone.

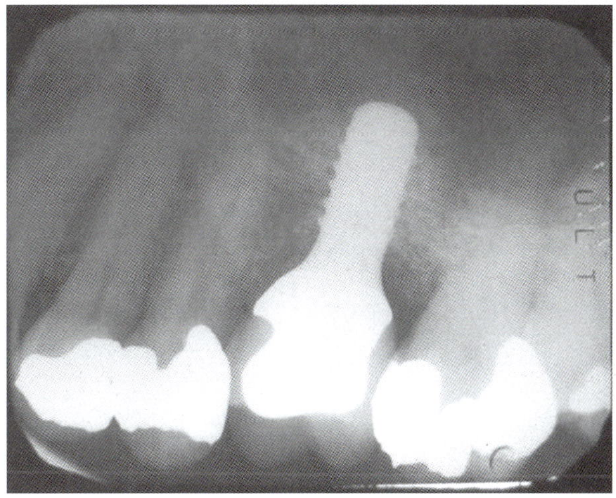

Figure 8.32 A radiograph taken eight-plus years in function demonstrates stable peri-implant crestal bone.

TREATMENT PLANNING CASE # 3

A 61-year-old male presented with a decayed, fractured, and hopeless maxillary first molar (Figure 8.34). A large buccal fistula was present. Radiographically, significant destruction to the buccal alveolar plate was evident. This destruction had approached but not yet reached the distal surface of the second bicuspid. However, the bone remaining on the distal surface of the second bicuspid, which both helped support the tooth and protect the entrance to the distal furcation, was

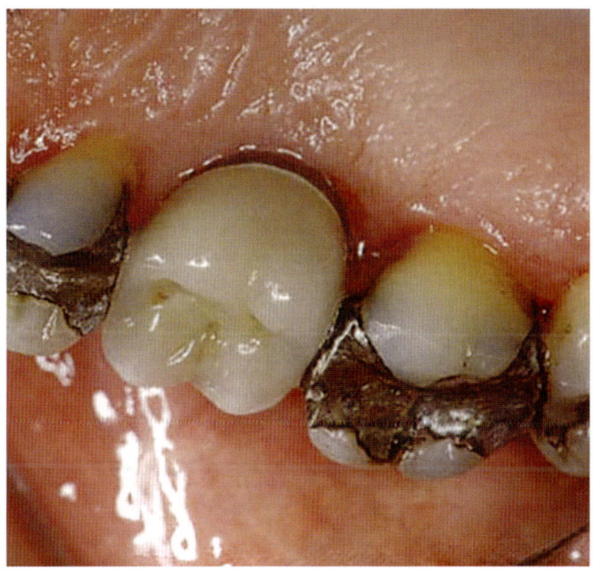

Figure 8.33 A clinical view of the restored implant.

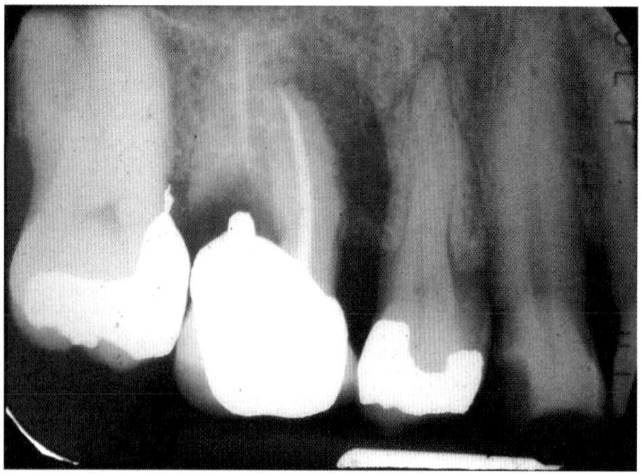

Figure 8.34 A patient presents with a fractured and hopeless maxillary first molar. A large buccal fistula is present, and the inflammatory lesion is approaching the distal aspect of the second bicuspid.

thin and at risk. Potential treatment approaches include:

- Extraction of the first molar with defect debridement, without concomitant regenerative therapy or subsequent tooth replacement: This treatment option represents a number of significant compromises. Failure to perform regenerative therapy at the time of tooth removal will result not only in significant resorption of the bone in the extraction socket area, necessitating sinus augmentation therapy if eventual implant placement is to be carried out, but will also place the thin patina of bone on the distal aspect of the second bicuspid at risk. At best, some resorption of the crestal aspect of this bone will occur, affecting the distal furcation of the second bicuspid and compromising its long-term prognosis. This treatment approach also represents a compromise in patient function.
- Extraction of the first molar without concomitant regenerative therapy, followed by fabrication of a three-unit fixed splint from the second molar to the second bicuspid: This treatment option represents a number of significant compromises. As already discussed, failure to perform regenerative therapy at the time of tooth removal will result in significant resorption of the bone in the extraction socket area, and will place the bone on the distal aspect of the second bicuspid at risk. In addition, due to the presence of extensive amalgam restorations in both the second molar and second bicuspid, the likelihood of either one or both of these teeth requiring endodontic intervention and post and core build-up is high. The net result of such treatment would be increases in both the complexity and cost of care. Finally, the second molar, which would undoubtedly be compromised as a result of postextraction bone resorption, would be ill suited to serve as a terminal abutment for a three-unit fixed splint.
- Extraction of the first molar without concomitant regenerative therapy, followed by fabrication of a four-unit fixed splint: All of the compromises in therapy previously detailed would result from this course of therapy. Inclusion of the first bicuspid in the fixed splint due to the compromised nature of the second bicuspid as a result of postextraction bone resorption would represent both an increase in the cost and complexity of care, and compromise of the integrity of the first bicuspid.
- Extraction of the first molar without concomitant regenerative therapy, followed by sinus augmentation therapy six-month postextraction and subsequent implant placement: In addition to the aforementioned concerns with postextraction bone resorption, the need to perform subsequent sinus augmentation therapy represents performance of another surgical procedure, and significantly increases the cost and complexity of care. In addition, the second bicuspid may have to be replaced in the future due to its compromised prognosis.
- Removal of the first molar with concomitant regenerative therapy, without subsequent implant placement: While such a treatment option does regenerate all damaged bone, and preserves the bone on the distal aspect of the second bicuspid, it represents a compromise in patient function.
- Extraction of the first molar with concomitant regenerative therapy, followed by a three-unit fixed prosthesis from the second molar to the second bicuspid: This treatment option does regenerate damaged bone and preserve bone on the distal aspect of the second bicuspid. However, as previously mentioned, the likelihood of endodontic therapy and post and core buildup on the second molar and/or second bicuspid if they are to be employed as

abutments for a fixed prosthesis is high, thus increasing the complexity and cost of care.

- Extraction of the first molar with implosion of the interradicular bone, performance of regenerative therapy at the time of tooth removal, and subsequent implant placement and restoration: This treatment option regenerates all lost bone, increases the apicocrestal dimension of the regenerated bone, and preserves the bone on the distal aspect of the second bicuspid. In addition, the final treatment result does not necessitate further regenerative surgical therapies, nor involve the second molar and the second bicuspid in prosthetic therapy and the possibility of endodontic treatment and post and core buildup. As previously discussed, the excuses of inadequate diagnosis, poor understanding of treatment capabilities, or technical insufficiencies are not appropriate rationales for therapeutic selection.

Treatment Performed

Six months following regenerative therapy, significant bone regeneration in the extraction socket area and preservation of bone on the distal aspect of the second bicuspid were evident radiographically (Figure 8.35). The titanium strut of the reinforced membrane and a fixation tack were also noted radiographically. Following completion of bone regeneration, an implant was placed and restored.

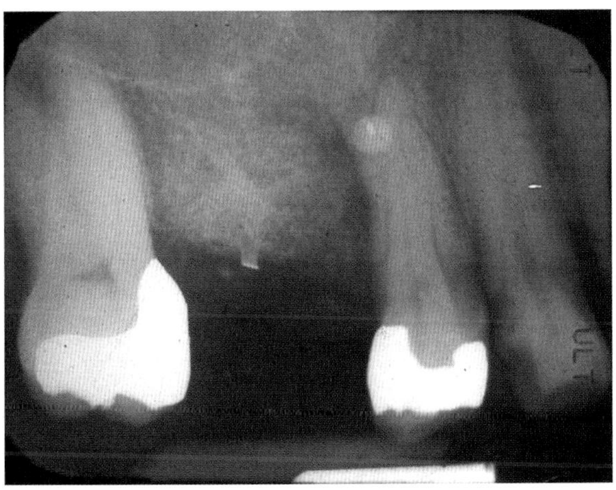

Figure 8.35 Following tooth extraction, core implosion and regenerative therapy, the regenerating alveolar bone is evident, as are the titanium strut of the membrane and the titanium fixation tack.

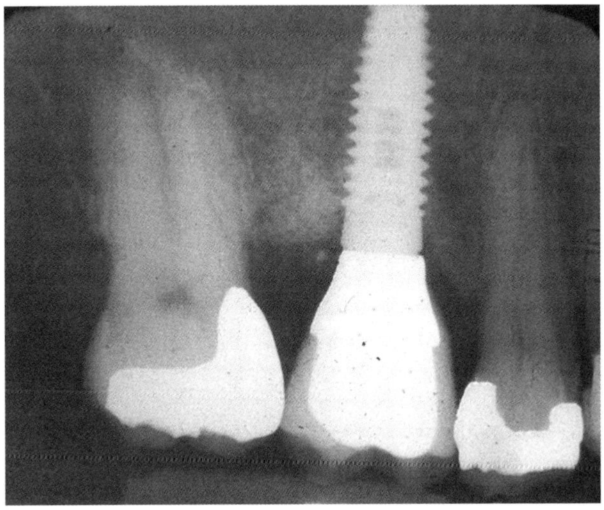

Figure 8.36 Following completion of bone regeneration, an implant has been placed and restored. A radiograph taken after 10-plus years in function demonstrates preservation of the bone both on the distal aspect of the second bicuspid and around the implant.

A radiograph taken of the restored 13-mm-long replace select implant in function for 10-plus years (Figure 8.36) demonstrated preservation of both the supporting bone around the implant and the bone on the distal aspect of the second bicuspid, which was protecting the entrance to the distal furcation of this tooth.

The advantages to the patient of multidimensional regenerative therapy performed at the time of tooth removal cannot be overemphasized. Such a paradigm shift represents a significant advancement in patient care.

TREATMENT PLANNING EXERCISE # 4

A 51-year-old female presented with a hopeless prognosis for a maxillary left first molar, which was a terminal abutment for a three-unit fixed splint (Figure 8.37). A palatal periodontal infrabony defect was noted around the first bicuspid. The crown on the first bicuspid displayed intact, healthy margins. The patient was esthetically satisfied with the crown on the first bicuspid and wished to maintain it. Treatment options include the following:

- Sectioning of the existing fixed splint on the distal aspect of the first bicuspid, and extraction of the first molar and the pontic in the

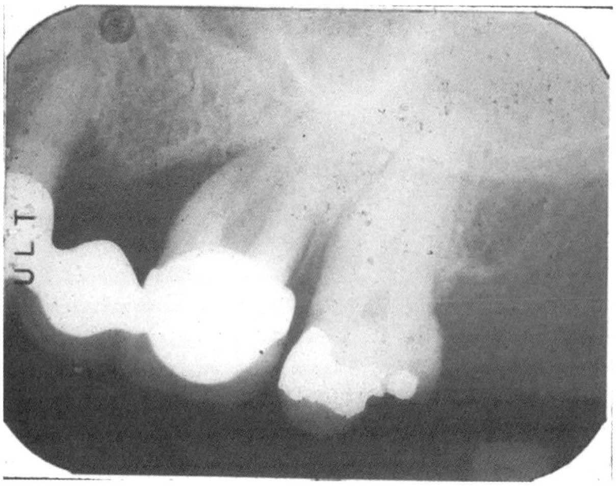

Figure 8.37 A patient presents with a hopeless prognosis for a maxillary first molar, the terminal abutment for a fixed splint.

position of the second bicuspid, without concomitant regenerative therapy, followed by fabrication of a four-unit fixed splint: Although this approach may at first seem to be the simplest manner by which to address the patients' concerns, it does not offer an acceptable long-term prognosis. Failure to perform regeneration at the time of removal of the first molar will result in loss of the interproximal bone between the first and second molars, thus potentially compromising the long-term support of the second molar. In addition, the second molar is ill suited to serve as a terminal abutment for a four-unit fixed splint due to its periodontal condition and tapered root form. Finally, the first bicuspid is a poor candidate for utilization as a terminal abutment for a four-unit fixed splint due to the significant periodontal destruction which has occurred around it, and its relatively short root.

- Sectioning of the existing fixed splint on the distal aspect of the first bicuspid, followed by extraction of the first molar and pontic in the position of the second bicuspid, and fabrication of a five-unit fixed splint without concomitant regenerative therapy: Many of the compromises inherent in this treatment approach have been discussed above. The need to include the cuspid in the planned fixed prosthesis due to the compromised nature of the first bicuspid also represents a significant compromise in care. Finally, this treatment approach mandates a greater financial commitment.
- Sectioning of the existing fixed splint on the distal aspect of the first bicuspid, followed by extraction of the second molar and the pontic in the position of the second bicuspid, and concomitant regeneration: The area will subsequently be restored with a four-unit fixed splint. While this treatment option will preserve the bone on the mesial aspect of the second molar, thus enhancing its long-term prognosis, the compromises already discussed regarding fixed splint fabrication still apply.
- Sectioning of the existing fixed splint on the distal aspect of the first bicuspid, followed by extraction of the second molar and the pontic in the position of the second bicuspid, with concomitant regeneration and subsequent restoration with a five-unit fixed splint: This treatment option will preserve the bone on the mesial aspect of the second molar, thus enhancing its long-term prognosis. However, the compromises already discussed regarding splint fabrication still apply.
- Sectioning of the existing fixed splint on the distal aspect of the first bicuspid, followed by extraction of the second molar and the pontic in the position of the second bicuspid without concomitant regenerative therapy: A sinus augmentation procedure will be performed in a second surgery, followed by eventual placement of two implants and their restoration with single crowns. This treatment approach eliminates the involvement of adjacent teeth in a fixed prosthesis, with the attendant aforementioned problems. Unfortunately, the net result of treatment is still a loss of bone on the mesial aspect of the second molar, thus potentially compromising its long-term prognosis. In addition, the patient must now undergo an additional surgical procedure to effect sinus augmentation therapy in the area. The net result is an increase in both the complexity and cost of care.
- Sectioning of the existing fixed prosthesis on the distal aspect of the first bicuspid, with extraction of the second molar and the pontic in the position of the second bicuspid, followed by concomitant regeneration including implosion of the residual interradicular bone and utilization of graft materials and membranes as previously described. The area will

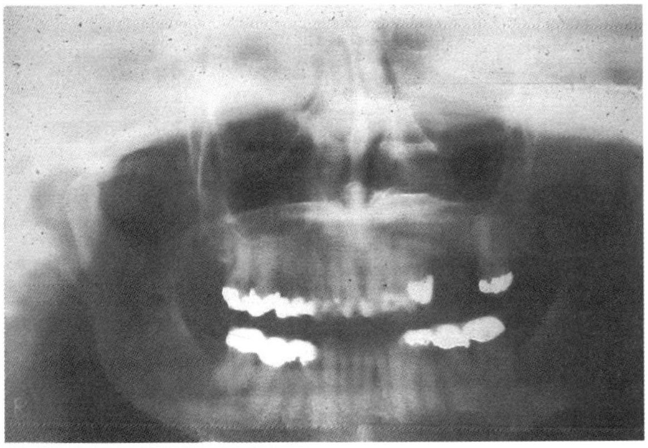

Figure 8.38 Six months following prosthesis sectioning, tooth extraction, core implosion, and appropriate regenerative therapy, extensive bone regeneration is evident.

subsequently be treated with two implants which will be restored with single crowns: This treatment option affords a number of advantages. By performing regenerative therapy at the time of extraction of the first molar, the supporting bone on the mesial aspect of the second molar is preserved. In addition, the need to involve adjacent teeth in fixed prosthetics is eliminated. Finally, the number of surgical visits necessary to effect implant placement and restoration is lessened, as a separate sinus augmentation procedure is not necessary.

Treatment Performed

Six months following sectioning of the bridge, extraction of the hopeless first molar, implosion of the interradicular bone, and guided bone regeneration therapy as previously described, regeneration of significant alveolar bone was evident radiographically (Figure 8.38). This regenerated bone was of adequate dimension to easily accept two Straumann implants (Figure 8.39). These implants will be ready for restoration approximately 3–6 weeks after insertion, depending upon which implant surface is utilized. Implant surfaces will be discussed in a subsequent chapter.

Implant Placement at the Time of Maxillary Molar Extraction

If it is determined following tooth sectioning, root extraction and defect debridement that adequate interradicular bone is present to effect implant placement in an ideal restorative position, both

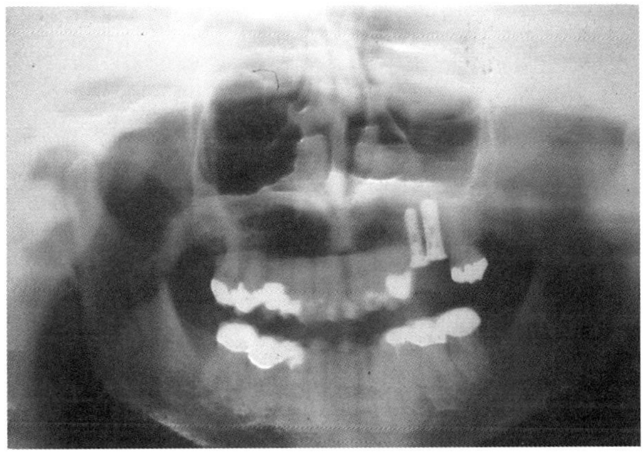

Figure 8.39 Two implants have now been placed in the regenerated bone. Depending upon the implant surface utilized, the implants may be restored 3–8 weeks after insertion.

the interradicular bone morphology and the need or lack of need for additional bone height must be assessed. Therapy will then proceed in one of four manners depending upon these considerations (4, 5).

If no additional alveolar bone height is required:

(a) In the presence of a wide interradicular septum, with wide being defined as a septum which will completely cover the rough surface of the implant following its manipulation, a 2.0- or 2.2-mm guide drill is utilized to prepare the initial osteotomy to its final depth, depending upon which implant system will be employed. Tapered osteotomes, of sequential diameters, which correspond to the drilling sequence for a given implant system, are utilized to spread the interradicular bone. As this spreading occurs, the most crestal aspect of the interradicular bone may split or be lost. This is of no consequence. The aim of this interradicular bone manipulation is to afford both an osteotomy of sufficient dimension to accept the planned implant, and bone of adequate dimension and density to stabilize the most apical portion of the implant upon its insertion. Following interradicular bone site preparation, either a parallel-walled wide platform Straumann implant or a tapered implant with a 4.8-mm-wide "apex" and a 6.5-mm-wide platform is inserted, depending upon the final morphology of the manipulated interradicular bone.

If utilization of a tapered implant will result in loss of significant portions of the interradicular bone as it broadens in its most crestal third, a parallel-walled implant will be placed. The advantages to tapered end implant use are both greater obliteration of the residual extraction socket defect surrounding the implant, and an increased implant surface area available for osseointegration. Particulate materials and the appropriate secured covering membrane are placed around the implant, and the flaps are manipulated as previously described to ensure passive primary closure throughout the course of regeneration.

(b) If a narrow interradicular bony septum is evident following tooth sectioning and extraction, with narrow being defined as a septum which will not wholly encompass the rough surface of the implant body following its manipulation, different site preparation protocols and implant selection are employed. A round bur is utilized to notch the most crestal aspect of the interradicular bone, thus providing a set point for use of a tapered osteotome. A tapered osteotome is employed to the final depth of the planned osteotomy. Sequentially widening

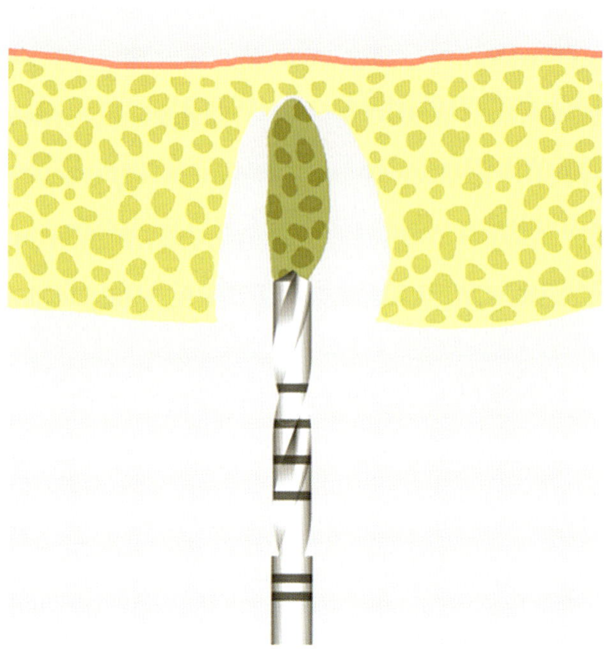

Figure 8.41 The most crestal aspect of the interradicular bone is notched with either a bur or a piezosurgery unit.

tapered osteotomes, whose diameters correspond to the drilling sequence of the implant system to be utilized, are tapped to the final osteotomy depth, spreading and shaping the residual interradicular bone. However,

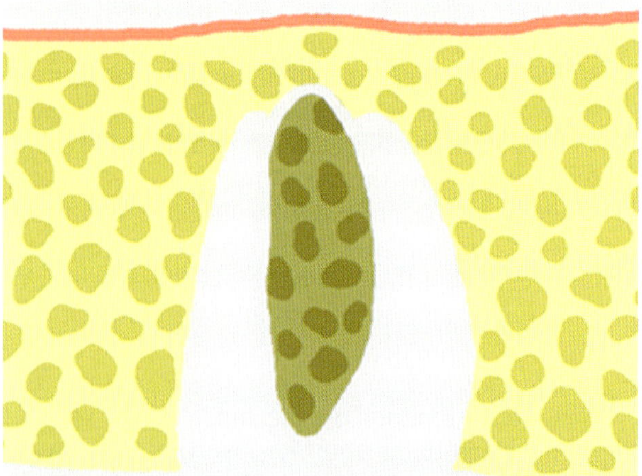

Figure 8.40 A maxillary molar is trisected and its roots are removed, with care being taken to preserve the interradicular bone.

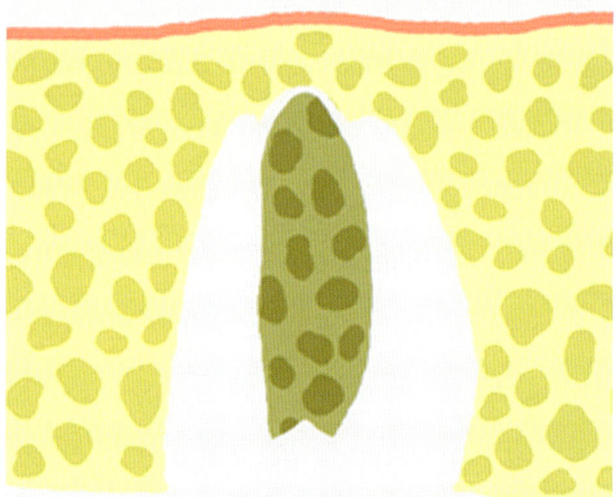

Figure 8.42 A view of the notched interradicular bone.

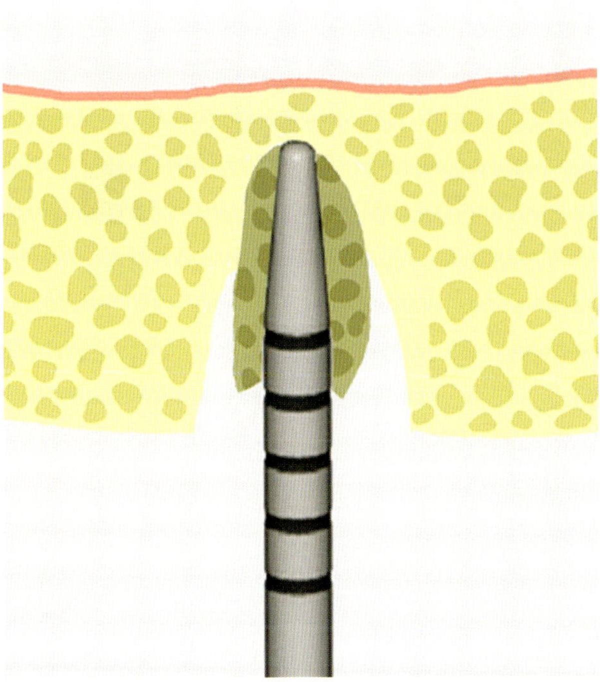

Figure 8.43 A tapered end 2.2-mm-wide osteotome is utilized to spread the interradicular bone.

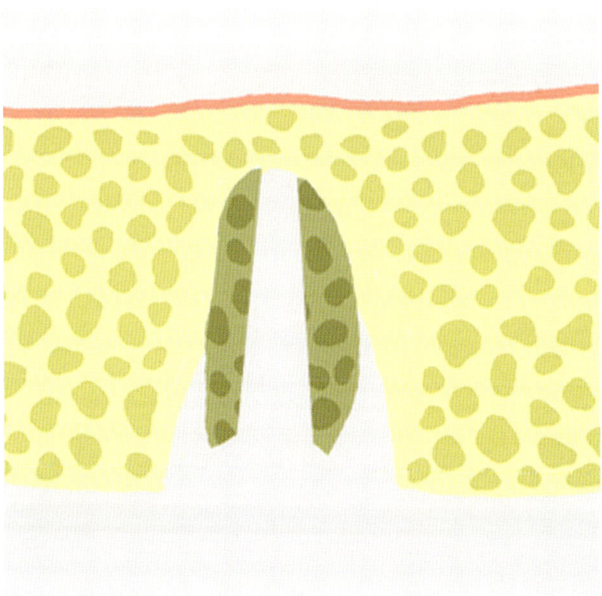

Figure 8.44 Sequentially sized osteotomes are employed to spread the interradicular bone to 3.5 mm.

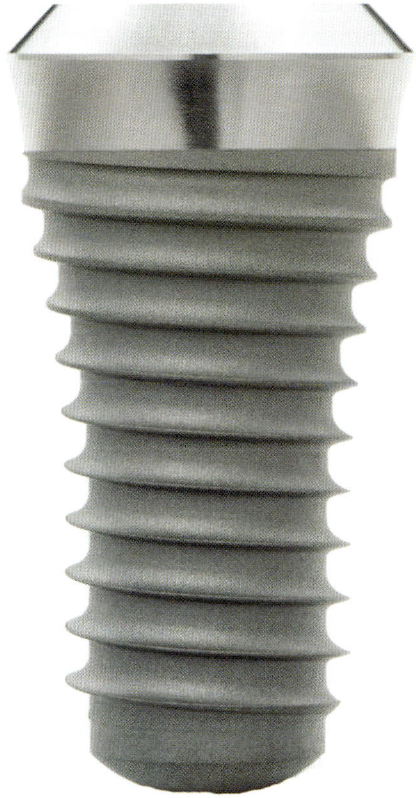

Figure 8.45 A tapered end implant with a 4.1-mm base and a 6.5-mm restorative platform is inserted into the manipulated interradicular bone.

rather than widening the osteotomy to 4.2 mm as would be necessary for placement of a parallel-walled or tapered end conventional wide platform implant, the osteotomy is only widened to 3.5 mm. A specific implant design is utilized which demonstrates a 4.1-mm-wide "apex" and a 6.5-mm-wide platform. This implant configuration affords the opportunity to place the implant into the manipulated interradicular bone and attain primary stability without unduly widening this interradicular bone and potentially causing loss of its integrity and thus its stabilizing function. In addition, although the narrower apical implant diameter facilitates placement in such situations, there are no inherent restorative compromises, as the implant presents with a 6.5-mm-wide restorative platform. Appropriate regenerative materials and a fixated covering membrane are placed, and flap designs are utilized to ensure maintenance of soft tissue primary closure. This approach allows ideal implant positioning in previously untenable areas (Figures 8.40–8.45).

Clinical Example Three

A 53-year-old female presented with a hopeless prognosis for her maxillary right first and second premolars and her maxillary right first molar. Her maxillary right second molar will be restored. Following extraction of the first and second premolars, and sectioning and extraction of the roots of the first molar, the extraction socket morphologies and preserved interradicular bone were evident (Figure 8.46). The osteotomies were prepared in the first and second premolar positions, and a 2.2-mm-wide osteotome was employed to begin shaping the interradicular bone in the first molar position (Figure 8.47). Following osteotome use, the interradicular osteotomy was completed to a width of 2.2 mm (Figure 8.48). A 2.8-mm osteotome followed by a 3.5-mm osteotome were employed, completing the osteotomy in the interradicular bone (Figure 8.49).

Following completion of the osteotomy, a tapered end Straumann implant, with a 4.1-mm wide "apex' and a 6.5-mm-wide platform will be inserted (Figure 8.50). As previously mentioned, all implant insertion is accomplished utilizing a handpiece attachment to help minimize generation of lateral torque to the supporting bone during implant placement (Figure 8.51).

The implant was inserted to depth at 30 RPM. The ideal buccopalatal position of the implant was

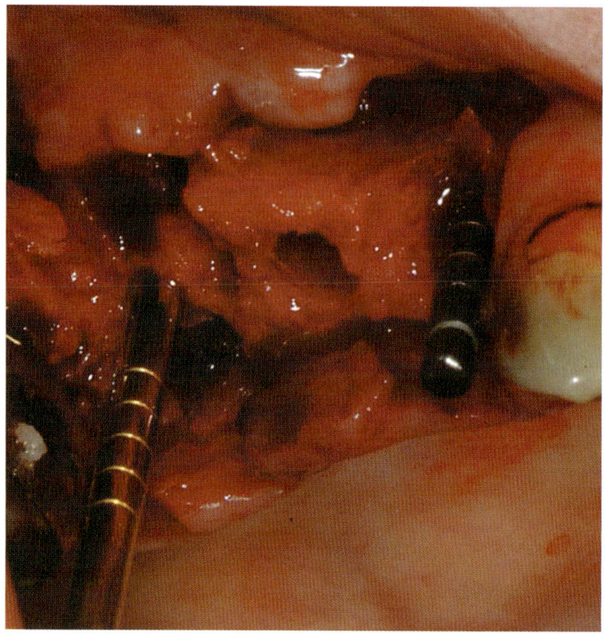

Figure 8.47 A 2.2-mm-wide osteotome is utilized to spread the interradicular bone.

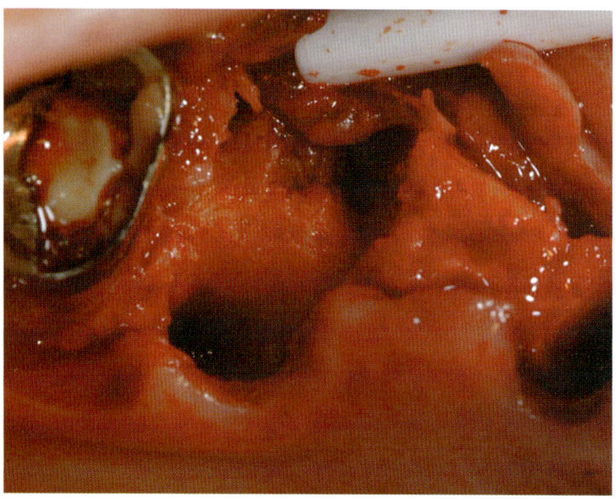

Figure 8.46 The hopeless maxillary right first and second bicuspids and first molar have been extracted. Note the intact interradicular bone in the first molar area.

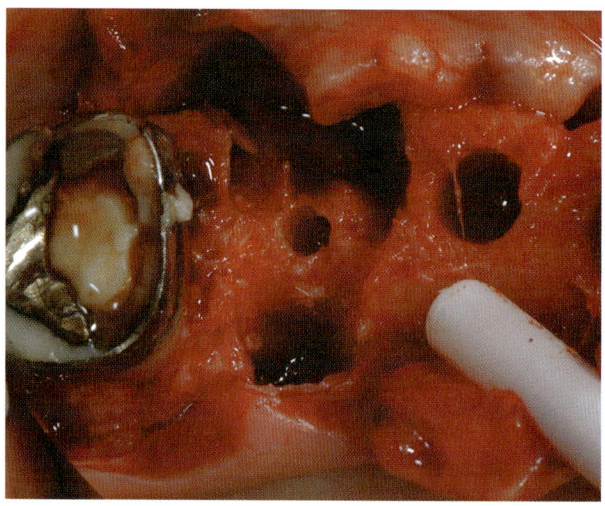

Figure 8.48 A view of the interradicular bone in the first molar area following use of the 2.2-mm-wide osteotome. Note the 3.5-mm-wide osteotomy in the second bicuspid site.

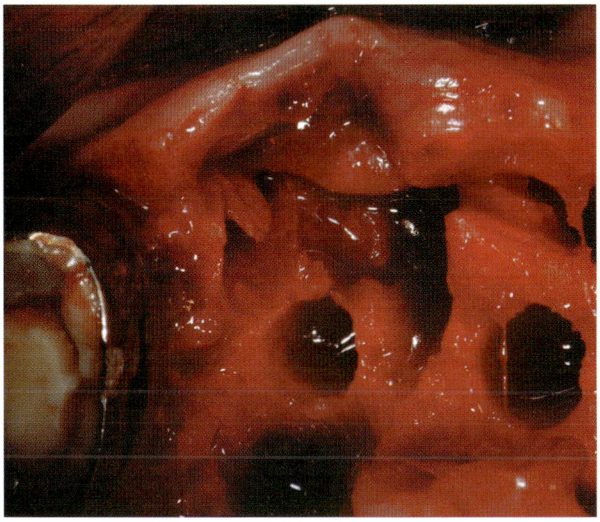

Figure 8.49 The interradicular bone osteotomy is expanded to 3.5 mm.

evident in Figure 8.52. A buccal view (Figure 8.53) demonstrated loss of the most crestal aspect of the interradicular bone. Such loss is of no consequence. The implant was inserted at 50 Ncm and was brought to a halt at the appropriate depth, due to the density of the surrounding bone.

Autogenous bone collected in a bone trap during osteotomy preparation was packed around the

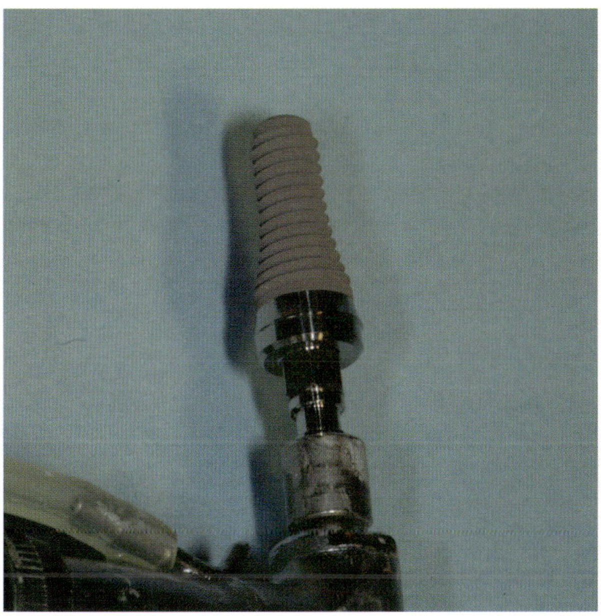

Figure 8.50 A tapered end implant with a 4.1-mm base and a 6.5-mm restorative platform is brought to the mouth on a handpiece carrier.

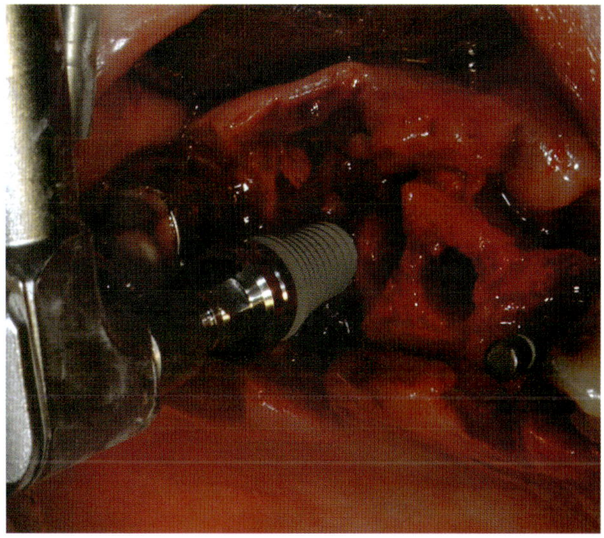

Figure 8.51 Implant insertion begins utilizing a handpiece carrier, at 30 RPMs.

implant, filling the residual extraction socket defect (Figures 8.54 and 8.55). This area will be covered with the appropriate secured membrane, and passive soft tissue primary closure will be attained and maintained throughout the course of regeneration.

Buccal and occlusal clinical views of the final restorations demonstrate ideal restorative contours, made possible through appropriate implant positioning at the time of tooth removal

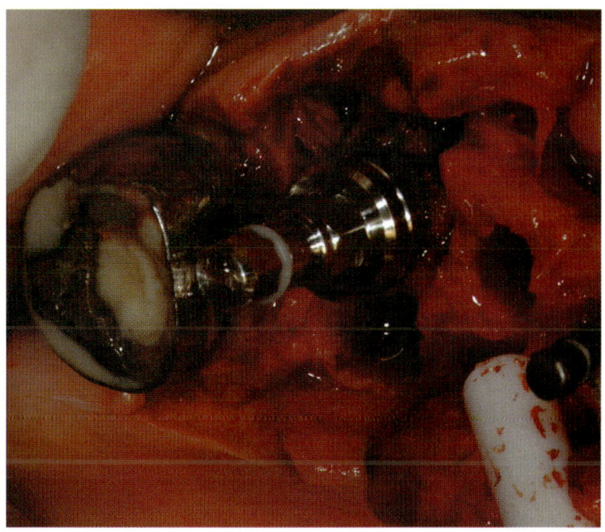

Figure 8.52 The implant is inserted to the appropriate depth.

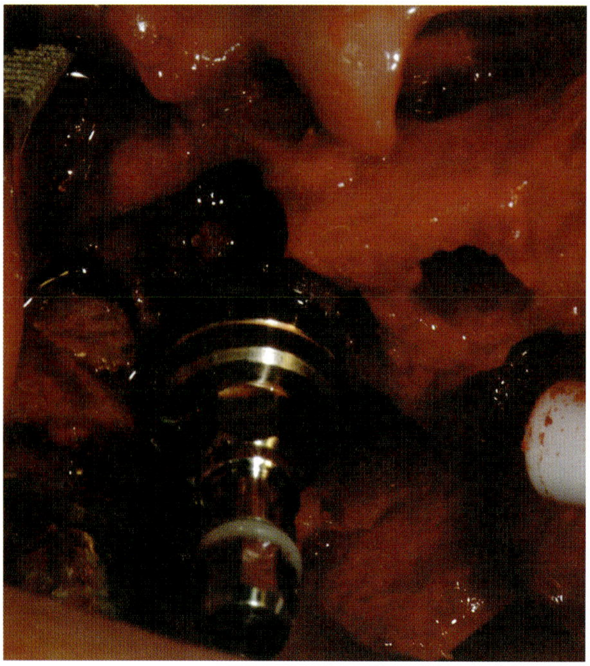

Figure 8.53 A buccal view demonstrates the compromised buccal alveolar ridge around the implant. Note the ideal positioning of the implant.

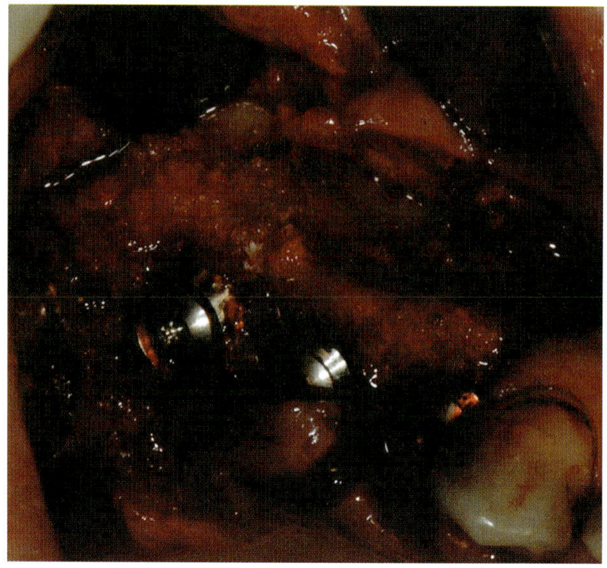

Figure 8.55 A view of the filled extraction socket defect. An appropriate membrane will now be placed and secured with tacks.

(Figures 8.56 and 8.57). A six-month radiograph demonstrated complete bone regeneration around the implant in the first molar position (Figure 8.58). A radiograph taken after more than six years in function demonstrated preservation of the crestal-supporting bone around the three implants (Figure 8.59). The combination of conventional and innovative implant and regenerative techniques afforded the opportunity to greatly simplify therapy while ensuring the appropriate high level of predictability of care.

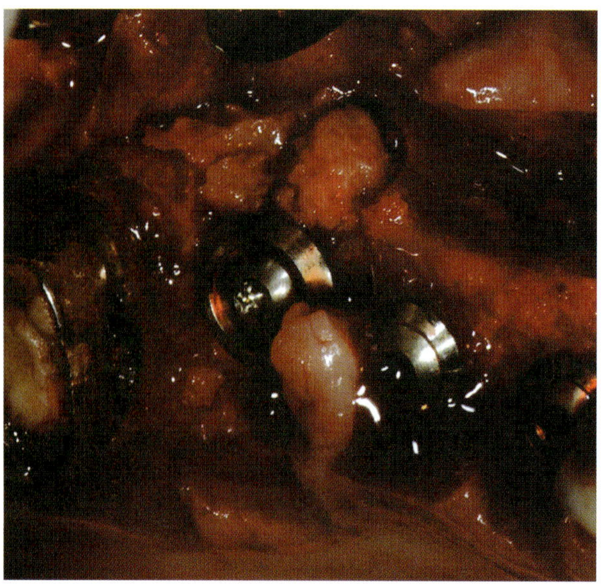

Figure 8.54 Osseous coagulum is packed in the residual extraction socket defect surrounding the implant.

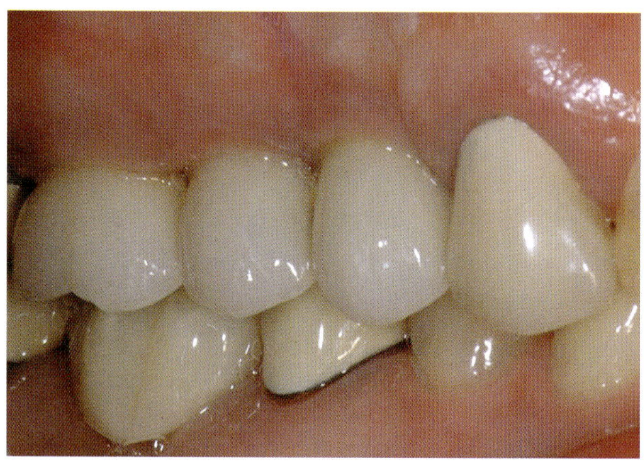

Figure 8.56 A buccal view of the completed restorations of the implants in the first molar and first and second bicuspid positions.

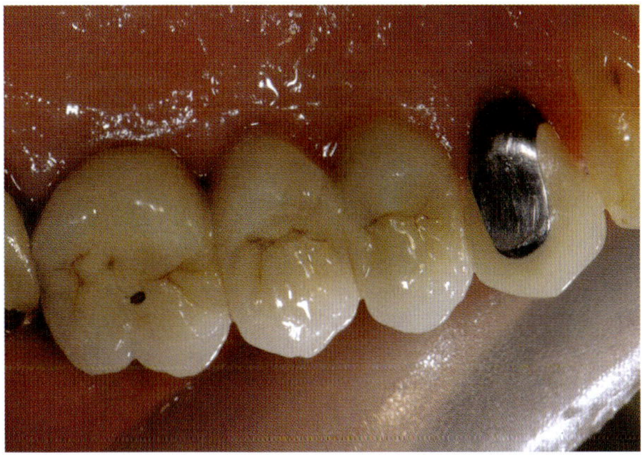

Figure 8.57 An occlusal view of the completed restorations. Note the normal-sized occlusal tables of the implant restorations.

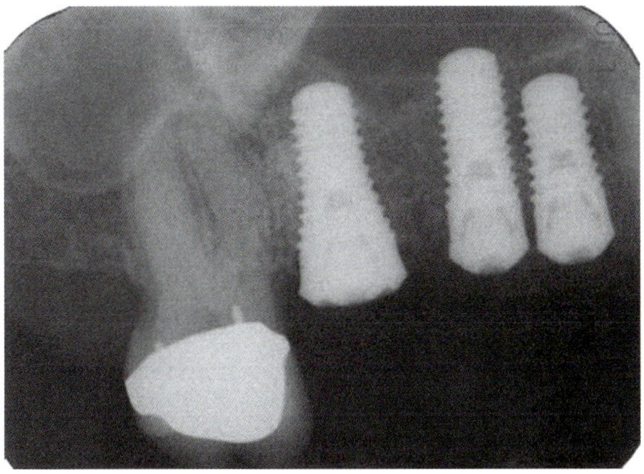

Figure 8.58 A radiograph taken six months posttherapy demonstrates complete bone fill around the implants.

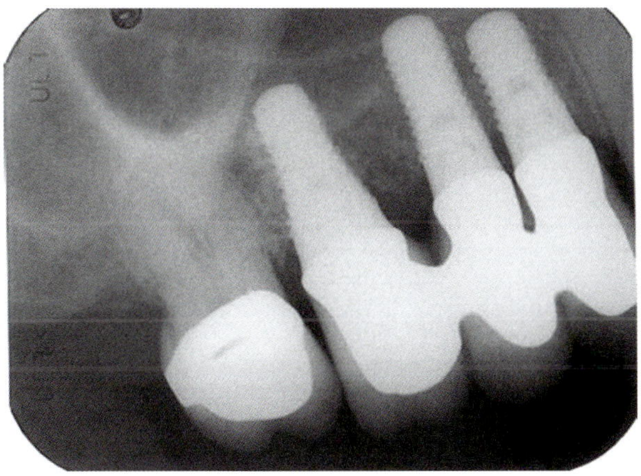

Figure 8.59 A radiograph taken more than six years after restoration demonstrates stable crestal bone around the implants. These implants would not be splinted today.

Clinical Example Four

A 58-year-old female presented with hopeless prognoses for the fractured maxillary right second bicuspid and first molar, and a missing maxillary right second molar (Figure 8.60). Radiographically, a significant periapical lesion was noted around the mesial root of the first molar. Clinically, a buccal fistula was evident in this region. Following extraction of the hopeless second bicuspid and first molar, therapy proceeded as follows: The residual bone crestal to the floor of the sinus was imploded following an osteotome and trephine technique, and an undersized osteotomy was prepared as previously described in Chapter 6. A 10-mm-long parallel wall, wide platform Straumann implant was inserted. Following sectioning and extraction of the first molar, the extraction socket defect was debrided, the interradicular bone was shaped, and a 10-mm-long tapered end Straumann implant with a 4.8-mm-wide "apex" and a 6.5-mm-wide restorative platform was inserted. A standard diameter tapered end Straumann implant was placed in the position of the second bicuspid following tooth sectioning, removal of the interradicular bone, and implant placement, as already described. Finally, demineralized bone matrix paste was utilized beneath a covering resorbable membrane secured with fixation tacks to effect regeneration in the small residual extraction socket defects

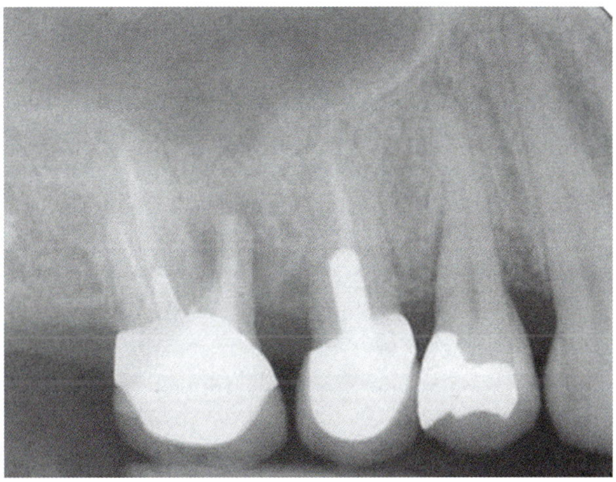

Figure 8.60 A patient presents with hopeless prognoses for a fractured maxillary right second bicuspid and first molar, and a missing maxillary right second molar.

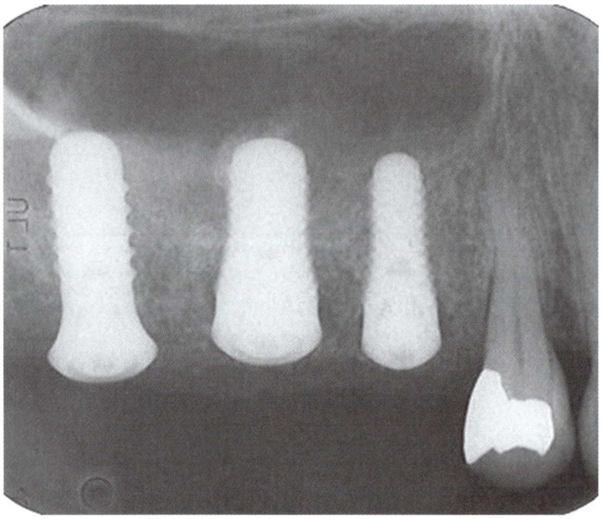

Figure 8.61 A radiograph taken six months after tooth extraction, implosion of a bone core with simultaneous implant placement in the second molar position, manipulation of the interradicular bone with simultaneous implant placement in the first molar position, and immediate implant placement in the second bicuspid position, demonstrates excellent bone healing around the implants.

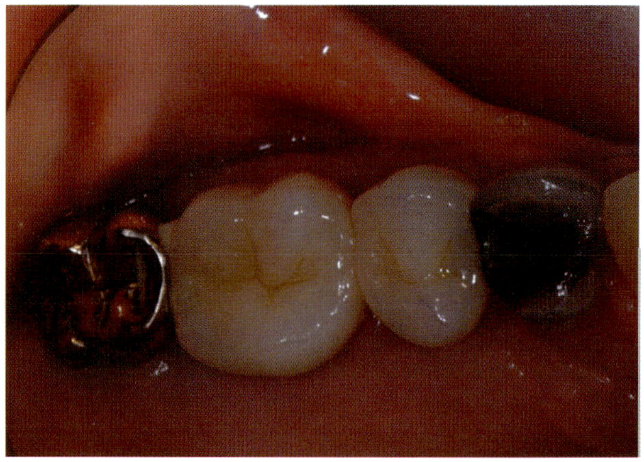

Figure 8.62 An occlusal view of the implant restorations after over four years in function.

surrounding the implants in the positions of the second bicuspid and first molar.

A radiograph taken six months after implant and regenerative therapy had been performed demonstrated complete regeneration of bone in the previously present residual extraction socket defects, and consolidation of bone around the "apex" of the implant in the second molar position (Figure 8.61). Occlusal and buccal views of the implant restorations after over four years in function demonstrate ideal prosthetic form and healthy peri-implant soft tissues (Figures 8.62 and 8.63).

If additional bone height is required in the interradicular area: When inadequate alveolar bone height is present crestal to the floor of the sinus, and 2x-2 is an adequate dimension for the length of the desired implant, therapy proceeds in one of two manners, depending upon the morphology of the interradicular bone:

(c) If a wide interradicular septum is present: A 2.2-mm-wide trephine and flat-ended osteotome are utilized to implode the interradicular bone, utilizing techniques already described. The osteotomy site is widened with sequentially sized osteotomes, whose diameters correspond to the drilling sequence for the implant system to be utilized. Each osteotome is brought to the desired depth, with care once again being taken to ensure that the most crestal millimeter of the imploded interradicular core still rests within the apical confines of the residual alveolar bone. Once the desired osteotomy site has been prepared, either a straight-walled implant with a 6.5-mm-wide platform or a tapered end implant with a 4.8-mm-wide "apex" and a 6.5-mm-wide restorative platform is placed, depending upon the final morphology of the manipulated alveolar bone, as previously discussed.

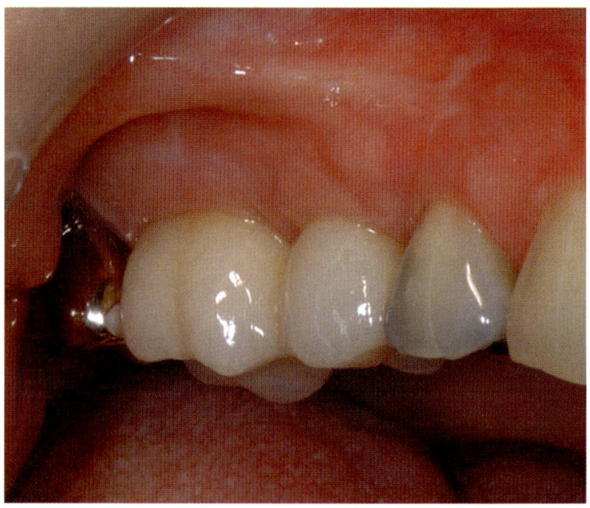

Figure 8.63 A buccal view of the implant restorations after over four years in function.

The need to attain additional bone height should not be seen as a contraindication to manipulation of the interradicular bone and implant placement at the time of sectioning and extraction of multirooted maxillary teeth.

Clinical Example Five

A 61-year-old male presented with an intrafurcal fracture of a maxillary first molar (Figure 8.64). Following tooth sectioning and root removal, the interradicular osteotomy was prepared utilizing a 2.2-mm-wide twist drill followed by sequentially widening flat-ended osteotomes. Due to the broad nature of the residual interradicular alveolar bone, it was determined that a 10-mm-long tapered end Straumann implant could be placed, which had a 4.8-mm-wide "apex" and a 6.5-mm-wide restorative platform. The imploded bone core apical to the implant base, which was repositioned due to the inadequate interradicular bone height which was present, was evident radiographically (Figure 8.65). A radiograph taken four years post-tooth extraction, implant placement, regenerative treatment and restoration demonstrated both complete bone fill of the residual extraction socket defect surrounding the implant, and consolidation of the imploded bone above the implant "apex" (Figure 8.66).

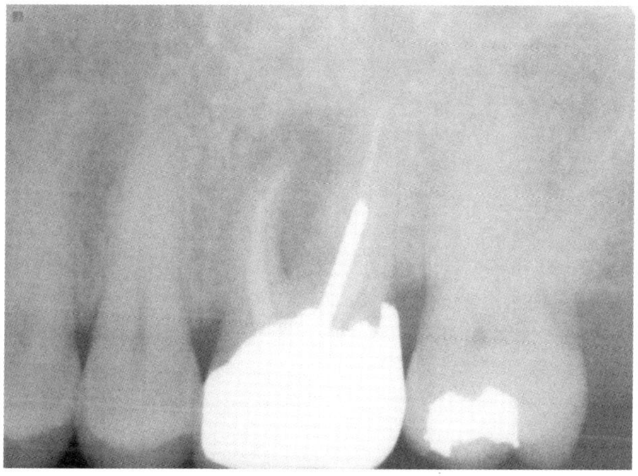

Figure 8.64 A patient presents with a vertically fractured maxillary first molar. Radiographically, inadequate bone appears to be present for implant placement at the time of tooth removal. However, the radiograph only shows the bone between the buccal roots. The radiograph gives no indication of the quantity of bone between the buccal roots and the palatal root.

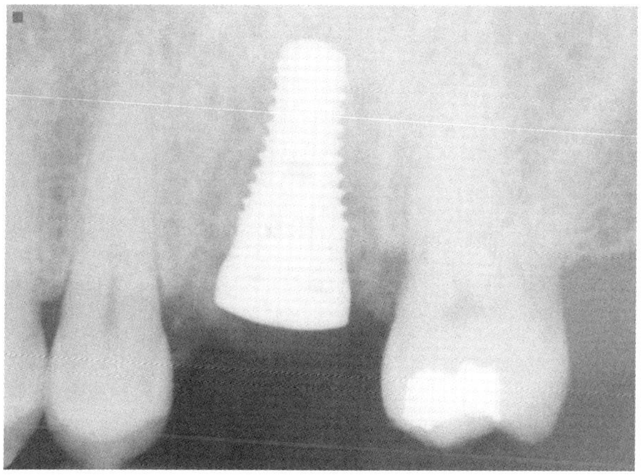

Figure 8.65 A radiograph taken six months post-interradicular bone manipulation and implosion, implant placement, and concomitant regenerative therapy, demonstrates complete bone fill around the implant.

(d) If a narrow interradicular septum is present: Sequentially widening tapered end osteotomes are utilized to both implode the interradicular bone coronal to the floor of the sinus and to widen the interradicular bone in anticipation of accepting the previously described tapered and implant with a 4.1-mm-wide "apex" and a 6.5-mm-wide restorative platform. The interradicular osteotomy is widened to 3.5 mm and the implant is inserted as previously described. Appropriate regenerative materials and flap designs are employed as already discussed.

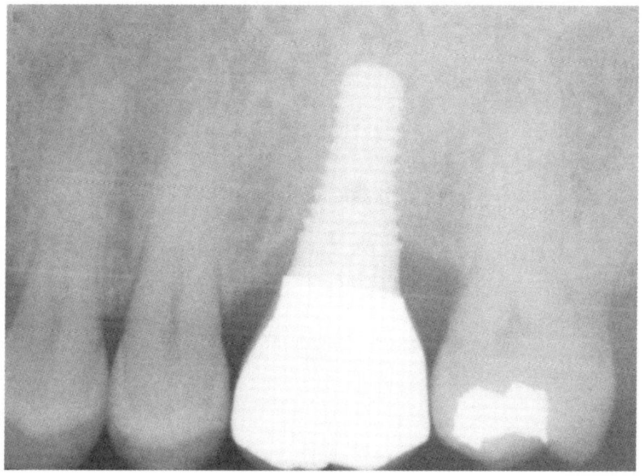

Figure 8.66 A radiograph taken seven years post-restoration demonstrates stable peri-implant bone levels.

Appropriate diagnosis of the morphology and health of the residual interradicular bone cannot usually be carried out prior to tooth sectioning and root removal. The only view afforded to the clinician by a periapical radiograph is the interradicular bone morphology and quantity between the mesiobuccal and distobuccal roots of the first molar. As such, this view offers limited information and should not be relied upon to make final treatment decisions.

While a periapical radiograph may mislead the clinician into believing more interradicular bone is available for implant stabilization than is actually present, the opposite may also be true. If care is not taken to delay the selection of the appropriate treatment modality until tooth sectioning and root removal has been carried out, the clinician may eliminate from consideration a number of valuable treatment options.

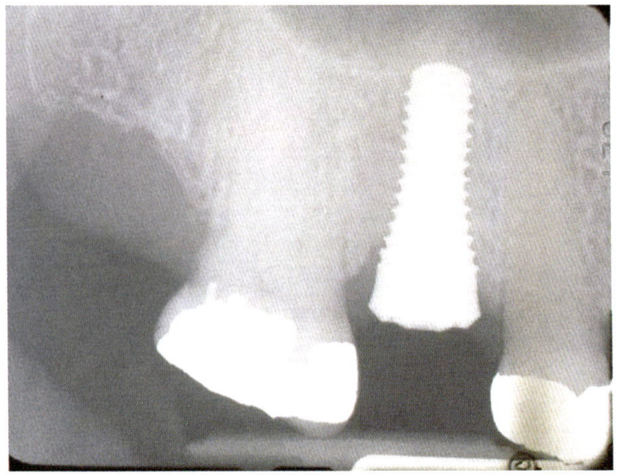

Figure 8.68 Following tooth trisection and extraction, debridement and manipulation of the interradicular bone, a 10-mm-long tapered end implant with a 4.1-mm-wide "apex" and a 6.5-mm-wide restorative platform has been placed. Appropriate regenerative materials will now be utilized.

Clinical Example Six

A 51-year-old male presented with a vertically fractured maxillary first molar (Figure 8.67). Minimal interradicular alveolar bone is evident radiographically. However, it is imperative to realize that this periapical radiograph affords a view of the interradicular bone between the mesiobuccal and distal buccal roots. Following tooth sectioning and root extraction, interradicular bone was present of the adequate dimensions to support the tapered implant with a 4.1-mm-wide "apex" and a 6.5-mm-wide restorative platform. It was determined that approximately 2 mm of additional apical height would be required to the interradicular bone, due to the limitation in available sizes of this implant configuration. The shortest available implant is 10 mm in length. Following implosion and shaping of the interradicular bone as previously described, the implant was inserted and concomitant regenerative therapy was performed. A radiograph taken six months posttreatment demonstrates complete bone regeneration in the residual extraction socket defect surrounding the implant, and consolidation of bone at the "apex" of the implant where the alveolar bone core was imploded (Figure 8.68). Maintenance of both the crestal and "apical" bone around the implant is evident on a radiograph taken after over seven years in function (Figure 8.69).

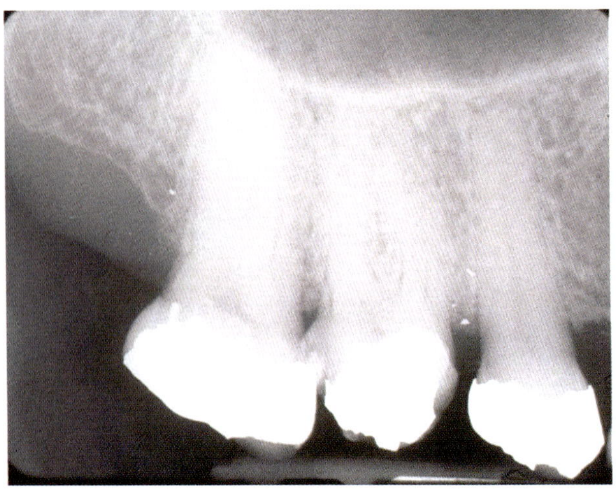

Figure 8.67 A patient presents with a fistulating and hopeless maxillary first molar.

If adequate bone height is not present crestal to the floor of the sinus and 2x-2 is not an adequate dimension for the desired length of the implant to be placed, a lateral window sinus augmentation procedure is performed, with simultaneous augmentation of the extraction socket area utilizing the appropriate particulate materials and secured covering membrane.

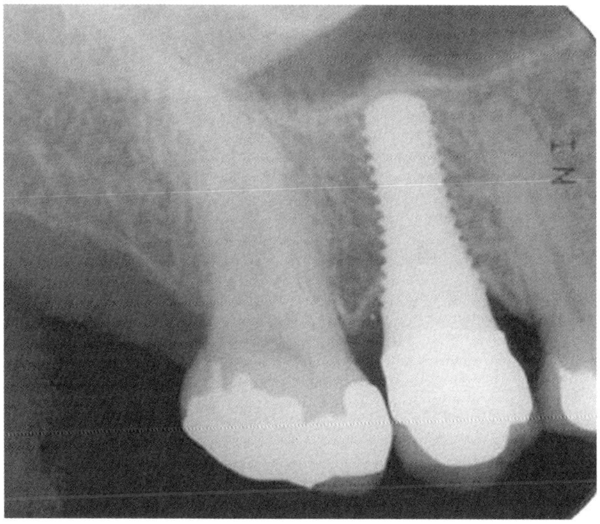

Figure 8.69 A radiograph taken 38 months after implant restoration demonstrates the stability of the crestal peri-implant bone.

Conclusions

The above outlined treatment approaches and decision trees afford a framework within which to predictably augment the posterior maxilla, with or without simultaneous implant placement, in a variety of clinical situations. While it is certainly possible to obtain more dramatic results by "stretching the envelope," both clinical experience and published literature demonstrate a significant decrease in therapeutic predictability in such instances. It is difficult to justify risk-taking when highly predictable, proven treatment options exist.

References

1. Lazzara RJ. 1989. Immediate implant placement into extraction sites: Surgical and restorative advantages. *Int J Periodontics Restorative Dent* 9:333–343.
2. Schwartz-Arad D, Grossman Y, and Chaushu G. 2000. The clinical effectiveness of implants placed immediately into fresh extraction sites of molar teeth. *J Periodontol* 71:839–844.
3. Fugazzotto PA. 2002. Implant placement in maxillary first premolar fresh extraction sockets: Description of technique and report of preliminary results. *J Periodontol* 73:669–674.
4. Fugazzotto PA. 2006. Implant placement at the time of maxillary molar extraction: Technique and report of preliminary results of 83 sites. *J Periodontol* 77:302–309.
5. Fugazotto PA. 2008. Implant selection and treatment protocols at the time of maxillary molar extraction: Rationale and report of results. *J Periodontol* 79:216–223.

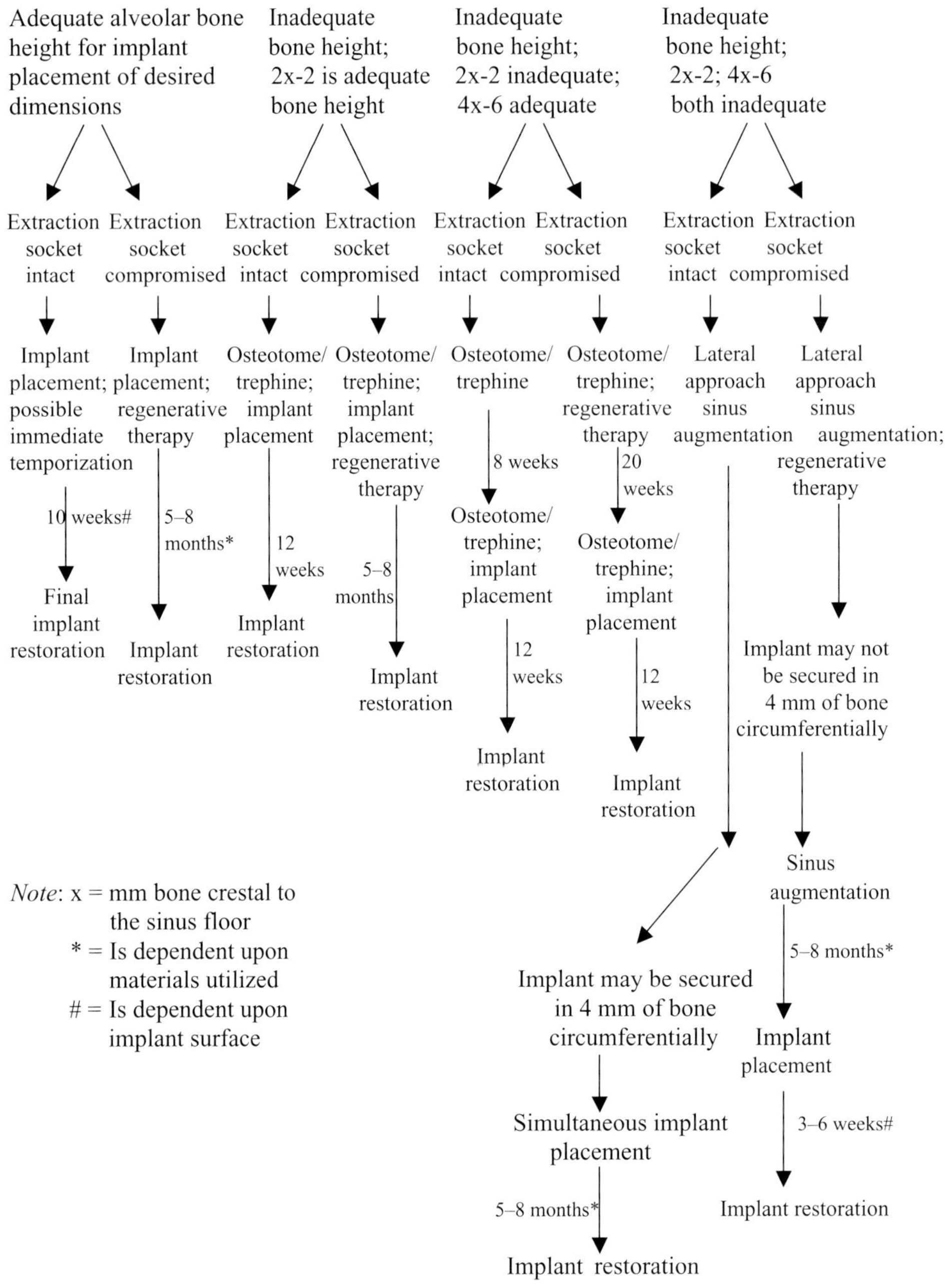

Flow chart 8.1 Treatment selection following extraction of a two-rooted maxillary bicuspid.

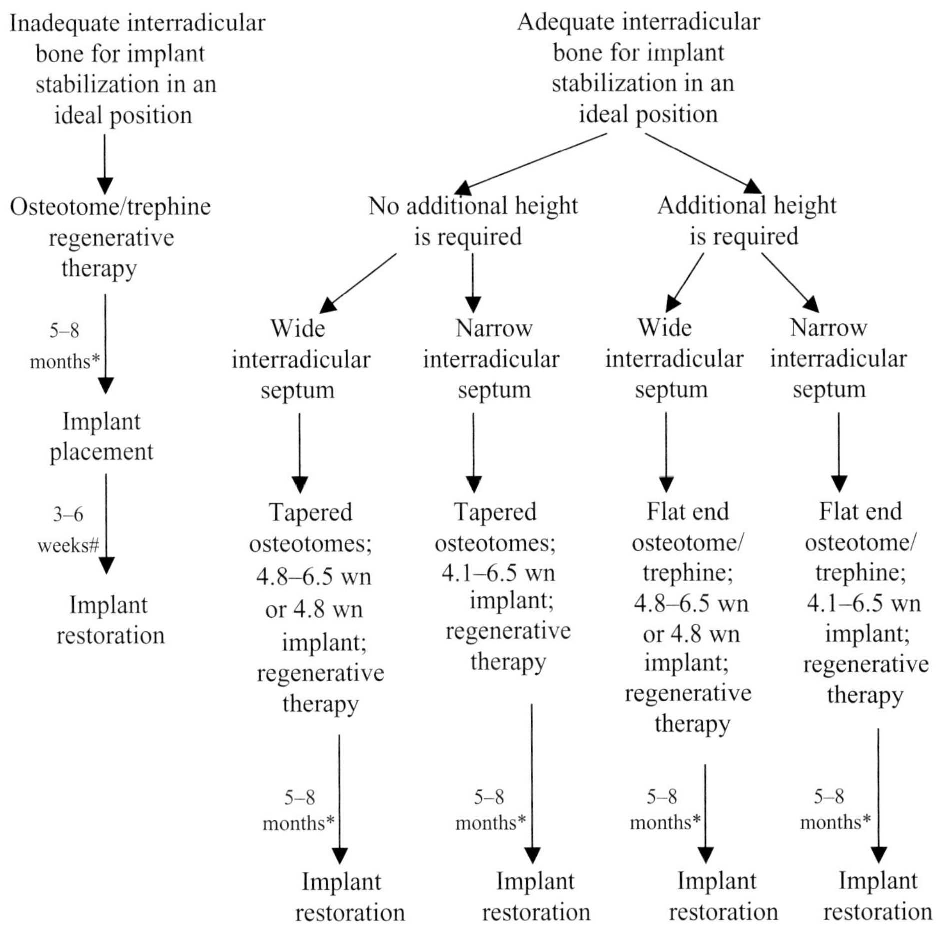

Note:

* = Is dependent upon graft materials utilized

= Is dependent upon implant surface

Flow chart 8.2 Treatment selection following extraction of multirooted molars.

Chapter 9

Decision Making at the Time of Treatment of Furcated Mandibular Molars: Roles of Resective, Regenerative, and Implant Therapies

Paul A. Fugazzotto, DDS

Outline

Definition of the Problem

The need to extract mandibular molars due to extensive caries, fracture, or other concerns, discussed in Chapter 1 when developing treatment algorithms, will not be reviewed here. However, a number of additional variables must be considered when designating a mandibular molar as needing removal due to periodontal breakdown in the furcation area. Assuming that all other pocketing around a given molar may be eliminated through appropriate periodontal osseous resective surgery, can the buccal and/or lingual furcation involvements of the tooth be treated in a like manner? Is it even necessary to eliminate these furcation involvements? These questions must be answered before determining the fate of the mandibular molar in question.

If an effort is to be made to retain a furcated mandibular molar, it is important to first decide upon an appropriate definition of therapeutic success. Such success cannot be characterized by short-term clinical health and immediate gratification. Truly successful periodontal therapy must boast an ease of patience maintenance and long-term predictability. Predictability following periodontal therapy is defined as stable attachment levels, no continuing loss of supporting bone or periodontal attachment, and no deepening of clinical probing depths around the teeth in question.

Specific patient considerations may impact upon this definition of success. When considering a patient of advanced age, or one whose medical status is a contraindication to performing the desired therapy, compromises in the above definitions of success must be accepted. However, for the purpose of our discussion, we will assume no medical contraindications to therapy, and will ignore actuarial considerations.

The challenges confronting the concerned clinician when considering periodontal health, whether he or she is a periodontist or a restorative dentist, are well documented. Deeper pocket depths are less conducive to plaque control efforts and the maintenance of oral health than shallower pocket depths. The literature has demonstrated that deeper pocket depths should be viewed as having greater potential for future periodontal breakdown than shallower pocket depths. Furcation involvements have been shown to represent a unique and challenging area of potential plaque accumulation and rapid periodontal breakdown.

Numerous authors have demonstrated that the presence of furcation involvements may be utilized as a predictor for future attachment loss around the tooth in question.

As discussed in Chapter 1, a comprehensive review of the literature conclusively demonstrates that reduction of post therapeutic pocket depths and the establishment of a stable, predictable attachment apparatus will result in improved long-term periodontal success with regard to the maintenance of oral health and the prevention of repocketing and reinitiation of periodontal disease processes.

An appropriate review of the literature also underscores the inadequacy of most therapies in the predictable treatment of the furcated tooth. "Maintenance" care, open flap and closed flap debridement of the furcation, chemical treatment of the root surfaces facing the involved furcation, and placement of various particulate materials without covering membranes have failed to demonstrate predictable success in the treatment of the periodontally involved furcation.

Use of covering nonresorbable and resorbable membranes to treat involved furcations has traditionally met with a varying degree of success, although strict diagnostic criteria and a number of technical modifications to the conventional techniques will yield a high degree of success in the treatment of many Class II buccal furcation involvements. Finally, the use of platelet-derived growth factors and a number of other growth factors shows great promise in effecting regeneration of damaged bone and attachment apparatus in the periodontal involved furcation. However, this is not the forum in which to discuss such therapies.

It is nevertheless critical to realize that some therapeutic approaches are simply inadequate in the treatment of furcations of varying degrees of involvement, while other approaches are predictable and straightforward in resolving the problems associated with early furcation involvement.

There is no doubt that periodontally involved furcations may not be predictably "maintained" through root planning and curettage and repeated maintenance care sessions. In a longitudinal study of patients who refused active periodontal therapy and underwent only continuing maintenance care, Becker et al. (1) reported an overall rate of tooth loss of 9.8% in the mandible and 11.4% in the maxilla. Patients demonstrated a rate of tooth loss of 22.5% for mandibular furcated teeth, and 17% for maxillary teeth with furcation involvements. These findings underscore the fact that teeth with furcation involvements proved less amenable to maintenance care than their single-rooted counterparts.

Goldman et al. (2) assessed tooth loss in 211 patients treated in periodontal private practices and maintained for 15–34 years on 3 or 6 months recall schedule. Patients were treated with root planning and curettage, and open flap debridement. No efforts were made to eliminate furcation involvements. The overall rate of tooth loss experienced over the course of patient care was 13.4%. However, the incidence of tooth loss of maxillary and mandibular teeth with furcation involvements was 30.7 and 24.2%, respectively. Teeth that exhibited furcation involvements were lost at a greater rate than nonfurcated teeth following therapy which did not eliminate the furcations, and continued maintenance care.

McFall (3) reported on tooth loss in 100 treated patients with periodontal disease, who were maintained for 15 years or longer following active periodontal therapy. Once again, therapy did not eliminate the furcation involvements which were present. About 11.3% of all teeth were lost over the course of observation. Maxillary teeth which demonstrated furcation involvements were lost at a rate of 22.3% over the course of this study. Mandibular furcated teeth were lost at a rate of 14.7%.

Similar findings are repeated throughout the literature (4–6).

As with other therapies, appropriate treatment of involved furcations depends upon many factors which are common to all aspects of dentistry. These include proper patient selection, establishment of adequate plaque control, formulation of a comprehensive overall treatment plan, and other factors previously discussed. However, a periodontally involved furcation also presents unique challenges which demand innovative treatment approaches and realistic assessment of when to maintain a furcated tooth and when it must be removed and replaced. A study by Fleischer et al. (7) underscores the fallacy of believing that total debridement of a periodontally involved furcation may be accomplished utilizing curettes and ultrasonic instrumentation. Fifty molars were treated through either closed curettage or open flap debridement. All teeth were treated by experienced operators. The teeth were then extracted and stained for the presence of plaque and/or calculus. Assessment of the extracted and stained teeth demonstrated that only 68% of the tooth surfaces facing the involved furcation were calculus free.

While there is no doubt that the utilization of microscopy and appropriate instrumentation will greatly improve upon this level of efficacy of furcation debridement, the three-dimensional structure of the involved furcation will remain. The net result will be repopulation of this area by plaque, and reinitiation of a periodontal inflammatory lesion. Such an approach will "slow down" the progression of bone and attachment loss, and may prove valuable in an older patient or one who does not wish to undergo more comprehensive therapy. It is not a desired treatment end point in most clinical scenarios. Therapy must be aimed at eliminating the periodontally involved furcation and providing the patient with a milieu which is amenable to appropriate plaque control efforts.

The treatment approach chosen, whether it be resection, regeneration, a combination of resection and regeneration, or tooth removal and implant placement, is dependent upon the involved furcation morphology. It is therefore critical that easy to use, clinically applicable definitions of furcation involvements be employed to aid in the development of appropriate treatment algorithms.

Furcation defects are described as a function of the extent of periodontal destruction in both the horizontal and vertical dimensions.

Horizontal furcation involvements:

(a) Class I: The entrance into the furcation proceeds less than half of the horizontal dimension of the tooth (Figure 9.1).

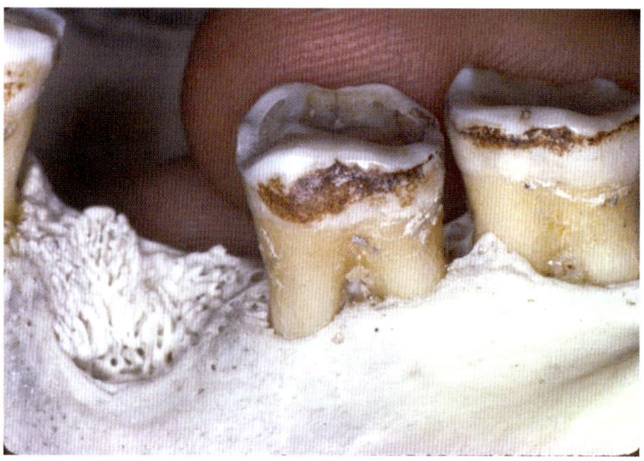

Figure 9.1 Class I furcation involvements are noted on both molars.

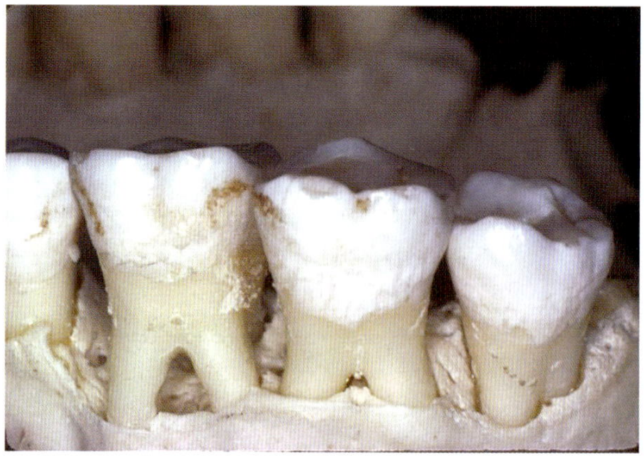

Figure 9.2 Class II furcation involvements are present on both the first and second molars. The greater vertical component to the furcation involvement on the first molar renders treatment of this area more problematic than the Class II furcation on the second molar.

(b) Class II: Entrance into the furcation proceeds greater than half of the horizontal dimension of the tooth, but less than the full horizontal dimension of the tooth (Figure 9.2).
(c) Class III: Entrance into the furcation proceeds along the complete horizontal dimension of the tooth, connecting both the buccal and lingual furcation entrances (Figure 9.3).

Vertical furcation involvements:

(a) Loss of attachment apparatus along less than 25% of the vertical component of the furcation of the tooth.

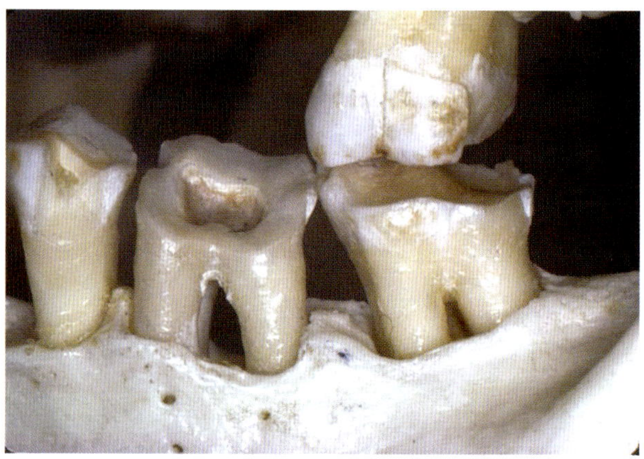

Figure 9.3 Class III furcation involvements are noted on both the first and second molars.

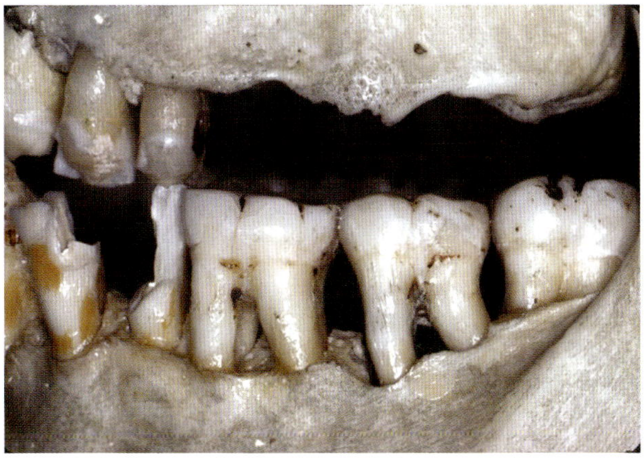

Figure 9.4 The morphology of the root surfaces facing a periodontally involved furcation on a mandibular molar renders appropriate debridement difficult if not impossible.

(b) Loss of attachment apparatus along more than 25% but less than 50% of the vertical component of the furcation of the tooth.
(c) Loss of attachment apparatus along more than 50% of the vertical component of the furcation of the tooth.

While the vertical component of furcation involvement has significant ramifications in the treatment of Class II furcations, it plays no role in the treatment of Class I furcations, unless this involvement extends to such a degree that it either renders attainment of appropriate osseous morphologies impossible, or reaches the apices of the tooth in question. In such situations, molar extraction and implant placement must be effected, as will be subsequently discussed.

Examination of the root morphologies facing involved periodontal furcations demonstrates the difficulty, and often futility, in attempting to thoroughly debride these areas through the use of curettes and/or ultrasonic instrumentation, either through a closed or open flap approach (Figure 9.4). Mandibular molars presenting with additional roots, whether they be fully formed or vestigial in nature, pose an even greater challenge to the treating clinician (Figure 9.5).

Cementoenamel projections represent another potential compromise in both periodontal health and periodontal treatment outcomes. Cementoenamel projections prevent the establishment of a connective tissue attachment to the root surface, as connective tissue attachment to enamel is not possible. As a result, these enamel projections are a potential "funnel" for bacteria into the entrance of the furcation, as the only barrier to such bacterial penetration is an overlying junctional epithelial adhesion. Epithelial adhesion has been shown to "unzip" in the face of a plaque front and the resultant inflammatory insult. A Class I cementoenamel projection, which extends less than 25% of the root trunk toward the furcation entrance, poses little concern with regards to periodontal health (Figure 9.6). However, a Class II cementoenamel projection, which extends more than 50% of the dimension of the root trunk toward the furcation entrance but does not actually reach the furcation entrance, should be viewed as a weak link to the fiber attachment periodontal defense system (Figure 9.7). A Class III cementoenamel projection, which by definition extends to or into the entrance of the furcation, is an absolute compromise to periodontal health, as no connective tissue attachment is present between the gingival sulcus and the entrance to the furcation (Figure 9.8). Patients with such an abnormality are literally born with furcation involvements (Figure 9.9). Failure to treat these areas in a timely and effective manner often

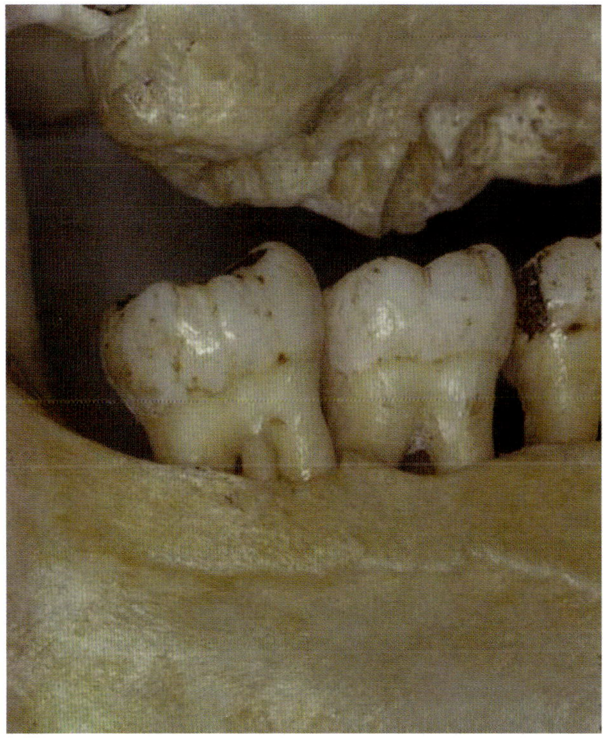

Figure 9.5 The presence of an additional root complicates debridement of the periodontally involved furcation of the second molar.

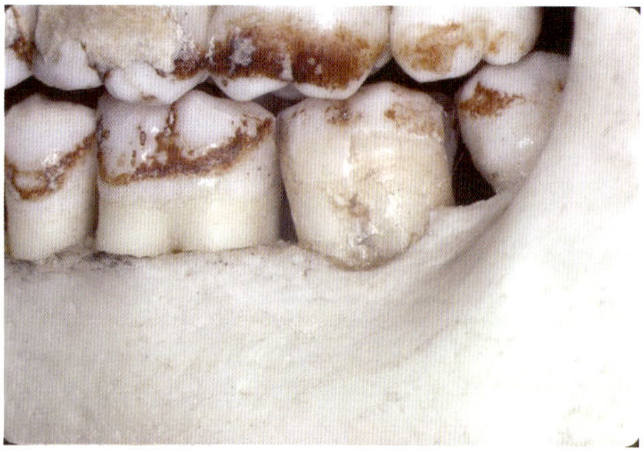

Figure 9.6 A Class I cementoenamel projection is present on the first molar.

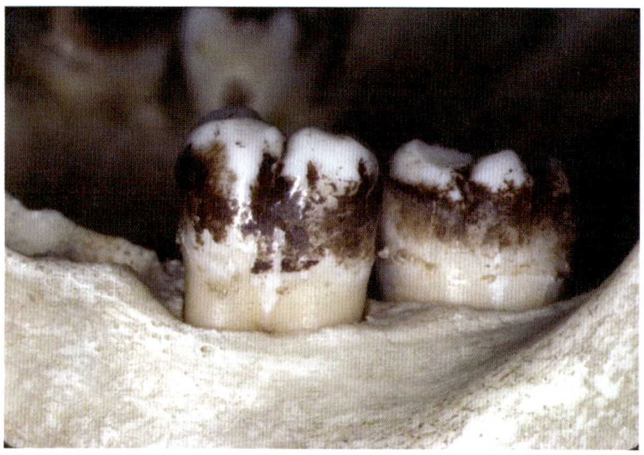

Figure 9.7 A Class II cementoenamel projection is present on the first molar.

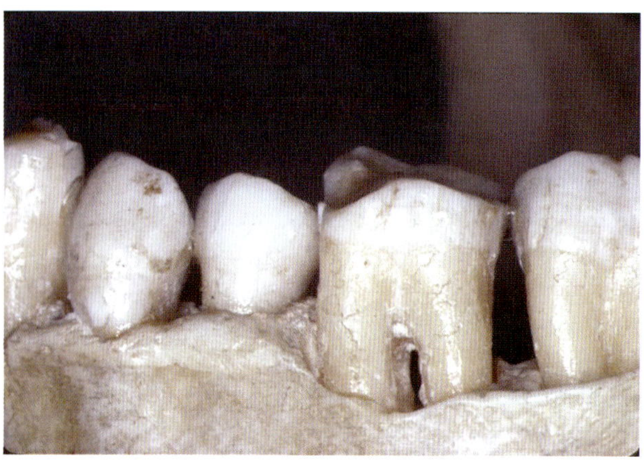

Figure 9.8 A Class III cementoenamel projection is present on the first molar.

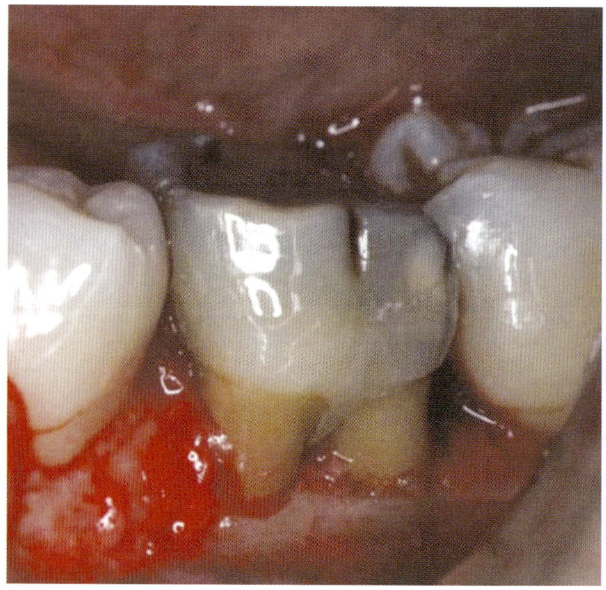

Figure 9.9 Flap reflection reveals a Class III cementoenamel projection with the expected furcation involvement. The inability of the body to develop a connective tissue attachment to enamel renders this tooth highly susceptible to continued periodontal breakdown in the furcation area.

leads to significant progression of periodontal disease problems in the furcation area, and premature loss of the molar in question.

Enamel pearls are also a concern (Figure 9.10). They represent both an area devoid of connective tissue attachment to the root surface and a morphology which is conducive to plaque accumulation.

Class I furcation involvements may be predictably treated through odontoplasty (Flow chart 9.1). The roof of the furcation is recontoured to eliminate the plaque trapping cul de sac which is present. The newly established tooth contours are then carried onto the radicular surfaces of the tooth to create a continuous, smooth morphology conducive to patient plaque control efforts (Figures 9.11 and 9.12). This therapy is performed in conjunction with osseous resection and apically positioned flaps. The end result of treatment is elimination of deeper pocket depths and Class I furcation involvements. The definitions of success after such therapy has been performed are no probing depths in excess of 3 mm, and no entrance of a probe into the furcation of the tooth. Coincidental to the aforementioned odontoplasty is the elimination of all cementoenamel projections and/or enamel pearls.

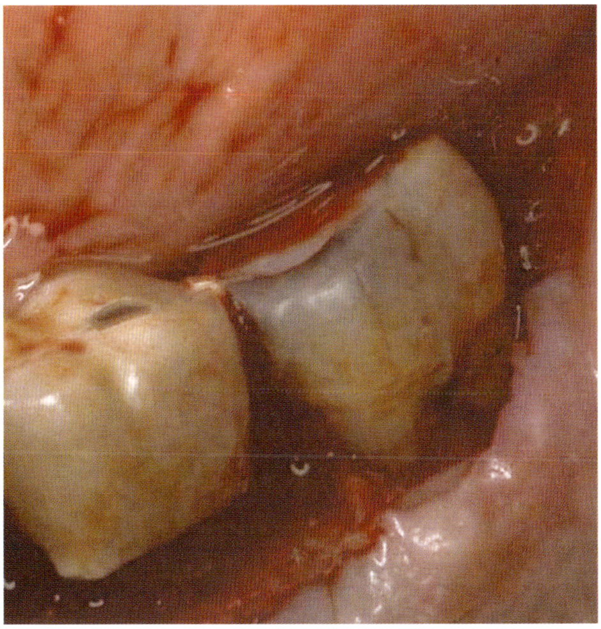

Figure 9.10 The enamel pearl in the furcation area of the second molar not only prohibits development of connective tissue attachment in the region, but also serves as a nidus for plaque and calculus accumulation.

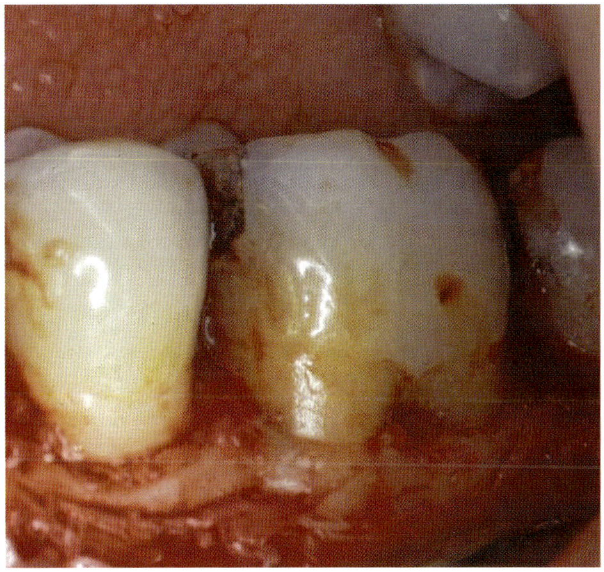

Figure 9.11 The patient presents with a Class I buccal furcation involvement and a Class II cementoenamel projection.

Odontoplasty is highly predictable and may be carried out in either the presence or absence of a prosthetic commitment. After having performed such odontoplasty thousands of times in conjunction with periodontal surgical intervention, only one instance has been encountered where the patient demonstrated continued tooth sensitivity in the area of odontoplasty beyond a two-week period, in a tooth in which endodontic intervention was not already planned.

Failure to eradicate early furcation involvements through odontoplasty will result in continued periodontal breakdown and attachment loss in the furcation area, and eventual tooth loss. Figure 9.13 demonstrates a patient who presented with a Class III cementoenamel projection and was not treated through appropriate resective therapy. The result was continued periodontal breakdown. A Class III furcation involvement is now present on the tooth in question, which has a hopeless prognosis. Appropriate and timely intervention would have avoided such a development.

Aggressive treatment of Class I furcation involvements must be viewed as conservative therapy. In a hypothetical situation, a 25-year-old patient presents with excellent home care and mini-

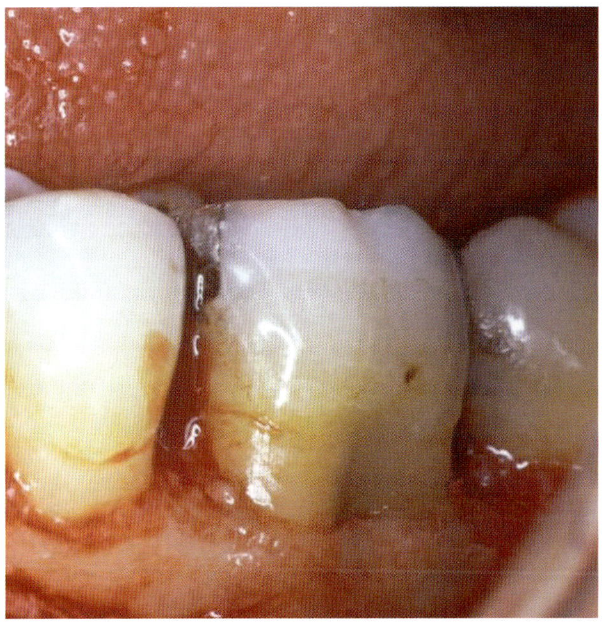

Figure 9.12 Following appropriate odontoplasty, the cementoenamel projection has been removed and the Class I furcation involvement has been eliminated. Mucoperiosteal flaps will now be sutured at osseous crest. The end result of treatment will be an area which is easily maintained by the patient.

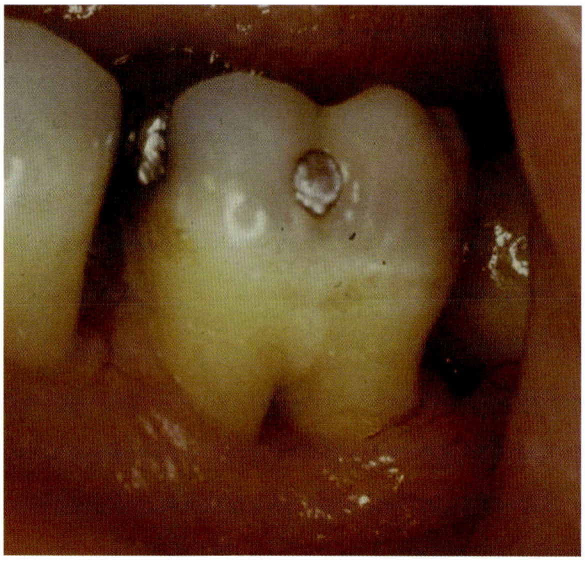

Figure 9.13 Failure to treat a Class III cementoenamel projection in a timely and effective manner has resulted in the development of Class III furcation involvement and a hopeless prognosis for a mandibular first molar.

mal probing depths. During examination, it is noted that the soft tissues in the buccal furcation area of a lower first molar are retractable. Further examination demonstrates the presence of a Class III cementoenamel projection. The clinician must now make a decision between two treatment approaches:

(a) The patient could be placed on a strict maintenance schedule and attempts could be made at "maintaining" the area in question through repeated professional prophylaxis visits and appropriate patient home care efforts. While this approach would at first appear enticing, the net result of the failure to perform the appropriate therapy will be periodontal attachment loss and/or the development of a furcation involvement.

(b) A periodontal surgical approach could be utilized which is characterized by conservative flap reflection and odontoplasty to eliminate the cementoenamel projection and any early furcation involvement which had developed. The result of this treatment approach will be elimination of the anatomical factors contributing to periodontal breakdown at the furcation area, and the establishment of hard and soft tissue morphologies which are conducive to both development of an appropriate attachment apparatus, and effective home care efforts.

Timely intervention in either areas of Class I furcation involvements or Class III cementoenamel projections is a means by which to preserve alveolar bone and attachment apparatus on a given tooth, and to eliminate the need for more aggressive therapies at a later date.

Class II furcation involvements cannot be eliminated through the use of odontoplasty. The resultant tooth contours, characterized by a deep notch in the treated furcation area, would harbor plaque and not be conducive to effective home care measures. When faced with Class II furcation involvements, if the tooth is to be maintained either resective techniques involving root resection or tooth sectioning, or regenerative techniques employing membranes, graft materials, growth factors or other substances must be employed. There is no doubt that root resective and tooth sectioning techniques are highly effective if performed correctly in the appropriate cases. However, as already discussed in Chapter 1, such a therapeutic approach is diagnosis and technique sensitive, and mandates a significant financial commitment. The question is whether such a commitment is warranted when we are now able to predictably utilize ossseointegrated implants to replace compromised molars.

Nevertheless, it is important to understand the high-degree of predictability attainable through appropriately performed furcation resection therapy.

Nabers et al. (8) treated 1,530 patients with severe periodontal disease and followed them for an average time of 12.9 years posttherapy. All patients were treated with resective periodontal therapy, including furcation elimination through root resection or tooth sectioning. An average of 0.29 teeth was lost over the observation time of the study.

Carnevale et al. assessed the results of resective therapy of 500 sectioned teeth restored and followed for 3–11 years posttreatment. About 94.3% of these teeth were periodontally healthy and functioning successfully at the end of the observation period.

A paper published in 2001 documented the success and failure of 701 root-resected molars followed for up to 16 years with a mean time in function of 8.1 years (9). The cumulative success rate of the root-resected molars, with success being defined as periodontal stability with no further attachment loss or increase in probing depth, was 96.8%.

If such levels of predictability are attainable through root resection, endodontic therapy, and tooth restoration, it is imperative that other treatments be considered, such as tooth replacement with an implant and crown, at least match this level of success.

As root resection and endodontic and restorative intervention have become less desirable, due to either a lack of facility with the techniques, financial considerations, or both, various regenerative approaches have been championed for treatment of Class II furcation involvements.

Unfortunately, preliminary positive results utilizing either membrane-assisted guided tissue regeneration or other types of grafting and regenerative techniques have led some researchers and clinicians to hail a given regenerative approach as a guaranteed means of eliminating Class II furcation involvements. Each approach in turn has been offered as a method for easily attaining reattachment and closure of periodontally involved furcations.

As successive products and techniques have fallen short of this claim upon subsequent examination, many clinicians have been all too ready to condemn specific treatment approaches as short-term solutions at best. The truth undoubtedly lies between the two extremes.

Numerous materials and techniques have demonstrated great promise in regenerating alveolar bone and attachment apparatus in Class II furcation areas. While each of these approaches requires further study and clinical documentation, they should not be completely abandoned.

Regardless of which material and approach are utilized to attempt regeneration in a periodontally involved furcation, the following diagnostic and technical modifications to conventional techniques undoubtedly prove helpful and worthwhile.

All furcations should be debrided with either microscope-assisted instrumentation or rotary burs. Periodontal regeneration in the presence of residual plaque and calculus is highly unpredictable. If all root surfaces bordering a given furcation cannot be accessed for appropriate debridement, regenerative therapy should not be attempted.

Odontoplasty should be performed on all Class II furcations to an extent which would eliminate the horizontal component of a Class I furcation for the tooth in question. Decreasing the horizontal component of the involved furcation places a lesser demand on the regenerative procedure to effect furcation closure. This fact is especially important when employing time sensitive materials such as resorbable membranes, or nonresorbable membranes which must be removed 6–8 weeks after insertion due to plaque accumulation and/or host response.

An in-depth discussion of various materials now being tested and utilized to effect periodontal regeneration in Class II furcations is not the purpose of this chapter.

Regenerative therapy performed in Class III furcations is wholly predictable, but discouraging. Therapy is never successful. To date no techniques have proven effective in regenerating lost alveolar bone and attachment apparatus, and attaining furcation closure when treating Class III furcations.

Implant Placement at the Time of Mandibular Molar Extraction

Modifications and combinations of existing surgical techniques now afford the opportunity to ideally position implants in mandibular molar sites at the time of tooth extraction. Concomitant bone regenerative therapy is often performed around the implant at the time of placement, obviating the need for a second surgical session and significantly contracting the overall length of therapy. Replacement of hopeless or missing mandibular molars with implant restorations has undergone significant evolution since the introduction of osseointegrated implants in the early 1980s. Treatment approaches advocated at various times in the last 25 years have included:

1. **Tooth extraction, defect debridement, and implant placement approximately 12 months following resolution of any "inflammatory lesions in" the bone:** While this approach agreed with the original protocols concerning implant placement in "infected sites," it presented a number of disadvantages. In addition to significantly protracting the course of therapy, the degree of alveolar ridge resorption postextraction was unpredictable, often resulting in less than ideal alveolar bone at the receptor site for eventual implant placement.
2. **Tooth extraction and defect debridement followed by immediate placement of two**

implants in the root extraction sockets: This approach helped to avoid postextraction bone resorption, and permitted the clinician to affect implant placement in a fresh extraction socket of sufficient dimension. Unfortunately, the final prosthetic result of two "bicuspids" was less than ideal. The concept of "bicuspidization" of a mandibular molar presenting with a deep furcation involvement was developed for utilization during resective periodontal therapy and periodontal prosthetic reconstruction. This concept is inherently flawed. The result of sectioning a mandibular molar is not two bicuspids. If the ratio of the mesiodistal dimension to the buccolingual dimension of the created "interproximal space" is examined, it does not approach the ratio of the space between mandibular bicuspids. As a result, unless the roots of the mandibular molar are more dramatically flared than normal, or orthodontic therapy is employed to separate the sectioned roots, the result is an interproximal space which heals with a nonkeratinized, concave soft tissue col form, posing a significant challenge to home care efforts (Figures 9.14–9.17). While the ossseointegrative bond has been shown to be less susceptible to extension of an inflammatory lesion from the gingival sulcus than its natural tooth counterpart, it is by no means impervious. A treatment approach which results in a potential area for greater plaque accumulation, and difficulty in plaque control efforts, should not be considered ideal.

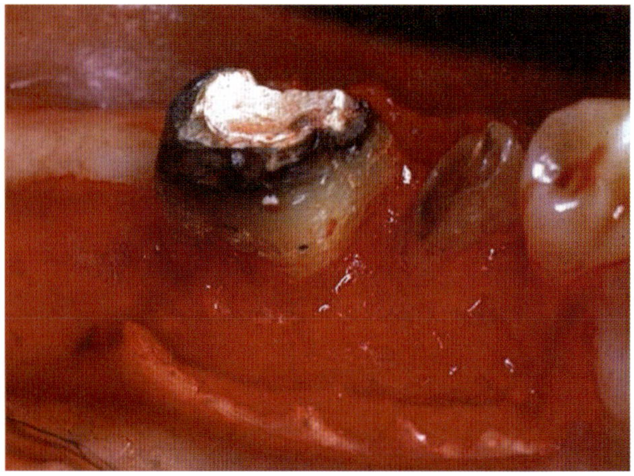

Figure 9.15 A lingual view demonstrates no periodontal involvement of the lingual furcation of the first molar.

3. **Extraction of a hopeless mandibular molar, defect debridement, and placement of an implant in one of the root sockets, followed by restoration with a molar-sized crown:** This approach eliminated the aforementioned concern of two implants placed closely together in the root extraction sockets. However, the final treatment result was by no means ideal, resulting in a mesial cantilever

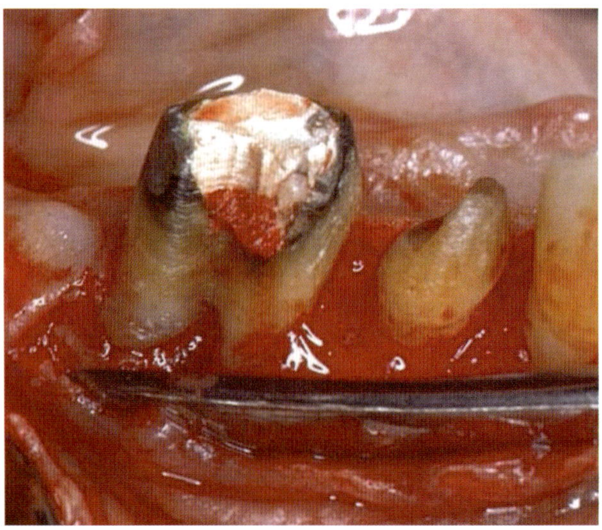

Figure 9.14 A Class II buccal furcation involvement is present on a mandibular first molar.

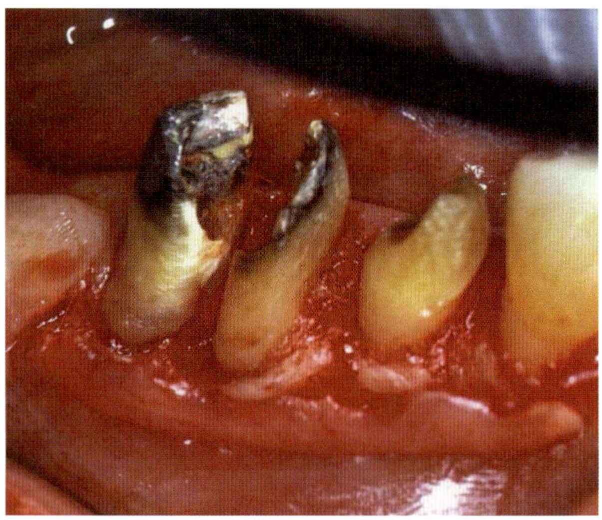

Figure 9.16 A mandibular first molar has been sectioned. This "bicuspidization" does not result in two bicuspids.

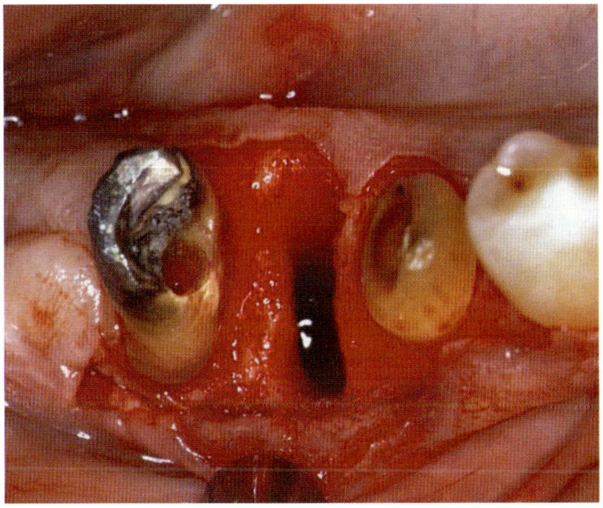

Figure 9.17 Following extraction of the mesial root of the mandibular first molar, it is evident that a ratio of the bucco-lingual to mesiodistal dimensions of the interradicular bone between the sectioned roots of the mandibular molar would not have been equal to the same ratio between the two adjacent bicuspids. Retention of both roots of the sectioned mandibular molar would have resulted in an area of difficult maintenance for the patient.

of the implant restoration, and an area of potential plaque accumulation (Figure 9.18).

4. **Tooth extraction, defect debridement, and placement of particulate graft material in the extraction socket defects, followed by second-stage implant placement:** This approach has traditionally offered an incremental improvement in treatment outcomes over Option 1. However, as was discussed in Chapter 2, placement of particulate graft materials without the appropriate covering membrane, while effecting greater socket fill than tooth extraction with no graft material, results in a final alveolar bone quantity and morphology which is unpredictable.
5. **Tooth extraction followed by particulate graft placement and utilization of an appropriate covering membrane, as discussed in Chapter 2, with subsequent second-stage implant placement:** This approach affords the clinician the ability to predictably rebuild the desired alveolar ridge morphology in anticipation of eventual implant placement. Such an approach idealizes implant position, and allows selection of the desired implant morphology. The only disadvantage to this treatment approach is the need to perform a second surgical procedure (Figures 9.19 and 9.20).
6. **Tooth extraction and immediate implant placement in an ideal restorative position, without the use of concomitant regenerative materials:** The greatest challenge to performing this therapy is the ability to ideally position an implant of the desired dimension in the area of the interradicular bone. All too

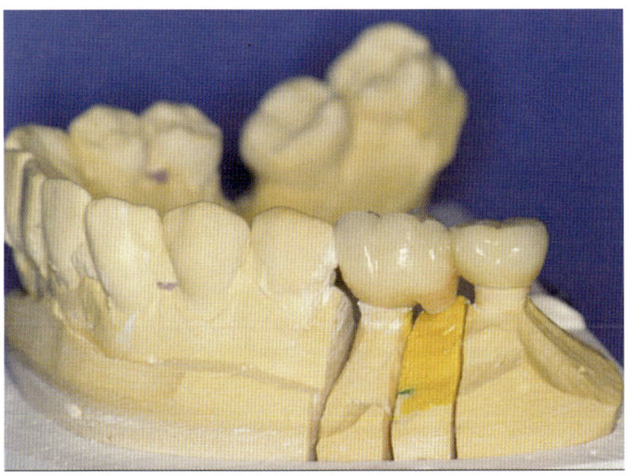

Figure 9.18 An implant has been placed in the mesial root socket of a mandibular first molar by a previous practitioner. The restoration recreated a "furcation" in the area, representing a hindrance to proper patient plaque control.

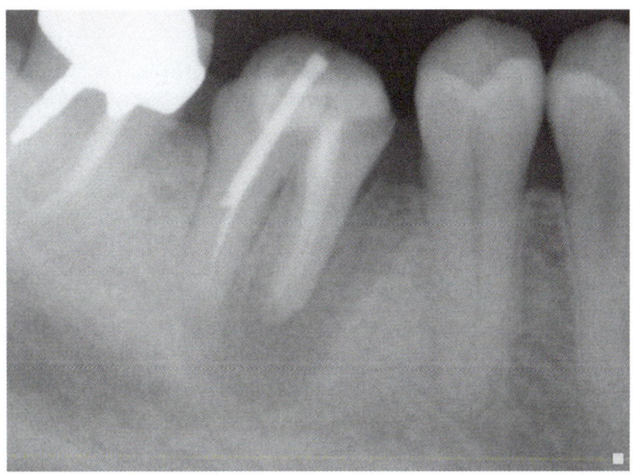

Figure 9.19 Extensive alveolar bone loss is noted around a fractured and hopeless mandibular first molar. As a result of this bone destruction it was determined that an implant could not be placed in an ideal position at the time of tooth removal.

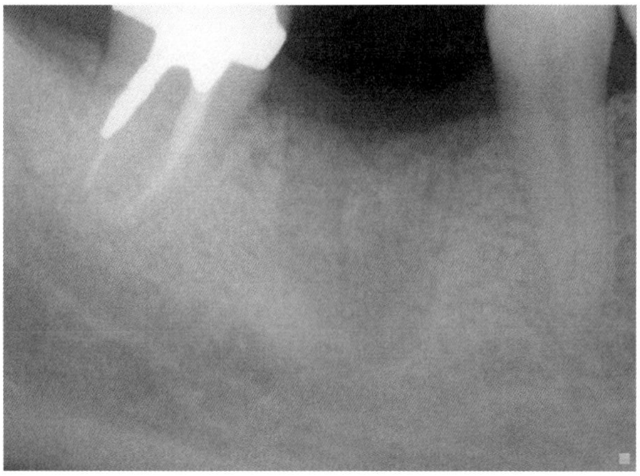

Figure 9.20 Following tooth extraction, defect debridement, and utilization of particulate material and a covering titanium membrane, a prepathologic ridge morphology has been regenerated in anticipation of implant placement.

often a clinician chooses to either place the implant into one of the extraction sockets, or utilizes a narrower implant than ideally desired in order to anchor it in the residual interradicular bone. Either approach represents a compromise in treatment outcomes. Assuming that the ideal implant position of a fixture of the desired dimensions and morphology has been attained, the failure to perform concomitant regenerative therapy represents another potential treatment compromise. There is no doubt that an implant placed in a mandibular molar extraction socket without concomitant therapy will attain osseointegration. However, Becker et al. have demonstrated that significant socket remodeling will occur, resulting in loss of buccolingual socket dimension and crestal height to varying degrees.

7. **Tooth extraction followed by ideal implant positioning and concomitant regenerative therapy:** This treatment approach should not be employed unless an implant of the desired dimension and morphology can be placed in an ideal restorative position. If such placement may be effected, the use of concomitant regenerative therapy will result in both preservation of all remaining alveolar bone in the extraction socket area, re-establishment of prepathologic alveolar ridge morphology, and bone buccal and lingual to the implant of sufficient thickness to withstand functional forces over time. The need for a second surgical session is thus eliminated.

Should there be doubt about the ability to attain primary stability of an appropriately sized implant in an ideal restorative position at the time of mandibular molar extraction, such therapy should not be attempted. Rather, appropriate regenerative techniques should be employed to regenerate prepathologic alveolar ridge morphology in anticipation of eventual implant placement.

Clinical Example One

A patient presented with a vertically fractured mandibular left first molar (Figure 9.21). At the time treatment was performed, techniques were not available to predictably place an implant of the desired dimension in an ideal restorative position in such a site. As a result, the tooth was sectioned and extracted, and particulate material and a covering membrane were utilized to regenerate the damaged alveolar bone in the region. A radiograph taken six months posttherapy demonstrates bone regeneration in the extraction socket region (Figure 9.22). A Straumann implant with a 4.8-mm-wide body and a 6.5-mm-wide restorative platform was placed and restored with a solid abutment and single crown. Six years postrestoration, a radiograph

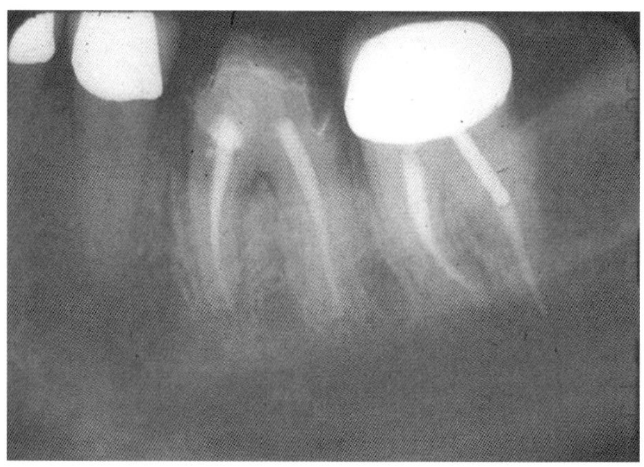

Figure 9.21 The mandibular first molar is hopeless due to the presence of a vertical fracture. At the time when treatment was performed, techniques were not available to ideally position an implant of desired dimension at the time of mandibular molar extraction.

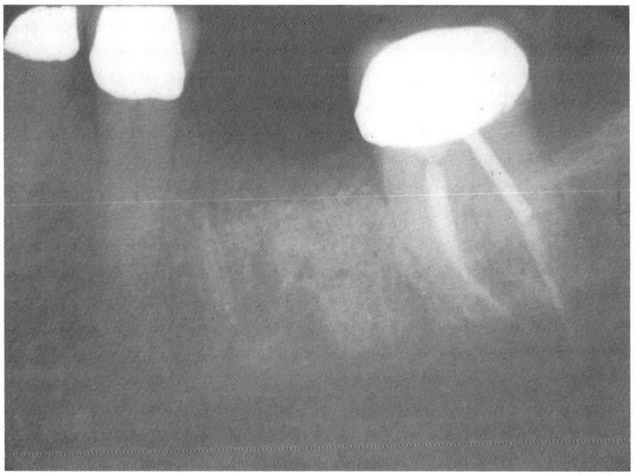

Figure 9.22 Following tooth sectioning and extraction, defect debridement and utilization of appropriate regenerative materials, extensive bone regeneration is noted in the area of the first molar. An implant of the desired dimension may now be placed in an ideal prosthetic position.

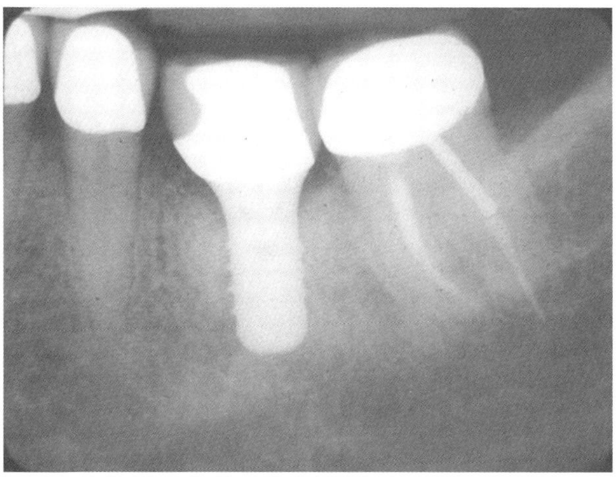

Figure 9.23 An implant with a 4.8-mm-wide body and a 6.5-mm-wide restorative platform has been restored with an abutment and crown, and has been in function for over five years.

demonstrates stability of the peri-implant alveolar bone (Figure 9.23).

INTRAOPERATIVE SITE ASSESSMENT

While most multirooted mandibular teeth may be removed and replaced with an implant in one surgical session, it is important to assess the surgical site after tooth removal and defect debridement has been accomplished (Flow chart 9.2).

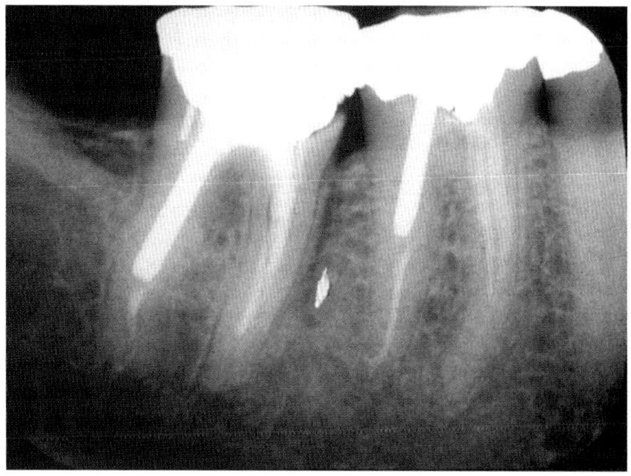

Figure 9.24 A second molar presents with an intrafurcal fracture and a hopeless prognosis. During tooth extraction, repeated root fracture necessitated the use of rotary instruments, resulting in significant trauma to the residual alveolar bone. As a result, regenerative therapy was performed without implant placement.

All mandibular multirooted molars to be removed are hemisected (or trisected in the rare cases of three-rooted mandibular molars), and the roots are carefully removed one at a time so as to preserve all remaining interradicular bone. Occasionally, a tooth is encountered which has undergone significant endodontic and restorative therapy, and which fractures repeatedly during the extraction process. Should this be the case, excessive trauma and/or the use of high-speed instrumentation may be necessary to effect removal of tooth fragments. It is then prudent to perform guided bone regeneration therapy with the appropriate graft materials and covering membrane rather than to place an implant in a site of overly traumatized bone (Figures 9.24 and 9.25). The site will be re-entered following maturation of the regenerated hard tissues to place the planned implant in an ideal prosthetic position.

The presence of a periodontal and/or periapical inflammatory lesion around the tooth to be extracted is not a contraindication to immediate implant placement with concomitant regenerative therapy. However, the extent and morphology of alveolar bone destruction as a result of the aforementioned infection may preclude immediate implant placement.

Figure 9.26 demonstrates a tooth which was to be hemisected and removed. Implant placement was anticipated during the same visit, following defect debridement. However, after hemisection and

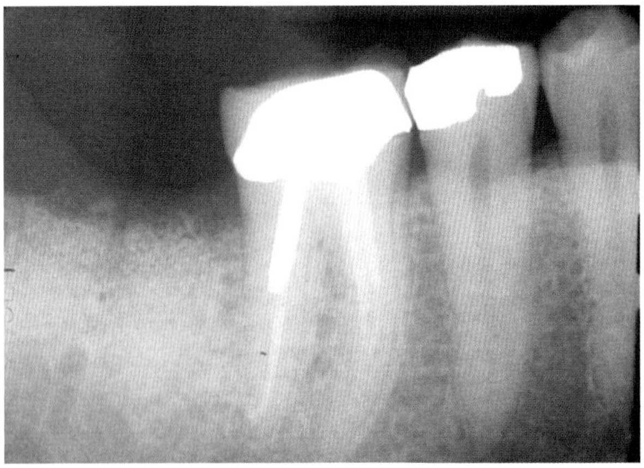

Figure 9.25 Six months after tooth removal and appropriate regenerative therapy, more than adequate bone regeneration has occurred to allow ideal positioning of an implant of the desired dimensions and morphology.

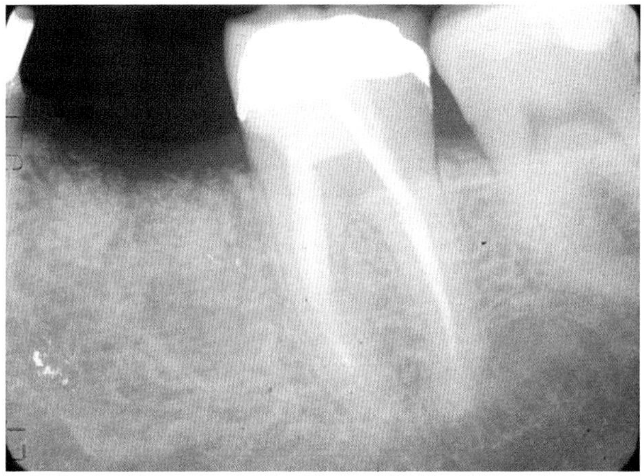

Figure 9.27 Six months after the aforementioned regenerative therapy, more than adequate bone regeneration is evident for ideal positioning of an implant of the desired dimensions and morphology.

removal of tooth number 19 and debridement of the inflammatory lesion, inadequate alveolar bone remained to effect ideal implant positioning. The two inflammatory lesions at the apices of the mesial and distal roots communicated through the interradicular septum, undermining the septum and eliminating the bone necessary for attainment of primary implant stability in the proper position. As a result of these findings, guided bone regeneration was performed in the socket area at the time of tooth removal. Five and a half months postoperatively, more than adequate bone is present to effect implant placement in an ideal position (Figure 9.27).

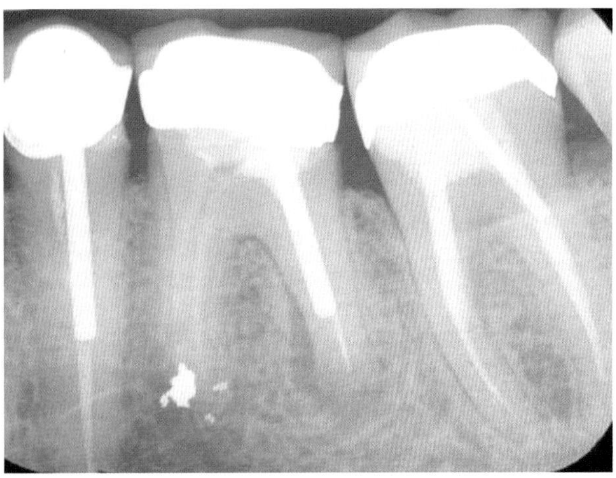

Figure 9.26 The first molar presents with a hopeless prognosis. Following tooth sectioning and extraction, and debridement of the periapical lesions which were present, the interradicular bone was undermined and incapable of supporting an implant in an ideal restorative position. As a result, regenerative therapy was performed without implant placement.

IMPLANT SELECTION

Most clinicians now advocate the use of a wider platform implant to replace a missing molar rather than two narrower implants, for reasons previously discussed. Figure 9.28 demonstrates two 6-mm-wide hex-headed fixtures restored with abutments and cemented crowns, utilized to replace missing first and second molars. Utilization of

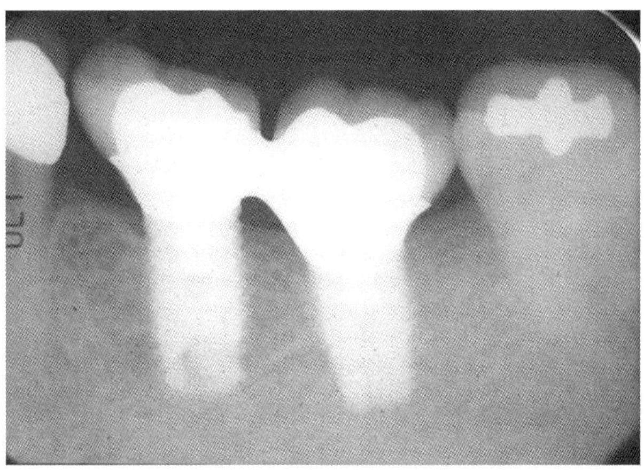

Figure 9.28 Two missing mandibular molars have been replaced with 6-mm-wide implants, abutments, and cemented crowns.

narrower implants would have required either placement of additional implants, resulting in increased cost of therapy and more difficulty in patient home care efforts, or placement of two narrower implants which would have resulted in crowns with significant mesial and distal cantilevers.

While the advent of various implant dimensions and morphologies offers a number of functional and aesthetic advantages in the replacement of individual teeth throughout the mouth, it is imperative that this plethora of available designs not be seen as a substitute for appropriate diagnosis and execution of therapy as needed, but rather as an adjunct to the care to be performed.

The introduction of wider diameter implants, and their widespread use to replace missing molars in atrophic alveolar ridges, initially led to a number of untoward results. Numerous authors reported a loss of buccal bone around these implants under function over time, in the absence of inflammatory lesions. There is no doubt that this observed phenomenon was due to the implants having been placed in areas which resulted in very thin residual buccal alveolar plates. As previously discussed, such thin alveolar bone is highly labile, and susceptible to resorption under functional load. This is especially true around implants, as the forces placed upon the implants are distributed primarily to the crestal bone region.

When considering implant placement in an area where a mandibular molar has been missing for quite some time, it is important to assess the amount of ridge atrophy which has occurred (Figure 9.29). While it is theoretically possible to place the implant in a more lingual position so as to preserve what atrophic buccal bone remains, such a treatment approach is far from ideal. An implant of the desired dimension should instead be placed in an ideal restorative position (Figure 9.30), and concomitant regenerative therapy carried out at the time of implant placement as necessary, to ensure regeneration of bone of adequate dimension to withstand functional forces over time on the buccal aspect of the implant (Figure 9.31).

Atrophic molar areas present a unique challenge when contemplating utilization of a wider platform implant to support a restoration. In such

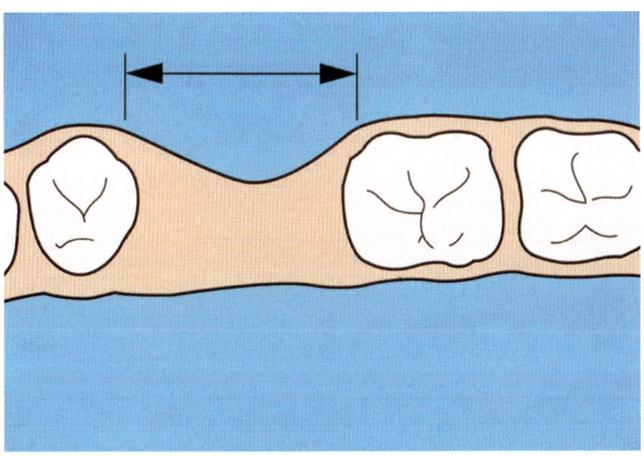

Figure 9.29 Significant ridge atrophy has occurred following loss of a mandibular molar.

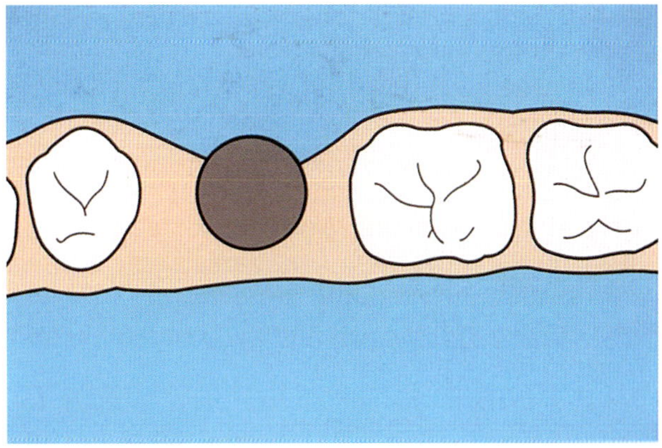

Figure 9.30 Placement of a wide implant in an ideal prosthetic position in this atrophic ridge has resulted in a significant buccal dehiscence.

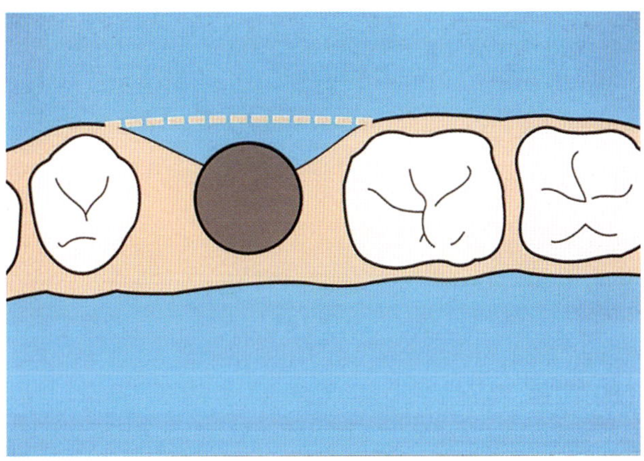

Figure 9.31 Regenerative therapy must be performed to rebuild buccal alveolar bone of sufficient dimension to withstand functional forces over time.

areas, specific implant designs offer tangible benefits over other morphologies.

In general, two wide platform implant designs are available for use in such situations. The first is a tapered implant which presents with a 6- or 6.5-mm-wide restorative platform, and tapers to a narrower "apical" diameter. The second design is one with a nontapering body, and flares to the desired wider restorative platform supracrestally. The results attained utilizing each implant design are not the same.

If a mandibular molar has been missing for some time and significant ridge atrophy has occurred, a threaded implant is utilized with a 4.8-mm-wide straight-walled body and a 6.5-mm-wide restorative platform. The implant flares from 4.8 to 6.5 mm in width in the supracrestal area, between the bone crest and the implant collar (Figure 9.32). Utilization of this design affords the advantages of a wider restorative platform, while still preserving the maximum thickness of bone possible on the buccal and lingual aspects of the implant.

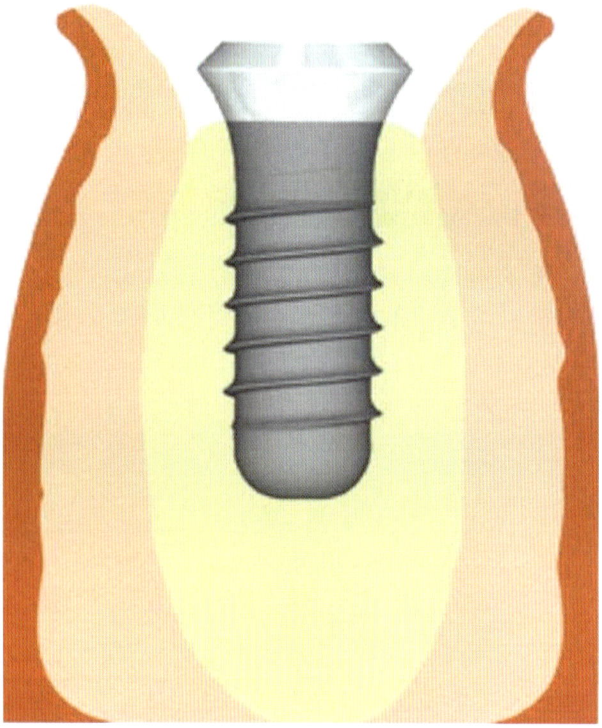

Figure 9.32 An implant has been placed in an atrophic mandibular ridge. Utilization of an implant design with a straight-walled 4.8-mm-diameter body, a 6.5-mm-wide restorative platform, and a flare of the implant supracrestally from the body diameter to the restorative platform diameter results in maximum preservation of residual alveolar bone on the buccal and lingual aspects of the implant.

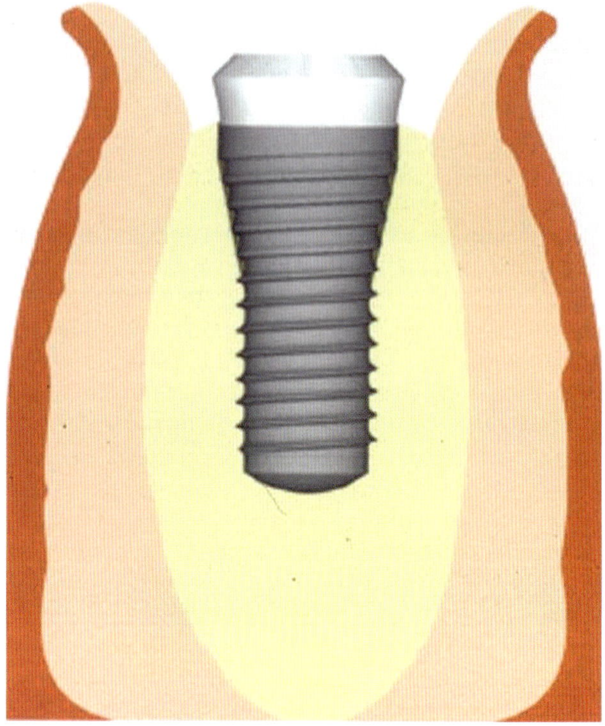

Figure 9.33 Placement of a tapered implant with a 4.8-mm apical diameter and a 6.5-mm restorative platform diameter, which begins to broaden subcrestally as it expands to the restorative platform diameter in an atrophic ridge, results in thinner residual buccal and lingual alveolar bone than the utilization of the implant design in Figure 9.32.

In contrast, if a more conventional tapered implant design is employed, which is 4.8 mm wide at its base and has a 6.5-mm-wide restorative platform, but begins to flare to the final restorative dimension subcrestally as the diameter of the implant increases, the residual alveolar bone thickness on the buccal and lingual aspects of the implant is significantly reduced (Figure 9.33). This thinner bone is more susceptible to resorption under functional load than the thicker bone preserved through the utilization of the previously described implant morphology.

Such considerations do not come into play if an implant is being placed at the time of mandibular molar sectioning and extraction, as no ridge atrophy has occurred, and the buccolingual

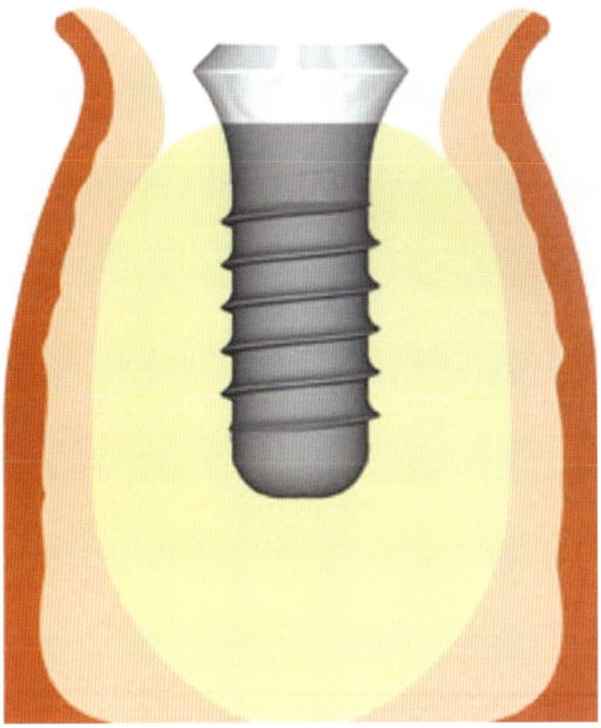

Figure 9.34 Placement of an implant at the time of mandibular molar extraction with appropriate regenerative therapy results in more than adequate buccal and lingual bone thickness to withstand functional forces over time.

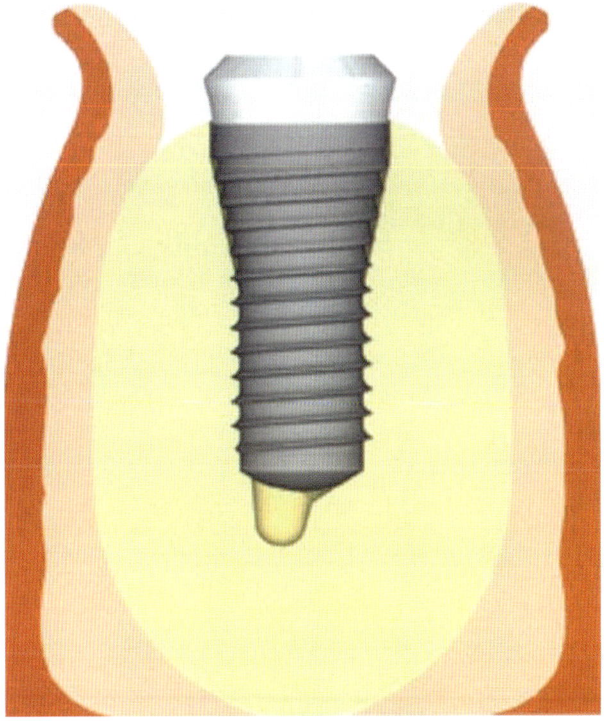

Figure 9.35 Utilization of a tapered design implant, which begins to broaden subcrestally to the final restorative platform diameter at the time of mandibular molar removal, with appropriate regenerative therapy, also results in more than adequate buccal and lingual bone thickness to withstand functional forces over time. Implant design selection is dependent upon the ability to attain primary stability in the desired position, rather than the impact of implant design on the residual buccal and lingual alveolar bone width.

dimension of the extraction socket is significantly greater than the buccolingual ridge width encountered in an area where a mandibular molar has been missing for some time.

When placing an implant at the time of mandibular molar extraction, utilization of either implant design with the appropriate concomitant regenerative therapy will result in bone of adequate thickness buccally and lingually to withstand functional forces over time (Figures 9.34 and 9.35).

The primary determining factor in choosing one implant design over the other when placing a fixture at the time of mandibular molar extraction is the ability to attain primary stability in the residual interradicular bone, in an ideal restorative position. It is for this reason that a third implant design is also utilized in these situations. This implant is characterized by a 4.1-mm-wide base, and a 6.5-mm-wide restorative platform. The implant does not begin to flare toward the 6.5-mm-wide neck diameter until the midpoint of the implant length is reached. This implant is especially useful for placement at the time of molar extraction if a narrower implant "apex" is required to anchor the implant in thinner residual interradicular bone (Figure 9.36).

Concomitant Tooth Extraction and Implant Placement

Technical Variations

Following tooth sectioning and delicate removal of each root independently, implant placement proceeds in one of the following manners:

If the most crestal aspect of the interradicular bone is at least 3-mm-wide mesiodistally: A 2.2-mm-wide guide bur is drilled to the

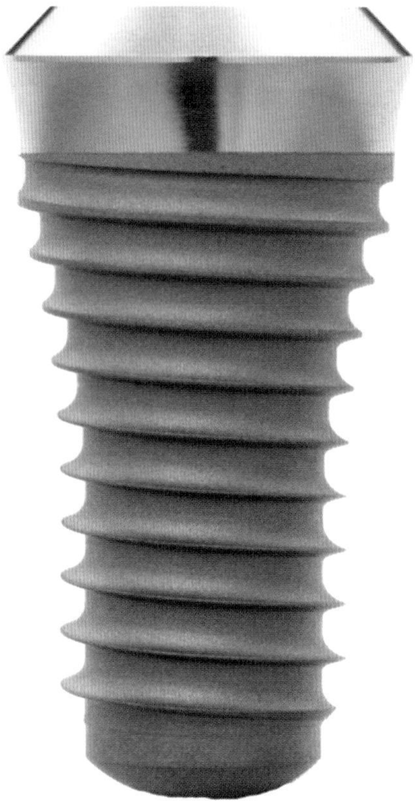

Figure 9.36 An implant design with a 4.1-mm apical diameter and a 6.5-mm restorative platform is often employed for simultaneous implant placement at the time of mandibular molar removal in areas of thin residual interradicular bone.

appropriate depth. A guide pin is inserted and a radiograph is taken (Figure 9.37). If necessary, the initial osteotomy is extended apically. A tapered osteotome is inserted into the osteotomy and moved mesiodistally and buccolingually to expand the osteotomy site. A 2.8-mm bur is used to prepare the osteotomy to depth. A 2.8-mm-wide tapered osteotome is inserted in the osteotomy and once again utilized in mesiodistal and buccolingual directions to expand the osteotomy site. If the mesial and distal aspects of the interradicular bone are still intact at this point, a 3.5-mm-wide osteotome is inserted into the osteotomy and utilized in the manner already described. A decision is made as to whether to place a tapered implant with a 4.1-mm-wide base and a 6.5-mm-wide neck, or to utilize a 4.8-mm-wide bur and prepare the osteotomy to depth, in anticipation of placement of an implant

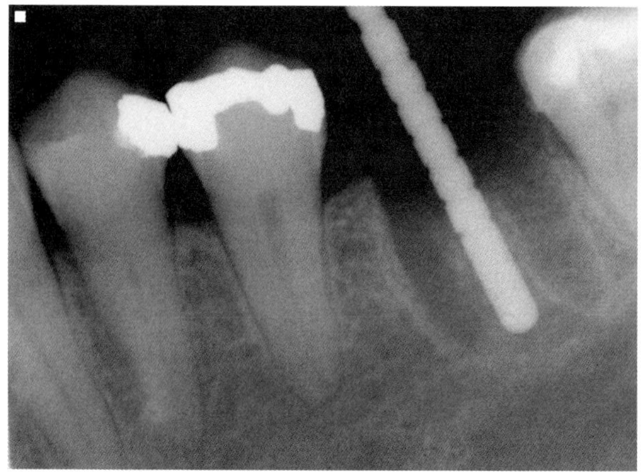

Figure 9.37 Following removal of a mandibular first molar, an osteotomy was performed in the interradicular bone. A guide pin has been placed and a radiograph taken.

with a 4.8-mm-wide parallel wall body and a 6.5-mm-wide platform. The chosen implant is then inserted into the osteotomy (Figure 9.38). Appropriate regenerative materials are placed, and the flaps are sutured. Following maturation of the regenerating hard tissues, the implant is ready for restoration (Figure 9.39). A radiograph taken 54 months after implant restoration demonstrates stability of the peri-implant crestal bone (Figure 9.40).

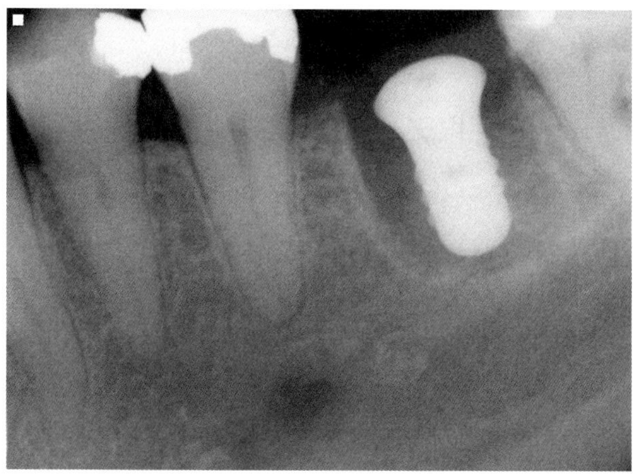

Figure 9.38 A straight-walled implant with a 4.8-mm body diameter and a 6.5-mm restorative platform diameter has been placed in the interradicular bone following tooth sectioning and removal. Primary stability has been attained.

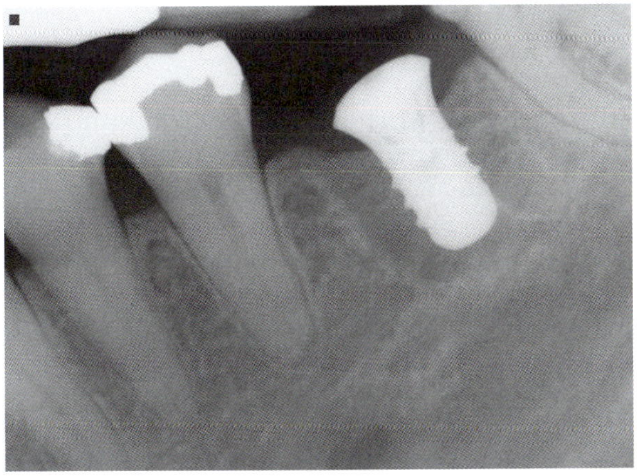

Figure 9.39 Following manipulation of the interradicular bone, implant placement, and performance of concomitant regenerative therapy, the hard tissues are mature and the implant is ready for restoration.

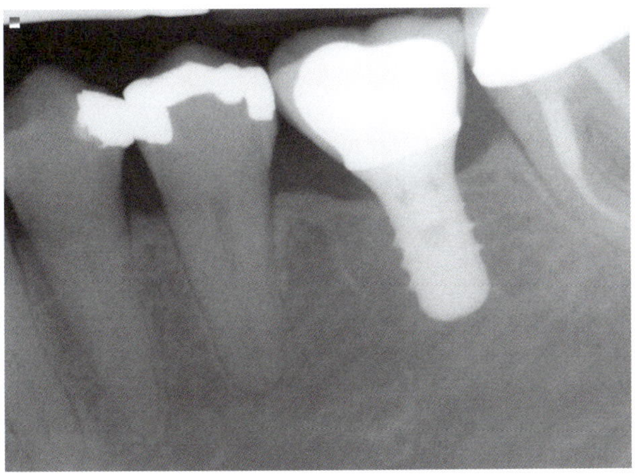

Figure 9.40 A radiograph taken 54 months after implant restoration demonstrates the stability of the crestal peri-implant bone.

If the interradicular bone does not demonstrate a mesiodistal dimension of at least 3 mm, or if the mesial and/or distal aspects of the interradicular septum are lost during site preparation, the following modifications are employed: Once the tooth has been hemisected and removed, the depth and position of a guide pin are verified by a radiograph. If continued site preparation will result in loss

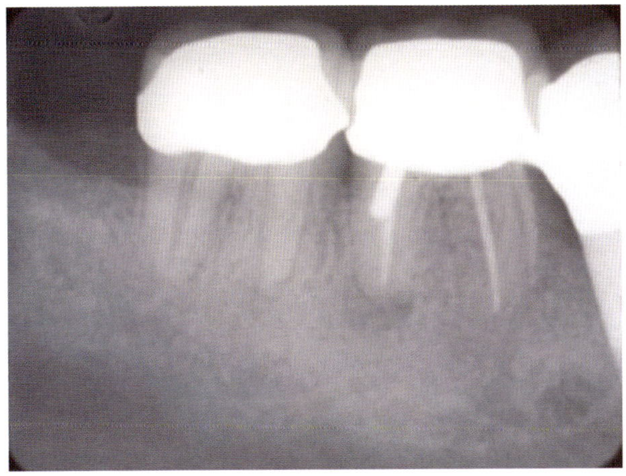

Figure 9.41 The mandibular second molar is fractured. Note the periapical lesions around this tooth.

of the mesial and/or distal aspects of the interradicular bone (Figures 9.41 through 9.44), it is imperative that final preparation of the osteotomy be accomplished in the appropriate position. The challenge to the clinician is the tendency of the bur to chatter and "walk out of" the osteotomy into one of the root sockets, due to loss of the mesial and/or distal bony retaining wall(s). Precise osteotomy preparation

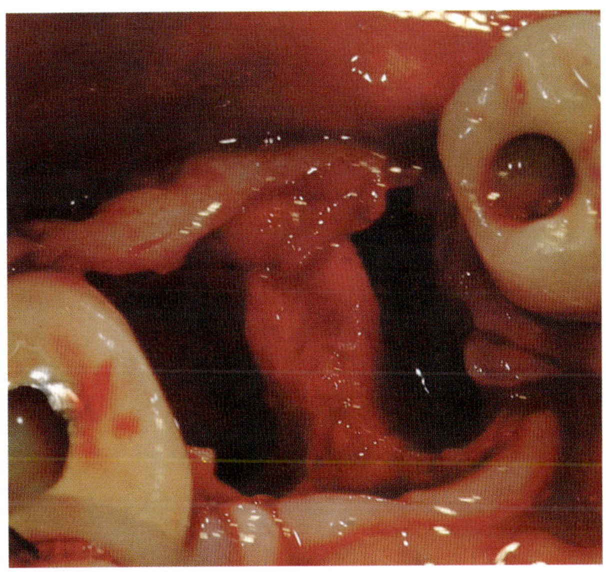

Figure 9.42 The first molar has been extracted and hemisected without damaging the interradicular bone.

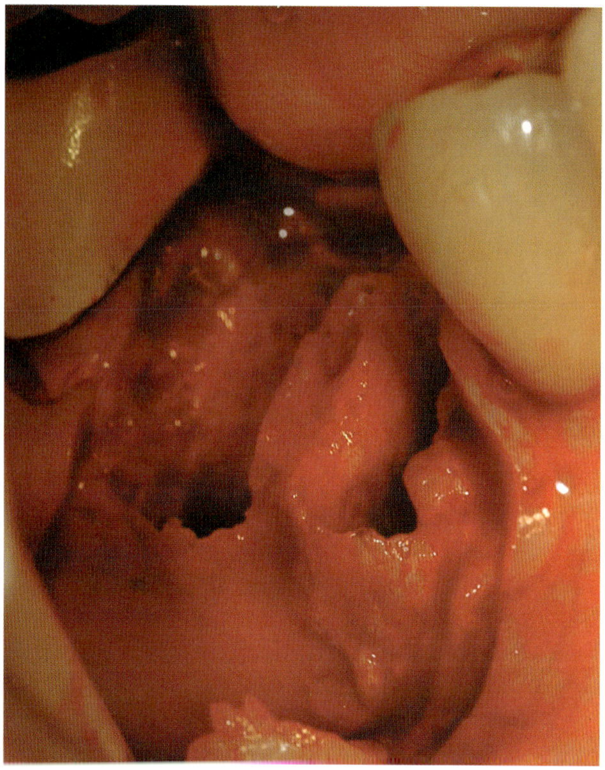

Figure 9.43 An initial osteotomy has been prepared in the interradicular bone utilizing a 2.2-mm-wide bur.

in such a situation is accomplished through the use of a modified drilling technique, employing differential pressure. The bur enters the interradicular bone at an angle, with the base of the bur engaging the lateral wall of the most apical extent of the osteotomy preparation. As the bur achieves a set point in the interradicular bone, it is straightened up and osteotomy preparation is begun. Osteotomy preparation continues in the same manner, with each subsequent bur requiring a less acute initial angle of entry. Upon completion of the osteotomy, the implant is placed in an ideal restorative position (Figures 9.45 and 9.46). Following bone regeneration and osseointegration, the implant is ready to be restored with a single crown. A radiograph taken after the implant has been in function for over seven years demonstrates stable peri-implant crestal levels (Figure 9.47).

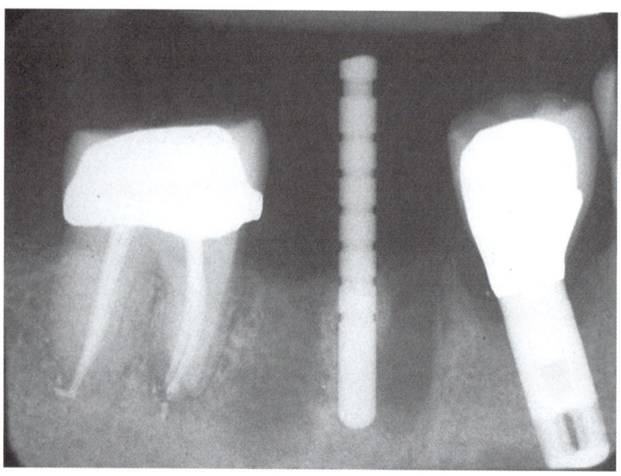

Figure 9.44 A radiograph of a guide pin in the prepared osteotomy.

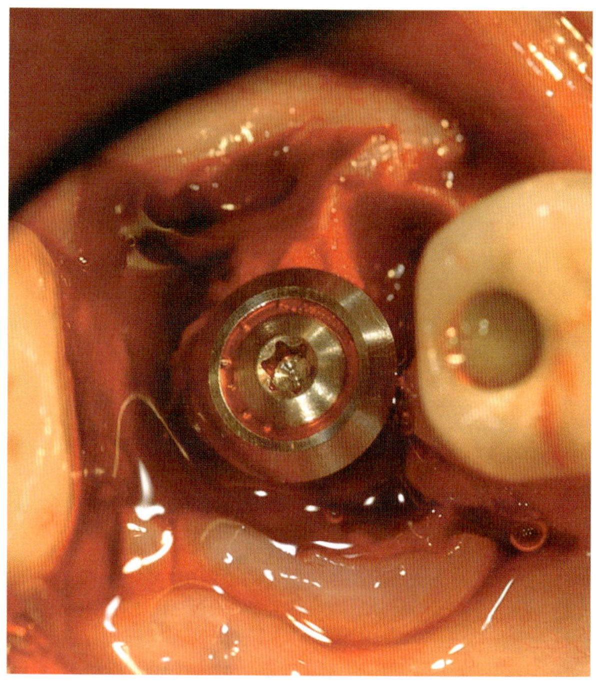

Figure 9.45 An implant with a parallel wall 4.8-mm-wide body and a 6.5-mm-wide restorative platform has been placed in the interradicular bone following appropriate preparation.

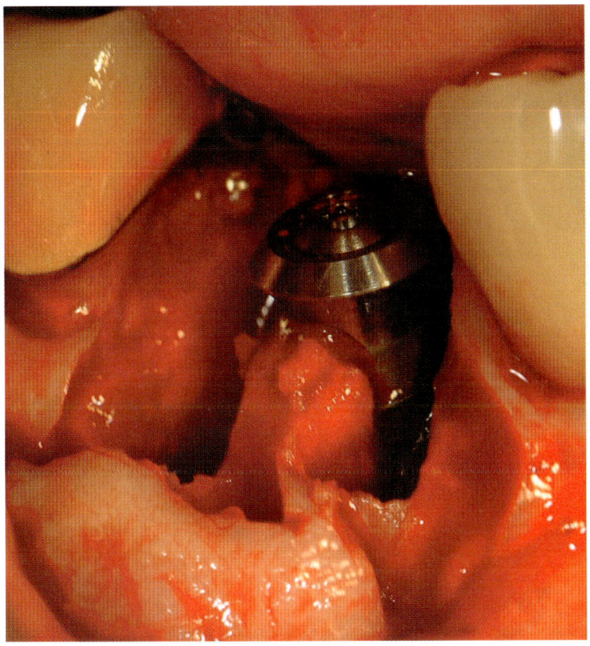

Figure 9.46 Another view of the implant in the interradicular bone. Note that the mesial and distal aspects of the interradicular septum have been lost. The implant attained primary stability from the buccal and lingual aspects of the interradicular bone.

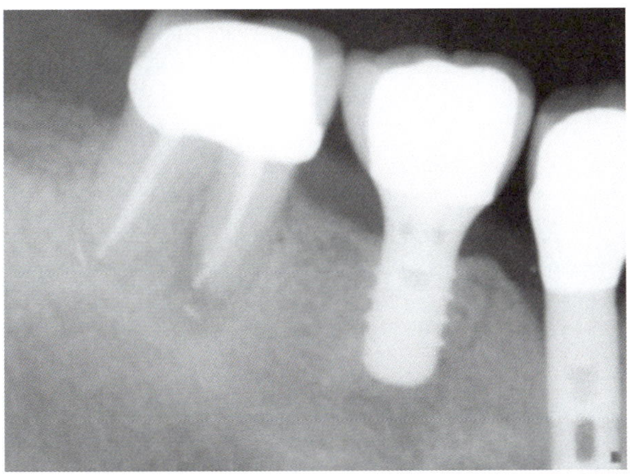

Figure 9.47 A radiograph of the restored implant taken after more than seven years in function demonstrates stable peri-implant crestal bone levels.

Clinical Example Two

A 65-year-old female presented with a missing mandibular left second molar, and a decayed and periodontally hopeless first molar (Figure 9.48). Following hemisection and extraction of the hopeless first molar, initial osteotomies were prepared in the molar sites and guide pins were inserted (Figure 9.49). Manipulation of the interradicular bone in the area of tooth number 19 was completed, and two parallel-wall 4.8-mm-diameter implants with 6.5-mm-diameter platforms were placed in the molar positions. Appropriate regenerative materials were utilized. Soft tissue primary closure was attained and maintained throughout the course of regeneration. A radiograph taken six months after therapy was performed demonstrated consolidation of the regenerating bone around the implant in the position of the first molar (Figure 9.50). The stability of the peri-implant crestal bone after more than 42 months in function is evident radiographically (Figure 9.51).

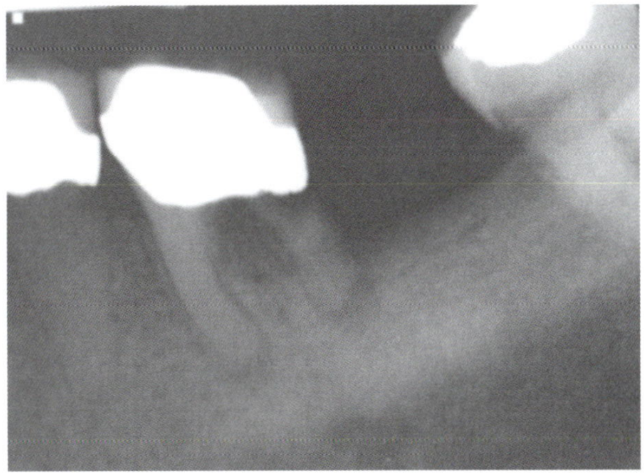

Figure 9.48 The mandibular second molar is missing and the mandibular first molar is hopeless.

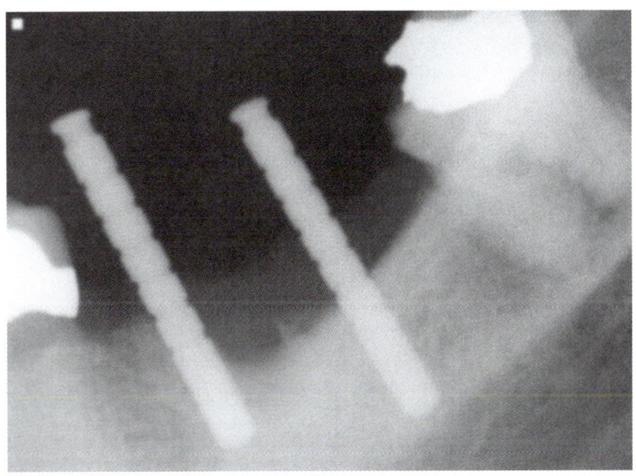

Figure 9.49 Following hemisection and extraction of the first molar, initial osteotomies have been performed and measuring pins inserted.

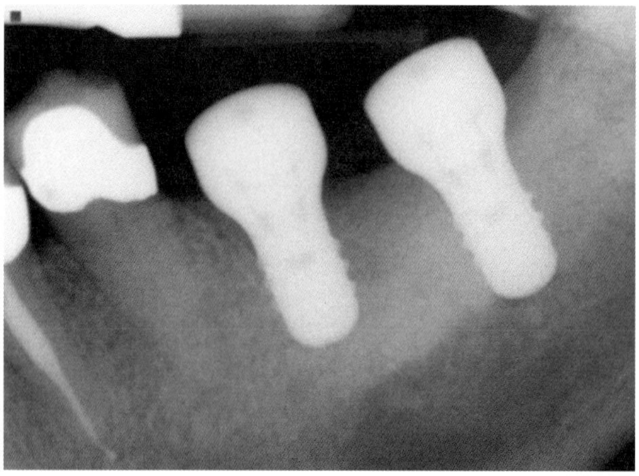

Figure 9.50 Six months after implant and regenerative therapy, consolidation of the regenerating bone around the implant in the first molar position is evident.

Clinical Example Three

A 61-year-old male presented with a fractured and hopeless mandibular second molar, the terminal abutment for a three-unit fixed splint (Figure 9.52). Following hemisection and extraction of the first molar, the interradicular bone was manipulated and prepared. Due to the position of the interradicular bone, it was crucial that a modified drilling technique be used for osteotomy preparation. If the angulation of the osteotomy was followed, the positioning of this implant would have been nonideal. Rather, the bur entered the distal aspect of the interradicular bone at the point which represented the center of the desired implant placement. A drilling technique was then utilized which employed the side of the bur to help prepare the osteotomy against the distal aspect of the interradicular bone. This variable pressure drilling technique allowed for ideal positioning of the bur as it prepared the interradicular bone at the desired angle. Once the bur passed through the interradicular bone, and engaged the bone apical to the

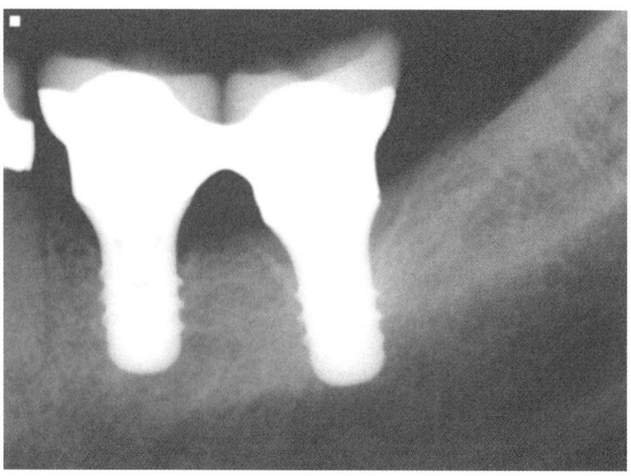

Figure 9.51 A radiograph taken after 42 months in function demonstrates the stability of the crestal peri-implant bone around both implants.

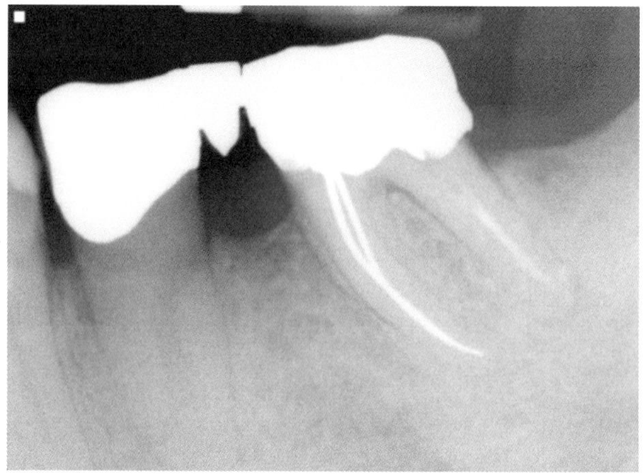

Figure 9.52 The mandibular left second molar is fractured and hopeless.

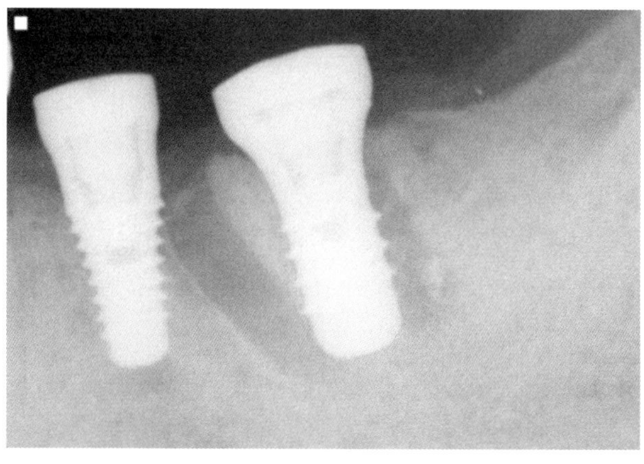

Figure 9.53 Following hemisection and extraction of the hopeless molar, implants are placed in the first and second molar positions, utilizing specific interradicular bone preparation techniques. Note the positioning of the implant in the second molar site so as to provide adequate dimension for ideal placement of an implant in the first molar area.

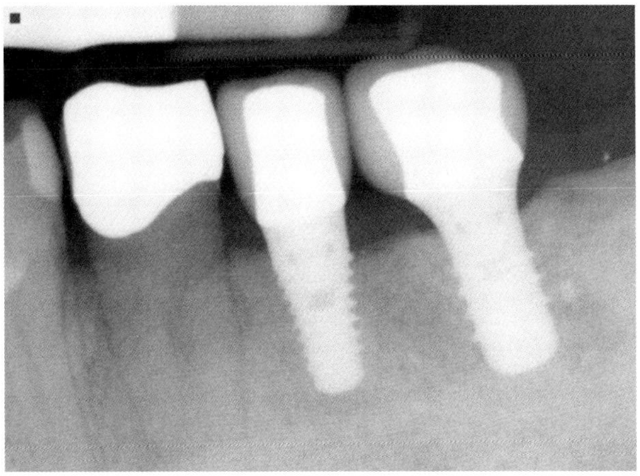

Figure 9.54 A radiograph taken after 46 months in function demonstrates the stability of the crestal peri-implant bone around both implants.

interradicular bone, the site preparation took on a more conventional nature. Implants were placed in the first and second molar positions (Figure 9.53). Note the positioning of the most distal implant so as to provide adequate dimension for appropriate placement of an implant in the first molar position. A radiograph taken after 46 months in function demonstrates the stability of the crestal peri-implant bone around both implants (Figure 9.54).

Conclusions

The described techniques are highly predictable, and help ensure ideal implant positioning at the time of mandibular molar extraction. A total of 341 implants have been placed and subsequently restored utilizing these techniques. Two hundred four of the implants are 4.8-mm-wide parallel wall implants with a 6.5-mm-wide restorative platforms, and 137 are tapered implants with a 4.1-mm-wide base and a 6.5-mm-wide restorative platform. Two implants were lost during the initial stages of healing. No implants have been lost in function, yielding a cumulative success rate of 99.1%. The implants have been in function for up to 5 years with a mean time in function of 30.7 months (10).

References

1. Becker W, Becker BE, Berg L, et al. 1998. New attachment after treatment with root isolation procedures. Report for treated class III and class II furcations and vertical osseous defects. *Int J Periodontics Restorative Dent* 8:8–23.
2. Goldman MJ, Ross IF, and Goteiner D. 1986. Effect of periodontal therapy on patients maintained for 15 years or longer. A retrospective study. *J Periodontol* 57:347–353.
3. McFall WT. 1982. Tooth loss in 100 treated patients with periodontal disease—a long-term study. *J Periodontol* 53:539–549.
4. Wood WR, Greco GW, and McFall WT Jr. 1989. Tooth loss in patients with moderate periodontitis after treatment and long-term maintenance. *J Periodontol* 60:516–520.
5. Hirschfeld L and Wasserman B. 1978. A long-term study of tooth loss in 600 treated periodontal patients. *J Periodontol* 49:225–237.
6. Wang HL, Burgett FG, Shyr Y, et al. 1994. The influence of molar furcation involvement and mobility of future clinical periodontal attachment loss. *J Periodontol* 65:25–29.
7. Fleischer HC, Mellonig JT, Brayer WK, Gray JL, and Barnett JD. 1989. Scaling and root planning efficacy in multi-rooted teeth. *J Periodontol* 60:402–409.
8. Nabers CL, Stalker WH, Esparza D, et al. 1988. Tooth loss in 1,535 treated periodontal patients. *J Periodontol* 59:297–300.
9. Fugazzotto PA. 2001. A comparison of the success of root resected molars and molar position in implants in function in a private practice: Results of up to 15 plus years. *J Periodontol* 72:1113–1123.
10. Fugazzotto PA. 2008. Implant placement at the time of mandibular molar extraction: Description of technique and preliminary results of 341 cases. *J Periodontol* 79:737–747.

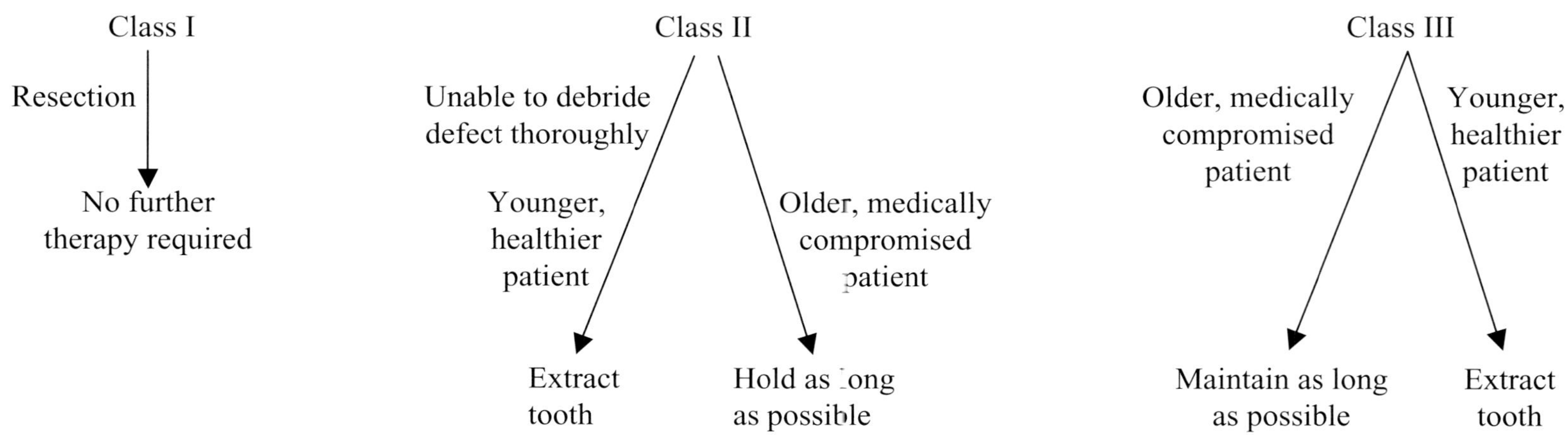

Flow chart 9.1 Treatment decisions for mandibular furcations.

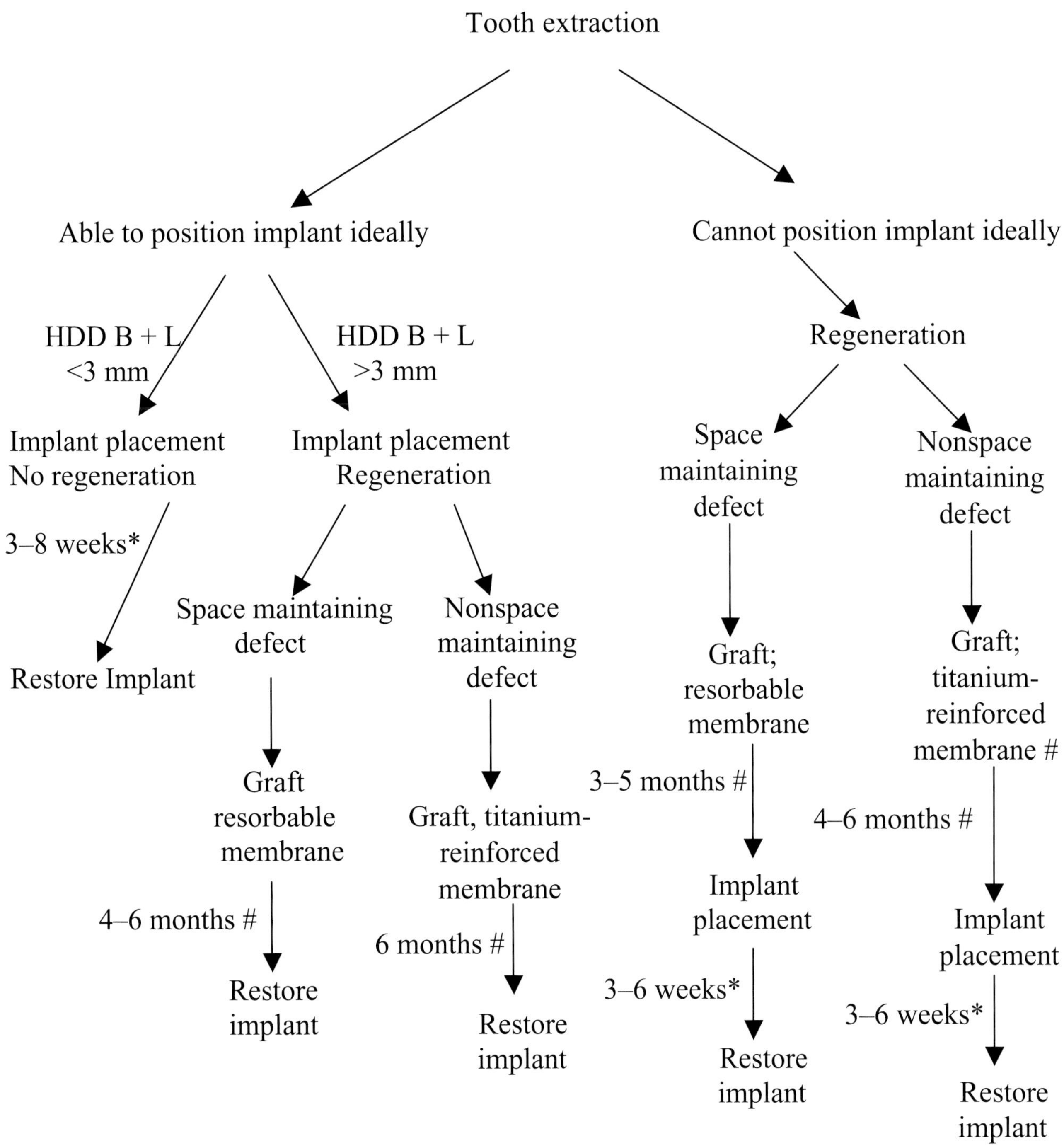

* Dependent upon implant surface
# Dependent upon regenerative materials utilized

Flow chart 9.2 Treatment decisions following mandibular molar extraction.

Chapter 10

Alveolar Bone Preservation Following Tooth Extraction in the Esthetic Zone

Philip R. Melnick, DMD, FACD and
Paulo M. Camargo, DDS, MS, MBA, FACD

Outline

Introduction

Any discussion of alveolar ridge or socket preservation following tooth extraction in the esthetic zone must proceed within the context of implant dentistry as a primarily prosthetic treatment. The therapeutic targets of comfort, function, and predictability are desirable and achievable goals with implant-supported restorations. High success rates have been attained in both fully edentulous (1) and partially edentulous situations (2). However, implant dentistry in the esthetic zone takes on added importance. Treatment outcomes that are functionally successful but esthetic failures are potential catastrophes (3) (Figure 10.1). For that reason, an interdisciplinary team effort is required to maximize treatment outcomes. An implant team consisting of the restoring dentist, surgeon, orthodontist, laboratory technician, and patient is often necessary to bring about a desired treatment outcome.

The Esthetic Concept

Esthetic criteria proposed for dental implant restorations have been inspired by those applied to natural teeth with respect to circumdental soft-tissue contours, which include bilaterally symmetrical gingival heights, intact interdental papillae, and naturally occurring root convexities (4–8) (Figure 10.2). However, fulfilling these esthetic criteria may be in conflict with the technical challenges posed by tissue inadequacies. For example, deep implant placement, excessive countersinking, and buccal angulation in an effort to compensate for insufficient bone dimensions can result in undesirable treatment outcomes such as tissue recession, elongated crowns or incomplete papillae (4, 8, 9) (Figure 10.3).

Classical implant protocols suggested tooth removal followed by at least a 12-month healing period before implant placement (10). However, hard and soft tissue changes that occur following tooth extraction often result in inadequate alveolar ridge dimensions for proper implant placement. In such

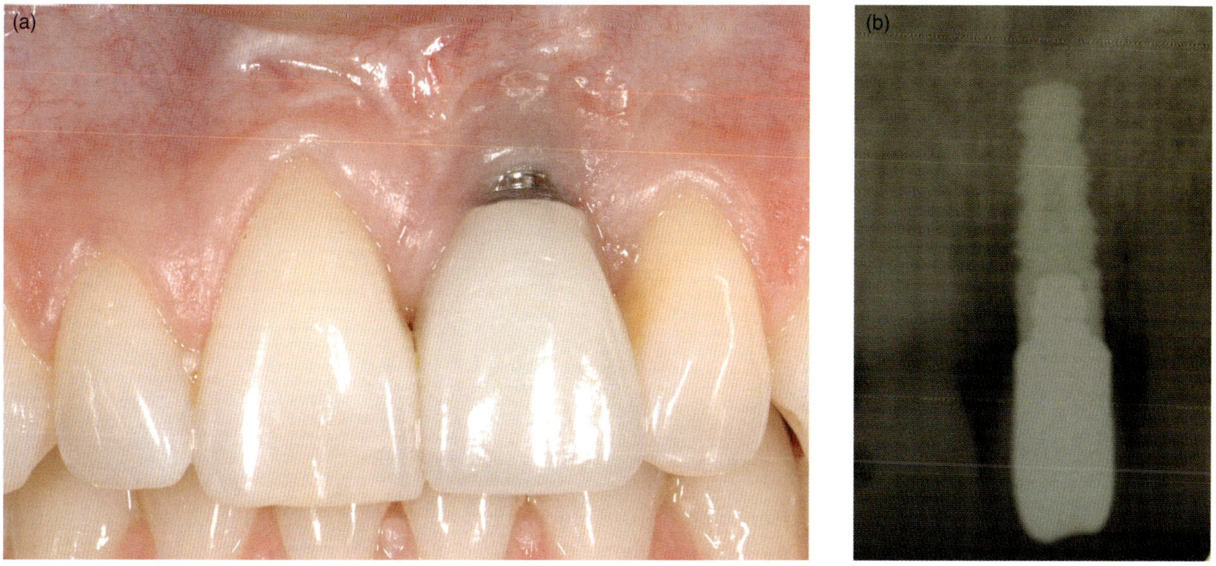

Figure 10.1 (a) An example of an adverse esthetic result on a single tooth implant in the area of tooth number 9. The patient initially presented with a highly scalloped periodontium, and developed gingival recession twelve months following restoration of the implant fixture. (b) A radiograph of the implant in the tooth number 9 position, showing evidence of osseointegration.

a scenario, preparatory ridge reconstruction should be undertaken (11, 12). Alveolar ridge preservation procedures have been devised to reduce the extent of postextraction modeling, and to promote both the efficiency and predictability of restoration-driven implant dentistry (13–17). Other treatment modalities have been introduced with the intention of reducing the number and intrusiveness of surgical interventions, and treatment duration. These developments include rough and bioactive implant surfaces (18, 19) which allow for earlier implant placement; the successful use of short implants (20, 21), which decreases the need for bone augmentation procedures; early-loading protocols; (22) and the use of growth factors intended to promote bone regeneration (16, 17).

External Dimensional Changes Following Tooth Extraction (Modeling)

It has long been acknowledged that the shape of the alveolar ridge is related to the presence and position of the teeth, and that there is a variable degree of bone resorption and remodeling following tooth loss (23–25). Numerous studies have documented significant dimensional changes in both height and width of the alveolus following tooth loss (13, 14, 25, 26). Approximately two-thirds of these changes were found to occur in the first few months of post-extraction healing (26, 27). Botticelli et al. (28) reported horizontal reduction of 56 and 30% of the buccal and lingual aspects of the ridge respectively, four months after tooth extraction. Schropp et al. (26), in a human study utilizing subtraction radiography, found that during the first 12 months

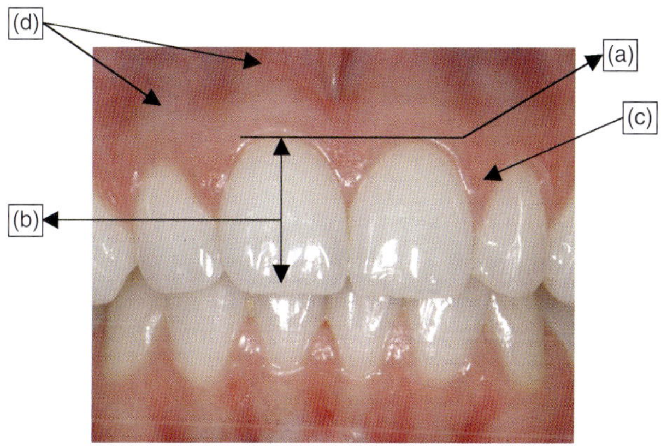

Figure 10.2 Clinical gingival characteristics of a harmonious smile include: (a) symmetry of the gingival line, (b) ideal apico-coronal/mesiodistal (golden) proportions of the clinical crown, (c) interdental papillae fully occupying the embrasures, and (d) naturally occurring root convexities.

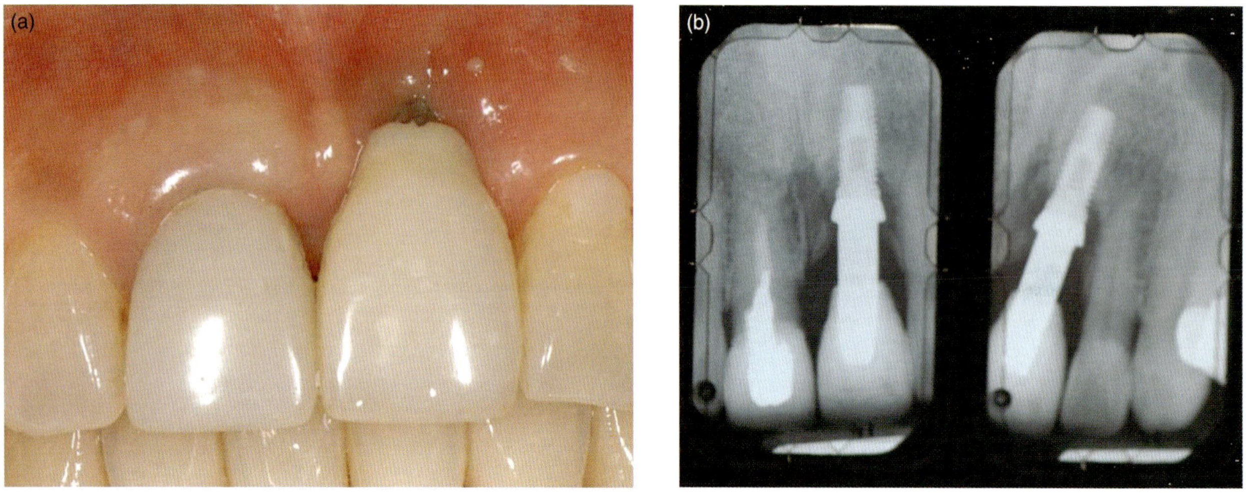

Figure 10.3 (a) Gingival recession and asymmetry of the gingival line are evident in the area of teeth numbers 8 and 9. (b) Radiographic examination revealed the platform of the implant fixture to be located approximately 10 mm apical to an imaginary line connecting the buccal cemento enamel junctions (CEJs) of the adjacent teeth. Ideally, the distance should be between 2 and 3 mm. Because of a significant hard tissue deficiency, the implant fixture was placed in an extremely apical position, resulting in an extensive area of nonbone-supported gingival tissue. Over time, the soft tissue receded, resulting in an esthetic dilemma for the treating dentist and the patient. The extraction area should have been treated with a ridge preservation procedure and/or ridge augmentation procedure to prevent this problem.

postextraction the alveolar ridge width was reduced by 50%. Pietrokovski and Massler (29), employing plaster casts, and Araujo et al. (25) in a dog model, demonstrated that postextraction alveolar bone changes were asymmetrical, with greater buccal than lingual bone resorption, resulting in a shifting of the ridge center toward the lingual/palatal. Human and animal studies have shown a variable buccal vertical height reduction of up to 2 mm (25, 30, 31). Depending upon the corresponding lingual/palatal vertical changes, this buccal ridge height can result in a negative buccal slope (25, 30, 31).

The causes of bone modeling phenomena have been speculated upon by Araujo et al. (25), who suggested that bone modeling of the extraction socket occurs in two overlapping phases. The first phase includes the replacement of bundle bone by woven bone. The thinner buccal marginal bone crest consists exclusively of bundle bone. The lingual aspect of the crest consists of a combination of bundle bone and lamellar bone. Upon extraction, the bundle bone is deprived of its blood supply from the periodontal ligament (PDL) on the tooth side. This bone is quickly resorbed and is not replaced (Figure 10.4). Such a finding may help explain the asymmetrical dimensional ridge changes

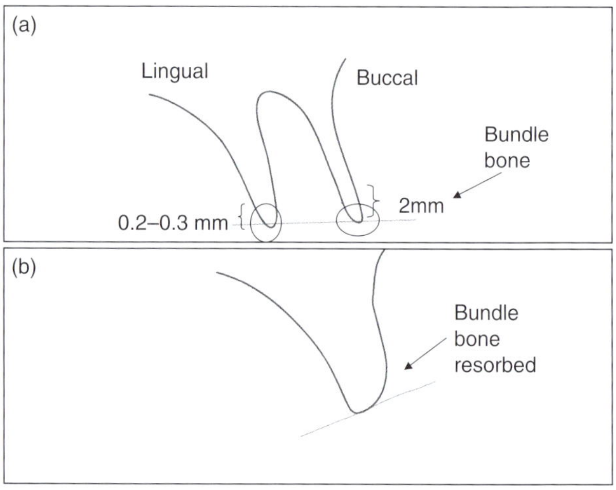

Figure 10.4 A diagrammatic view of the natural bone remodeling following tooth extraction. (a) The bundle bone that comprises most of the buccal plate resorbs due to inadequate blood supply. Blood supply is interrupted from the PDL and from the periosteum if a buccal flap is elevated. The average vertical loss of the buccal plate is 2 mm. The lingual plate, by virtue of containing a higher proportion of lamellar bone, is subject to less resorption (0.2–0.3 mm). (b) The healed ridge presents with more vertical resorption on the buccal than on the lingual (palatal) aspect. A "negative" slope is observed in the area.

Table 10.1 Stages of socket healing in humans (33).

Stage	Event	Time
I	Clot formation	Immediately
II	Granulation tissue formation	4–5 days
III	Connective tissue formation	14–16 days
IV-A	Osteoid tissue at socket base	7–10 days
IV-B	Trabeculae fill socket	6 weeks
V	Epithelial coverage	24–35 days

observed, which are related to the absence of bundle bone on the buccal aspect of the socket. The second phase of healing includes resorption of the outer walls of both the buccal and lingual surfaces. Inflammation resulting from surgical trauma and deprivation of blood supply by the separation of the periosteum from underlying bone by flap elevation may be responsible for these changes (32).

Internal Healing (Remodeling)

Bone formation within the socket (i.e., the space previously occupied by the root of the tooth) is referred to as remodeling. A number of studies have examined internal socket healing in animals (25) and humans (23, 33–35). Amler (33) described five distinct stages of the process: initial clot development, granulation tissue formation, connective tissue in-growth, osteoid and bone formation, and epithelial cover (Table 10.1). Bone restoration is most active between 5 and 10 weeks postextraction, and is complete by 4 months postextraction (36).

Rationale for Ridge Preservation

The modeling and remodeling processes following tooth extraction result in a net shrinkage of the alveolar ridge. Clinically, it is obvious that the position of the soft tissues moves in apical and palatal directions. It has been well established that the position of the soft tissues is determined by the presence and location of the underlying supporting bone. Therefore, such bone resorption can have significant long-term esthetic consequences (37–40). Several authors have suggested that, in order to maintain a stable peri-implant mucosal margin over time, a 1–4 mm of buccal bone thickness may be required (41, 42). Procedures aimed at socket preservation are performed in order to conserve bone volume and thus maintain the soft tissue position. Ideally, procedures aimed at ridge preservation should also assure bone quantity and position that make future implant placement possible without additional augmentation. However, even partially successful ridge preservation may facilitate earlier future implant placement. Ridge preservation techniques can significantly reduce postextraction dimensional change, lessening the extent of future alveolar bone reconstruction required (Figure 10.5). This concept is of particular merit if a delayed implant placement protocol (i.e., 4–8 weeks postextraction) is selected (36, 43).

Scientific Data Supporting Alveolar Ridge Preservation Following Tooth Extraction

Alveolar bone resorption after tooth extraction and the attendant morphologic-dimensional changes can make it difficult or impossible to place dental implants in an esthetically desirable manner (5–8). Consequently, attenuation of these changes via bone preservation is a desirable goal. Data from clinical trials provide evidence that surgical intervention after tooth removal can reduce negative bone changes when compared to untreated controls (13–17, 44).

In two clinical trials, Lekovic et al. (13, 14) advanced full thickness flaps for primary closure over sockets immediately after tooth extraction. In the first study, sockets were covered with nonabsorbable membranes while the second trial employed absorbable membranes. No bone grafting materials were utilized. The controls were treated by flap advancement without membranes. At six months postoperatively, horizontal ridge measurements were 5.57 mm for sockets treated with expanded polytetrafluorethylene (e-PTFE), and 6.06 mm for those treated with glycolide and lactide polymers. Horizontal measurements of the untreated controls were 2.57 and 2.94 mm, respectively. This 3.00 and 3.12 mm respective variance represents a 34 and 43% reduction in horizontal bone loss when compared to the controls. There was also 23 and 33% less loss of vertical dimension, as compared to the nonmembrane-treated controls. The resulting ridge dimensions found in the experimental sites of both studies would often be considered adequate for the placement of a 4.0-mm-diameter implant.

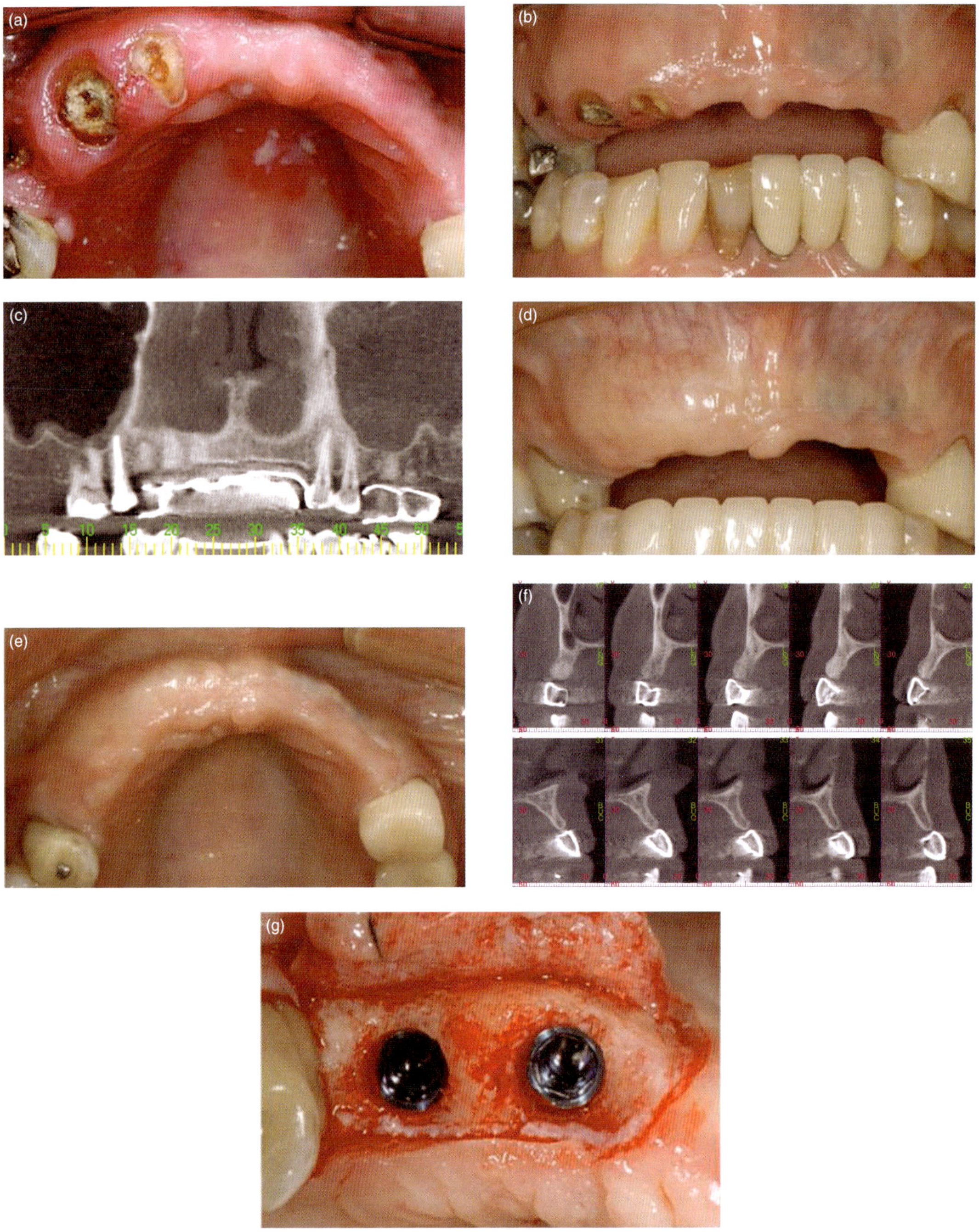

Figure 10.5 (a) An occlusal view of an upper anterior segment. The upper left anterior teeth had been extracted several years ago. No ridge preservation procedure was performed. The upper right anterior teeth are to be extracted due to caries. (b) A buccal view of the upper anterior segment. (c) The upper right anterior teeth were extracted. A preservation procedure, consisting of extraction socket grafting with a xenograft and guided bone regeneration with an absorbable membrane, was carried out. A panoramic radiograph was taken nine months after the extraction/preservation procedure. (d) A buccal view 12 months postextraction of the upper right anterior teeth. Note the more coronal position of the gingival margin in the upper right segment as compared to the upper left. (e) An occlusal view 12 months postextraction of the upper right anterior segment. The increased buccolingual dimension of the ridge on the right as compared to the left side is evident. (f) A CT scan of the upper anterior segment confirms the increased dimensions of the alveolar ridge in the upper right anterior segment (top) as compared to the upper left anterior segment (bottom). Ideal implant position is more easily attainable when the dimension of the alveolar ridge is preserved through osseous grafting and/or guided tissue regeneration at the time of tooth extraction. (g) A clinical view of the upper right anterior segment demonstrates the ideal buccolingual dimension of the preserved alveolar ridge. Note the presence of at least 2 mm of bone on the buccal aspect of both implants.

Iasella et al. (15) combined a bone allograft with a collagen membrane as preservative treatment for extraction sockets in a nonsubmerged approach (no flap advancement). Control sites received neither a bone graft nor a membrane. Flaps were sutured back to their original positions. The experimental sites showed 1.4 mm or 16% less horizontal ridge resorption and 2.2 mm more residual vertical ridge height than the control sites. This study design does not lend itself to direct comparison to the effects of the membrane or bone graft use separately, but rather only to comparison with an empty socket. However, the treatment result and benefits are similar to those of Lekovic et al. (13, 14), albeit less dramatic, due no doubt in part to failure to attain soft tissue primary closure over the grafted sites.

Zubillaga et al. (44) examined the combination of a bone allograft and a collagen membrane under advanced full thickness flaps. There were no controls. After four months, the authors concluded that the study protocol did not prevent or preserve the original ridge dimension. However, the data presented demonstrated that the experimental sites had outcomes similar to the experimental sites reported in previous papers.

Fiorellini et al. (17) treated extraction sockets with buccal wall vertical deficiencies of greater than or equal to 50% with rhBMP-2 on collagen sponges. The control sites received collagen sponges alone. About 86% of the experimental sites were able to receive dental implants with no additional grafting procedures. Only 45% of the control sites were able to receive dental implants without additional grafting procedures. The newly induced bone's density and histology were identical to that of native bone.

Nevins et al. (16) treated immediate extraction sockets with a xenograft, and flap advancement to achieve primary wound closure. The control sites received no grafts under the advanced flaps. Computerized tomographic scans were utilized to assess changes in the dimensions of the buccal plates. At three months postoperatively 79% of the sockets receiving the xenograft showed less than 20% loss of the buccal plate, while 71% of the control sockets demonstrated more than 20% loss of the buccal plate. At reentry, control sites showed more loss of buccal bone height than the experimental sites, 5.24 mm versus 2.42 mm. About 71% of the control sites presented with less than the minimal (i.e., 6 mm) ridge width required for implant placement, while only 16% of the experimental sites demonstrated less than 6 mm of ridge width.

Analysis Before Tooth Extraction

Before tooth removal, the surgeon must anticipate the future placement of the dental implant in a three-dimensional manner (5–7). Careful pre- and intraoperative assessment should be undertaken to determine whether an implant will be immediately placed (with or without concomitant regenerative procedures), or ridge preservation procedures will be employed.

The decision to accept or reject the immediate placement of a dental implant into a fresh extraction site in the esthetic zone is based on many factors. This process is described in detail in Chapter 11. Martin et al. (45) delineated a number of situations which could negatively influence a successful treatment outcome. Conversely, contraindications for immediate implant placement may serve as indications for ridge preservation and delayed implant placement (Table 10.2).

Prior to tooth removal, and in anticipation of future dental implant placement, it is important to identify factors that could both positively and negatively affect treatment outcome. This pretreatment evaluation includes factors related to both the patient and surgical site (45–48).

Table 10.2 Indications for ridge preservation may be relative contraindications for immediate implant placement in the esthetic zone (45).

	Condition/finding
I	Immune compromise
II	Heavy smoker (>10 per day)
III	High patient expectation
IV	High lip line
V	Highly scalloped, thin biotype
VI	Triangular crowns
VII	Acute infection
VIII	>7 mm to contact point
IX	Restored neighboring teeth
X	2 or more teeth
XI	Soft tissue defects
XII	Vertical bone deficiency

Orthodontic History

The patient's orthodontic history should be considered. Orthodontic tooth positioning toward the buccal can have a profound effect on soft tissue thickness, and underlying osseous profiles (49). Rapid arch expansion has been found to result in a reduction in thickness of the buccal plate, and increase the likelihood of bone dehiscences. Garib et al. (50), utilizing CT scans, found a 0.6–0.9 mm reduction in buccal plate thickness and dehiscences of up to 7.0 mm. Consequently, it may be possible to "convert" a" thick-flat" into a "thin-scalloped" biotype, increasing surgical risk and postoperative hard and soft tissue resorption.

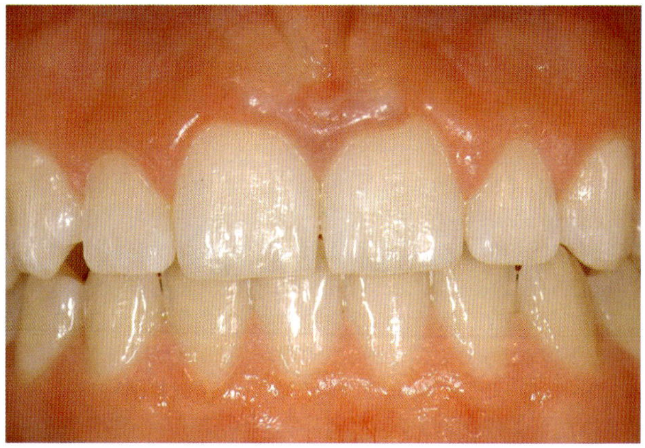

Figure 10.6 An example of a thick-flat periodontium. Note the buccolingual thickness of the gingival tissues, and the absence of gingival recession. The esthetic aspects of implant therapy on patients presenting with a thick-flat periodontium are easier to manage with respect to bone modeling and remodeling following tooth extraction, as more tissue volume (soft and hard) translates into a decreased incidence of gingival recession.

Periodontal Assessment

A comprehensive periodontal examination of the area of concern is requisite. It is important that periodontal infections be resolved as much as possible prior to surgical therapy. Where a variation of 1 or 2 mm in marginal tissue height can mean the difference between success and failure, resolution of soft-tissue inflammation should be sought before the clinician can accurately assess gingival contours and project the final treatment outcome.

Gingival recession is often reflective of an underlying bony dehiscence and should prepare the clinician for the possible need for enhanced reconstructive procedures. Significant gingival recession might also suggest the need for preparatory treatment such as orthodontic extrusion, to effect coronal movement of the gingival marginal tissues and bone, or soft-tissue enhancement procedures. A deep vestibule and an adequate zone of attached keratinized tissue facilitate flap advancement and tissue management, whereas a shallow vestibule and a lack of attached gingiva often require a more technically demanding procedure.

Increased tooth mobility may indicate reduced buccal bone thickness or dehiscences while tooth immobility could indicate ankylosis.

Esthetic Assessment

An esthetic assessment takes on special significance in the "esthetic zone." Smile line, gingival display, tooth position, and shape should all be noted and documented.

Of particular importance is the periodontal biotype (7, 51). Two distinct morphotypes have been most often described: thick-flat and thin-scalloped. The thick-flat variety (Figure 10.6) is characterized by a relatively square crown form, long flat contact points, broad zones of attached gingiva, short interdental papilla, thick gingival tissue, and a thick alveolar housing. The thin biotype (Figure 10.7) is distinguished by a more triangular tooth form, short contact points, shallow zones of attached gingiva, long interdental papilla, thin, delicate gingival tissue, and thin supporting bone. Becker and colleagues, in a human dry skull study, described a third periodontal biotype, the "pronounced scalloped." They found that the bone scallop of the pronounced scalloped was almost twice that of the flat type (4.1 mm versus 2.1 mm) (52).

These anatomical variations often allow the clinician to predict the behavior of the periodontal tissues after tooth removal. The thick-flat morphotype appears to be more resistant to postextraction resorption. Alternatively, the thin-scalloped, and the pronounced-scalloped varieties are more labile, with greater susceptibility to resorptive changes (7, 53). Unfortunately, many patients present with blended morphotypical characteristics and are difficult to classify (51, 53). Consequently, the clinician must be prepared to treat every defect as if it were the "thin-scalloped" variety (53).

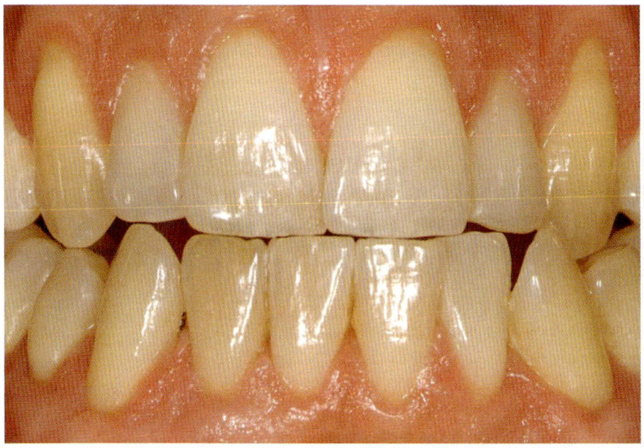

Figure 10.7 An example of a thin-scalloped periodontium. Note the accentuated scalloped form of the gingival line and the presence of gingival recession. Cases with a thin-scalloped periodontium are more prone to gingival recession, particularly when immediate implant delivery is attempted. Ridge preservation procedures play a crucial role in minimizing hard and soft tissue collapse after tooth extraction.

Anatomical Assessment

The anatomy of the surgical site deserves special attention. Such an evaluation should include the height of the alveolus, the thickness of alveolar housing, root placement within the alveolus, and trajectory (angle) of the alveolus.

Alveolar height: Adequate alveolar height must be present to allow the placement of a standard length implant. The distance between the point at which the implant circumference is engaged by the extraction socket walls and either the nasal floor or maxillary sinus should be sufficient to allow for implant stabilization (usually 3–5 mm) in the event that an immediate implant is considered. If residual bone is insufficient, ridge preservation and/or augmentation may be elected.

Alveolar thickness: Alveolar thickness both overlying and apical to the root should be considered. Buccolingual bone dimension can be estimated by the use of bone mapping calipers and/or a CT scan. The ideal bone dimension is at least 7.0 mm in the event that a 4.0 mm implant is to placed, allowing for 2.0 mm of bone on the buccal and 1.0 mm on the lingual aspects of the implant. A deep canine fossa can also be indicative of a reduced bone thickness.

Root placement within the alveolus: Buccal or lingual root placement may indicate reduced alveolar thickness. Mesial or distal root placement may suggest encroachment on the contiguous root. A prominent root is more likely to have thin overlying soft and hard tissues than a less prominent root.

Trajectory of the alveolus relative to angle of the root: If the alveolus and the root are at sufficiently acute angles to one another, there is often an increased risk of perforation of the buccal plate during implant placement. This situation may indicate the need for buccal bone augmentation at the time of tooth removal, either as a separate procedure or at the time of delayed implant placement.

Surgical Technique

Once a clinical decision is made that extraction is the treatment of choice, that an immediate implant is not indicated and that ridge preservation is desirable, the clinician faces several options with respect to the execution of the surgical procedure and the selection of materials to be utilized in attempting to preserve the socket dimensions. The decisions to be made include no less than the following:

- The instruments, devices, and techniques used to extract the tooth.
- The elevation (or not) of a buccal flap.
- The option of an absorbable or a nonabsorbable barrier for guided bone regeneration.
- The choice of a bone graft or substitute to fill the socket space, as opposed to leaving the socket space to be occupied by a blood clot alone.
- The decision to attempt primary closure of the wound by advancing the flap, as opposed to employing a nondisplaced flap where soft tissue healing of the socket orifice occurs by secondary intention.
- The concomitant use of a soft tissue graft with the hard tissue ridge preservation procedure.

A decision tree describing the choices facing the clinician in cases of tooth extraction and ridge preservation is shown in Flow chart 10.1. A detailed description of the steps involved in executing these surgical procedures and their variations is given below.

TOOTH EXTRACTION

Tooth removal is a biologically traumatic event, resulting in the morphologic changes previously described. Reduced-trauma techniques are intended to attenuate these changes (46, 47). With decreasing extraction-associated trauma as a main objective of the surgical procedure, the clinician should assume that all extractions and ridge preservation procedures can be achieved without flap elevation until intraoperative findings dictate otherwise. In other words, tooth extraction should be conducted prior to the elevation of gingival flaps.

Following local anesthesia, an intrasulcular incision is made with a microsurgical scalpel or 15 c blade in order to detach the junctional epithelium from the tooth surface and to sever the supra-alveolar connective tissue fibers (Figure 10.8). This initial incision is made 360° around the tooth to be extracted with the tip of the blade making contact with the most coronal aspect of the alveolar bone.

In order to further minimize trauma during the extraction, the Periotome® (46) is the instrument to be utilized following the scalpel or the 15 c blade. The use of the Periotome® must precede the utilization of the extraction forceps, which is the most common method of tooth removal. The extraction forceps is used to forcefully expand the bony walls of the socket and overcome the resistance of the PDL fibers by a luxating movement of the tooth. This procedure can risk damage to the socket walls, resulting in more extensive bone destruction and/or a longer treatment course. The Periotome® is intended to facilitate tooth extraction with the forceps by minimizing the amount of digital pressure that needs to be applied with the forceps. The Periotome® works by severing the fibrous attachment of the PDL fibers between the bony socket walls and the root of the tooth. The Periotome® blade is oriented parallel to the long axis of the root. By virtue of being thin, it can be inserted into the sulcus and directed toward the PDL space at the mesial, distal, and lingual (palatal) aspects of tooth (Figure 10.9). Placement of the Periotome® into the buccal PDL space should be avoided in order to minimize mechanical damage to the buccal bony plate. The Periotome® blade insertion is achieved either with hand pressure or by light tapping with a surgical mallet. Once it is successfully inserted, a back and forth movement is utilized. The blade should be progressively inserted in an apical direction to a depth of 3–5 mm from the coronal bone level. After a 3–5 mm deep insertion is completed on one aspect of the tooth, the Periotome® is left in place for about 1 min before repeating the process on the opposite side, and then on the palatal surface of the tooth. In addition to severing the PDL attachment, this technique allows for slight expansion of the socket wall and enhances tooth displacement. The Periotome® insertion in the mesial, distal and lingual (palatal) PDL space should be performed in an alternating sequential mode (repeated many times on each

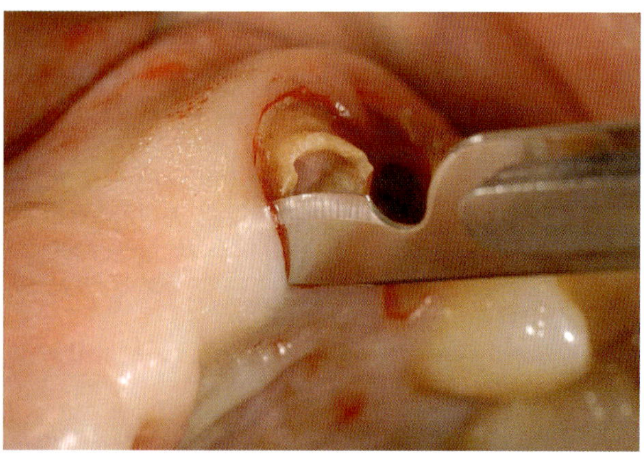

Figure 10.8 A number 15 c blade is inserted into the sulcus. This is the first step in tooth extraction. The blade should be inserted until its tip makes contact with the alveolar bone crest. The blade is then moved 360° around the tooth to be extracted.

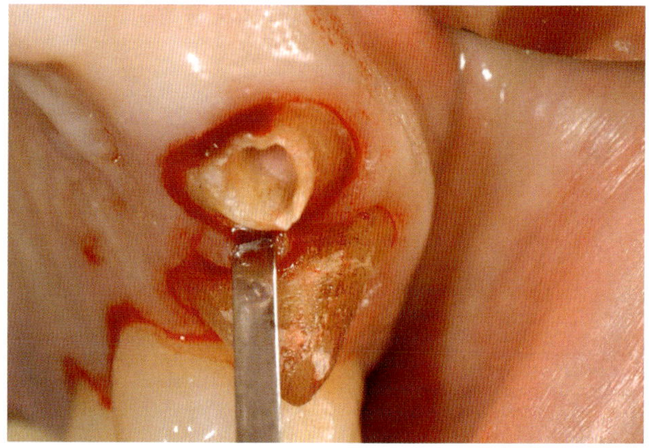

Figure 10.9 A Periotome® is inserted into the PDL space. The Periotome® should be inserted 3–5 mm apical to the bone crest level on the mesial, distal and lingual (palatal) aspects of the tooth to be extracted.

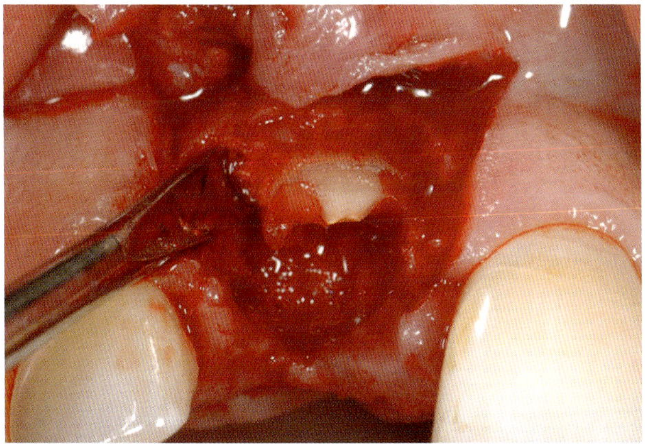

Figure 10.10 A small-tipped elevator is in position to elevate the tooth to be extracted. Application use of a small-tipped elevator is preceded by Periotome® use.

aspect of the root), with each insertion deeper than the previous, until the tooth exhibits increased mobility and can be easily removed with a forceps. Care must be exercised not to bend or twist the thin Periotome® blade to avoid permanent deformation or breakage of the instrument.

A small elevator can also be applied for tooth extraction. As small elevators are larger than the Periotome® they will allow for a higher degree of leverage. The clinician must be careful to avoid causing trauma to the surrounding alveolar bone. A sharp small-tipped elevator or a number 2 Molt curette can be employed in place of the Periotome® (Figure 10.10). The principles of operating small elevators are the same as those of a Periotome®. The straight shank is placed parallel to the long axis of the root and the blade is inserted into the PDL space. Digital force is directed apically and the blade is twisted, alternating among the mesial, distal, and lingual (palatal) surfaces until the tooth is mobilized and luxated. As with the Periotome®, the blade should never be inserted into the buccal aspect of the PDL in order to minimize the risk of traumatizing the buccal bony plate. The Proximator® is an instrument that combines some of the best features of the Periotome® and the elevator. It has a relatively thin sharp blade on a stiff shank. It is also inserted into the PDL space, can be carried further apically than the elevator, and allows for more rotating force application than the Periotome®.

Extended beak forceps may also be employed for tooth extraction. They allow for deep apical placement of the active end and a strong frictional grip to maximize leverage (Figure 10.11). The PDL that surrounds the root is narrow (approximately 0.2 mm in width) (54) and is easily ruptured. The forceps are rotated clockwise and counterclockwise mesially and distally in an alternating fashion until resistance is met, and then held for approximately 10–15 s. With a single-rooted tooth, no more than a few rotation motions are usually required before luxation of the tooth is achieved. Buccolingual movement is to be avoided to reduce the likelihood of damage to the thinner buccal plate. It is important to remember that the utilization of any forceps, including the ones with extended beaks, should be preceded by the use the Periotome® and/or small

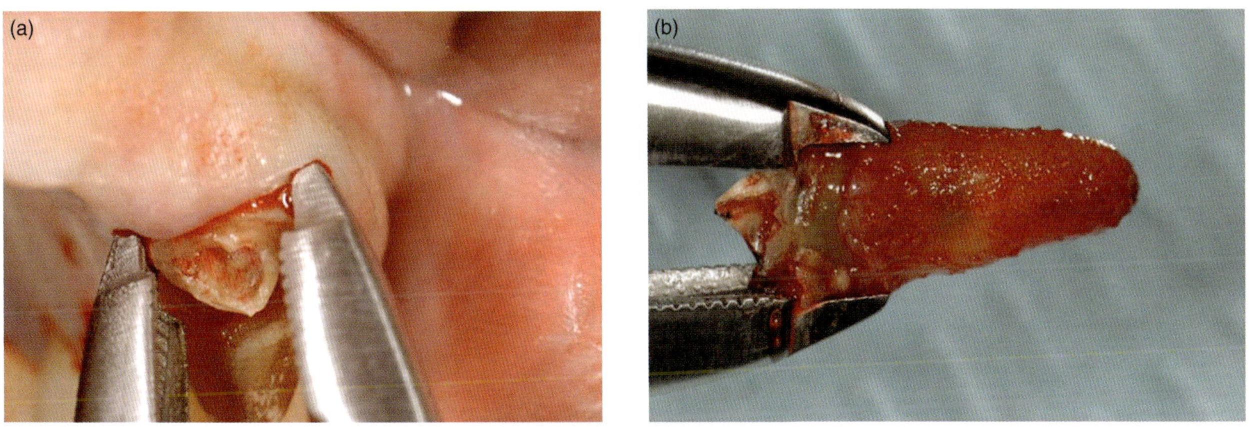

Figure 10.11 (a) Extended beak forceps are in place. Rotational movement, clockwise and counterclockwise, is employed. Buccolingual movement should be avoided, as it can cause fracture of the buccal bony plate. (b) A detailed view of the extended apical reach of the extended beak forceps.

elevators, so as to greatly reduce the force required for tooth removal, and minimize the possibility of fracturing the extraction socket walls.

The vertical extraction device has recently been introduced as an alternative device to minimize trauma during tooth extraction. The vertical extraction device takes advantage of the conical root shape. The crown is excised from the root and the threaded mechanical traction device is placed into the root canal space (Figure 10.12). Using the contiguous teeth for leverage, the root is pulled in a coronal direction, which results in its rapid withdrawal from the intact socket. This rapid extrusional delivery is particularly useful with teeth demonstrating severe coronal destruction, as it avoids both flap reflection and the use of more traumatic elevators and forceps.

Roots can also be separated from the alveolus by piezo ultrasonic surgical instruments (55). Specifically designed to cut hard tissue only, the piezo surgical tip is placed into the PDL space and the tooth is separated from the alveolus at the expense of the root. When utilizing the piezo ultrasonic device, the clinician must exercise care to keep the active end of the insert against the root surface. If the active end of the insert is applied against bone, iatrogenic bone destruction may occur, which constitutes an undesirable effect of the surgical procedure.

SOCKET DEBRIDEMENT

Once the root of the tooth has been removed, a careful inspection of the socket area for the presence of granulation tissue should be conducted. If granulation tissue remains in the socket area, it can serve as a source of cells for the regrowth of soft tissue in the extraction area. The regrowth of soft tissue in the early phases of healing may inhibit

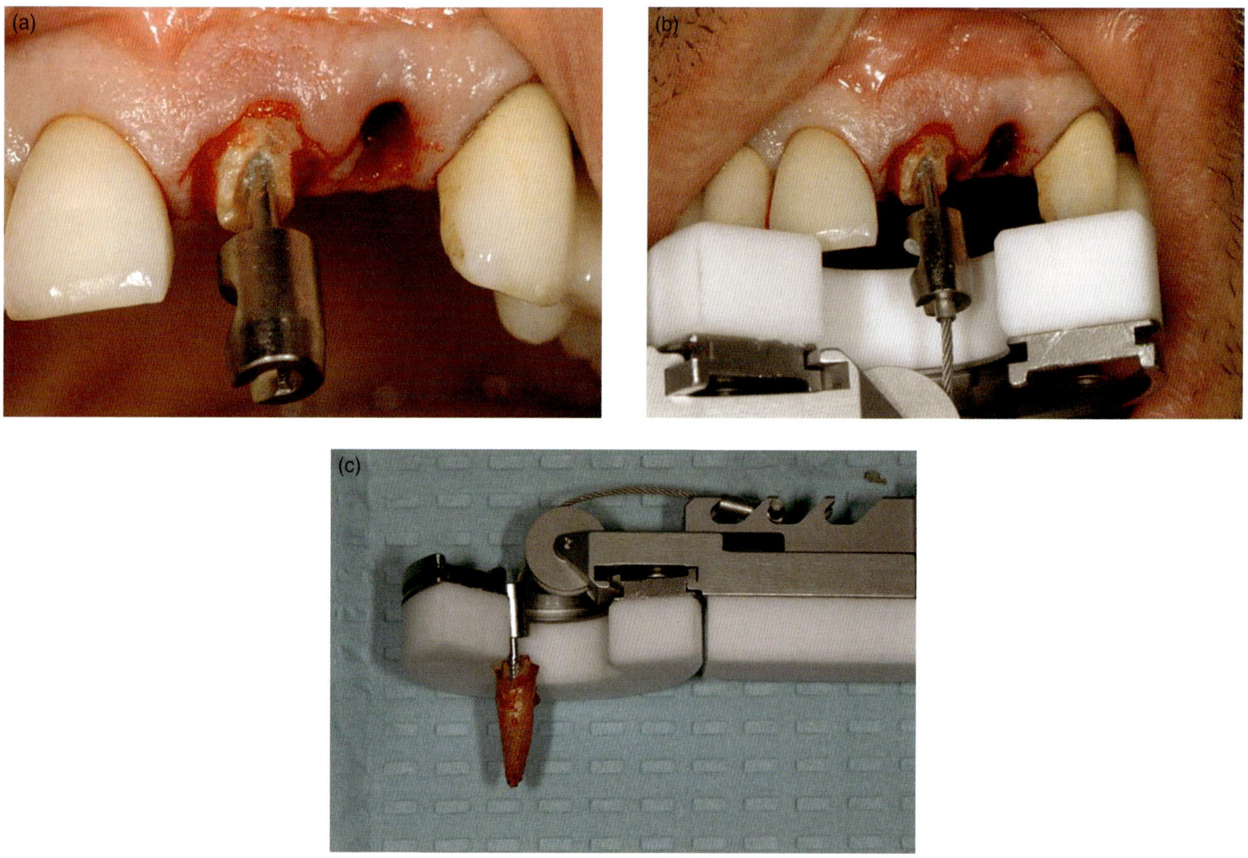

Figure 10.12 A vertical extraction device. (a) Following coronectomy, the active end of the vertical extraction device is inserted into the root canal space of the tooth to be extracted. (b) Extraction force leverage is obtained from the adjacent teeth. (c) A view of the extracted root attached to the active end of the vertical extraction device.

the formation of hard, mineralized tissue in the socket and compromise future implant placement (56). Moreover, as granulation tissue is usually in close anatomical proximity with the source of infection on the root surface, the presence of residual granulation tissue can serve as a bacterial reservoir and contaminate the graft and/or mechanical barrier used to treat the socket, which in turn can result in the infection of those devices (57).

Removal of granulation tissue from the socket area is usually achieved with the progressive use of hand curettes from larger to smaller sizes. Ultrasonic units such as the magnetostrictive or piezoelectric devices can be used to curette the socket, so that small tags of granulation tissue are loosened from bone and can be removed by curettes. The end point for socket debridement includes the exposure and visualization of all bony walls of the socket being treated. In the event that the socket walls are highly cortical and therefore nonbleeding, small round burrs or narrow drills can be used to open vascular channels and improve blood supply to the surgical site (58).

ELEVATION OF BUCCAL AND LINGUAL FLAPS

Once the socket has been curetted and its remaining bony walls inspected, it is important to determine the extent to which the buccal bony wall is present. If the vertical loss of the buccal wall is minimal, elevation of a buccal flap should be avoided (Figure 10.13) (53, 59). The buccal bony plate is usually thin, mostly cortical in nature, it receives blood supply from the PDL on its inner aspect and from the periosteum on its outer surface. Given that the root has been extracted, the blood supply from the PDL is no longer present. If a buccal flap is elevated, the periosteal blood supply is also discontinued, further enhancing the resorption of the buccal cortical plate. As explained below, in clinical situations where the a buccal flap is not elevated, a membrane can be adapted against the internal aspect of the socket buccal wall so as to prevent the migration of cells of the gingival epithelium and connective tissue into the socket area.

In situations where more than 5 mm of the vertical dimension of the buccal plate is missing, elevation of a buccal flap is necessary to allow for placement of a barrier membrane (Figure 10.14). The elevation of a buccal flap also allows for definitive degranulation of the socket on its buccal aspect, a step that might be difficult in deeper areas of the socket with the buccal soft tissues in place. The design of the buccal flap includes slightly divergent vertical incisions initiated on the proximal line angles of the teeth adjacent to the socket. The vertical incisions should be extended apical to the mucogingival junction. Horizontal incisions are made at the crest of each papilla, and a full thickness flap is carried out to expose the perimeter of the buccal bony dehiscence. Once the extent of the buccal bony margin is fully identified, a periosteal releasing incision at the base of the flap can be performed. These surgical maneuvers are performed to preserve blood supply to the flap and to facilitate flap advancement, which is critical to attainment of primary wound closure.

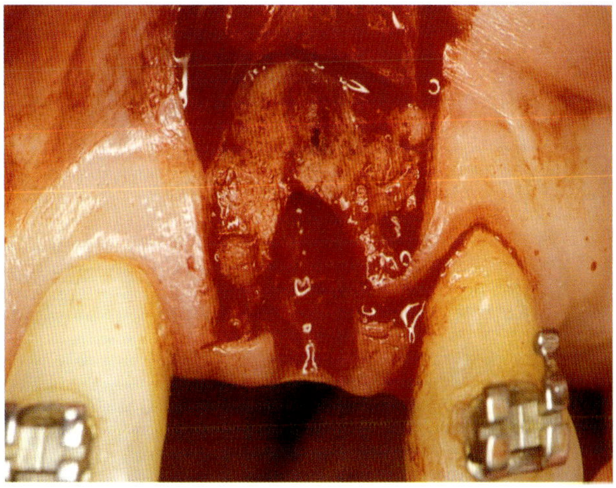

Figure 10.13 A view of a socket in which the elevation of a buccal flap is not indicated. Minimal destruction of the extraction socket walls has occurred.

The need to elevate lingual (palatal) flaps follows the same clinical judgment criteria. However, such a need is less frequent than that for buccal flaps, because the lingual (palatal) bony plate is often thicker and tends to be absorbed to a lesser extent in the course of pathologic processes. Elevation of the lingual (palatal) flap is performed for adaptation, immobilization of membranes used for guided bone regeneration.

The elevation of a buccal flap is also necessary in cases where a combination of extraction socket preservation and ridge augmentation are required to enable the placement of dental implants. This combined therapeutic modality is the treatment of

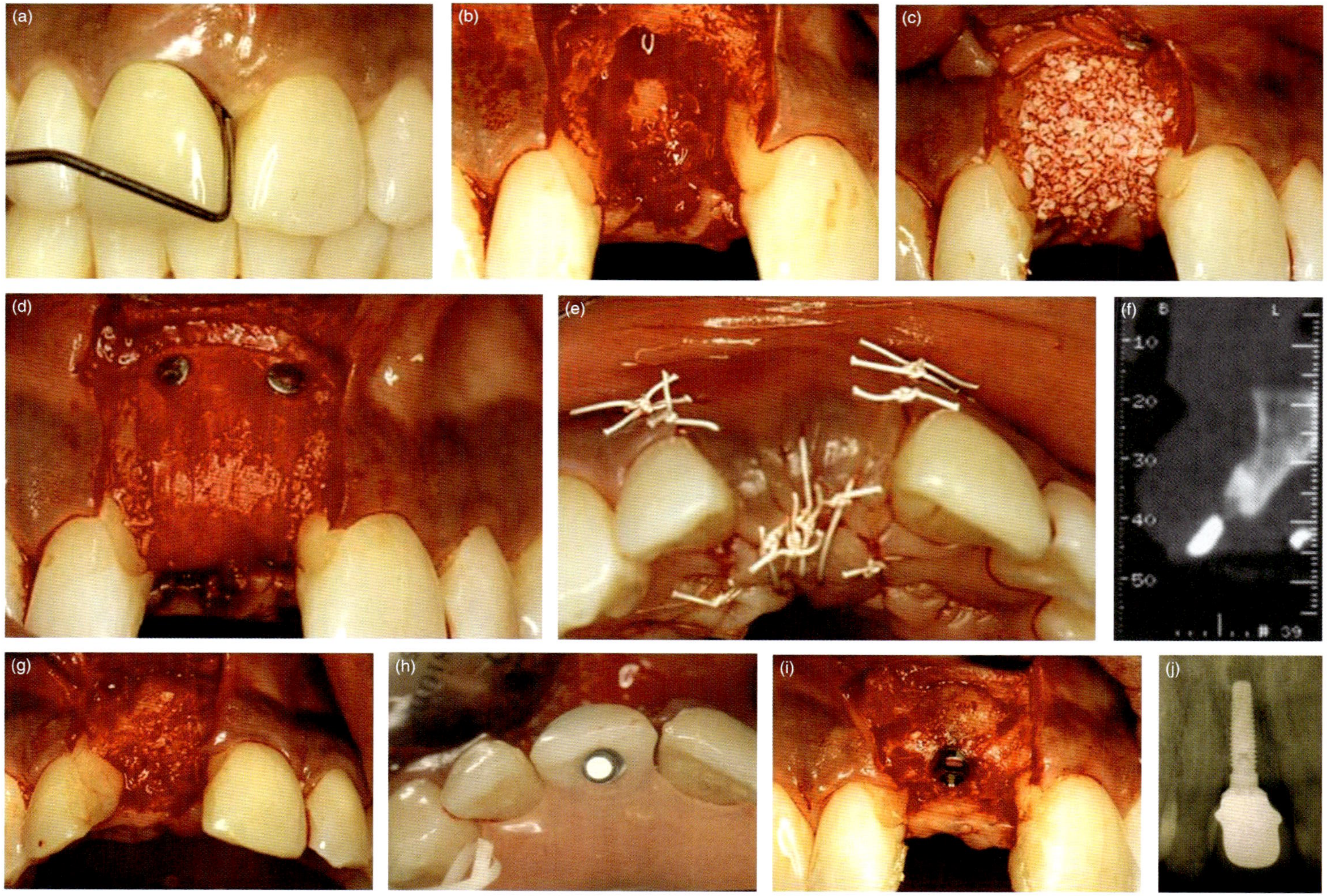

Figure 10.14 Elevation of a buccal flap is necessary when the vertical loss of the buccal bony wall exceeds 5 mm. (a) A preextraction view of the upper right central incisor, which presents with a vertical root fracture. (b) A view of the extraction socket following soft tissue degranulation and elevation of a buccal flap. (c) The socket was loosely packed with bovine porous bone mineral. (d) An absorbable (collagen) membrane was adapted over the buccal aspect of the buccal bony wall, and secured with press-fit titanium tacks. (e) The buccal flap was advanced to achieve tension-free, soft tissue primary closure of the wound. (f) A CT scan of the area 18 months postoperatively demonstrated the ridge to be in a harmonious relationship with the radiopaque maker, determining ideal implant position. (g) A view of surgical exposure of the treated area 18 months postoperatively. (h) A transoperative view of the implant osteotomy site. (i) Implant exposure is carried out 18 months following the ridge preservation procedure. Note the hard tissue surrounding the implant. (j) A radiograph of the implant following its final restoration.

choice in two situations: cases where a severe buccolingual concavity is present on the buccal aspect of the apical area of the extraction socket (preservation and augmentation of the same site need to be performed), and cases where ridge augmentation is necessary in sites that were previously edentulous and are adjacent to teeth which need to be extracted and socket preservation is to be performed.

There are situations in which preservation of the original extraction socket dimensions, even if fully accomplished, is not sufficient to enable the placement of a dental implant. This challenge is often observed in patients who present with a thin biotype, where the natural teeth are located in an accentuated buccal position in relation to the alveolar housing (60). Naturally occurring bone dehiscences and fenestrations are often observed on the buccal aspects of such teeth. Accentuated buccolingual concavities may be present on the apical areas of the alveolar bone of these teeth. When implant fixtures are utilized to replace anterior teeth, particularly in the upper arch, they often need to be placed in a more upright position than those of natural teeth. The palatal placement of the implant head in these particular cases can result in the apical portion of the fixture being more buccal than the root of the natural tooth that previously occupied the space. Therefore, a significant area of the implant fixture may be out of the alveolar bone. In such cases, the extraction socket needs to be preserved, and the bone volume augmented in the buccal direction (Figure 10.15) (6).

Augmentation of the edentulous ridge in the buccal direction may be the treatment goal for a previously edentulated area adjacent to a tooth or teeth that need to be extracted, where the treatment objective for the extraction socket(s) is preservation of its dimensions (56). These clinical situations also require the elevation of a buccal flap, followed by the placement of a titanium-reinforced nonabsorbable membrane. Preservation of the extraction socket dimensions is carried out as previously described.

MEMBRANE APPLICATION FOR GUIDED BONE REGENERATION

Any extraction socket in the esthetic zone for which preservation of its dimensions is desirable should be treated with a physical barrier (e.g., membrane) for guided bone regeneration. The clinically superior outcomes of treating a socket with a membrane as opposed to not utilizing a barrier have been clearly demonstrated (13, 14). The steps involved in the application of membranes for guided bone regeneration over extraction sockets are depicted in Figure 10.16.

The first decision the clinician needs to make is related to selecting a titanium-reinforced nonabsorbable or an absorbable membrane (56). Membranes do not tolerate exposure to the oral cavity well during healing, which dictates the need for a tension-free, primary closure of the wound. The main advantage of nonabsorbable membranes is that they are not subject to a variable rate of absorption as compared to absorbable membranes. Nonabsorbable membranes manufactured with a titanium-reinforcing frame allow for a more effective maintenance of space and a more precise control of the shape of the alveolar ridge to be developed during healing (Figure 10.17).

In cases when a buccal flap is elevated, the membrane is adapted over the external aspect of the buccal bony wall and tacked under the lingual (palatal) tissue, again covering the occlusal aspect of the socket (Figure 10.14).

SOCKET FILL

When a buccal flap is elevated, if sufficient bony walls remain around the socket space so that a blood clot can be stabilized and a membrane for guided bone regeneration immobilized without collapsing into the socket space, fill of the extraction socket is optional. Nonabsorbable membranes, particularly the ones manufactured with titanium reinforcement, lend themselves to providing the socket with such a "tent" effect in the absence of a bone graft or substitute. From the wound-healing standpoint, it makes sense to expect faster bone formation in the absence of a bone graft or substitute material, as the latter needs to be absorbed in the course of healing prior to the formation of new bone. In sockets in which the destruction of the bony walls is more severe, particularly the buccal wall, socket fill is necessary if a blood clot cannot be stabilized or if a membrane does not have enough rigidity and support to stand on its own, and it tends to collapse into the socket space. When utilizing an absorbable membrane for guided bone regeneration, there is a need for physical support from a bone graft or substitute because absorbable

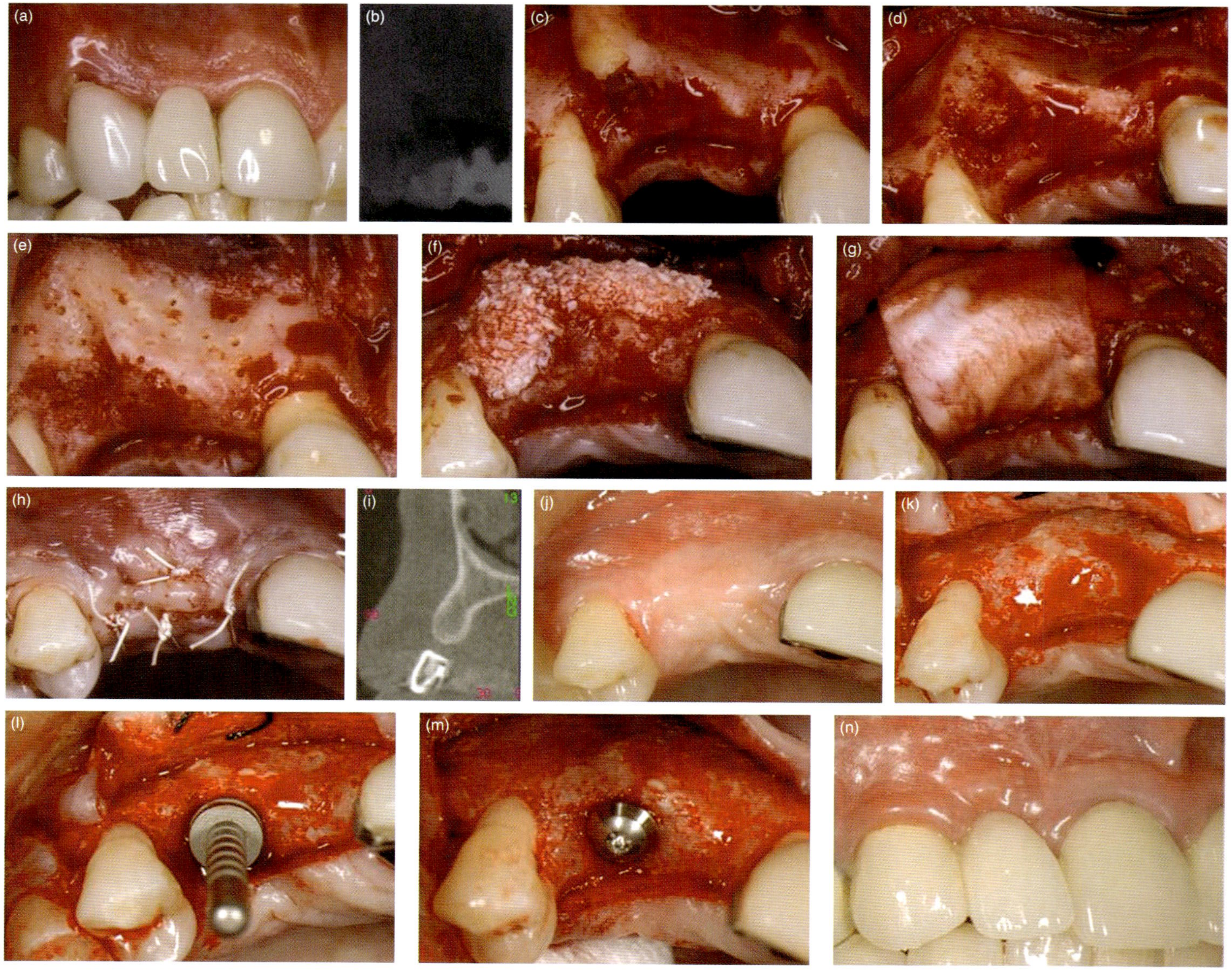

Figure 10.15 Upper right canine extraction socket preservation and augmentation, combined with ridge augmentation of the upper right lateral incisor edentulous area was carried out. (a) A clinical view of a three-unit fixed partial denture replacing the lateral incisor. (b) A periapical radiograph showing extensive root resorption of the canine. (c) Following elevation of a buccal flap the residual root of the canine was exposed. (d) A view of the surgical area after extraction of the root. (e–f) Following multiple perforations of the buccal cortical plate to enhance blood supply, the extraction socket and edentulous ridge areas were augmented with bovine porous bone mineral. (g) An absorbable (collagen) membrane was adapted, to protect the xenograft. (h) The flap was advanced to achieve a tension-free, primary closure of the wound. (i) A CT scan of the surgical area taken 12 months after the surgical procedure had been performed demonstrated the buccolingual dimension of the augmented edentulous ridge in the canine area. (j) A clinical view of the treated area 12 months after surgery, immediately prior to implant placement. (k) Flap elevation demonstrated the attained contours of the edentulous ridge, as compared to Figure 10.15 d. (l) A direction indicator in place highlighted the favorable future position of the fixture. (m) The implant fixture was delivered. (n) Final restoration of the implant, including a cantilevered tooth number 7, was carried out six months after placement of the implant.

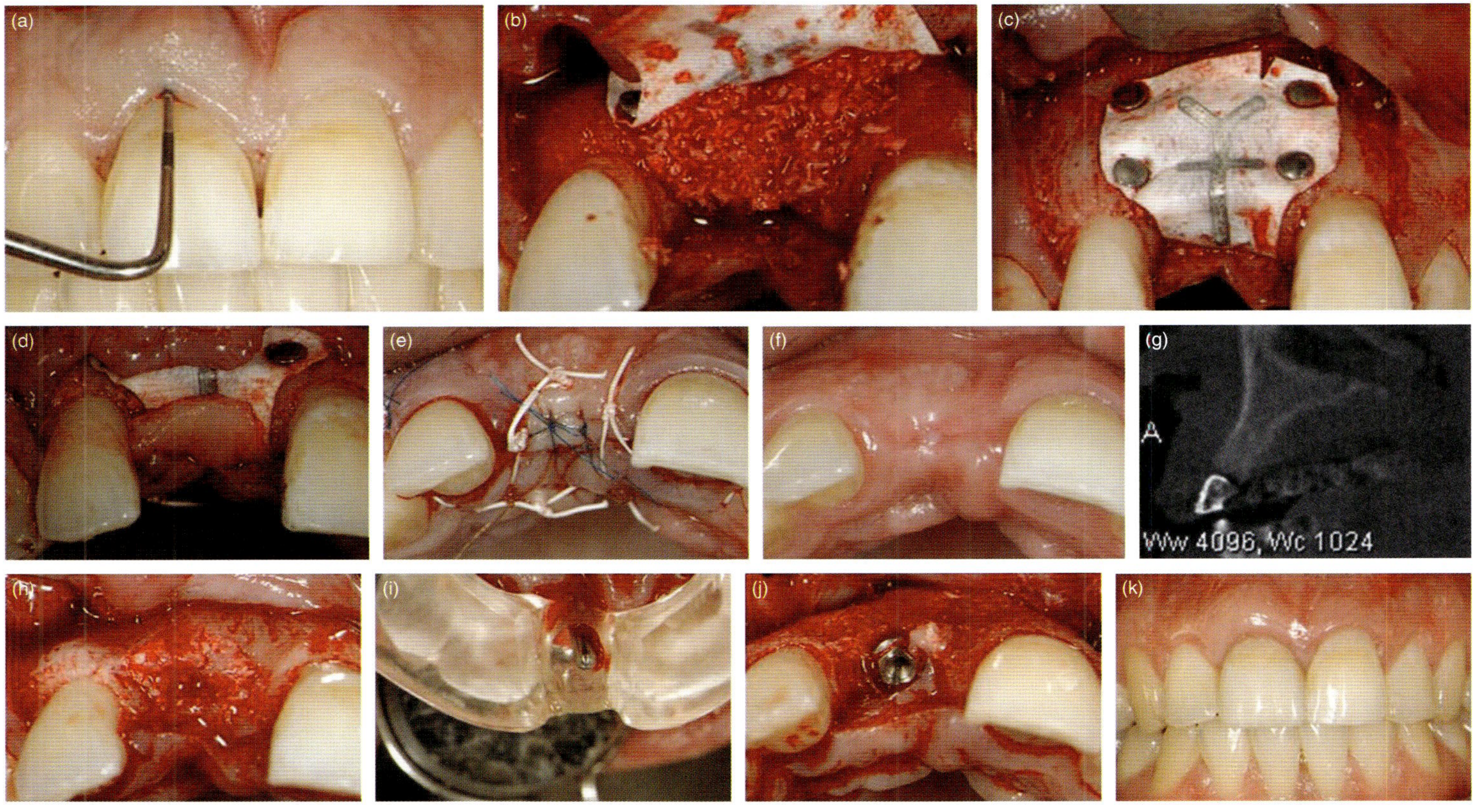

Figure 10.16 Ridge preservation with a titanium-reinforced nonabsorbable (extended polytetrafluorethylene) membrane was carried out. (a) A hopeless central incisor required extraction due to external root resorption. (b) Following tooth extraction, elevation of a buccal flap and soft tissue degranulation of the socket, bovine porous bone mineral was placed. (c) A titanium was reinforced membrane was secured with press fit titanium tacks; the titanium reinforcement ensuring predictability of the future alveolar ridge shape. (d) A connective tissue autograft was sutured along the incision line to help provide a biological barrier to the exposure of the membrane to the oral cavity during healing. (e) Tension-free, primary closure of the wound was achieved. (f) A clinical view of the treated area nine months after treatment. (g) A CT scan of the treated area, taken nine months postoperatively. (h) A clinical view of the alveolar ridge prior to implant osteotomy preparation. (i) A view of the implant osteotomy. (j) Implant placement allowed the access of the restoration screw through the cingulum. (k) A view of the implant final restoration six months after implant placement.

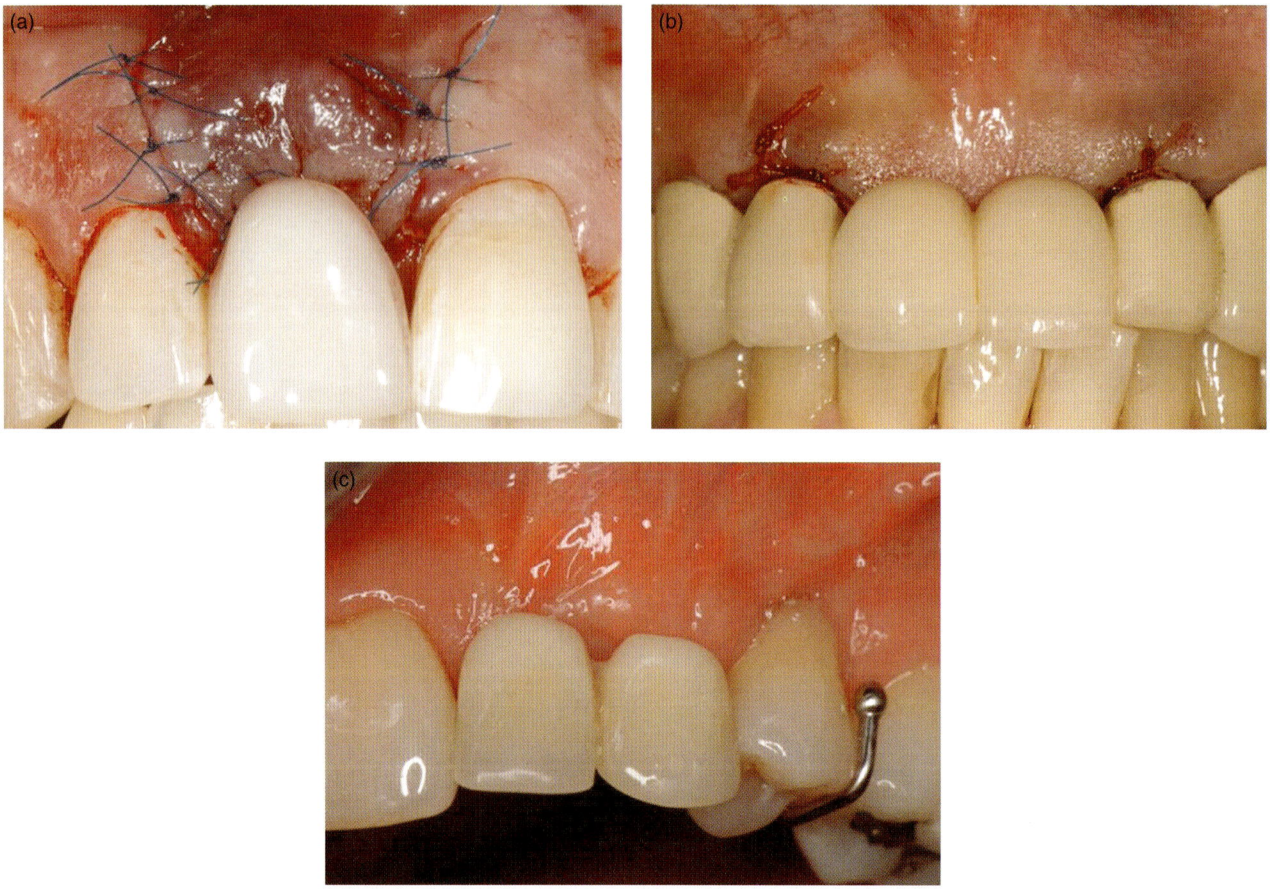

Figure 10.17 Management of temporary restorations following a ridge preservation procedure: Direct pressure over the treated area should be avoided by relieving the most apical aspect of the pontic. (a) A view of a removable temporary restoration. (b) A view of a fixed temporary restoration. (c) Once healing of the soft tissues is complete and all surgical edema has subsided, relining of the pontics is carried out to enhance esthetics of the temporary restoration. Excessive pressure over the surgically treated area should be avoided at all times.

membranes tend to be soft and flexible and are inclined to collapse into the socket space (56).

When selecting a bone graft or substitute to fill an extraction socket, autogenous bone has long been considered the "gold standard," as it is both osteoinductive and osteoconductive. However, as the amount of bone needed to fill extraction sockets is usually relatively large, harvesting the adequate amount of bone requires a second surgical site, adding time, trauma, and morbidity to treatment. While there is some evidence suggesting that the use of autogenous bone as treatment for extractions sockets results in greater bone formation than other types of bone grafts or substitutes (61), the clinical superiority of autogenous bone for this purpose has not been demonstrated through large clinical trials.

Several bone grafts and bone substitutes other than autogenous bone have been studied as fillers for extraction sockets. There are reports showing effective socket preservation with allografts (i.e., calcified and decalcified freeze-dried bone) (62–64), xenografts (i.e., bovine porous bone mineral) (65), and synthetic materials (i.e., bioactive glass) (66). These materials are primarily osteoconductive in nature, work as space maintainers in the socket space, and afford a scaffold for osteogenesis. There are no direct comparative studies in the literature identifying a superior material among the available alternatives.

When selecting a bone graft or substitute, the speed by which the material is absorbed during the healing process may be relevant, as its slow turnover may limit the amount of natural bone being formed. Despite the fact that the rate of graft absorption appears to be relevant in the formation of new bone and have an effect on the outcome of implant therapy, no studies have been conclusive in determining the ideal rate of absorption for a bone graft or substitute. Theoretically, the ideal material should last long enough to prevent collapsing of the extraction socket walls early in the course of healing, but should be absorbed as soon as enough natural healing has occurred so that newly formed mineralized tissue can support the original bony walls.

When utilizing any bone graft or substitute, the clinician should avoid dense packing of the material. Such a practice can decrease the space for osteoprogenitor cells to migrate into the socket area and increase the time involved in graft turnover and new bone formation. Graft packing should be performed loosely (Figures 10.15–10.17). Overfilling of the socket should be avoided, as adaptation of the membrane can be difficult and primary soft tissue closure of the defect prevented. Recently, bone grafts mixed with a collagen matrix have become commercially available. This modality of graft preparation can be useful in avoiding over condensation and ensuring the existence of spaces that allow for angiogenesis and osteogenesis.

Recently, bioactive molecules such as recombinant human bone morphogenetic protein 2 (rhBMP-2) have been proposed as osteoinductive agents for extraction sockets (17). rhBMP-2 has been shown to be effective when used in the absence of guided bone regeneration in preserving the dimensions of extraction sockets where primary closure of the wound was achieved by flap advancement. More research is necessary to assess how effective bioactive molecules are in preserving the dimensions of extraction sockets when used in combination with guided bone regeneration, and in comparison with other modalities of therapy.

SUTURING OF THE SURGICAL WOUND

In cases where no buccal flap has been elevated, a free gingival graft has been suggested to cover the membrane as it may work as a biological dressing for the wound (67). However, the free gingival graft may or may not survive.

Primary closure of the wound in a tension-free mode is mandatory. In order to achieve such a passive closure, the vertical incisions need to be carried well beyond the mucogingival junction and the periosteum released in the apical area of the surgical wound (Figures 10.14 and 10.17). Additional flap release can be achieved by making cut-back incisions into the buccal mucosa or by making horizontal incisions in directions opposite to that of the flap at the most apical ends of the vertical incisions (68).

A connective tissue graft can be placed between nonabsorbable or absorbable membranes and the advanced flap (Figure 10.16) (69). The connective tissue graft may work a second biological barrier in cases where wound dehiscences occur early in the course of healing, allowing more time for soft tissue formation to occur without exposure of the membrane to the oral cavity. The graft also provides increased soft tissue volume.

Once the buccal flap has been mobilized, the coronal aspect of the wound is sutured first. Interrupted or mattress sutures may be placed with a less reactive nonabsorbable material (i.e., expanded polytetrafluoroethylene or polypropylene). Mattress sutures are preferred by virtue of everting the edges of the wound. The vertical incisions are sutured last with U-shaped interrupted sutures.

ADJUSTMENT OF TEMPORARY RESTORATIONS AND POSTOPERATIVE CARE

Any mechanical pressure exerted by temporary restorations must be avoided as it can compromise healing. Bonded restorations are preferable. If properly adjusted, they will not come into contact with the wound during mastication. If a removable partial denture is the temporary restoration of choice, relief must be provided in the edentulous area so that the pontic does not make contact with the surgical area when the patient is at rest, or during mastication. It is often helpful to provide "stops" such as occlusal rests on the prosthesis to prevent impingement upon the surgical site.

Bacterial contamination of the wound in the early phase of healing must be avoided, as it may negatively affect the outcome of therapy (14). In order to avoid such contamination, patients should be placed on systemic antibiotics (amoxicillin

500 mg tid or clindamycin 300 mg qid) and 0.12% chlorhexidine rinses (15 milliliter of the solution for 30 s bid) until the wound is completely covered with soft tissue.

Sutures are removed 7–14 days after surgery.

HEALING TIME

There are no well-established protocols for the time that should elapse between an extraction socket preservation procedure and placement of a dental implant. Factors that should be considered by the clinician include the overall size of the extraction socket, the extent to which the buccal bone was lost, the relative percentage of the implant area that will be in contact with native (preexisting) bone, if a bone graft or substitute was utilized in the preservation procedure, the type of bone graft or substitute employed and its expected turnover, and the general health and age of the patient.

In the absence of hard tissue grafting, extraction socket preservation with guided bone regeneration showed that bone-like tissue was present six months after surgery (13, 14). These findings were consistent with both nonabsorbable and absorbable membranes that remained submerged in the course of healing. In the presence of a bone graft or substitute, new bone formation tends to occur more slowly, as absorption of the graft material requires extra time (63–65). Histological studies have shown that graft particles remain in the treated area 6–12 months after the extraction socket preservation procedure was performed, regardless of the material used. The question as to what role nonviable graft material plays in the integration and long-term success of dental implants remains unanswered. The percentage of viable bone that needs to be in contact with the dental implant for sustained osseointegration, also remains unanswered. Using clinical common sense and looking at wound healing from the bone turnover standpoint, with a material that has a low substitution rate, "one cannot wait too long" for the extraction socket preservation procedure to heal. However, practicality plays a role in patient care. It appears reasonable to wait between 9 and 12 months after an extraction socket preservation procedure is performed and placement of a dental implant. It should be emphasized, that this suggestion is based upon clinical observations and experience rather than on research data. Osteoinductive materials have the potential to shorten the healing period.

It has been shown that remodeling of the buccal bone often occurs following placement of an implant fixture (70). The buccal bone over the implant fixture, when thin at the time of placement, may be subject to absorption during initial healing or following its loading with the resultant loss of vertical height. Such bone absorption may result in the gingival tissue being in direct contact with the buccal aspect of the implant fixture. Such a situation may not be stable, and might result in pocketing or soft tissue recession. In order to avoid the risk associated with these clinical situations, it has been suggested that the buccal bone should be at least 2 mm thick (buccolingual direction) immediately following implant placement (40). While this dimension is of primary importance on the most coronal aspect of the implant fixture, it can also be of clinical relevance in the mid or apical aspects of the implant because bony fenestrations may develop. If buccal bone is less than 2 mm in thickness, the area should be secondarily augmented with a bone graft combined with guided bone regeneration. If secondary augmentation is necessary, the implant fixture should be submerged for healing. Implant exposure will need to be conducted in the future.

Conclusions

Existing data demonstrate conclusively that bone resorption is a predictable consequence of tooth loss. Proper three-dimensional implant placement, implant retention, and the stability of peri-implant tissues are to a great degree reliant on the quantity and position of buccolingual and apico-coronal surrounding bone. Therefore, preservation procedures aiming at minimizing bone resorption following tooth extraction are valuable in enhancing the esthetic outcomes of implants placed in the upper anterior segment. Grafting of the extraction socket with a slowly resorbing material sheltered by a barrier membrane is an effective method of reducing the extent of postextraction bone loss. Bone preservation techniques following tooth extraction are routinely recommended in cases where immediate implant placement is contraindicated, in the esthetic zone.

References

1. Adell R, Eriksson B, Lekholm U, et al. 1990. Long-term follow-up study of osseointegrated implants in the treatment of totally edentulous jaws. *Int J Oral Maxillofac Implants* 5:347–359.
2. Lindhe T, Gunne J, Tillberg A, and Molin M. 1998. A meta-analysis of implants in partial edentulism. *Clin Oral Implants Res* 9:80–90.
3. Hürzeler MB, Fickl S, Zuhr O, and Wachtel H. 2006. Clinical failures and shortfalls of immediate implant procedures. *Eur J Esthet Dent* 1:128–140.
4. Buser D, Martin W, and Belser U. 2004. Optimizing esthetics for implant restorations in the anterior maxilla; anatomic and surgical considerations. *Int J Oral Maxillofac Implants* 19(Suppl):43–61.
5. Grunder U, Gracis S, and Capelli M. 2005. Influence of the 3-D bone-to-implant relationship on esthetics. *Int J Periodontics Restorative Dent* 25:113–119.
6. Garber DA and Belser UC. 1995. Restoration driven implant placement with restoration generated site development. *Compend Contin Educ Dent* 16: 796–804.
7. Kois JC. 2004. Predictable single tooth peri-implant esthetics: Five diagnostic keys. *Compend Contin Educ Dent* 25:895–900.
8. Salama H, Salama M, and Garber D. 1998. The interproximal height of bone: A guidepost to predictable aesthetic strategies and soft tissue contours in anterior tooth replacement. *Pract Periodontics Aesthet Dent* 10:1131–1141.
9. Jemt T. 1997. Regeneration of gingival papillae after single-implant treatment. *Int J Periodontics Restorative Dent* 17:327–333.
10. Lekholm U. 1983. Clinical procedures for treatment with osseointegrated dental implants. *J Prosthet Dent* 50:116–120.
11. Jovanovic SA. 1997. Bone rehabilitation to achieve optimal esthetics. *Pract Periodontics Aesthet Dent* 9:41–52.
12. Jovanovic SA. 2006. Esthetic therapy with standard and scalloped implant design: The five biologic elements for success. *J Calif Dent Assoc* 33:873–880.
13. Lekovic V, Camargo PM, Klokkevold PR, et al. 1998. Preservation of alveolar bone in extraction sockets using bioabsorbable membranes. *J Periodontol* 69:1044–1049.
14. Lekovic V, Kenney EB, Weinlaender M, et al. 1997. A bone regenerative approach to alveolar ridge maintenance following tooth extraction. Report of 10 cases. *J Periodontol* 68:563–570.
15. Iasella JM, Greenwell H, Miller RL, et al. 2003. Ridge preservation with freeze-dried bone allograft and a collagen membrane compared to extraction alone for implant site development: A clinical and histologic study in humans. *J Periodontol* 74:990–999.
16. Nevins M, Camelo M, De Paoli S, et al. 2006. A study of the fate of the buccal wall of extraction sockets of teeth with prominent roots. *Int J Periodontics Restorative Dent* 26:19–29.
17. Fiorellini JP, Howell TH, Cochran D, et al. 2005. Randomized study evaluating recombinant human bone morphogenetic protein-2 for extraction socket augmentation. *J Periodontol* 76:605–613.
18. Cochran DL. 1999. A comparison of endosseous dental implant surfaces. *J Periodontol* 70:1523–1539.
19. Chiese R, Giavaresi G, Fini M, et al. 2007. In vitro and in vivo performance of a novel surface treatment to enhance osseointegration of endosseous implants. *Oral Surg Oral Med Oral Pathol Oral Radiol Endod* 103:745–756.
20. Fugazzotto PA, Beagle JR, Ganeles J, et al. 2004. Success and failure rates of 9 mm or shorter implants in the replacement of missing maxillary molars when restored with individual crowns: Preliminary results 0–84 months in function. A retrospective study. *J Periodontol* 75:327–332.
21. Deporter D, Todescan R, and Caudry S. 2000. Simplifying management of the posterior maxilla using short, porous-surfaced dental implants and simultaneous indirect sinus elevation. *Int J Periodontics Restorative Dent* 20:476–485.
22. Attard NJ and Zarb GA. 2005. Immediate and early implant loading protocols: A literature review of clinical studies. *J Prosthet Dent* 94:242–258.
23. Amler MH, Johnson PL, and Salman I. 1960. Histological and histochemical investigation of human alveolar socket healing in undisturbed extraction wounds. *J Am Dent Assoc* 61:32–44.
24. Atwood DA and Coy WA. 1971. Clinical, cephalometric, and densitometric study of reduction of residual ridges. *J Prosthet Dent* 26:280–295.
25. Araujo MG and Lindhe J. 2005. Dimensional ridge alterations following tooth extraction. An experimental study in the dog. *J Clin Periodontol* 32:212–218.
26. Schropp L, Kostopoulos L, and Wenzel A. 2003. Bone healing following immediate versus delayed placement of titanium implants into extraction sockets: A prospective clinical study. *Int J Oral Maxillofac Implants* 182:189–199.
27. Johnson K. 1969. A study of the dimensional changes occurring in the maxilla following closed face immediate denture treatment. *Aust Dent J* 14:371–376.
28. Botticelli D, Berglundh T, and Lindhe J. 2004. Hard-tissue alterations following immediate implant placement in extraction sites. *J Clin Periodontol* 31:820–828.
29. Pietrokovski J and Massler M. 1967. Alveolar ridge resorption following tooth extraction. *J Prosthet Dent* 17:21–27.
30. Covani U, Bortolaia C, Barone A, et al. 2004. Buccolingual crestal changes after immediate and delayed implant placement. *J Periodontol* 75:1605–1612.

31. Covani U, Cornelini R, and Barone A. 2007. Vertical crestal bone changes around implants placed into fresh extraction sockets. *J Periodontol* 78:810–815.
32. Wilderman MN. 1963. Repair after a periodontal retention procedure. *J Periodontol* 34:487–494.
33. Amler MH. 1969. The time sequence of tissue regeneration in human extraction wounds. *Oral Surg Oral Med Oral Pathol* 273:309–318.
34. Boyne PJ. 1966. Osseous repair of the post extraction alveolus in man. *Oral Surg Oral Med Oral Pathol* 21:805–813.
35. Evian CI, Rosenberg ES, Cosslet JG, et al. 1982. The osteogenic activity of bone removed from healing extraction sockets in human. *J Periodontol* 53:81–85.
36. Chen ST, Wilson TG Jr, and Hammerle CF. 2004. Immediate or early placement of implants following tooth extraction: Review of biologic basis, clinical procedures, and outcomes. Consensus statement. *Int J Oral Maxillofac Implants* 19(Suppl):12–28.
37. Tarnow D, Elian N, Fletcher P, et al. 2003. Vertical distance from the crest of bone to the height of the interproximal papilla between adjacent implants. *J Periodontol* 74:1785–1788.
38. Grunder U, Polizzi G, Goene R, et al. 1999. A 3-year prospective multicenter follow-up report on the immediate and delayed-immediate placement of implants. *Int J Oral Maxillofac Implants* 142:210–216.
39. Grunder U. 2000. Stability of the mucosal topography around single-tooth implants and adjacent teeth: 1-year results. *Int J Periodontics Restorative Dent* 20:11–17.
40. Grunder U, Gracis S, and Capelli M. 2005. Influence of the 3-D bone-to-implant relationship on esthetics. *Int J Periodontics Restorative Dent* 25:113–119.
41. Spray JR, Black CG, Morris HF, et al. 2000. The influence of bone thickness on facial marginal bone response: Stage 1 placement through stage 2 uncovering. *Ann Periodontol* 5:119–128.
42. Leblebicioglu B, Rawal S, and Mariotti A. 2007. A review of the functional and esthetic requirements for dental implants. *J Am Dent Assoc* 138:321–329.
43. Nemcovsky CE and Artzi Z. 2002. Comparative study of buccal dehiscence defects in immediate, delayed, and late maxillary implant placement with collagen membranes: Clinical healing between placement and second-stage surgery. *J Periodontol* 73: 754–761.
44. Zubillaga G, Von Hagen S, Simon BI, et al. 2003. Changes in alveolar bone height and width following post-extraction ridge augmentation using a fixed bioabsorbable membrane and demineralized freeze-dried bone osteoinductive graft. *J Periodontol* 74:965–975.
45. Martin WC, Morton D, and Buser D. 2007. Preoperative analysis and prosthetic treatment planning in esthetic implant dentistry. In: Belser U, Martin W, Jung R, Hämmerle C, Schmid B, Morton D, and Buser D (eds), *ITI Treatment Guide*. Berlin: Quintessence, pp. 9–24.
46. Garber DA, Salama MA, and Salama H. 2001. Immediate total tooth replacement. *Compend Contin Educ Dent* 22:210–216.
47. Kan JYK and Rungcharassaeng K. 2001. Site development for anterior single implant esthetics: The dentulous site. *Compend Contin Educ Dent* 22:221–231.
48. Sonick M and Hwang D. 2007. Tooth extraction—an opportunity for site preservation. *Contemp Esthet* 2:36–41.
49. Wennström JL. 1996. Mucogingival therapy. *Ann Periodontol* 1:671–701.
50. Garib DG, Henriques JF, Janson G, et al. 2006. Periodontal effects of rapid maxillary expansion with tooth–tissue–borne and tooth–borne expanders: A computed tomography evaluation. *Am J Orthod Dentofacial Orthop* 129:749–758.
51. Olsson M and Lindhe J. 1991. Periodontal characteristics in individuals with varying form of the upper central incisors. *J Clin Periodontol* 18:78–82.
52. Becker W, Ochsenbein C, Tibbetts L, and Becker BE. 1997. Alveolar bone anatomic profiles as measured from dry skulls. Clinical ramifications. *J Clin Periodontol* 24.727–731.
53. Caplanis N, Lozada JL, and Kan JYK. 2005. Extraction defect assessment, classification, and management. *J Calif Dent Assoc* 33:853–863.
54. Fiorellini JP, Kim DM, and Ishikawa SO. 2006. The tooth-supporting structures. In: Newman MG, Takei HH, Klokkevold PR, and Carranza FA Jr (eds), *Carranza's Clinical Periodontology*. Philadelphia: Saunders, pp. 68–92.
55. Vercellotti T. 2004. Piezoelectric bone surgery in periodontology and implantology. New concepts and optimal dental practice. In: *The 8th International Symposium on Periodontics and Restorative Dentistry*. Boston, June 10, 2004.
56. Hämmerle CHF and Jung RE. 2003. Bone augmentation by means of barrier membranes. *Periodontology* 33:36–53.
57. Casap N, Zeltser C, Wexler A, Tarazi E, and Zeltser R. 2007. Immediate placement of dental implants into debrided infected dentoalveolar sockets. *J Oral Maxillofac Surg* 65:384–392.
58. Klokkevold PR and Jovanovic S. 2002. Advanced implant surgery and bone grafting techniques. In: Newman MG, Takei HH, and Carranza FA Jr (eds), *Carranza's Clinical Periodontology*. Philadelphia: Saunders, pp. 905–921.
59. Saadoun AP and Landsberg CJ. 1997. Treatment classifications and sequencing for postextraction implant therapy: A review. *Pract Periodontics Aesthet Dent* 9:933–941.

60. Funato A, Salama MA, Ishikawa T, et al. 2007. Timing, positioning, and sequential staging in esthetic implant therapy: A four-dimensional perspective. *Int J Periodontics Restorative Dent* 27:313–323.
61. Becker W, Clokie C, Sennerby L, et al. 1998. Histologic findings after implantation and evaluation of different grafting materials and titanium micro screws into extraction sockets: Case reports. *J Periodontol* 69:414–421.
62. Wang HL and Tsao YP. 2007. Mineralized bone allograft-plug socket augmentation: Rationale and technique. *Implant Dent* 16:33–41.
63. Brugnami F, Then PR, Moroi H, et al. 1996. Histologic evaluation of human extraction sockets treated with demineralized freeze-dried bone allograft (DFDBA) and cell occlusive membrane. *J Periodontol* 67:821–825.
64. Smukler H, Landi L, and Setayesh R. 1999. Histomorphometric evaluation of extraction sockets and deficient alveolar ridges treated with allograft and barrier membrane: A pilot study. *Int J Oral Maxillofac Implants* 14:407–416.
65. Artzi Z, Tal H, and Dayan D. 2000. Porous bovine bone mineral in healing of human extraction sockets. Part 1: Histomorphometric evaluations at 9 months. *J Periodontol* 71:1015–1123.
66. Norton MR and Wilson J. 2002. Dental implants placed in extraction sites implanted with bioactive glass: Human histology and clinical outcome. *Int J Oral Maxillofac Implants* 17:249–257.
67. Landsberg CL. 1997. Socket seal surgery combined with immediate implant placement: A novel approach for single-tooth replacement. *Int J Periodontics Restorative Dent* 17:141–149.
68. Fugazzotto PA. 2006. Maintaining primary closure after guided bone regeneration procedures: Introduction of a new flap design and preliminary results. *J Periodontol* 77:1452–1457.
69. Tal, H. 1999. Autogenous masticatory mucosal grafts in extraction socket seal procedures: A comparison between sockets grafted with demineralized freeze-dried bone and deproteinized bovine bone mineral. *Clin Oral Implants Res.* 10:289–296.
70. Araujo MG, Sukekava F, Wennstrom JL, and Lindhe J. 2005. Ridge alterations following implant placement in fresh extraction sockets: An experimental study in the dog. *J Clin Periodontol* 32:645–652.

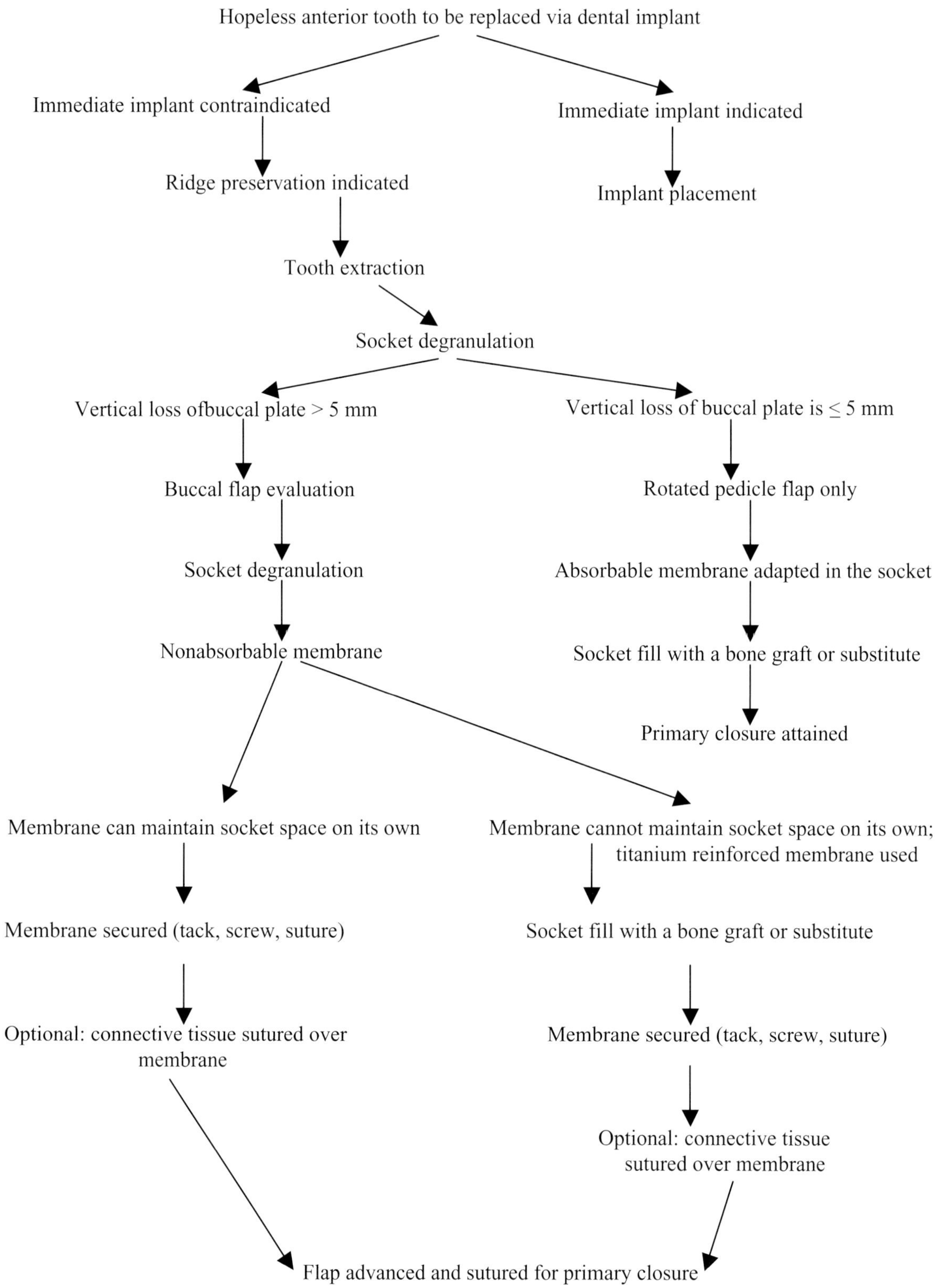

Flow chart 10.1 Decision tree summarizing the clinical choices associated with tooth extraction and ridge preservation procedures.

Chapter 11

Immediate Implant Placement in Esthetic Single Tooth Sites

Sergio De Paoli, MD, DDS and Paul A. Fugazzotto, DDS

Outline

The continued evolution of implant surface technology and restorative options have made implant therapy the treatment modality of choice in many, if not most, clinical situations. It is therefore only natural that the role of immediate implant therapy continues to expand. Proponents of immediate implant therapy advocate its use at the time of tooth removal, or in a partially or fully edentulous arch, to meet a variety of clinical challenges (1–10).

The goal of this chapter is to discuss the clinical realities of single tooth immediate implant therapy, and how best to utilize such treatment in daily practice.

Definitions

When discussing immediate implant therapy, it is important to differentiate between immediate placement at the time of tooth removal, immediate temporization of implants (in either fresh extraction sockets or previously edentulous areas without functional occlusion), and immediate functional loading of implants placed in fresh extraction sockets or previously edentulous areas. Each of these scenarios presents with its own unique challenges and demands for maximization of functional and esthetic outcomes of treatment.

Patient Examination and Workup

Prior to the initiation of immediate implant therapy, it is imperative that appropriate examination, diagnosis, and case workup be performed.

As previously discussed, a patient who presents with a fractured maxillary incisor (and an otherwise intact dentition with no periodontal or occlusal concerns), may require nothing more than a clinical and radiographic examination prior to the initiation of immediate implant therapy. However, patients demonstrating a greater degree of dental pathology, whether it is carious, periodontal, endodontic, orthodontic, or occlusal in nature, must undergo a thorough examination and assessment, including facebow-mounted models. The periodontist and restorative dentist are able to examine these models and, in conjunction with information gained from their clinical examinations, formulate a comprehensive, treatment outcome.

For the purpose of our discussion regarding immediate implant therapy in single tooth sites, the assumption is made that the aforementioned examination has been carried out and that all other dental problems have been appropriately managed for the patient in question.

Site-Specific Examination and Treatment Planning

Soft tissue examination should include assessment of soft tissue health to ensure that active gingival inflammation is not present, as well as evaluation of soft tissue thickness and the dimensions of available attached keratinized tissue. These factors are important in assessing the expected stability of the soft tissues following implant placement, temporization, and final restoration. Hard tissue examination must include an assessment of both the quality and quantity of available bone for implant placement. In instances of immediate implant insertion, the amount of bone available apical to the extraction socket for implant stabilization is not as crucial as the extent of alveolar bone which will be engaged by the implant after its placement, including the lateral walls of the extraction socket at its most apical extent where the diameter of the implant will exceed that of the extracted tooth.

At least as important as the above outlined assessment criterion is the patient's biotype. Tissue biotype defines the envelope of postoperative response. A patient with a blockier, less-scalloped biotype demonstrates thicker hard and soft tissues macroscopically than its thinner, highly scalloped counterpart (Figures 11.1 and 11.2). The histologic makeup of the soft tissues in a patient with a blockier, less-scalloped biotype demonstrates a larger percentage of dense gingival connective tissue, and a lesser percentage of epithelium and rete pegs (Figure 11.3), than a patient with a more highly scalloped biotype.

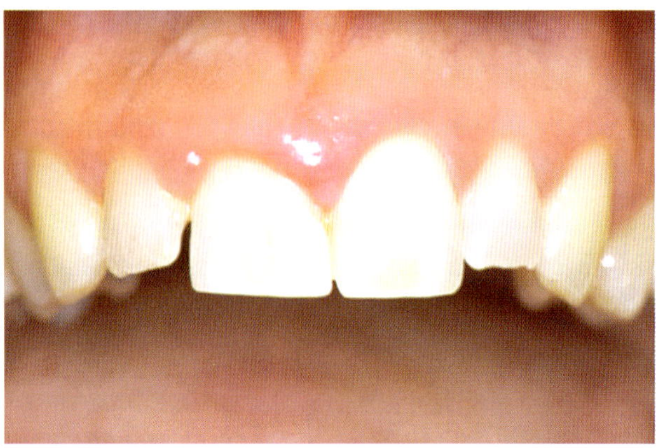

Figure 11.1 A patient presents with a hopeless prognosis for the fractured tooth number 8 and fairly thick, gently scalloped soft tissues.

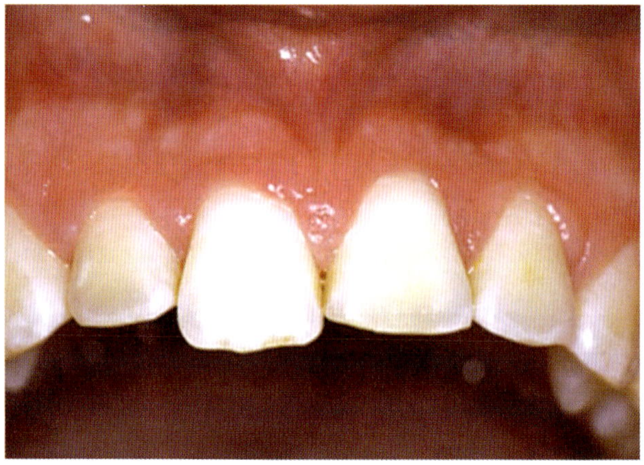

Figure 11.2 A patient presents with a hopeless prognosis for tooth number 8. Note the thinner, more highly scalloped tissues than those of the patient in Figure 11.1. These tissues are much more labile following surgical insult.

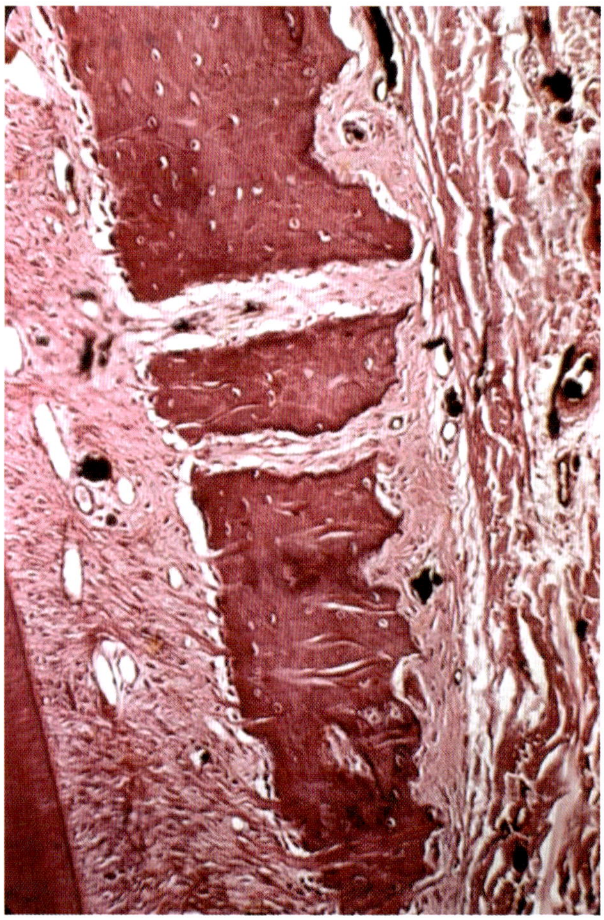

Figure 11.3 An example of thin delicate, hard and soft tissues on the buccal aspect of a prominent tooth. The tooth is to the left. The buccal alveolar bone septum is thin and cannot be expected to be maintained following tooth removal.

The alveolar bone in patients with a blockier, less-scalloped biotype demonstrates both a greater thickness and a larger percentage of marrow than its thinner, highly scalloped counterpart, which presents with thinner, more delicate bone and a lesser marrow component.

As a result of the differences in histologic characteristics between the two biotypes, the postoperative response of the blockier, less-scalloped biotype is characterized by greater hard and soft tissue stability and less resorption than its labile, more highly scalloped counterpart. Such considerations are important when contemplating tooth extraction and immediate implant insertion in the esthetic zone.

Extraction Technique

All single-rooted teeth should be extracted without reflecting a mucoperiosteal flap. This goal is attainable utilizing piezosurgery and appropriate periotomes, or a bone-extraction system which utilizes a posttapped into a fractured root, impression taking, and removal of the root through extrusion of the post with a torque system.

Assessing the Extraction Socket

Once the tooth has been removed, a 15 blade is utilized to achieve sharp dissection to the bone crest, removing approximately 1 mm of the internal lining of the soft tissue circumferentially. A molt curette is employed along the full extent of the internal aspect of the extraction socket, allowing removal of all residual soft tissues as one entity. This enucleation technique avoids development of soft tissue tags which may be difficult to completely remove. The integrity of the extraction socket is examined internally utilizing the small end of the molt curette. The extent and pattern of bone destruction which has occurred as a result of any periapical or periodontal inflammatory lesions which were present is determined.

The Question of Infection

The presence or absence of periapical or periodontal infection at the time of tooth removal does not preclude immediate implant placement. The clinician must instead consider the extent and severity of the infection. If the periodontal or periapical infection which was present has undermined the bone necessary to attain ideal implant positioning, the tooth is removed and appropriate regenerative therapy is performed. An implant is then placed in a second stage procedure.

If the infection which is present has undermined bone crucial to the maximization of esthetic treatment outcomes, or should the soft tissues which are present be unstable due to a fistula, the tooth is once again removed and appropriate regenerative therapy is performed without immediate implant placement.

In each instance, passive soft tissue primary closure is attained, utilizing previously described techniques.

The presence or absence of periapical or periodontal infection is never a contraindication to regenerative therapy at the time of tooth removal following appropriate debridement. Failure to perform the necessary regenerative therapy will result in significant resorption and hard and soft tissue changes, esthetic compromise, and the need for additional surgical interventions. The literature has conclusively demonstrated that guided bone regeneration (GBR) therapy may be successfully performed in the presence of periodontal and/or periapical infection.

The techniques and materials utilized to effect appropriate regenerative therapy in the esthetic zone are wholly dependent upon the residual extraction socket morphology. The goal of such regeneration is not merely to attain adequate bone for implant placement. Rather, complete regeneration of prepathologic bone morphology must be seen as the only acceptable treatment outcome. In order to predictably attain this goal, the clinician must understand the indications, contraindications, and limitations of various regenerative approaches.

Selecting the Appropriate Treatment Approach

If the buccal alveolar wall of the extraction socket is intact, and the extraction socket as a whole represents a space-maintaining defect (i.e., the morphologies of the extraction socket walls are such that they can support a membrane without collapse), therapy proceeds as follows:

A full thickness palatal flap is reflected which extends one tooth mesial and distal to the tooth to be extracted, and is palatal to the papillae. Releasing incisions are placed on the mesial and distal aspects of the palatal flap. A full thickness buccal flap is reflected approximately 2–3 mm past the buccal crest of the ridge without compromising the interproximal papillae, utilizing the small end of a molt curette. A resorbable membrane is shaped and placed over the extraction socket, and tucked beneath the small area of buccal flap reflection. The membrane extends beyond the extraction socket approximately 4 mm on its palatal aspect. The membrane is secured with palatal fixation tacks. A rotated palatal pedicle flap is now reflected, as described in previous publications (11–13). The area is sutured with two plain gut resorbable sutures, palatally. The advantage to this approach is that there has been no disruption of the interproximal papillae, or of the position of the marginal buccal soft tissue, while still attaining passive soft tissue primary closure. Maintenance of passive primary closure is crucial to maximization of regenerative outcomes, and assurance of an adequate soft tissue cover of the regenerated bone to provide appropriate esthetics in the final treatment outcome. While some authors advocate taking a tissue graft from the distal wedge area or the palate, and placing it over the extraction socket so as to avoid flap reflection, the lack of nutrition to this small gingival graft often results in sloughing of part if not all of the graft, and an unpredictable final soft tissue contour.

Placement of bone grafting materials without ensuring soft tissue coverage is ill advised. The extent of bone regeneration will be compromised, as the healing soft tissues impregnate the crestal 2–3 mm of the bone graft material. A membrane may not be utilized to prevent this problem, as its exposure will result in soft tissue complications and a less than ideal final soft tissue result.

If the buccal alveolar bone of the extraction socket is intact, but the extraction socket defect is not a space-maintaining defect due to extensive loss of the palatal and/or interproximal bone, therapy proceeds as follows:

Following flap reflection as previously described and placement of graft material, a titanium-reinforced membrane is trimmed and placed in a manner similar to that of the aforementioned resorbable membrane. It is crucial to use a titanium membrane in such a situation to ensure the regeneration of prepathologic alveolar ridge morphology. As discussed in Chapter 2, regardless of the consistency of the graft materials placed beneath the membrane, if the membrane is not titanium-reinforced and the defect is a nonspace maintaining, some membrane collapse will occur, compromising the final hard tissue regenerative result. The membrane is secured with palatal fixation tacks.

If the buccal alveolar wall of the extraction socket is compromised by small fenestration defect, therapy proceeds as follows:

The small end of a molt curette is placed through the fenestration from the internal aspect of the extraction socket, and utilized to reflect the periosteum and other soft tissues away from both the fenestration and the alveolar bone around the circumference of the fenestration for a distance of 2 mm. Regenerative therapy proceeds in one of the manners outlined above, depending upon the morphology of the extraction socket as a whole (i.e., space maintaining versus nonspace maintaining) (13).

If a dehiscence defect is present on the buccal wall of the extraction socket, therapy proceeds as follows:

A palatal flap is reflected as previously described. A buccal flap is reflected which employs mesial and distal releasing incisions, placed in such a way as to preserve the interproximal papillae. The buccal flap releasing incision designs, including horizontal incisions at their most apical extents, has been described in Chapter 2. A titanium-reinforced membrane is shaped and placed so as to cover both the dehiscence defect and the extraction socket. Two titanium fixation tacks are placed at the mesiobuccal and distobuccal aspects of the buccal apical border of the membrane to prevent membrane movement. A rotated palatal pedicle flap is utilized as previously described. The mucoperiosteal flaps are sutured with two to three interrupted plain gut sutures over the extraction socket, engaging the buccal and palatal flaps, and two to three interrupted plain gut sutures on each buccal releasing incision. The palatal releasing incisions are not sutured.

Implant Placement at the Time of Tooth Removal in the Esthetic Zone

Unless adequate bone is present apically and laterally to ensure primary stability of the implant, the implant must be angled in such a manner as to engage the palatal wall of the extraction socket and still exit the soft tissues within the desired restorative zone. Either approach, when performed appropriately, will result in an implant which is easily restored in an ideal manner, to help maximize esthetic treatment outcomes.

When the osteotomy is carried out toward the palatal wall to ensure appropriate implant stability and positioning, the osteotomy may result in the formation of a "buccal wall" independent of the actual buccal alveolar ridge at the most apical extent of the osteotomy.

The osteotomy is prepared utilizing as slow a speed as possible. The advantages to such an approach are:

- Less heat is generated during the preparation of the osteotomy, resulting in less trauma to the alveolar bone.
- Preparation of the osteotomy is more precise than when a higher speed is utilized, resulting in improved bone to implant contact.
- Utilization of a slower drill speed enhances the accumulation of autogenous bone in the "grooves" of the bur. This autogenous bone is immediately collected and placed in sterile saline. Such a collection approach is superior to the utilization of a bone trap, as it lessens the chances of collecting saliva, bacterial products, and other contaminants.

Implant selection is governed by the desired implant morphology, length, and width. A tapered implant morphology is chosen so as to attain a "wedging action" of the implant in the prepared extraction socket/osteotomy. The length of the implant is dependent upon a number of factors which have been previously enumerated.

The diameter of the chosen implant is not related to the width of the extraction socket following tooth removal. Rather, the diameter of the implant selected is related to the mesiodistal thickness of the interproximal alveolar septum, and the required mesiodistal width of the alveolar interproximal septum of bone which is needed around the implant following bone regeneration, osseointegration, and soft tissue healing.

If the implant is to abut a natural tooth, then a minimum of 2 mm of mesiodistal thickness of interproximal alveolar septum is required. Should the implant abut another implant, a minimum of 3 mm of mesiodistal width of the alveolar interproximal septum is necessary. At least 1.5–2.0 mm of alveolar bone thickness should be present buccally.

The precise course of therapy following implant placement is dependent upon a combination of patient biotype and defect morphology. When a patient presents with a blocky, less-scalloped biotype, and the alveolar buccal ridge is intact, two possibilities present themselves.

If the horizontal defect dimension (HDD), defined as the horizontal distance between the outer aspect of the implant and the buccal alveolar ridge, is less than 3 mm, no grafting materials are placed and the implant is temporized at the time of placement, unless other factors such as a deep overbite or a severe parafunctional habit preclude temporization. If immediate temporization is not accomplished, a healing cap is placed so that the implant is not submerged. In the vast majority of situations, this implant will be temporized at the time of placement.

If the HDD is greater than 3 mm, the implant is covered with a resorbable membrane following limited buccal and palatal pedicle flap reflection, as previously described. The implant is not temporized at the time of placement.

When the patient presents with a thin, highly scalloped biotype, the implant is placed and covered with a resorbable membrane, following flap reflection as previously described. This implant is submerged beneath the soft tissues following rotation of a palatal pedicle flap. Due to the labile nature of the hard and soft tissues in such a scenario, the implant is placed at the time of tooth removal but is never temporized immediately, regardless of the dimension of the HDD.

When a patient presents with a small buccal fenestration, the implant is placed following limited tissue reflection and graft placement at the site of the fenestration as previously described. The decision as to whether to immediately load the implant is now biotype dependent, as discussed above.

Clinical Example One

A patient presented with an externally resorbing maxillary central incisor with a hopeless prognosis (Figures 11.4 and 11.5). The tooth was extracted without raising a flap, in a minimally invasive manner (Figure 11.6). The inner aspect of the extraction socket was enucleated as previously described (Figure 11.7). The buccal wall of the extraction socket defect was examined internally to ascertain whether or not any buccal fenestration was present. A fenestration of approximately 3 mm in diameter was noted in the apical third of the extraction socket.

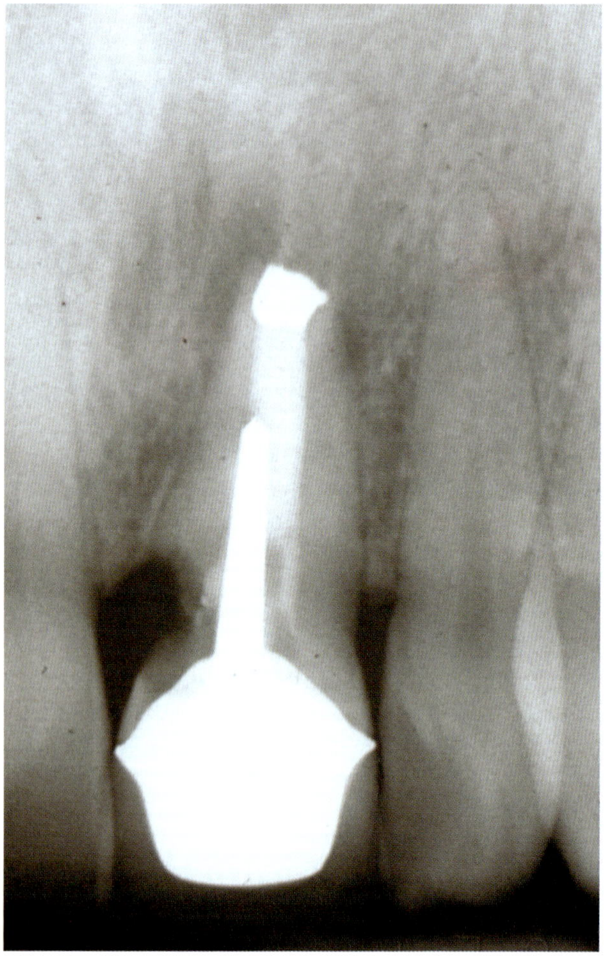

Figure 11.4 A central incisor demonstrates external resorption and a hopeless prognosis.

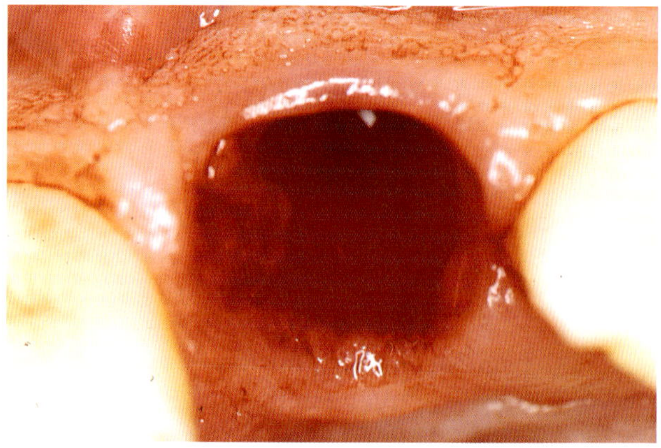

Figure 11.6 The central incisor has been extracted in a minimally traumatic manner.

Osseous coagulum was collected at slow speed during osteotomy preparation (Figure 11.8). This coagulum was placed into the extraction socket, over the area of buccal fenestration, following internal reflection of the buccal soft tissues away from the fenestration as previously described (Figure 11.9).

Following ideal implant positioning, microfibrillar collagen was placed around the implant, over the small expanse of HDD which was present (Figures 11.10 and 11.11). A temporary crown was placed during the same visit (Figure 11.12).

Twelve weeks after temporization, the soft tissues have adapted well to the contours of the provisional temporary crown (Figure 11.13). Removal of the temporary crown demonstrates the ideal soft tissue contours which have been obtained (Figure 11.14).

When a patient presents with a buccal alveolar ridge dehiscence which is 5 mm or less in

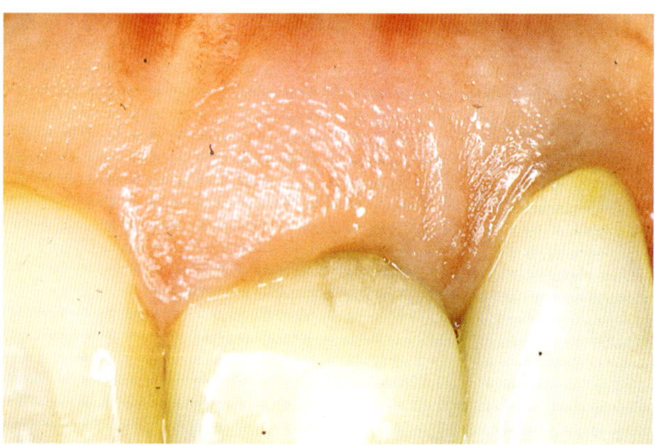

Figure 11.5 A clinical view of the hopeless central incisor.

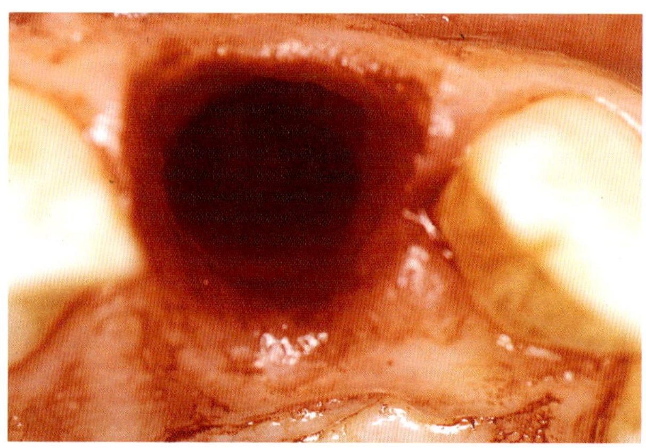

Figure 11.7 The extraction socket has been enucleated.

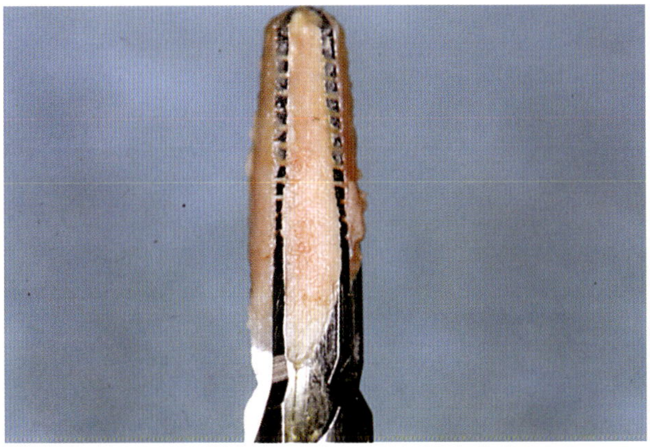

Figure 11.8 Osseous coagulum is collected during osteotomy preparation.

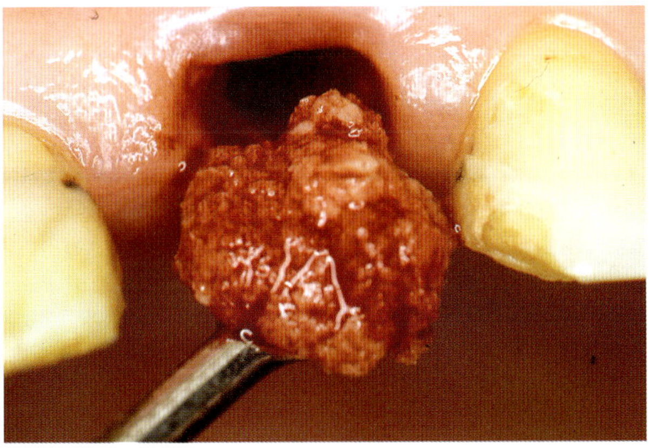

Figure 11.9 The osseous coagulum is brought to the mouth, to be utilized in the area of buccal alveolar bone fenestration, after "reflection" of the periosteum from within the socket.

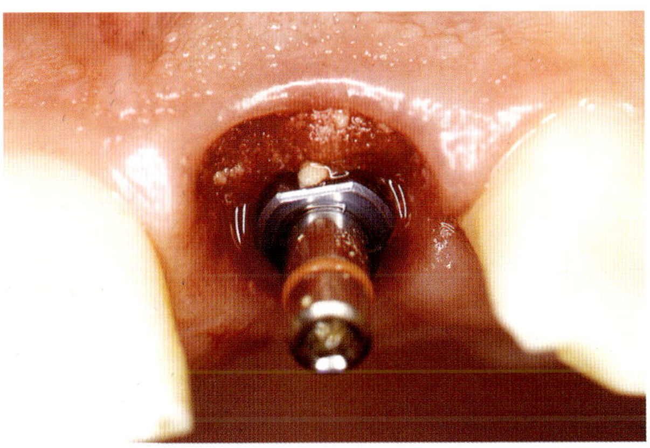

Figure 11.10 An implant has been placed and microfibrillar collagen has been inserted in the residual HDD.

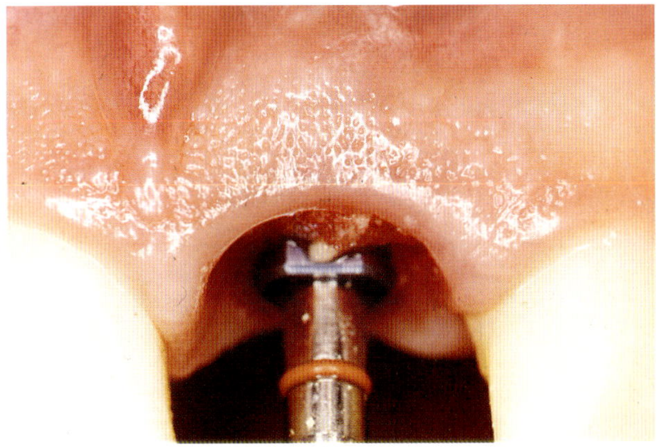

Figure 11.11 Another view of the inserted implant and microfibrillar collagen.

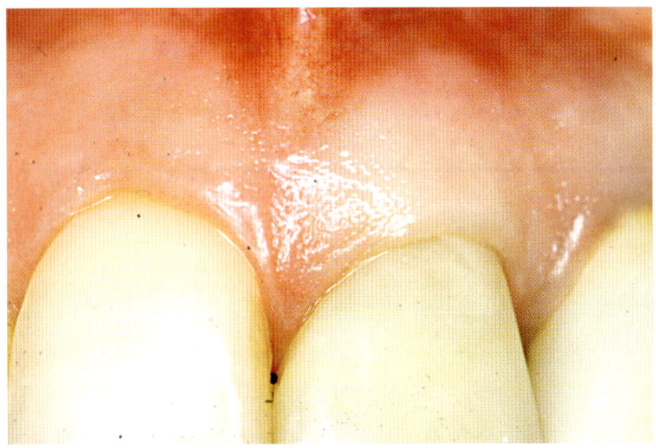

Figure 11.12 A temporary crown is appropriately contoured and inserted.

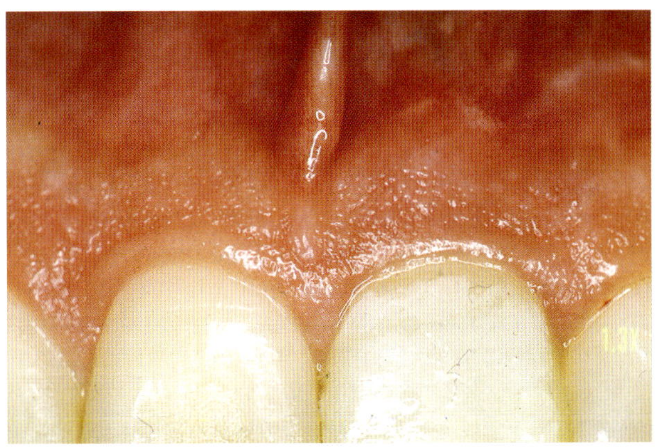

Figure 11.13 Twelve weeks after therapy has been performed, the soft tissues have adapted well to the contours of the temporary crown.

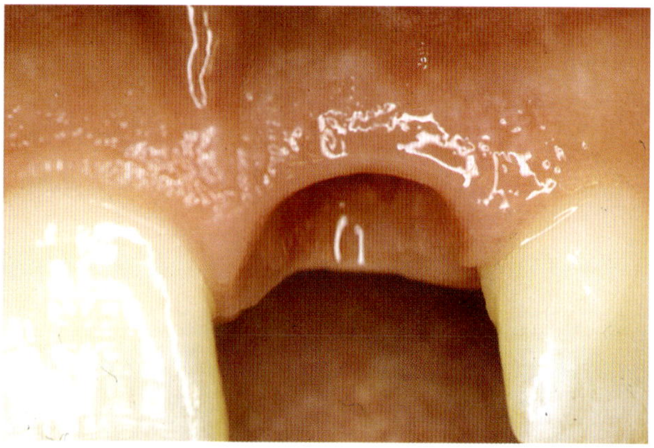

Figure 11.14 The developed soft tissue contours are evident following temporary crown removal.

mesiodistal expanse, the implant is placed at the time of tooth extraction, and graft material and a titanium-reinforced membrane are employed, following flap reflection and rotation of a palatal pedicle flap. The implant will be uncovered and temporized approximately six months after regenerative therapy has been performed. If the buccal dehiscence defect measures greater than 5 mm mesiodistally, regenerative therapy is performed without implant placement, and the implant is placed six months following regenerative therapy. In such a situation, the implant will most probably be temporized at the time of its placement.

Temporization is carried out utilizing a temporary meso abutment. This abutment is inserted into the implant, and the gingival margin is scribed with a sharp instrument. The meso abutment is placed on a laboratory analog and prepared as the clinician would prepare a tooth for acceptance of a single crown. The meso abutment is placed in the mouth, and a temporary crown is filled with acrylic and brought to the mouth. The meso abutment and temporary crown are removed from the mouth and placed on a laboratory analog. Final crown contours and marginal adaptation to the meso abutment are attained extraorally. The meso abutment is inserted into the implant, and the temporary crown is cemented onto the meso abutment following occlusion of the access hole of the meso abutment with a Skube and Panavia (Figures 11.22 through 11.26).

Use of the meso abutment allows the clinician to control the cement line of the temporary crown and easily remove excess cement following cementation. The method of temporization of choice is a single crown, so that the control of the pressures on the implant and surrounding soft tissues are minimized. The crown is slightly under contoured in its submerged profile, and attains normal emergence profile and contours as it exits the gingival sulcus, so as to provide more space for formation of soft tissue. The contours of the crown/meso abutment complex support the surrounding soft tissues, but do not impinge upon them. If the tissues blanche, adjustment of the provisional restoration is carried out. The cells to facilitate this soft tissue regeneration come from the surgically "freshened" surrounding soft tissues. This temporary crown remains in place for 8–12 weeks after implant insertion. An implant level impression is taken, and an abutment and crown are fabricated and inserted following accepted protocols.

Clinical Example Two

A patient presents with a resorbing, hopeless maxillary central incisor. The soft tissue papilla between the central incisors is inflamed and highly vulnerable (Figures 11.15 and 11.16). Following atraumatic flapless tooth extraction, debridement and assessment of the socket as previously described, and placement of an implant, a temporary meso abutment is shaped and inserted into the implant (Figure 11.17). A temporary crown is appropriately contoured and cemented over the meso abutment

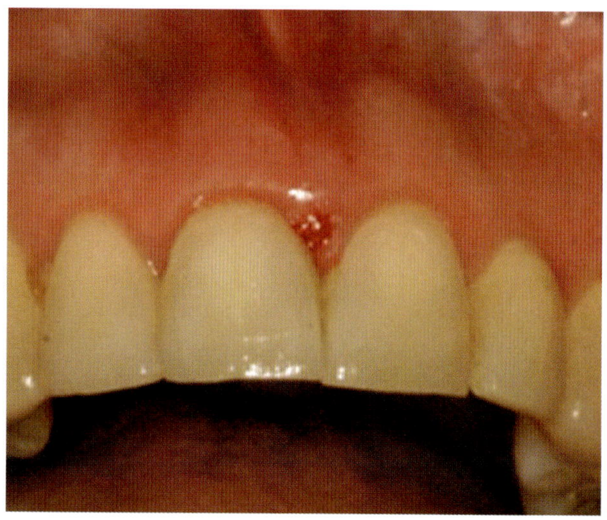

Figure 11.15 A patient presents with a fractured and hopeless tooth number 8.

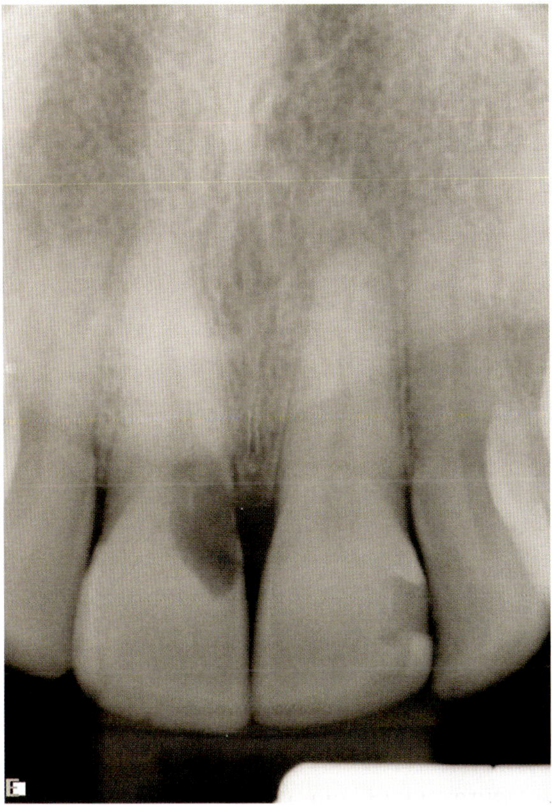

Figure 11.16 A radiograph demonstrates extensive resorption of the root of the hopeless tooth number 8.

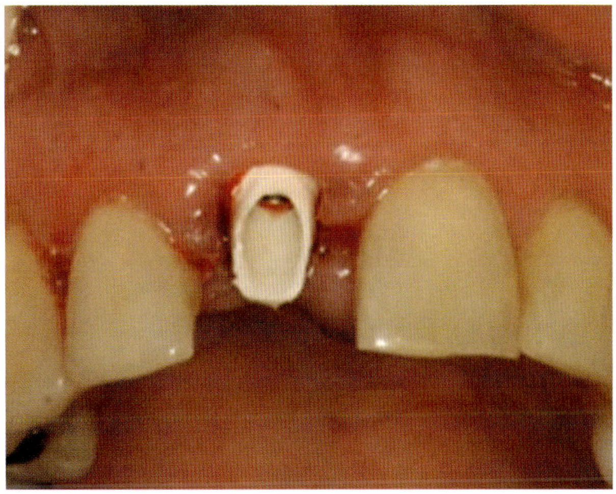

Figure 11.17 Following implant placement, a mesio abutment is contoured and inserted into the implant.

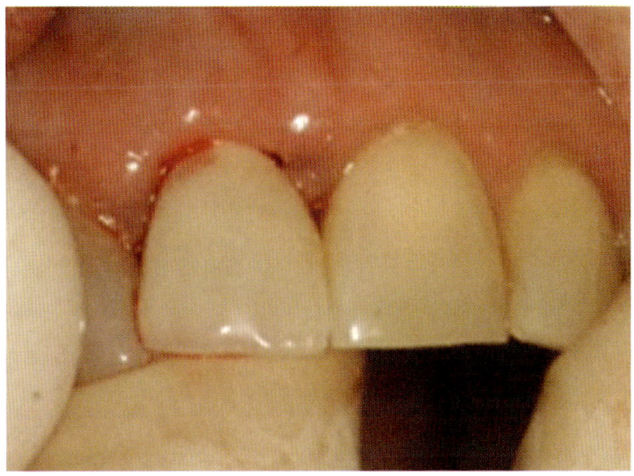

Figure 11.18 A temporary crown is shaped, relined, and cemented to the mesio abutment.

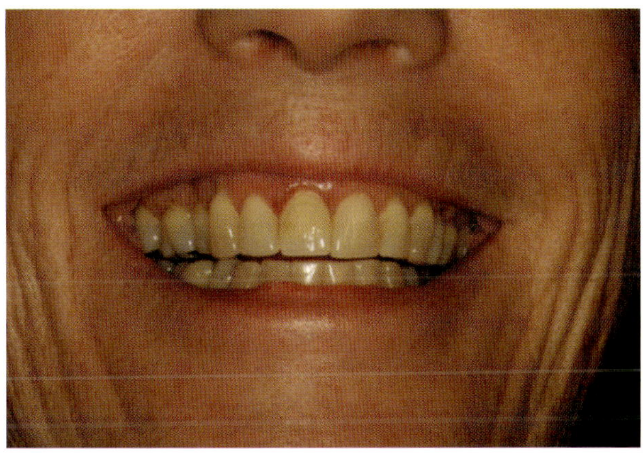

Figure 11.19 Seven days posttherapy, the preservation of the interproximal soft tissue papillae and the developing soft tissue contours around the temporary crown are evident.

with temporary cement (Figure 11.18). The temporary crown contours will provide immediate support for the delicate interproximal soft tissues between the central incisors, thus helping prevent tissue shrinkage and ensuring maximization of esthetic treatment outcomes.

One week posttherapy, the soft tissues are healing well around the temporary crown (Figure 11.19). Approximately 12 weeks after therapy has been performed the final restoration is placed (Figure 11.20).

Failure to appropriately diagnose, plan treatment, and manage the multifactorial challenges present when contemplating tooth extraction and simultaneous implant placement in the esthetic zone will lead to unesthetic and often irreparable final treatment outcomes. If a patient is congenitally missing a tooth, or it has been gone for quite some time and the hard and soft tissue papillae have resorbed, it may be impossible to reconstruct such tissues (Figure 11.21). However, when anticipating implant placement at the time of tooth extraction,

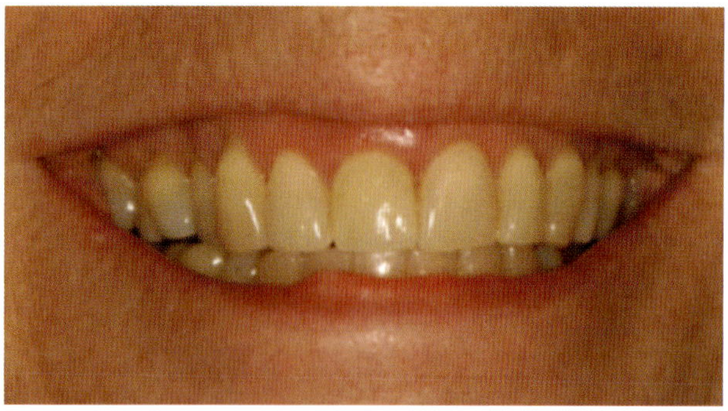

Figure 11.20 The final crown has been inserted.

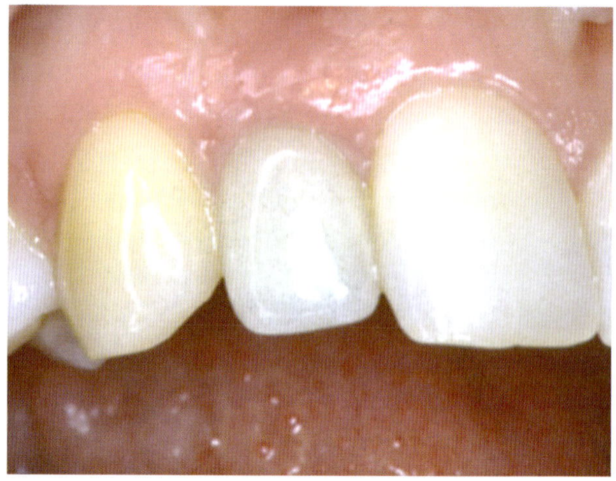

Figure 11.22 Following appropriate tooth extraction, implant placement, temporization, and final restoration of the implant in the position of the maxillary lateral incisor, the esthetic potential of therapy has been maximized.

appropriate care will help ensure regeneration of the alveolar bone in the residual extraction socket defect surrounding the implant, preservation of interproximal alveolar bone to support the soft tissues appropriately, and a satisfactory esthetic result (Figure 11.22).

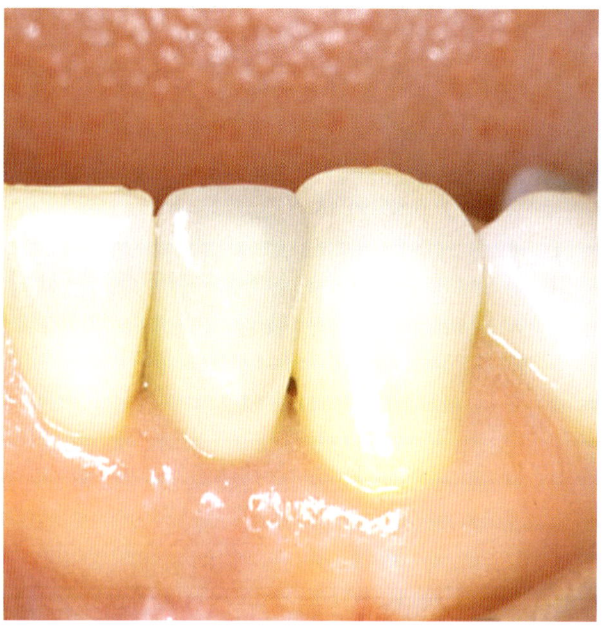

Figure 11.21 A congenitally missing mandibular lateral incisor has been replaced with an implant and crown. Note the lack of an interproximal papilla between the lateral incisor and cuspid.

Clinical Example Three

A patient presented with hopeless periodontal prognoses for the four maxillary incisors, and significant loss of supporting hard and soft tissues (Figures 11.23 and 11.24). Tooth extraction without concomitant regeneration would lead to further extensive bone loss due to the thin labial nature of the residual buccal plate and the inflammatory lesions which were present. Extraction of these teeth with or without concomitant regenerative therapy, in the absence of support of the remaining interproximal papillae, would further compromise the esthetic outcomes of treatment.

The teeth were extracted in a minimally traumatic manner (Figure 11.25), and the residual

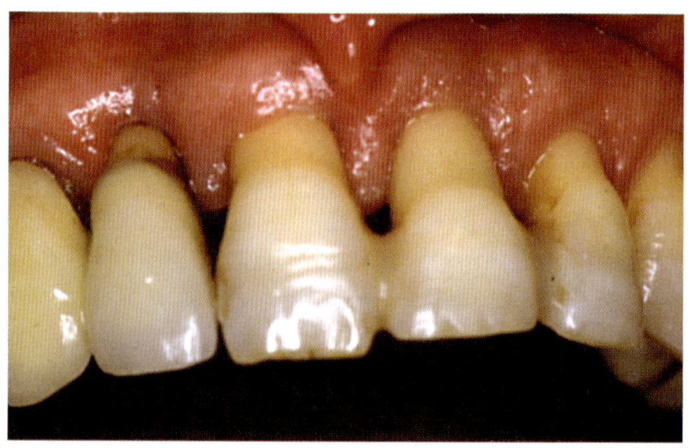

Figure 11.23 A patient presents with hopeless prognoses for the four maxillary central incisors.

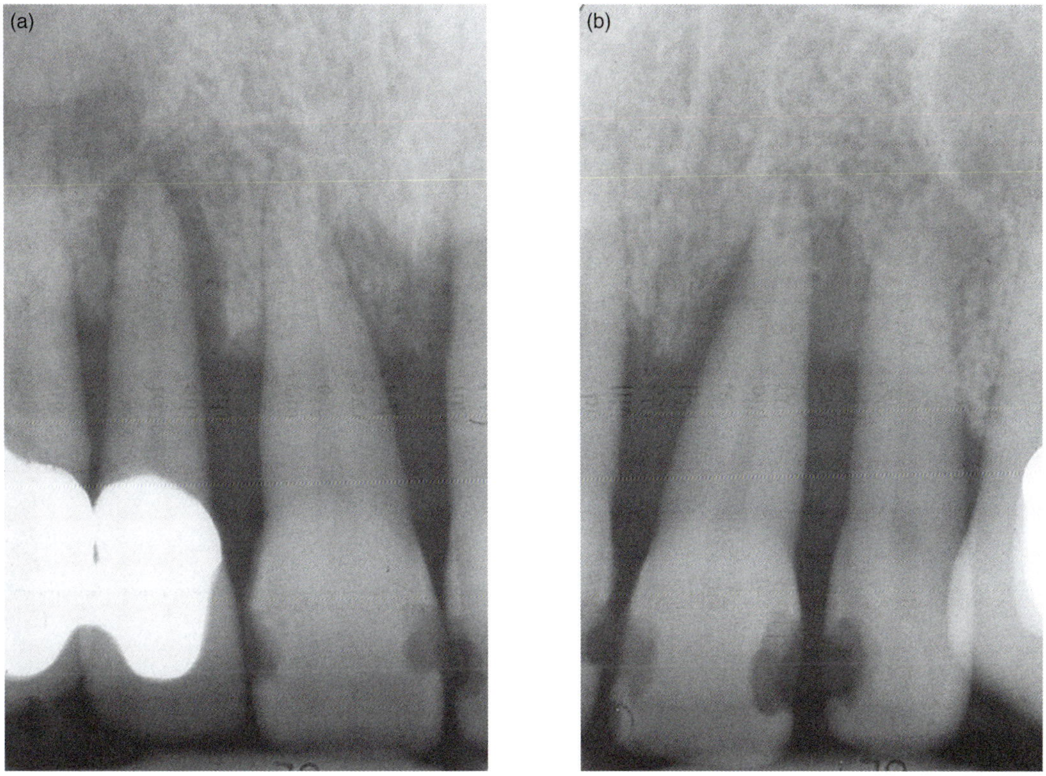

Figure 11.24 (a–b) Radiographs demonstrate the severe bone loss around the hopeless four maxillary central incisors.

extraction socket walls were examined internally. No fenestration or dehiscence defects were noted in the buccal alveolar walls of the extraction sockets.

The implants were placed utilizing previously detailed techniques (Figures 11.26 and 11.27), and osseous coagulum, covering microfibrillar collagen, and temporary crowns were inserted (Figure 11.28).

Six weeks after therapy had been performed, the soft tissues were adapting well around the provisional restorations (Figure 11.29). The developed soft tissue contours are evident following removal of the provisional restoration, 12 weeks postoperatively (Figure 11.30).

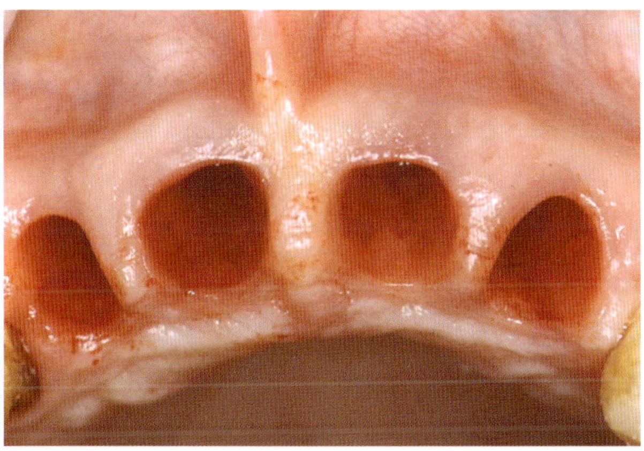

Figure 11.25 The incisors have been extracted in a minimally traumatic manner, and the sockets have been enucleated.

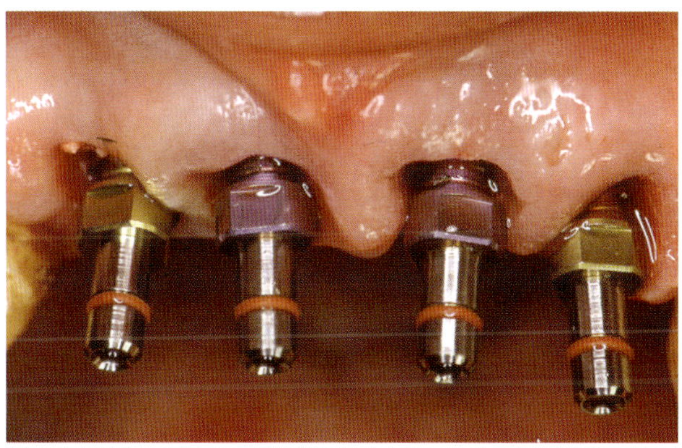

Figure 11.26 Four implants have been placed as previously described.

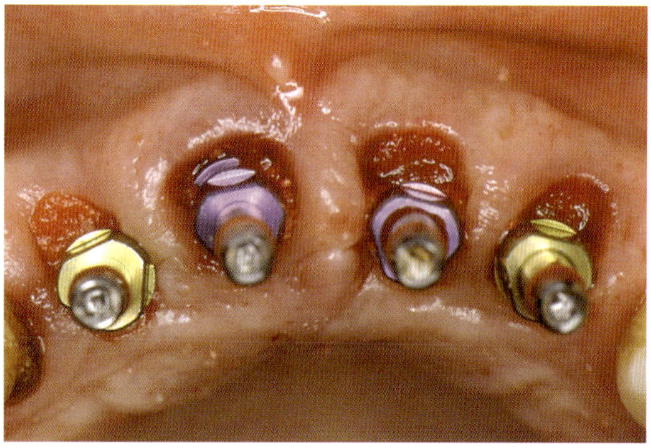

Figure 11.27 Osseous coagulum has been inserted in the residual HDDs and covered with microfibrillar collagen.

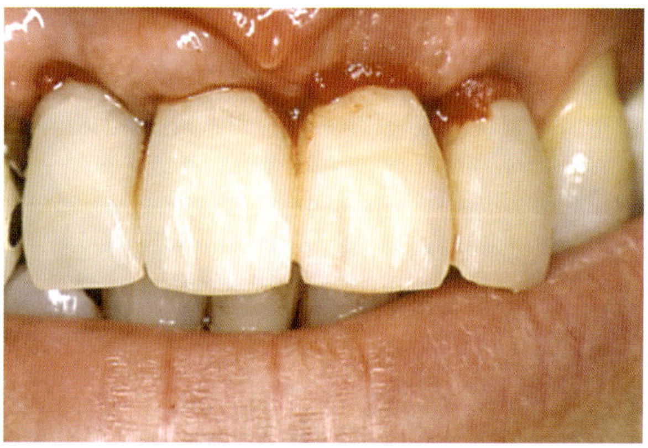

Figure 11.28 Temporary crowns are placed during the same visit.

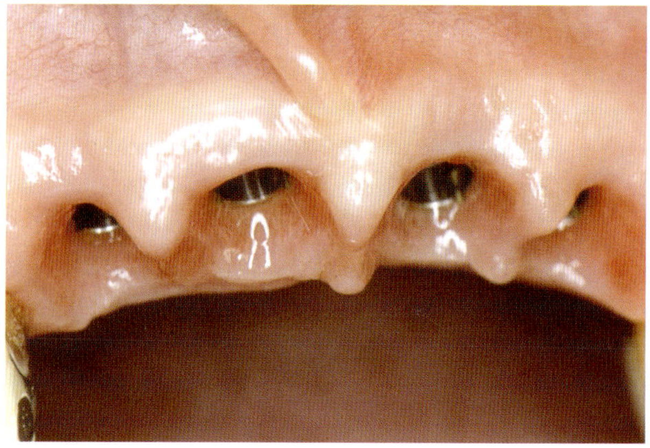

Figure 11.30 Following removal of the temporary restorations, the reattained soft tissue contours are evident.

THE INFLUENCE OF PATIENT BIOTYPE ON FINAL ABUTMENT SELECTION

Zirconia abutments offer significant esthetic advantages, especially in patients with thin, highly scalloped biotypes and the resultant thin buccal soft tissues. In addition to the greater translucency offered by such abutments and crowns over conventional metal abutments and porcelain fused to gold crowns, Zirconia abutments may be custom stained. This is especially important should any tissue recession occur at the crown margin. Such recession is certainly possible in a highly scalloped biotype patient, as the soft tissues are more labile than their less-scalloped counterparts.

In summary, care must be taken to preserve remaining alveolar bone, to recognize when such bone is missing, to identify sites which are at risk

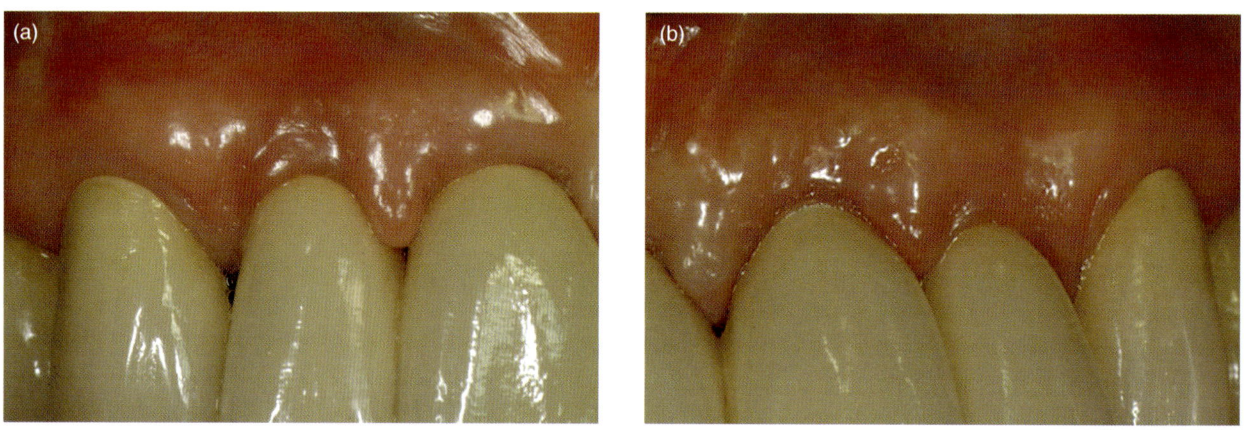

Figure 11.29 (a–b) Six weeks after therapy has been performed, the soft tissues are adapting well to the contours of the provisional restorations.

for loss of existing alveolar bone if certain treatment protocols are not utilized, and to regenerate lost bone appropriately. This is especially important in the interproximal areas. Once interproximal bone is lost, its regeneration in single tooth sites is unpredictable, and often leaves the restorative dentist having to perform "porcelain gymnastics" to fill the interproximal space, or requires the patient to understand the situation and accept unesthetic interproximal spaces.

IMPLANT PLACEMENT IN COMPROMISED SITES

While the aforementioned decision tree appropriately considers and manages variables at the time of tooth extraction when interproximal papillae are intact, such an "ideal" situation is not always encountered. When faced with papillary compromise at the site of tooth extraction, the risk factors and expected treatment outcomes of various therapeutic approaches must be carefully considered before developing appropriate treatment algorithms.

While the soft tissue papilla is the surrogate end point most often discussed, its existence and form are dependent upon the underlying bone and attachment apparatus to the adjacent tooth. A discussion which limits a determination of whether a papilla will be present to the distance between the contact point and bone crest fails to understand the dynamic three-dimensional nature of the interdental papilla, and its dependence upon bony contours apico occlusally, mesiodistally, and bucco lingually. The influence of such three-dimensional bony contours on the presence and shape of the dental papilla is well understood, having been established during the development of periodontal prosthetic principles.

Papillary bone may be compromised to varying degrees, apico occlusally, buccolingually/palatally, or mesiodistally (Figure 11.31). Greater esthetic risk is encountered as such compromise proceeds along each axis. The greatest risk is present when multiaxis compromise of the papillary bone is noted.

The presence or absence of an intact attachment apparatus on the tooth helping to support the papillary bone, and thus the soft tissue papilla, plays a crucial role in final papilla form and level. The pattern of periodontal attachment loss on the facing root surface of the adjacent tooth must also be considered.

Finally, the mesiodistal dimension of the papillary bone, and thus the overlying papillary soft tissues, must be assessed. Such assessment considers only if the mesial distal papillary bone is present or absent. Rather, the extent of mesiodistal compromise, and the pattern of bone loss, must also be evaluated.

Assessment of the aforementioned factors affords the opportunity to carry out an accurate three-dimensional evaluation of the preoperative papilla and the expected postoperative papillary form, thus aiding the development of treatment algorithms at the time of tooth extraction in the presence of papillary compromise (Flow chart 11.2). When treating a patient with a flat, bulky biotype, the papillary height may be intact, compromised by less than 2 mm, or compromised by greater than 2 mm.

If the papillary height is intact, the attachment apparatus on the adjacent teeth must then be assessed. Should this attachment apparatus also prove to be intact, the decision tree is utilized which has already been formulated for implant placement at the time of tooth extraction in the presence of intact mesial and distal papillae (Flow chart 11.1). However, should the attachment apparatus on the adjacent tooth or teeth be damaged in a patient demonstrating appropriate papillary height, regenerative therapy, most likely in the form of Emdogain, should be carried out at the time of implant placement. In such a situation, the implant is not temporized. Rather, primary soft tissue closure is attained over the implant, which will be uncovered and restored at a later date.

Should less than 2 mm of papillary height compromise be noted, and the attachment apparatus be intact, the implant is inserted following tooth extraction. A dermis connective tissue graft is then placed, and primary soft tissue closure is attained over the implant.

When papillary height is compromised less than 2 mm, but the attachment apparatus on the adjacent tooth is affected, the implant is not placed. Instead, periodontal and soft tissue regenerative procedures are carried out utilizing Emdogain and a dermis connective tissue graft. Primary soft tissue closure is attained, and implant placement is effected following appropriate healing. In such a situation, a flapless implant placement approach is often utilized.

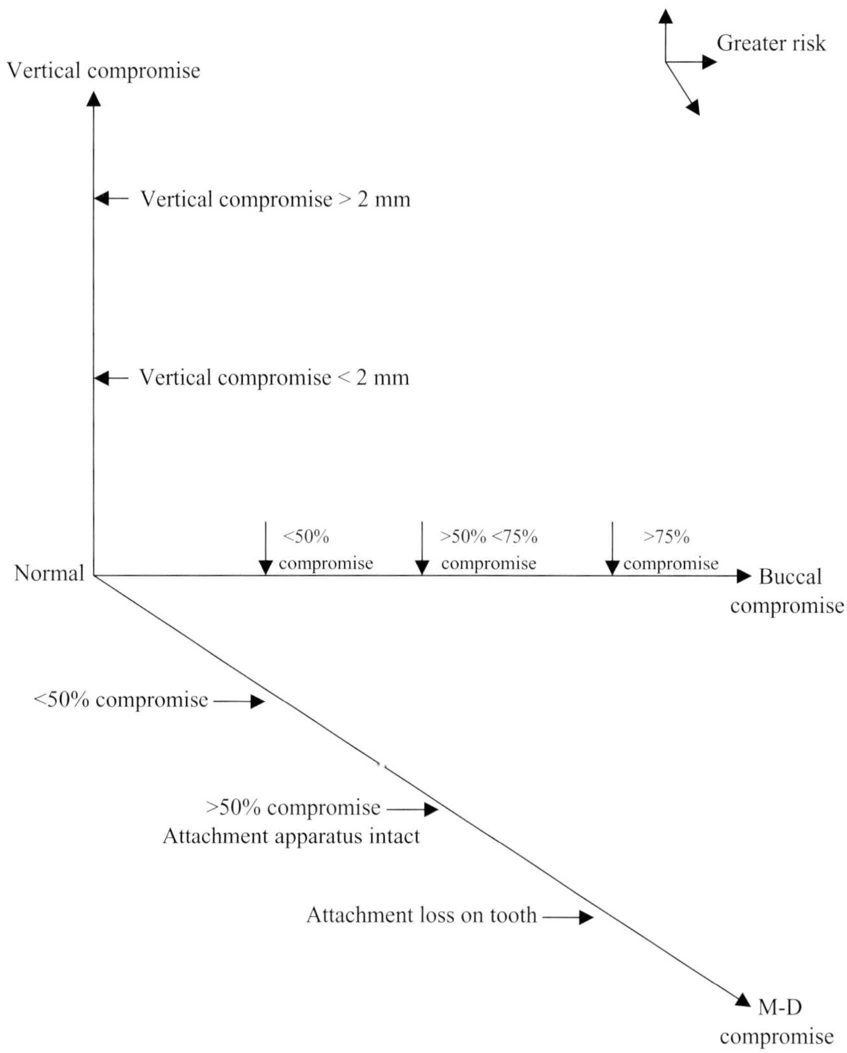

Figure 11.31 Assessing papillary bone.

Should papillary height damage of greater than 2 mm be noted in a flat, bulky biotype patient, Emdogain and a dermis graft are placed and primary soft tissue closure is attained without implant placement, regardless of whether or not the attachment apparatus is further effected on the adjacent tooth. Once again, the implant is placed at a second visit, often utilizing a flapless surgical approach.

Treatment decisions vary from those already described, when a tooth is extracted in a patient demonstrating a thin, highly scalloped biotype. In such a situation, if the papilla is wholly intact, the implant is placed as described in Flow chart 11.1 for implant placement at the time of tooth extraction, utilizing preparation rich in growth factors (PRGF) covering membrane, and obtaining primary soft tissue closure.

However, if papillary compromise is noted in a patient demonstrating a thin, highly scalloped biotype, one of two treatment approaches will be utilized.

When no damage has occurred to the attachment apparati of the adjacent teeth, the implant will be placed, and the area will be covered with a dermis connective tissue graft. Primary soft tissue closure will be attained.

Should the attachment apparatus of the adjacent tooth or teeth demonstrate compromise in a thin, highly scalloped biotype patient, Emdogain and a dermis connective tissue graft are placed, and primary soft tissue closure is attained. The implant is not placed at this time, but is inserted at a second surgical visit.

IMPLANT PLACEMENT IN SINGLE-TOOTH EDENTULOUS SITES

When implant placement is anticipated in a single-tooth edentulous space in the esthetic zone, the quality, quantity, and morphology of available bone must be carefully assessed (Figure 11.32). Such assessment includes both the bone which will house the implant, and the bone between the implant and the adjacent teeth. This papillary bone will play a significant role in determining the esthetic potential of implant therapy in the region.

Compromises may be noted in the vertical dimension of the bone, the horizontal dimension of the bone, and/or the adjacent papillae.

As papillary compromise increases, the likelihood of esthetic compromise becomes much more significant.

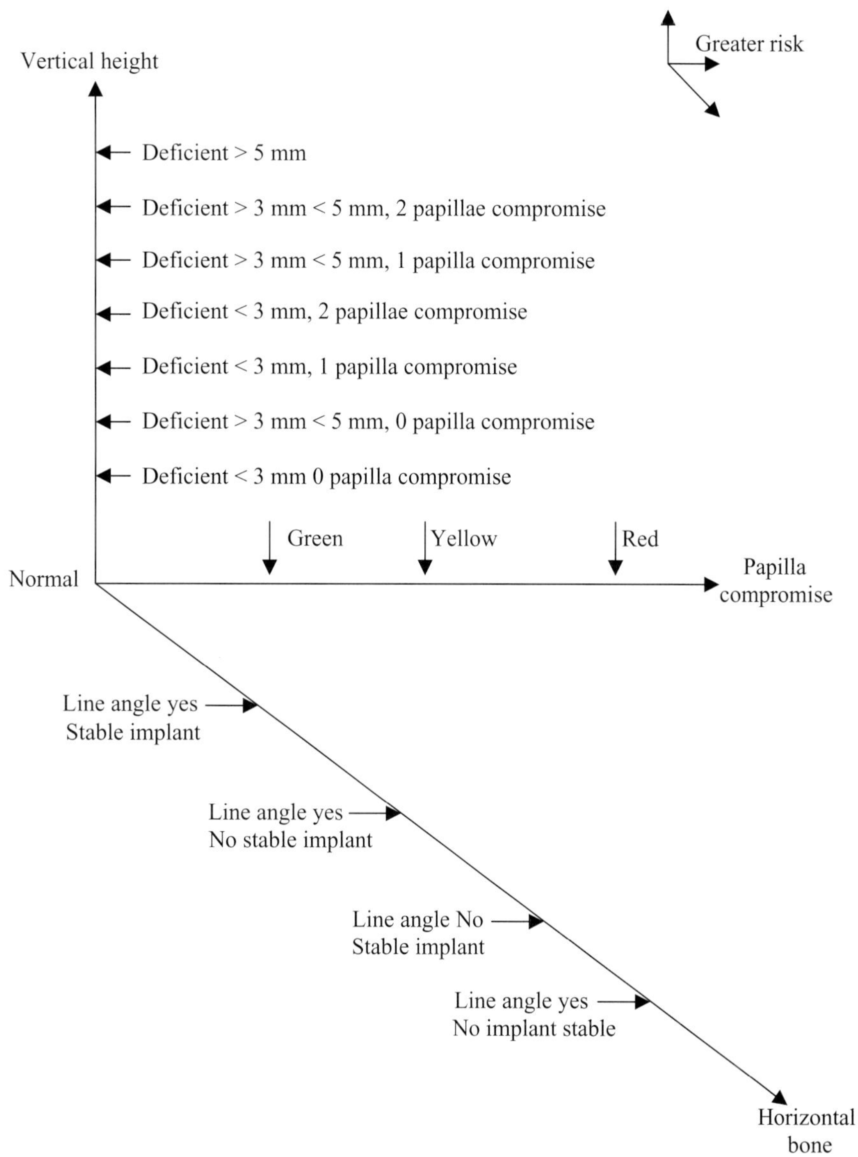

Figure 11.32 Assessing edentulous space bone.

Both the amount of available bone, and the presence or absence of the buccal line angle of bone, will play significant roles in both development of treatment algorithms and final esthetic treatment outcomes (Flow chart 11.3).

If the vertical dimension of bone in the edentulous space is uncompromised, the status of the adjacent papillae must then be assessed. When the papillae are intact, the presence or absence of an intact buccal alveolar bone line angle will be the determining factor in developing the appropriate treatment algorithm.

If the buccal line angle of bone is intact, and primary stability of the implant can be attained in the ideal position, the implant is placed, any necessary regenerative therapy is carried out, and primary soft tissue closure is attained. The selection of appropriate regenerative materials has been discussed in Chapter 2. If no regenerative therapy was necessary at the time of implant placement, the implant is temporized in infraocclusion during the same visit.

If the buccal line angle of bone is intact, but primary stability of the implant cannot be attained in an ideal position, a titanium-reinforced membrane is utilized over the appropriate graft materials, and primary soft tissue closure is attained. The implant is placed at a second surgical visit, following completion of bone regeneration.

When the papillae are intact in a patient with no vertical bone compromise, but the buccal line angle of bone is not intact, the patient's biotype plays a significant role in determining the appropriate treatment algorithm.

In a patient with a flat, bulky biotype, if primary stability can be attained in an ideal position, the implant is placed and appropriate regenerative therapy is carried out employing graft materials and a titanium-reinforced membrane. Primary soft tissue closure is effected over the implant.

If the implant cannot be stabilized in an ideal position, bone augmentation is carried out utilizing the appropriate grafting materials and a covering titanium-reinforced membrane. The implant is placed at a second surgical visit.

When the buccal line of bone angle is not intact in a patient with an uncompromised vertical dimension of bone in an edentulous site, in the presence of a thin, highly scalloped biotype, the implant is never placed at the time of bone regeneration. Rather, guided bone regenerative therapy is carried out utilizing the appropriate grafting materials beneath a titanium-reinforced membrane, and primary soft tissue closure is attained. The implant is placed at a second surgical visit.

If a patient presents with no compromise of the vertical dimension of bone in a single-tooth edentulous site, but the adjacent papilla or papillae are compromised, the patient's biotype determines the precise course of therapy. In such a situation, the same treatment algorithms are utilized which have been developed for decision making at the time of tooth extraction in the esthetic zone in the presence of papillary compromise (Flow chart 11.1).

When a patient presents with compromise of the vertical dimension of bone in a single-tooth edentulous site, the extent of the compromise is the prime determining factor in treatment algorithm development. Should less than 3 mm of vertical compromise be noted, and the papillae are uncompromised, the buccal line angle of bone is then assessed.

If the buccal line angle of bone is intact, and the implant can be stabilized in an ideal position, a bone level or Straumann design standard plus implant is placed in conjunction with a dermis connective tissue graft. Primary soft tissue closure is attained.

If the buccal line angle of bone is intact, but the implant cannot be stabilized in an ideal position, regenerative therapy is carried out utilizing a titanium-reinforced membrane over the appropriate grafting materials. Most often, a dermis connective tissue graft is placed at the same time, and primary soft tissue closure is attained. A bone level or standard plus implant is placed at a second stage visit. If necessary, a second dermis connective tissue graft is also placed at this time.

If the papilla or papillae are compromised in a patient demonstrating less than 3 mm of vertical bone compromise in a single-tooth edentulous site, the decision tree is employed which was utilized in the face of papillary compromise at the time of tooth extraction. Either a bone level or Straumann design standard plus implant is placed at the appropriate time.

When the line angle of the ridge is not intact, in an edentulous site which demonstrates less than 3 mm of vertical compromise, the same decision tree is employed as was utilized for patients with no vertical bone compromise, with the exception that a dermis connective tissue graft is always placed (Flow chart 11.3).

When a patient presents with between 3 and 5 mm of vertical bone compromise in a single-tooth edentulous site, the status of the adjacent papillae is first assessed. If the buccal line angle of bone is intact, and the implant can be stabilized in an ideal position, a Straumann design standard implant is inserted, regenerative therapy utilizing a bone graft beneath a PRGF membrane is carried out, and a dermis connective tissue graft is placed. Primary soft tissue closure is attained. The design of this implant, which offers 2.8 mm of additional implant crestal to the bony crest, helps support the regenerative materials which are placed, positions the implant abutment joint away from the crest of bone, and raises the abutment crown interface to a more manageable subgingival position.

Should the buccal line angle of bone be intact in a patient demonstrating between 3 and 5 mm of vertical bone compromise, but the implant cannot be secured in an ideal position, regenerative therapy is carried out utilizing a titanium-reinforced membrane over the appropriate graft materials. Primary soft tissue closure is attained. A bone level or Straumann design standard implant is placed at a second stage, in conjunction with placement of a dermis connective tissue graft. Primary soft tissue closure is once again attained.

When a patient demonstrates 3–5 mm of vertical bone compromise, as well as compromise of one or both of the adjacent papillae, the same treatment algorithms are utilized which have been developed for decision making at the time of tooth extraction in the face of papillary compromise (Flow chart 11.2), with the exception that a connective tissue dermis graft is always placed, and a bone level or Straumann design standard implant is employed.

When considering "normal" papillae or compromised papillae in situations where 3–5 mm of vertical bone compromise are noted, it is rare but not impossible to find the adjacent papillae intact. The clinician should expect to encounter compromised papillae, and ascertain how such an absolute compromise relates to the patient's perception of compromise and the desired treatment outcome.

In contrast, a patient demonstrating greater than 5 mm of vertical bone compromise almost always presents with significant papillary compromise.

In such a situation, if the attachment apparatus on the adjacent tooth is intact, regenerative therapy is carried out utilizing a titanium-reinforced membrane over the appropriate bone graft materials. A connective tissue dermis graft is placed and PRGF is utilized. A Straumann design standard implant is placed at a second stage. Another dermis connective tissue graft may be placed at this time.

If the attachment apparatus on the adjacent tooth is not intact when a patient presents with greater than 5 mm of vertical bone compromise, regenerative therapy is once again carried out, utilizing grafting materials beneath a titanium-reinforced membrane. Emdogain is also placed on the adjacent tooth's root surface in an attempt to effect reattachment, and a dermis connective tissue graft is placed over PRGF. Once again, a Straumann design standard implant is placed at a second stage surgical visit, with possible addition of another dermis connective tissue graft.

Conclusions

Utilized appropriately, immediate implant placement and temporization for replacement of single teeth in the esthetic zone is highly predictable and offers a plethora of patient advantages. The number of surgical insults and the overall time of therapy are decreased. Immediate implant temporization also affords the opportunity to support and control soft tissue healing, thus enhancing final esthetic treatment outcomes. However, it is imperative that appropriate case work up and diagnosis be carried out prior to the initiation of such therapy and that implant selection not be based upon manufacturer claims or financial considerations, but rather be grounded in sound biologic principles, independent research, and clinical reality.

References

1. Jaffin RA, Kumar A, and Berman CL. 2000. Immediate loading of implants in partially and fully edentulous jaws: A series of 27 case reports. *J Periodontol* 71:833–838.
2. Ganeles J, Rosenberg MM, Holt RL, and Reichman LH. 2001. Immediate loading of implants with fixed restorations in the completely edentulous mandible: Report of 27 patients from a private practice. *Int J Oral Maxillofac Implants* 16:418–426.

3. Cooper LF, Rahman A, Moriarty J, Chaffee N, and Sacco D. 2002. Immediate mandibular rehabilitation with endoseous implants: Simultaneous extraction, implant placement, and loading. *Int J Oral Maxillofac Implants* 17:517–525.
4. Norton MR. 2004. A short-term clinical evaluation of immediately restored maxillary TiOblast single-tooth implants. *Int J Oral Maxillofac Implants* 19: 274–281.
5. Cornelini R, Cangini F, Covani U, Barone A, and Buser D. 2004. Immediate restoration of single-tooth implants in mandibular molar sites: A 12-month preliminary report. *Int J Oral Maxillofac Implants* 19: 855–860.
6. Abboud M, Koeck B, Stark H, Wahl G, and Paillon R. 2005. Immediate loading of single-tooth implants in the posterior region. *Int J Oral Maxillofac Implants* 20:61–68.
7. Becker W, Sennerby L, Bedrossian E, Becker BE, and Lucchini JP. 2005. Implant stability measurements for implants placed at the time of extraction: A cohort, prospective clinical trial. *J Periodontol* 76: 391–397.
8. Becker W. 2005. Immediate implant placement: Diagnosis, treatment planning and treatment steps/or successful outcomes [Review]. *J Calif Dent Assoc* 33:303–310.
9. Quinlan P, Nummikoski P, Schenk R, et al. 2005. Immediate and early loading of SLA ITI single-tooth implants: An in vivo study. *Int J Oral Maxillofac Implants* 20:360–370.
10. Fugazzotto PA. 2005. Treatment options following single rooted tooth removal: A literature review and proposes hierarchy of treatment selection. *J Periodontol* 76:821–831.
11. Fugazzotto PA, DePaoli S, and Parma-Benfenati S. 1993. Flap design considerations in the placement of single maxillary implants. *Implant Dent* 2:93–95.
12. Fugazzotto PA. 1999. Maintenance of soft tissue closure following GBR procedures: Technical considerations and report of 723 cases. *J Periodontol* 70:1085–1097.
13. Fugazzotto PA. 2003. GBR using bovine bone matrix and resorbable and non-resorbable membranes. Part II: Clinical results. *Int J Periodontics Restorative Dent* 23:599–605.

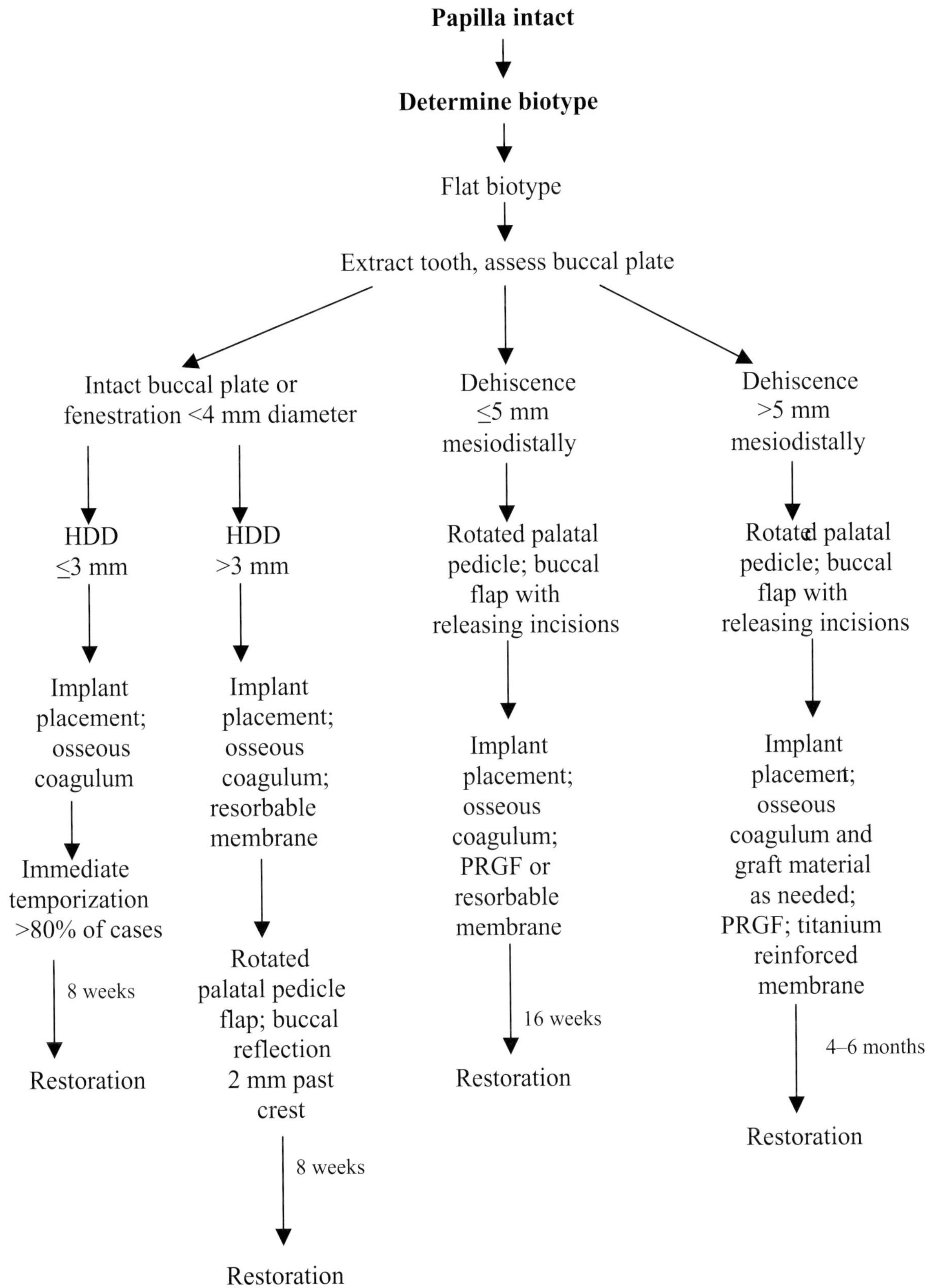

Flow chart 11.1 Decision making at the time of tooth extraction: The uncompromised site (Part 1 of 2)

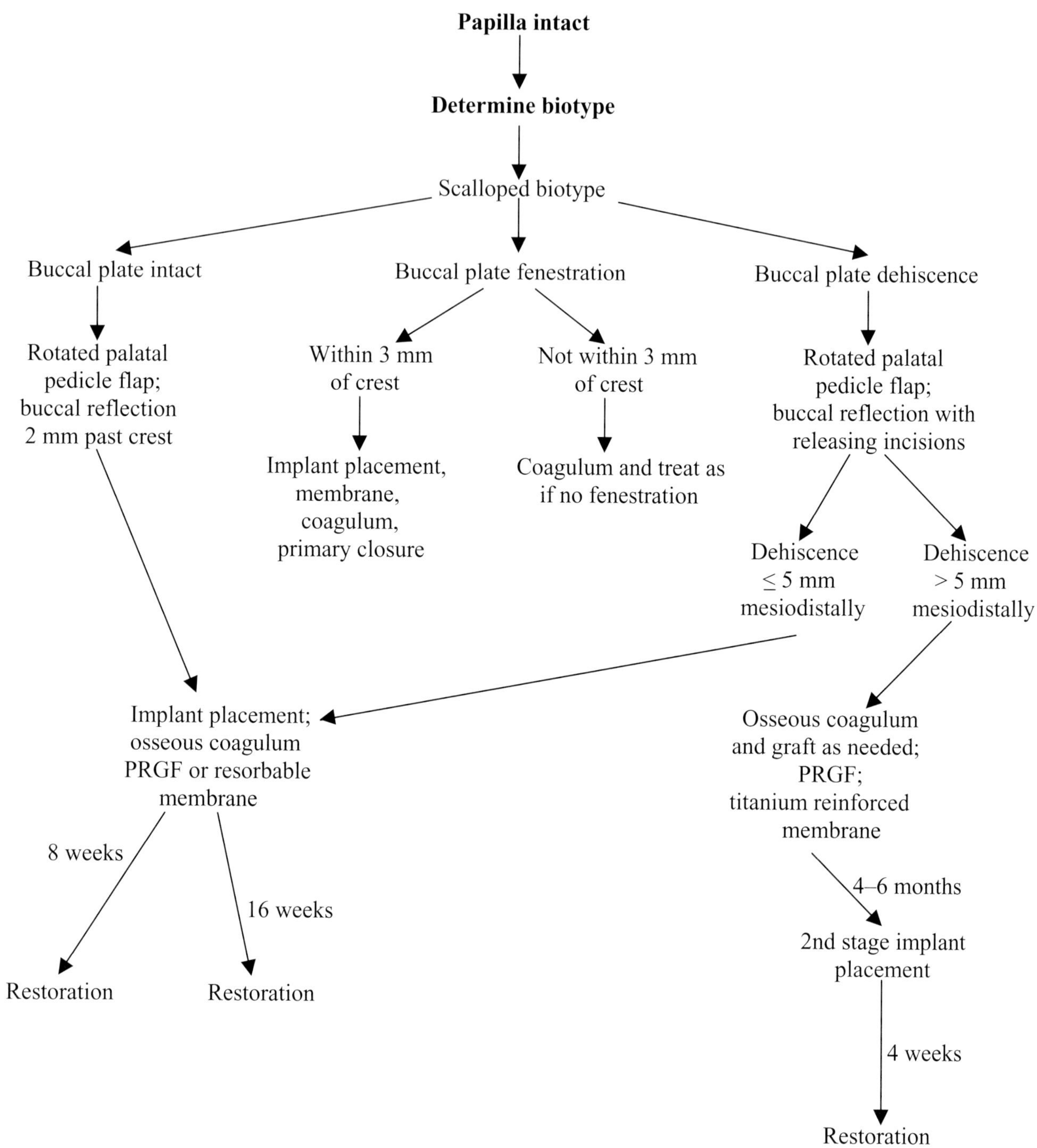

Flow chart 11.1 Decision making at the time of tooth extraction: The uncompromised site (Part 2 of 2)

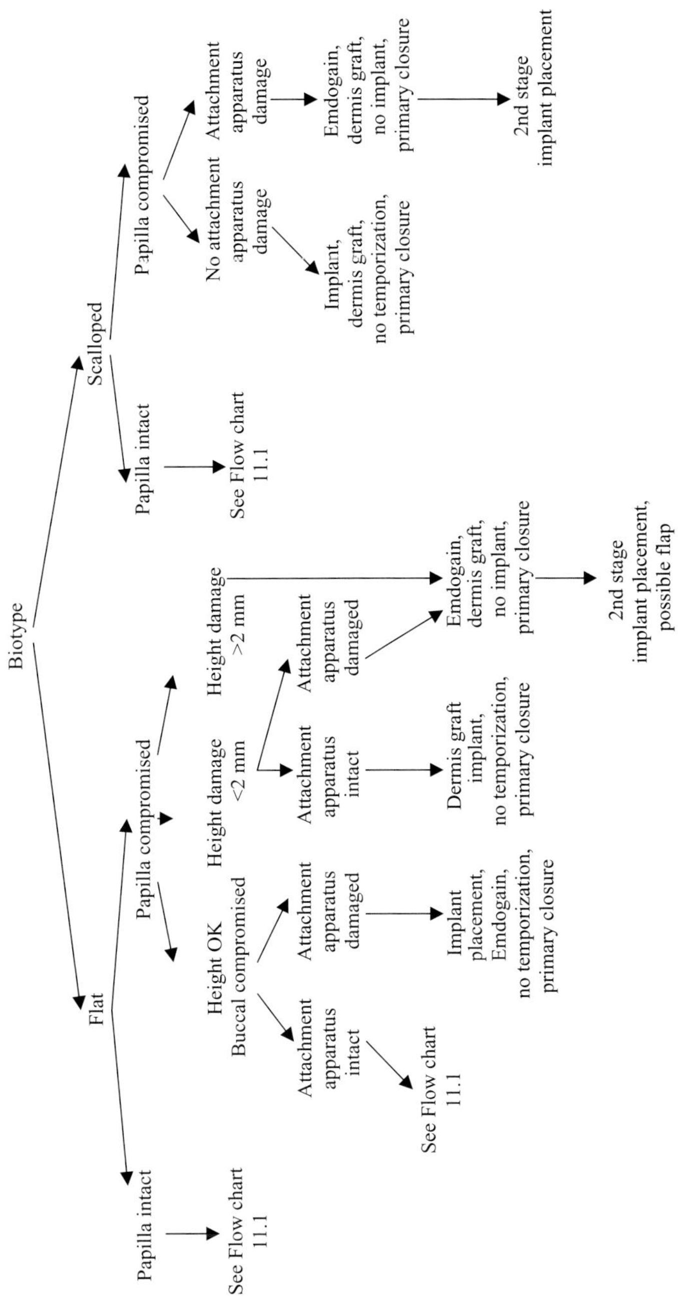

Flow chart 11.2 Decision making at the time of tooth extraction: The compromised site.

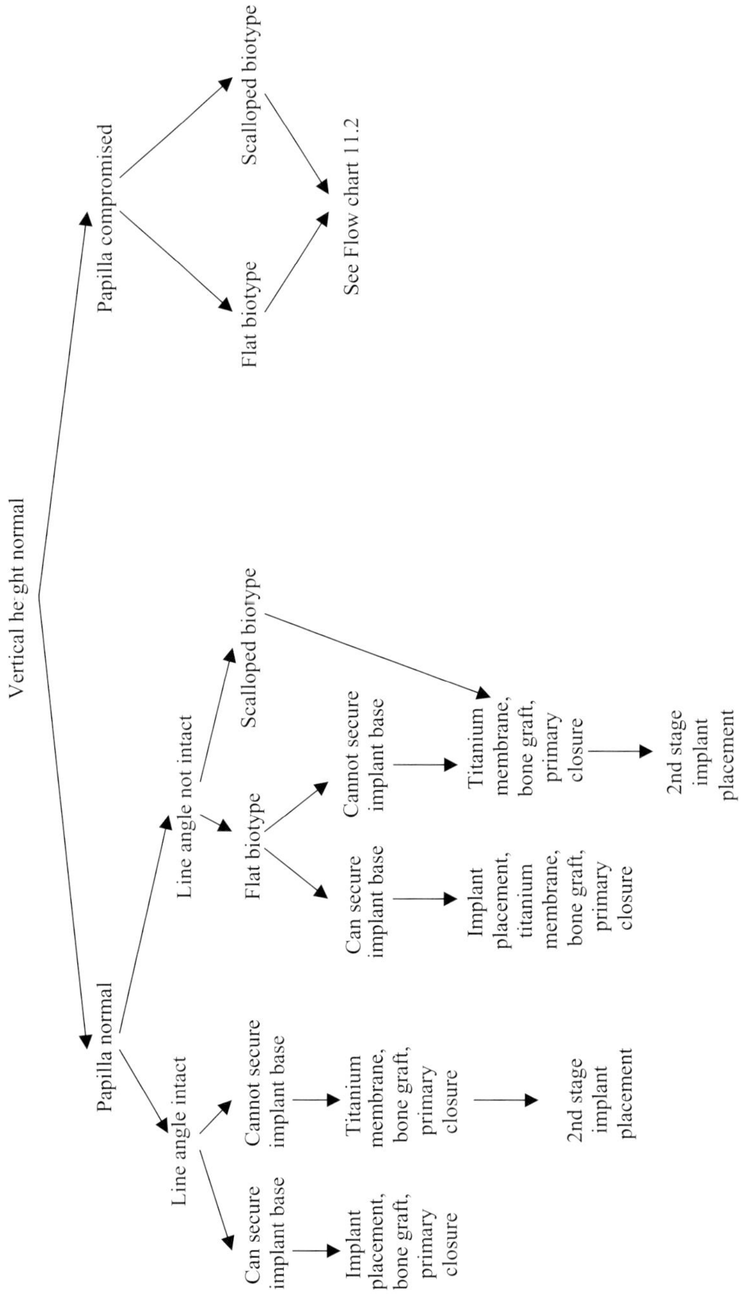

Flow chart 11.3 Implant placement in an edentulous site (Part 1 of 2).

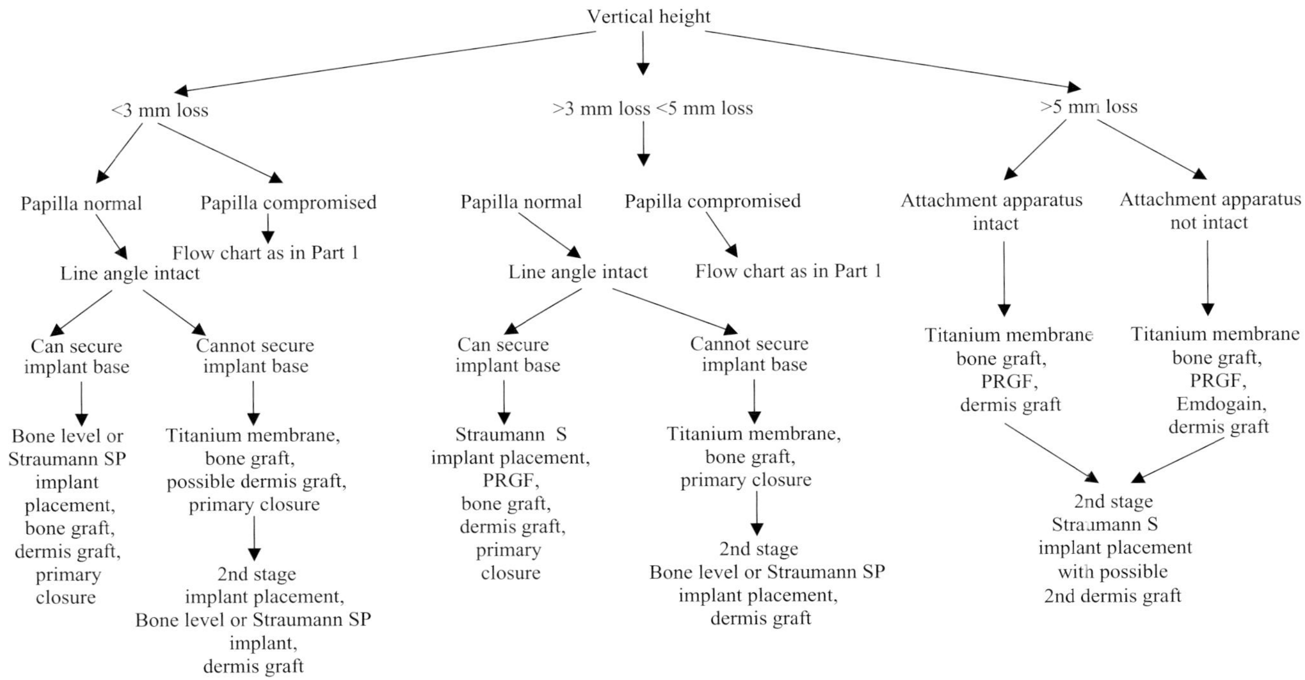

Flow chart 11.3 Implant placement in an edentulous site (Part 2 of 2).

Chapter 12

Immediate Loading of the Full Arch in Patients with a Failing Dentition

Robert Jaffin, DMD

Outline

Introduction

The use of implants to replace missing teeth has become the standard of care in most clinical situations. Their predictability, ease of placement for the patient, and longevity are some of the factors which have expanded implant utilization in clinical dentistry. Initially recommended for use in edentulous arches, implant placement has evolved to address almost all situations involving missing teeth.

Delayed loading of submerged implants was part of the initial treatment protocol, to allow for attainment of osseointegration before the implants were restored. This practice was developed both empirically and with a biologic basis (1). It was known that if implants moved during healing, they would not integrate (2). The concept of immediate loading of implants has been utilized since the mid-1990s (3). This treatment approach was developed to protect healing implants from micromotion by placing additional implants (which would eventually be removed) and loading them, allowing the submerged implants to heal without concern for overlaying force application. The concept of immediate implant loading has evolved so that many clinicians now employ such a treatment approach.

Implants installed into fresh extraction sockets (immediately placed implants) have also expanded our therapeutic options. Overall treatment times have been reduced, without a decrease in success rates or esthetic treatment outcomes (4).

Advances in implant designs and surfaces have further enhanced implant therapy. Implants no longer have to be submerged while healing. The use of single stage implants has eliminated the need for a second surgery. In addition, implant surface alterations afford faster, more predictable osseointegration.

Under specific circumstances, patients with a hopeless tooth or teeth may have implants installed in fresh extraction sockets, and teeth placed on the implants in the same day. This approach is utilized in situations ranging from a single tooth to a full arch. If the implant restoration is placed within 48 h of implant installation and is in occlusion, the implant is considered immediately loaded. If the inserted implant restoration is not in occlusal function, the term immediate temporization applies.

To appreciate these advances in implant therapy and how they relate to immediate loading, an understanding of the concepts of osseointegration are crucial. Factors such as the shape and surface of the implant, growth of bone onto the implant, and the manner in which applied forces are received by the implant are vital to predictably treating patients utilizing this mode of care.

The machined titanium surface was initially the gold standard for implants. It offered high success rates, but required healing periods of 3–6 months before loading. Roughened implant surfaces not only afford shorter healing times, but also demonstrate higher torque removal values and increased bone-to-implant contact at earlier time frames than their smooth-surfaced counterparts (5). Hydrophilic, micro-roughened surfaces have further reduced healing times (6). These advances can be traced to the cellular level. It has been demonstrated that roughened implant surfaces stabilize clot formation, which plays a key role in cell behavior and osseoinduction (7, 8). Since the clot was not as well attached to machined titanium, the cellular response was slower, thus requiring longer integration periods to achieve similar torque removal values and bone to implant contact as roughened surface implants. A roughened surface texture on the implant is beneficial when employing an immediate loading protocol, as more rapid osseointegration reduces the risk of implant loss.

The forces received by the implant and bone can be simulated utilizing finite element analysis (FEA) (9). In FEA, implants are placed in a material which simulates bone, and the forces placed on the "bone" by the implant are measured. Numerous studies demonstrate that most of the applied stresses are received by the crestal aspect of the implant, at the crestal bone (10). Increases in implant diameter lead to better stress reduction at the bone implant interface than do increases in implant length (11). Therefore, the concept of crown-to-implant ratio is not as relevant as when dealing with teeth. This fact has been validated in clinical studies that show high success rates with short implants, as discussed in Chapter 7 (12).

FEA have also established the fact that the implant abutment interface plays a key role in how occlusal forces are translated to surrounding bone. The implant/abutment interface (I/A) can be separated into two basic types: conical and flat-top (external hex). The peak interfacial shear stress is seen at marginal bone with both flat-top and conical I/A. However, axial stress is smaller and located deeper in the bone with the conical I/A interface than with the flat-top I/A, where the axial stress is located at the osseous crest. Therefore, the conical I/A resists larger axial loads than the flat-top I/A (13). It has also been demonstrated that the conical I/A resists axial bending forces much better than the flat-top I/A (14). As a result, the conical I/A offers a more advantageous situation in immediate loading.

Implants will integrate if micromotion of the implants does not exceed 150 μm during healing (2). This is a key element in the success of immediate loading of implants. Factors such as bone density, implant length, diameter, configuration and surface, as well as the number of implants placed, are all crucial to a successful treatment outcome. Numerous studies have demonstrated that osseointegration rates are generally lower in soft (type IV) bone with a machined titanium surface (15). However, roughened surface implants exhibit much greater bone to implant contact in type IV bone than their smooth surface counterparts (16).

The faster the implant integrates, the sooner concerns over external factors such as patient compliance are eliminated. The surface of the implant is a key determinant in this speed of integration. At installation, the primary stability of an implant is due to the screw's retention in the bone. Over time, bone grows onto the implant in the grooves between the threads, and bone resorption occurs in the area of primary stability. If bone growth can be accelerated, the duration of loss of primary stability will be diminished, and the implant will integrate sooner (Figure 12.1). Studies have

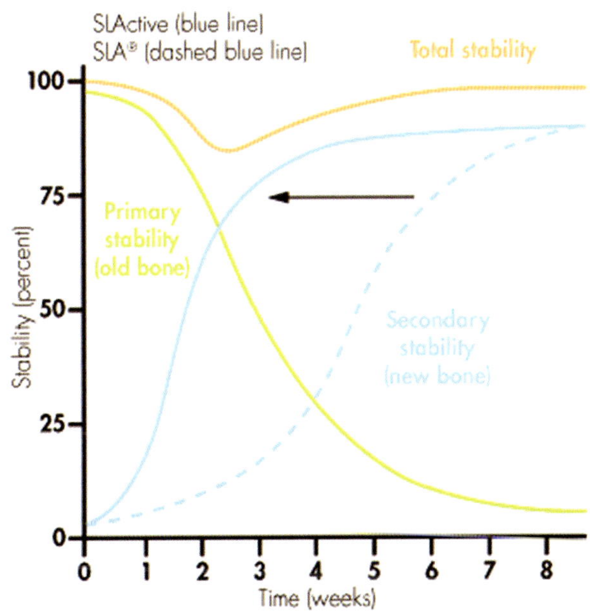

Figure 12.1 Graph demonstrating primary stability versus integration over time.

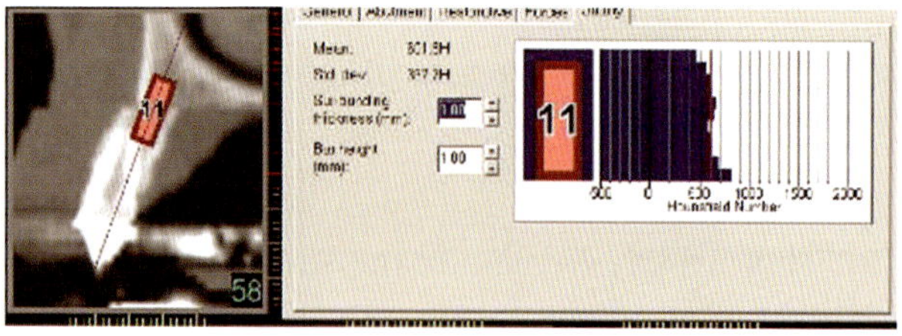

Figure 12.2 An oblique CT of an implant placed apical to the tooth, with density measures.

demonstrated increases in both bone apposition and density over time around implants (17). It was further shown that these increases occur more rapidly on a roughened than on a machined surface implant (18).

Since it is vital for the implant to be stable when immediately loaded, bone density becomes an important factor. Bone density readings can be obtained preoperatively with a CAT scan (Figure 12.2). If the bone density is less than 375–400 Hounsfield units, wider, longer implants must be considered. Tests for implant stability such as resonance frequency analysis (RFA) help determine the implant stability quotient (ISQ) at installation (19). These tests do not determine bone density but rather implant stability, which is a function not only of bone density but also of implant diameter, length, and configuration.

Utilizing this basic understanding of implant physiology and bone biology, a rationale for immediate loading has evolved. In order to load an implant at installation it must be stable enough to not move more than 150 μm under function. Bone density at the site of the implant should be determined in advance. If there is any question regarding implant stability, a wider implant should be selected before choosing a longer implant. The implant should have a micro-roughened surface and a conical I/A.

The key question that must be answered when contemplating immediate loading of a full arch is: Can a sufficient number of implants of adequate dimensions be placed in bone of adequate density to support an arch of teeth while the implants are integrating? If the answer to the above question is affirmative, the presurgical prosthetic planning stage may begin.

Treatment Planning

The determination of whether and when to extract or save teeth is based upon a host of factors. Of paramount importance is the patient's health. Can the patient tolerate the procedure? What are the ramifications of performing dental work on the patient? What medications is the patient taking? Will dental procedures interfere with the medications? Will the medications interfere with the dental procedure? Can the patient stop taking the medications? Once these questions have been answered, a general dental evaluation must be performed.

The patient's past dental history must be considered. Does the patient have a high caries rate? What is the patient's periodontal history? Has the patient had successful endodontics performed? Is there a history of root fracture? Has the patient been compliant? If there is a history of failure, are "heroics" indicated?

A thorough examination of the oral cavity should be performed. Each tooth must be evaluated regarding its long-term prognosis. An evaluation of periodontal support and restorability are necessary to determine whether a tooth is to be maintained. If the tooth has a good prognosis, does it aid in the long-term restoration of the arch?

With the high long-term success rates and stability of bone levels around implants, is there a benefit to maintaining natural teeth between implants? Is our primary goal as dentists to maintain the natural dentition in health, or to provide treatment which will offer the patient the best long-term prognosis, delivered over a realistic time interval, with the least amount of maintenance, for a reasonable fee? Patients do not want grief or aggravation. They also do not want to repeat therapy again and again and again. Therefore, when developing a treatment plan for a full arch rehabilitation, one must ask whether the retention of specific teeth will enhance or diminish the chances of attaining and maintaining the best long-term result.

Traditionally, patients who were losing their dentitions and were committed to having full arch implant supported restorations were either transitioned into full dentures while the implants were healing or underwent serial extractions. The problem with wearing a full denture over healing implants is that the denture can create

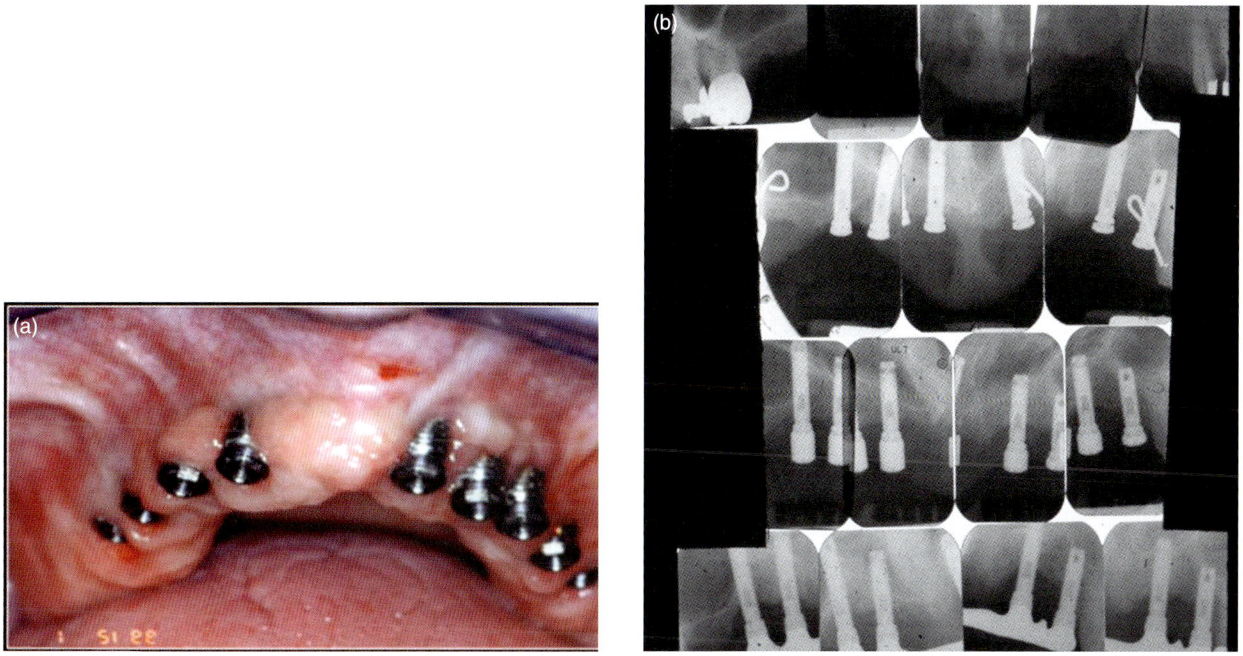

Figure 12.3 (a) Picture of implants that lost bone, under denture during integration. (b) A radiographic view of implants which lost bone during healing, under a denture.

micromotion, which may lead to implant and/or bone loss (Figures 12.3a–b).

Serial extraction involves saving enough teeth to place a full arch provisional fixed restoration, extraction of the remaining teeth and either installing implants in the sockets or permitting the sockets to heal and then placing implants. This treatment provides an ideal means by which to avoid the patient having to wear a denture. However, many disadvantages to this approach are evident. The selected abutment teeth frequently preclude the placement of all of the implants that are required, or placement of all implant in the desired positions. As a result, a second series of extractions and implant surgery become necessary. In such a situation, a second and sometimes third provisional restoration needs to be fabricated when the implants have integrated and the remaining teeth are extracted. These provisional restorations frequently require adjustment and/or repair. Multiple surgeries and provisional restorations add time (sometimes as long as two years) and additional fees to therapy.

The benefits of immediate implant loading are that the patient is converted from a failing dentition to a fixed dentition within 48 h, and that this approach eliminates the problems associated with serial extractions or full dentures. Success rates exceeding 90% in the treatment of full arches with immediately loaded implants have been reported (19–21).

Once it has been established that the dentition is hopeless, a series of steps must be followed to ensure that the planned day of surgery will run smoothly. Extensive presurgical planning by the restorative dentist and surgeon must be undertaken (Table 12.1)

The restorative dentist must perform a prosthetic evaluation. Esthetic parameters such as smile line, midline, tooth proportion, tooth position, lip support, phonetics, type of occlusion, and tooth

Table 12.1 Steps for presurgical planning.

- Mounted casts for occlusal evaluation and tooth position
- Radiographic evaluation
- Determine sites after wax-up
- Determine type of provisional (screw vs. cement and hybrid vs. crown and bridge)
- Fabricate template

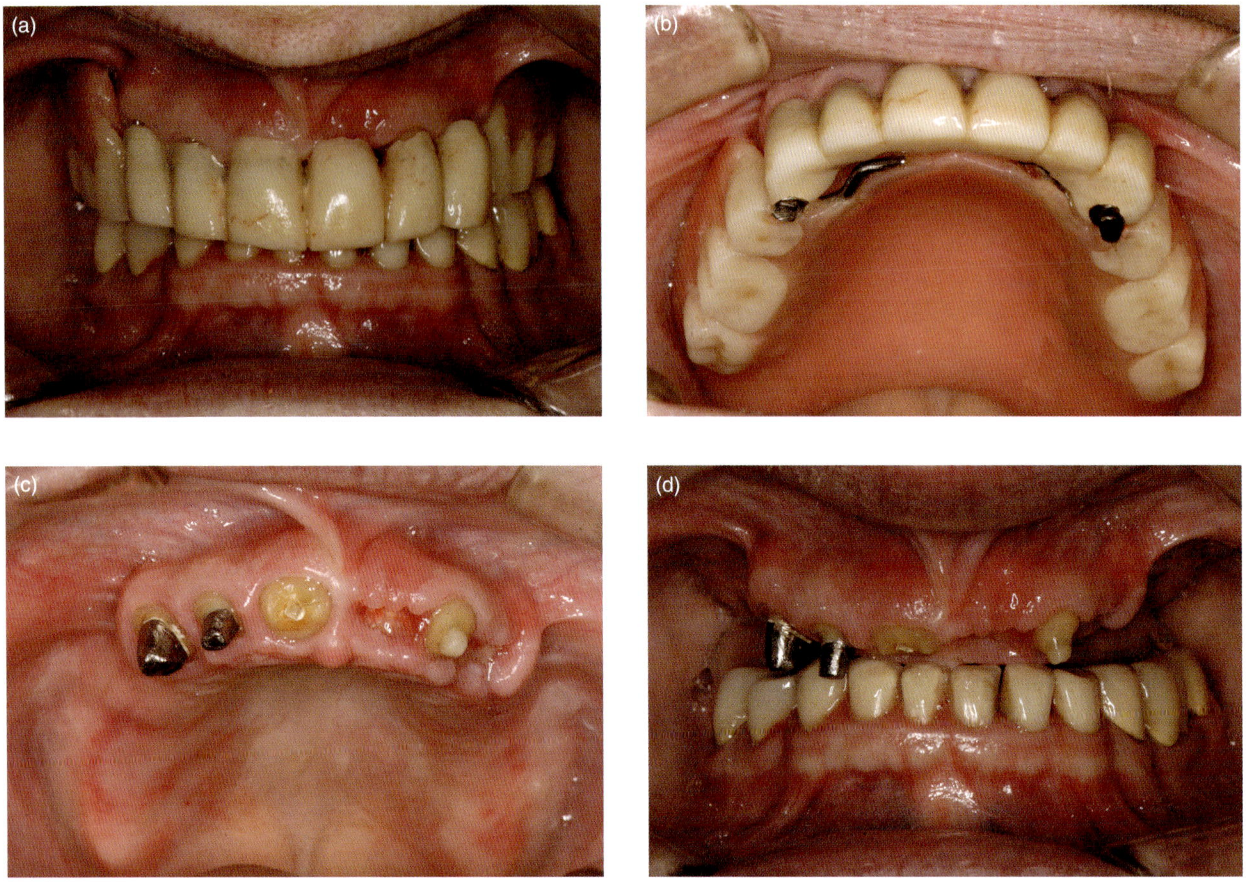

Figure 12.4 (a–d) A patient presents with a hopeless maxillary dentition.

length must be addressed. The amount of soft tissue loss and the patient's occlusal patterns and habits must be taken into consideration. The patient's esthetic expectations and psychological makeup must also be acknowledged. This pretreatment workup will determine whether the implants can be loaded immediately and whether a hybrid or crown and bridge-type prosthesis, cement- or screw-retained, or direct or indirect technique (where the implants must be indexed) will be utilized (Figures 12.4 and 12.5a–b).

Surgical templates must be fabricated. If the patient is going to be scanned, radio-opaque markers are added to the stent, so the patient can wear the stent during the CAT scan. The templates will be used during implant surgery. One template should be an omnivac shell which will cover the palate or have a positive seat in the mandible. The other stent should be reinforced with a nonpliable material, with the buccal halves of the teeth cut away and a 2-mm groove placed in the center of each tooth, where the bur can be placed (Figures 12.6a–c).

During the planning stages of therapy it is advisable to attempt to retain one tooth on each side of the arch during surgery, preferably a molar, to help stabilize the template and aid in taking a bite registration.

Radiographic evaluation should begin with a full series of parallel periapical radiographs. From these film, crestal bone levels, apical bone volume, root proximity, and periapical pathology can be observed (Figure 12.7). Anatomic structures such as the mandibular canal and maxillary sinuses can also be viewed. If the periapical radiographs do not reveal the above, a CAT scan is recommended.

The CAT scan is beneficial because it provides a more accurate assessment of the bone and teeth. Precise distances can be measured including tooth length, apical bone, distance to the mandibular canal and planned implant size. The density of the bone adjacent to the planned implant, a key

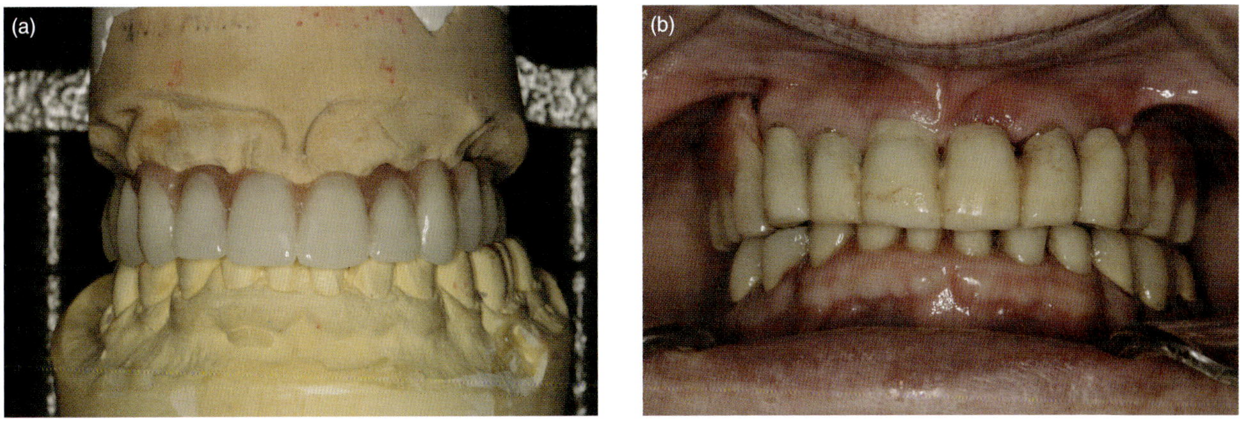

Figure 12.5 (a–b) A prosthetic wax-up of the case is carried out to determine proper tooth position.

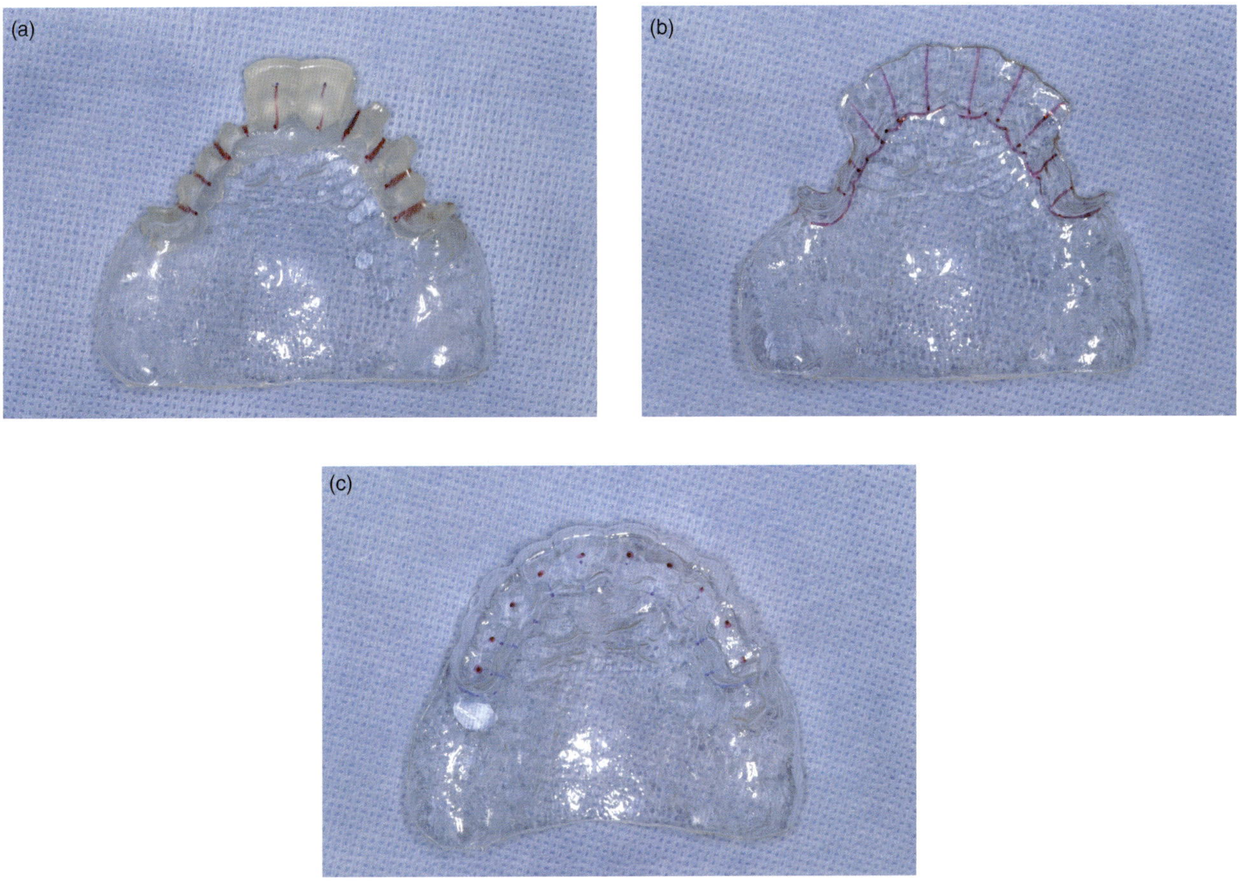

Figure 12.6 (a–c) Templates have been made from a wax-up. Note the buccal cut away, and clear vacuform with the entire tooth present.

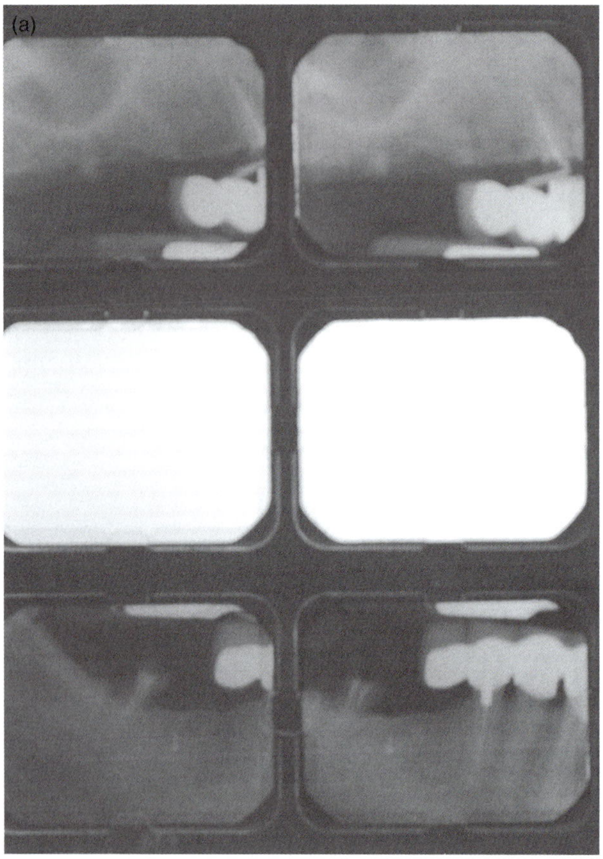

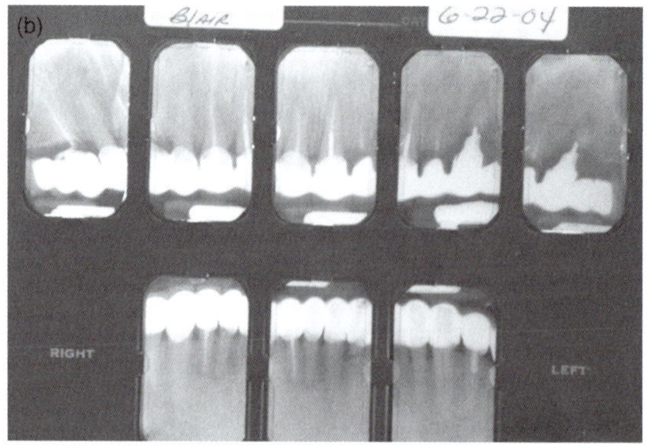

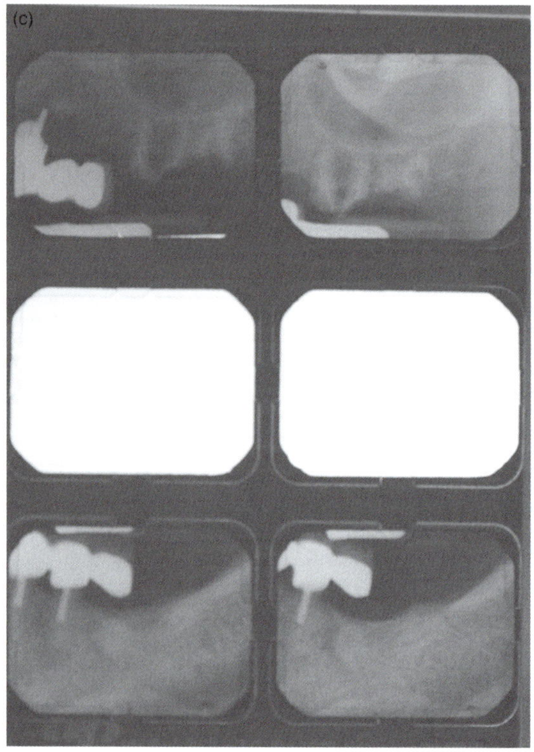

Figure 12.7 Periapical radiographs of the patient.

determinant for successful immediate loading, may be assessed. The inter-implant position, which will determine parallelism of the implants is also established. The entire case is planned beforehand to maximize predictability and success of therapy (Figures 12.8 and 12.9a–b).

Individual sites are selected which ensure at least 8 mm of implant will be embedded in bone with a density greater than 375–400 Hounsfield units, so as to offer adequate primary stability for the implants which are to be immediately loaded (Figure 12.10). Adjacent maxillary anterior implants are avoided, to reduce esthetic complications and restorative difficulties. A distance of 3 mm must be present between adjacent implant shoulders.

The primary goal of implant placement is to supply a foundation to support 10–12 teeth for both the immediately loaded and final restorations. In the maxilla, 6 implants are recommended; 4–6 implants are recommended in the mandible. Placing an insufficient number of implants will lead to

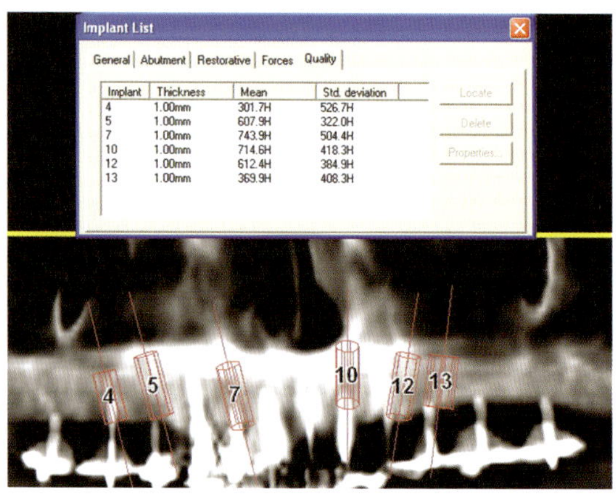

Figure 12.8 A panoramic view from the CT, with implants in place and density measurements.

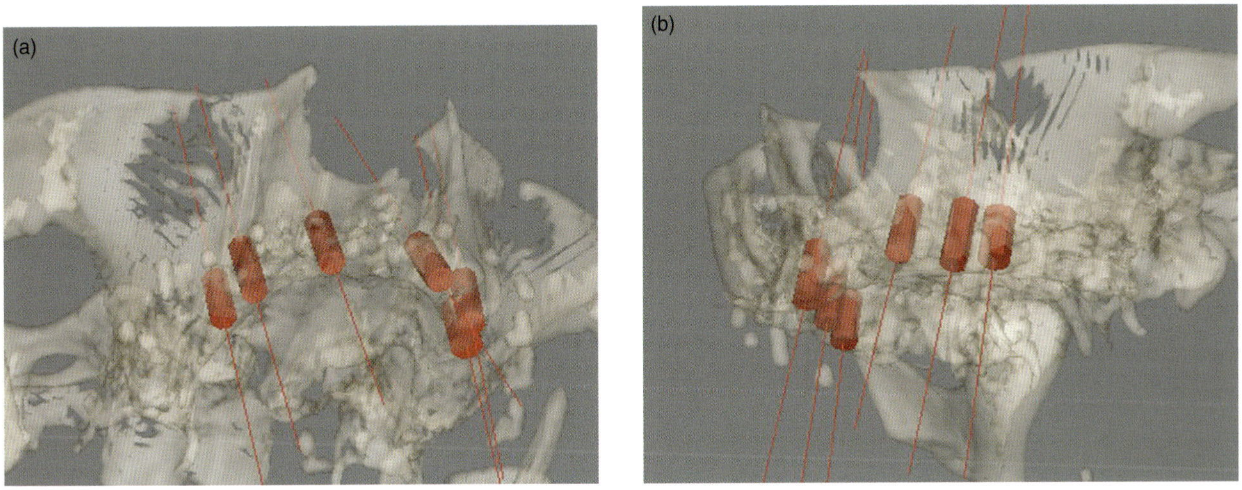

Figure 12.9 (a–b) Three-dimensional views from the CT with implants in place.

implant overload and implant loss. When installing more than 6 implants in an arch, attaining passivity of the provisional restoration becomes an issue (Figure 12.11).

The ideal positions for six implants in the mandible are first molars, first bicuspids, and lateral incisors; or first bicuspids and lateral incisors if four are to be placed. If the mandibular cuspid areas are fresh extraction sites, they are not considered primary implant sites due to the diameter and length of the root and the thin buccal alveolar plate. If the location of the mandibular canal precludes placing an implant of 8 mm in length, all implants are placed at least 5 mm anterior to the mental foramen to avoid the canal and anterior loop. Due to favorable anatomy, parallelism of the implants in full arch mandibular cases is generally achievable (Figures 12.12 and 12.13a–d).

In the maxilla, the first molar, first bicuspid, and lateral incisor sites are the ideal locations in which to place implants to produce a 12-tooth restoration. However, the first molar is rarely available as an implant location without augmentation. Therefore, the second bicuspid site is the most common distal implant position in maxillary immediate load cases. If the cuspid is a fresh extraction, the socket is generally wide, deep, and has a thin buccal alveolar plate. It offers a poor site for an immediately loaded implant. The lateral incisors offer the ideal anterior positions because they are not adjacent to each other, and the thick palatal wall

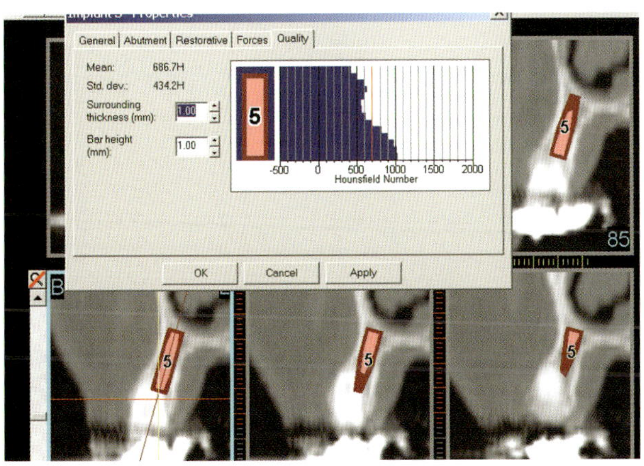

Figure 12.10 An oblique view of site 5, with density measurement (apical area).

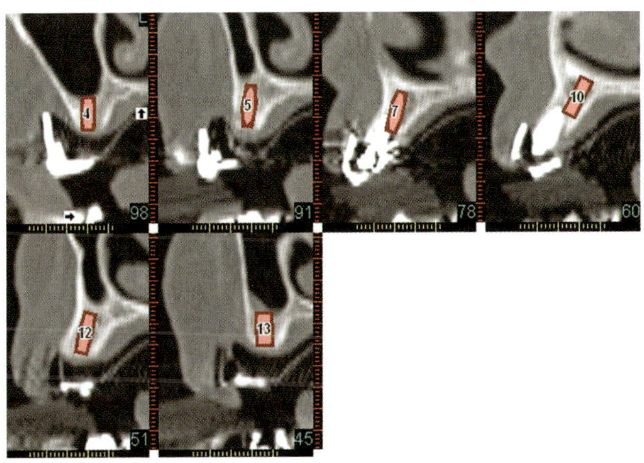

Figure 12.11 Oblique views of the six selected sites (4, 5, 7, 10, 12, 13).

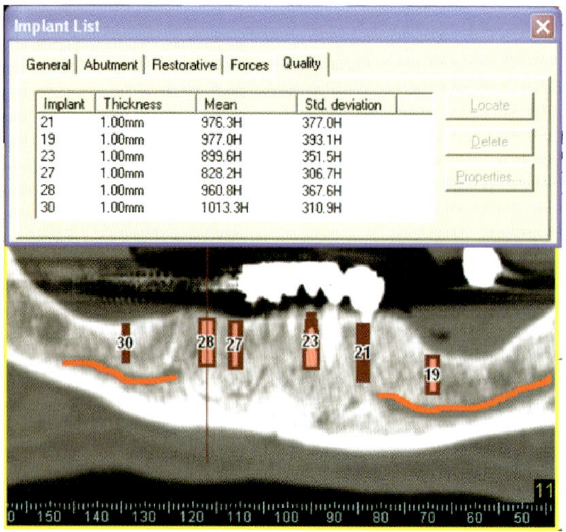

Figure 12.12 A mandibular panorex from the CT, with six sites selected, and bone density readings.

of the extraction socket affords excellent stability to the implant (Figures 12.14a–b).

Implant parallelism between the right and left sides of the arch is usually not achievable due to the resorptive patterns of the maxilla. This situation can be visualized using the three-dimensional view in the CAT scan program. There are many ways to compensate for this problem. If a cement-retained provisional restoration is planned, the implants on each side are installed parallel to each other, and the provisional restoration is fabricated in two pieces (right and left), then luted in the mouth at the midline (Figures 12.15a–b). If a screw-retained provisional restoration is planned, the implants at the lateral incisor sites are placed parallel to each other with the screw-access chambers in the cingulum. The implants placed in the posterior sites are parallel to each

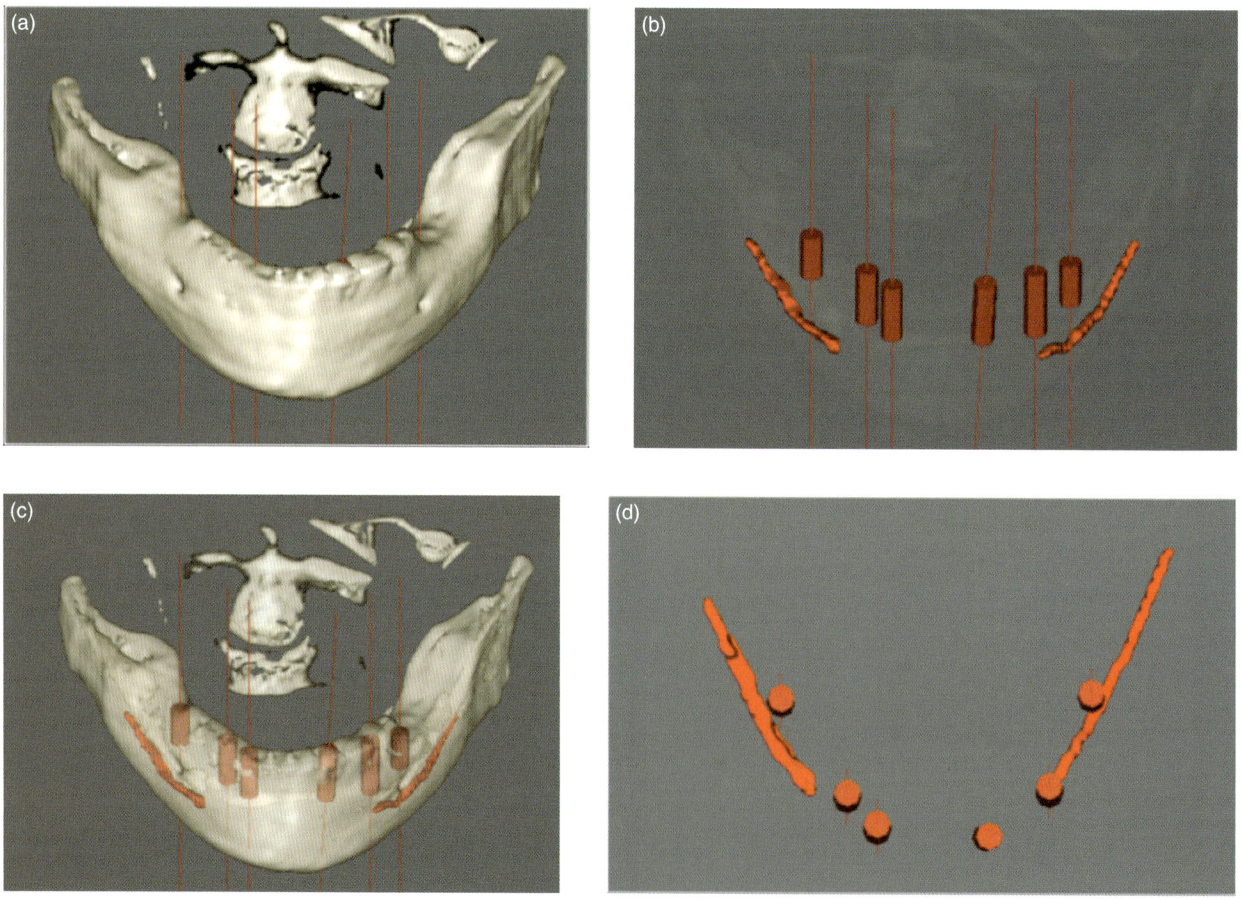

Figure 12.13 (a–d) Three-dimensional views of the mandible showing the mandibular canal and the implants.

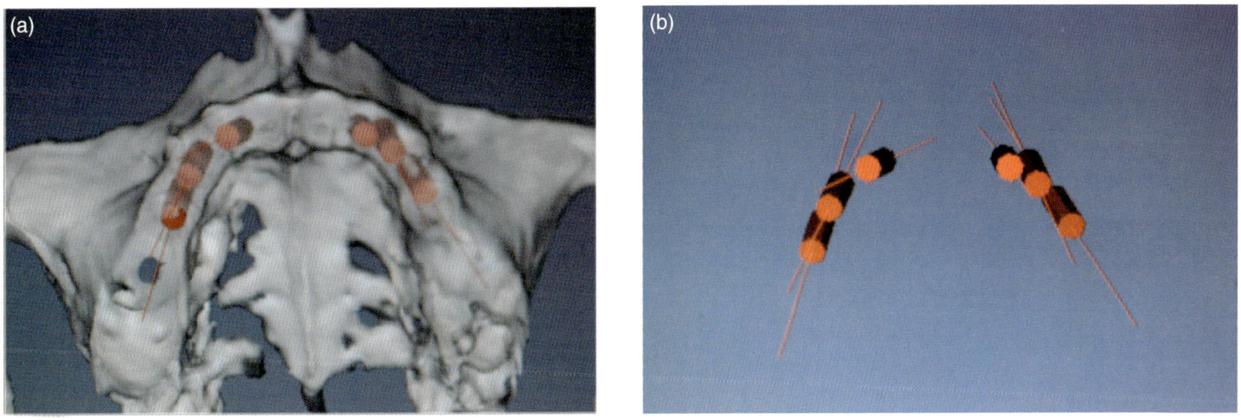

Figure 12.14 (a–b) Three-dimensional views of the maxilla demonstrating ideal implant positions and divergence of the implants from side to side.

other on each side, with the access channels placed in the central fossae. This fact will be important in the final restoration (Figures 12.16a–b). If a one piece, cemented provisional restoration is planned, the use of angled abutments will most likely be necessary.

In the presurgical planning phase, all contingencies must be anticipated. A patient who is dentate and having their teeth extracted expects to have a "new" dentition placed that day or soon thereafter. If there is any chance that the case may not be immediately loaded, a denture must be made ready as a standby (Table 12.2).

Implant sites are never prepared for the largest possible implant size, in the event that a "rescue" implant becomes necessary. Templates with sleeves are not used because, if there is a change in implant position or angulation due to complications at the planned site, the template would be rendered useless. Therefore, the template must accurately indicate tooth position without limiting implant angulation.

Before the patient is scheduled for surgery, the surgeon and the restorative dentist review the case a final time. The templates are verified in the patient's mouth. The inventory of implants and prosthetic components is checked. All contingencies are planned for. The goal is to have the day of immediate implant loading run as smoothly as a Beethoven symphony (Table 12.3).

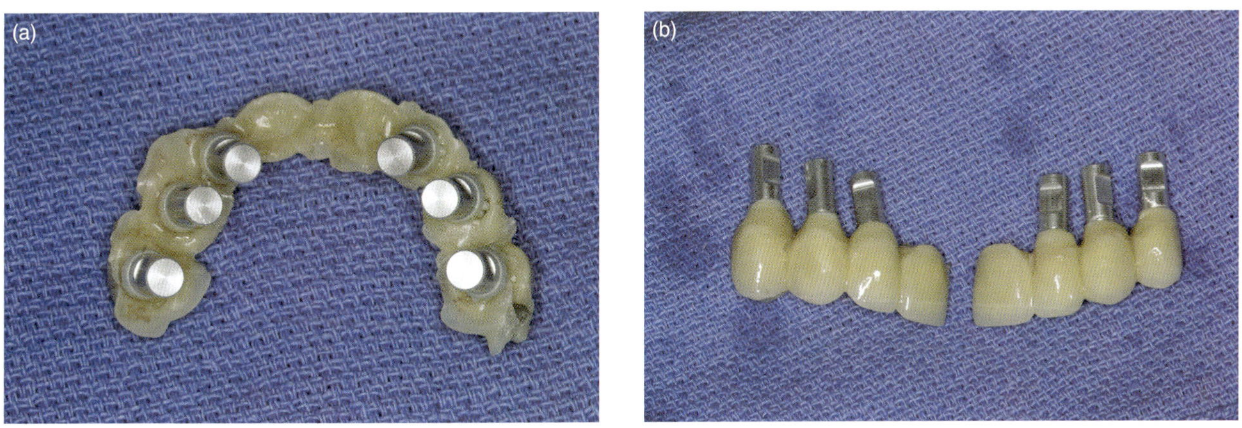

Figure 12.15 (a–b) Provisional restoration of maxilla demonstrates divergence of the implants from the right to left sides and appropriate contours of the carved provisional.

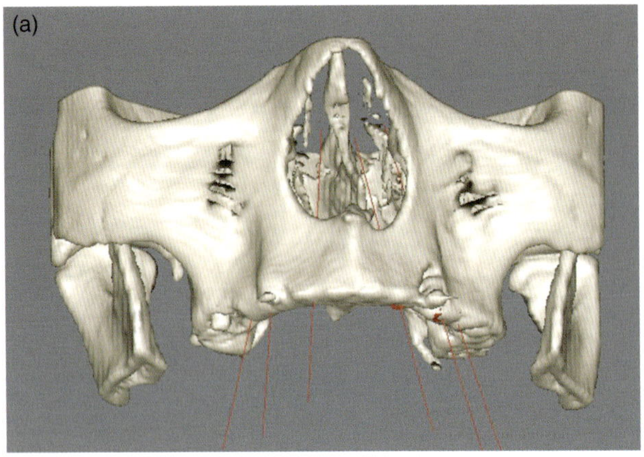

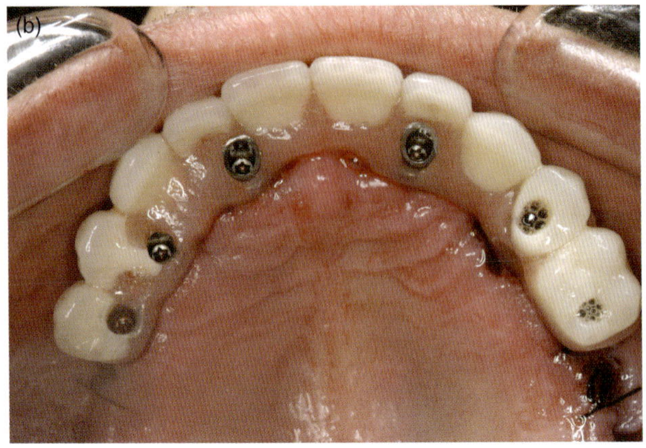

Figure 12.16 (a–b) Three-dimensional views of the maxilla demonstrating divergence of the implants and proper positioning of screw-access channels in the provisional.

Table 12.2 Criteria for immediate load therapy.

- Ability to place a minimum of four implants in the mandible and six in the maxilla, dispersed throughout the arch
- Implants must be secured in 8 mm of bone
- Density of bone must exceed 350–400 Hounsfield units
- Ability to place implants parallel to each other in the mandible
- Ability to place the implant shoulder at the buccal crest of bone
- Adjacent maxillary anterior implants are avoided
- Mandible site priority—if no bone is available superior to alveolar canal:
    - Intraforaminal placement
        - Four implants: anterior sites laterals, then cuspids; posterior sites second molars, then first molars
        - Five implants: central incisor implant placed first, then most posterior implant, usually second bicuspid if not first bicuspid, last two implants spaced between anterior and posterior implants
        - Six implants: posterior sites distal to mental foramen anterior sites—primary position—lateral incisor then cuspids; second site is generally first bicuspid; distal site either first molar or second bicuspid
- Maxilla
    - Six implants: anterior sites—ideal are; lateral incisors; if unusable then one central, one lateral, cuspids are third priority site; both centrals is last choice; middle site;—first bicuspid; distal site;—ideal is first molar but usually second molar
    - Bicuspid

Table 12.3 Criteria for type of immediate prosthesis.

- Evaluate esthetic profile
    - High smile, small teeth, thin biotype—hybrid
    - Multiple missing anterior teeth—hybrid
    - Lip support needed—hybrid
    - Any esthetic, tooth, hard or soft tissues deformities—hybrid

Surgery

The patient is premedicated with Amoxicillin 2 g or another appropriate antibiotic, 1 h before the scheduled treatment. An antiseptic scrub (Chlorhexidine gluconate 2%) is applied throughout the oral cavity. The templates are checked to verify a positive seat. The patient is draped for implant surgery.

Extractions are performed as atraumatically as possible. Molars are sectioned, and all sockets are thoroughly debrided following tooth removal.

As a general rule, selected sites should provide the most optimal bone available, while avoiding adjacent anterior implants. The anterior sites are prepared first. Sharp, new burs are employed to avoid chattering, which can shatter the supporting walls of a site. If all alveolar walls surrounding an implant are present, no augmentation will be required.

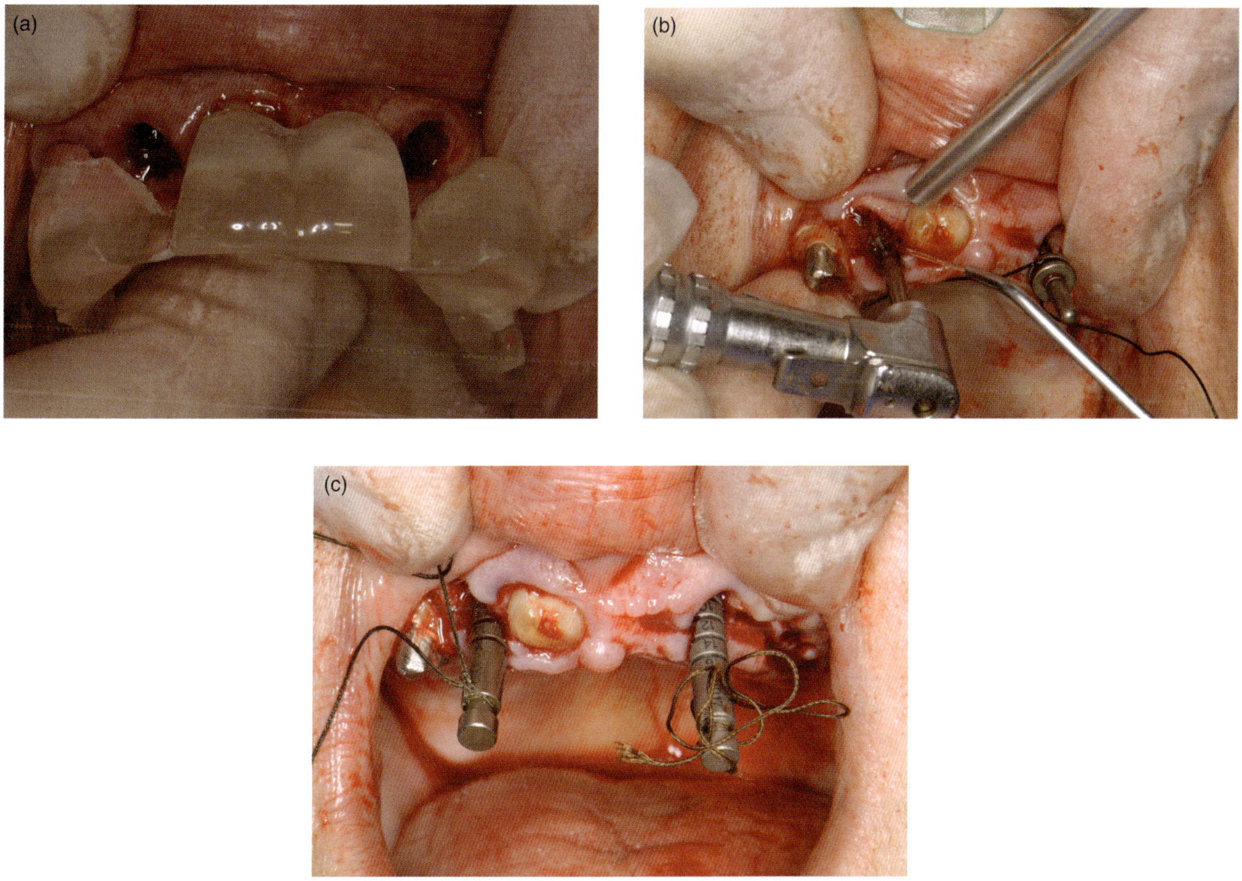

Figure 12.17 (a–c) A view of the maxillary surgery, demonstrating template utilization and parallel placement of the lateral incisor implants.

In the mandible, once the patient has been draped and the teeth have been extracted, the residual alveolar ridge is flattened to avoid ridge height discrepancies, and to help ensure that the implant shoulders will be at the same height. The template is placed in the mouth and the anterior sites are prepared. If the provisional restoration is going to be screw retained, the access holes will be placed on the cingulum. If a cement-retained prosthesis is planned, the implants should line up with the incisal edges of the prosthesis. This is verified with the clear omnivac stent.

The posterior sites are subsequently prepared utilizing the solid template with buccal grooves. Parallelism is generally attainable and can be verified with directional indicators and the clear template. Once the sites have been prepared and the implants installed, a visual check will determine whether bone covers any part of the implant shoulder. Should this occur, a bone profiler is used to eliminate the excess bone. Chisels may also be required if there is a significant scallop to the extraction socket.

In the maxilla, the surgery is generally more difficult in the anterior segment. The apices of the lateral incisors have a distal cant. Care must be taken to ensure that the implants do not emerge from the interproximal (lateral/central) areas. The initial access hole should be made in the palatal bone, approximately 2/3 of the way toward the apices of the sockets. The solid template with grooves is very helpful in determining these positions. If a screw-retained prosthesis is planned, the access holes must emerge from the cingula. If a cement restoration is planned, the solid abutments should line up with the incisal edges of the restoration. This fact is verified with the clear stent (Figures 12.17a–c).

Posterior implant placement will depend upon the type of restoration which will be

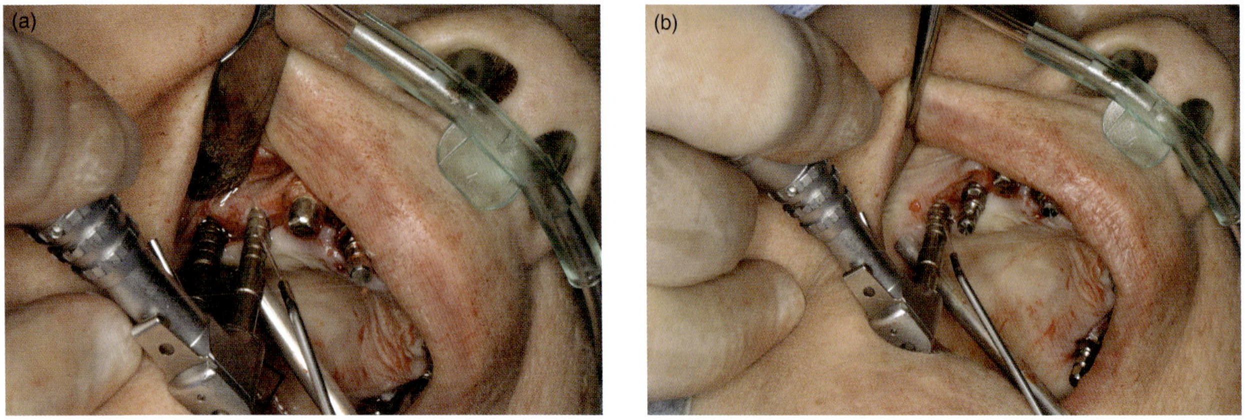

Figure 12.18 (a–b) A view of maxillary posterior implant placement with parallelism.

fabricated. If the restoration is to be cement retained, the posterior implants must be parallel to the anterior implant on a given side. Since there is a labial flare to the premaxilla, the posterior implants will either have an anterior tilt, or angled abutments will be employed. Screw-retained prostheses permit vertical placement of the implants in the posterior sockets, as a lack of parallelism can be compensated for in the restoration (Figures 12.18a–b, 12.19a–b, and 12.20a–b).

Since many of the implants are sitting in sockets that are scalloped, great care must be taken to remove any bone over the implant shoulders, as such bone could preclude proper seating of the impression or temporary cylinders. As previously discussed, this is accomplished through the use of a bone profiler (Figures 12.21a–b).

Prosthetics

SCREW-RETAINED PROVISIONAL RESTORATIONS

Once the implants have been placed, the shoulders and internal configurations of the implants should be free of tissue and blood. Solid abutments are loosely connected to the implants and a bite is taken with a very fast setting registration mousse (Figures 12.22a–b). If any teeth have been retained to help establish a bite and vertical dimension, they are now extracted. An implant level, open tray impression utilizing a heavy body material is taken (Figure 12.23). Large healing covers, lubricated with Neosporin or petroleum jelly, are gently affixed to the implants. The flaps are loosely sutured (Figure 12.24).

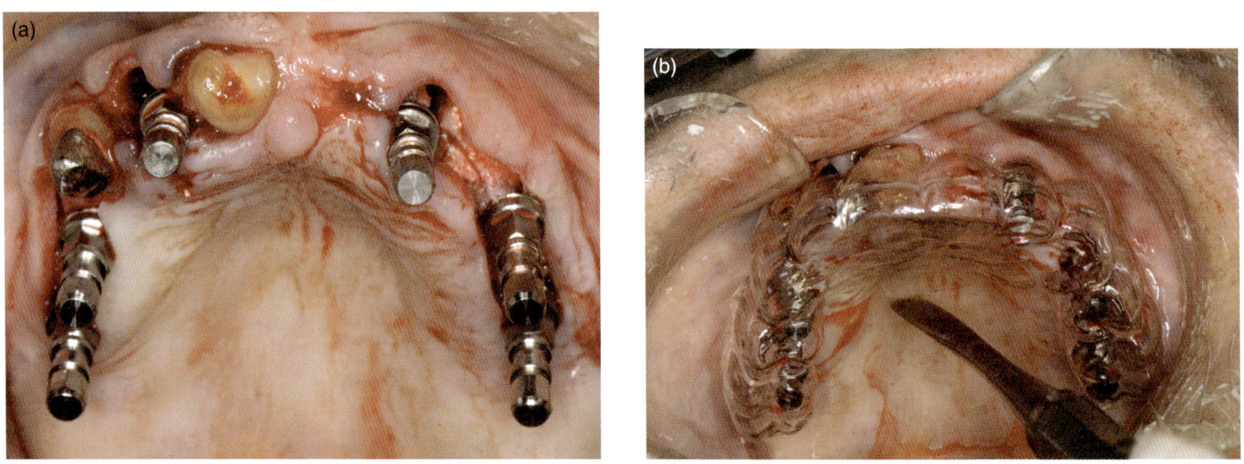

Figure 12.19 (a–b) Six implants are installed with the aid of surgical templates.

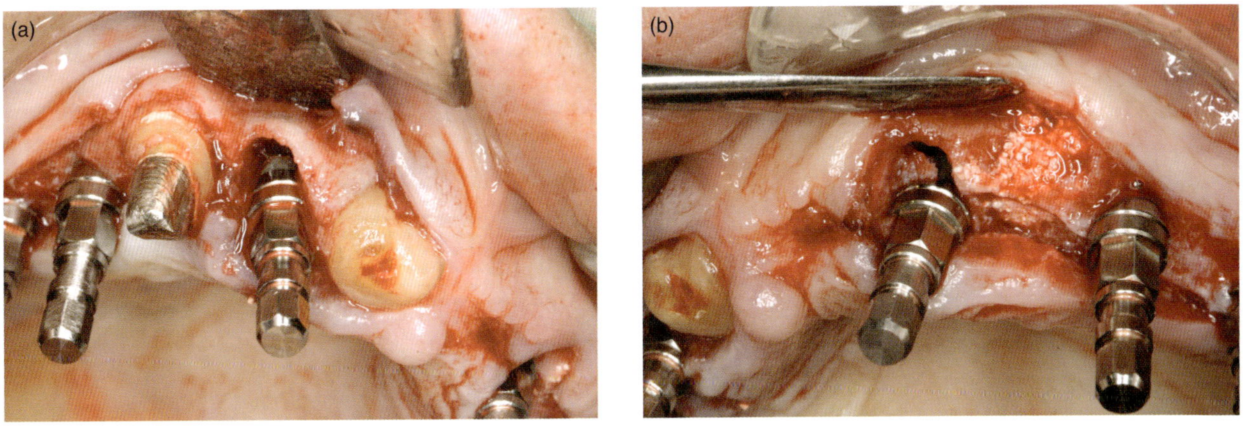

Figure 12.20 (a–b) A view of the implants in sockets, with the scalloped alveolar crest.

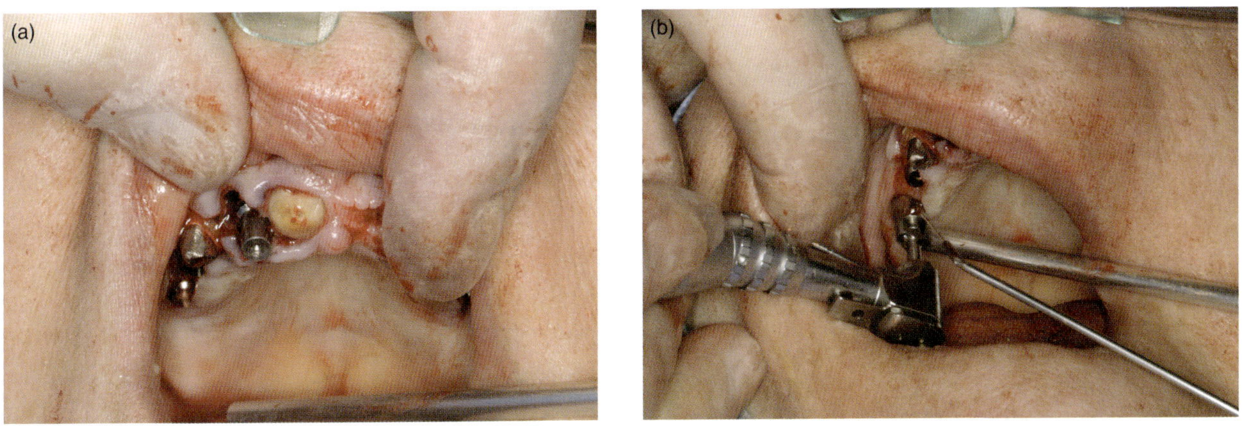

Figure 12.21 (a–b) Bone profiling is carried out to reduce excess interproximal bone, thus allowing seating of the impression coping or temporary cylinder.

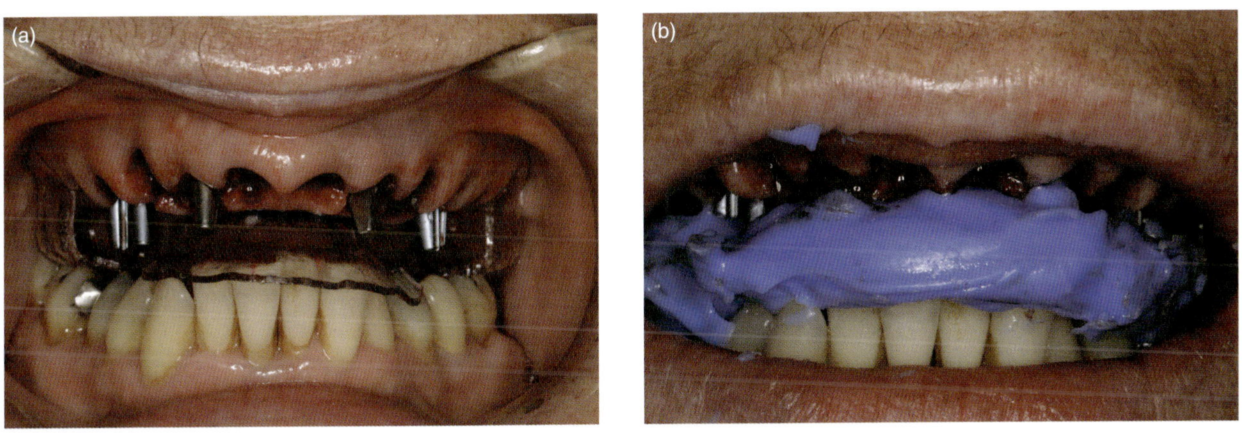

Figure 12.22 (a–b) A bite registration is taken with solid abutments, registration material, and the template.

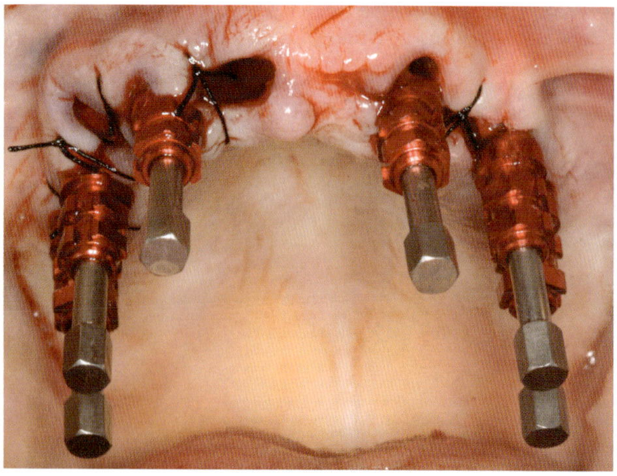

Figure 12.23 Sutures loosely approximate the tissues with the impression cylinders in place.

Analogs are connected to the impression cylinders and the model is poured. The casts are mounted with the aid of the solid abutments on the master cast. The solid abutments are removed and the temporary cylinders are screwed into the implants and trimmed to the appropriate heights. The provisional restoration is fabricated on the cylinders (Figures 12.25a–b, 12.26a–b, and 12.27a–b).

The patient returns to the dentist within 48 h. The healing covers are removed and the provisional restoration is seated (Figures 12.28a–b and 12.29a–b). Radiographs are taken to confirm complete seating. The screws are hand tightened, the access holes are covered with cotton and a temporary filling material. The occlusion is checked for bilateral simultaneous contact, with no interferences in lateral excursions.

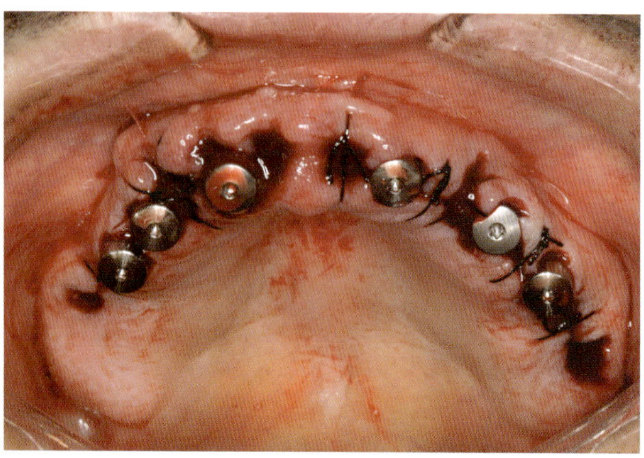

Figure 12.24 Lubricated healing covers are in place.

The patient is instructed to remain on a soft diet for six weeks. At one week, sutures are removed. The occlusion is rechecked over the next week. At the six-week postoperative visit, the bridge is removed and the implants are checked for integration. If the implants are firm and the patient is asymptomatic, they are told they may return to a normal diet. If any of the implants are loose, they are replaced with wider/longer implants and the bridge is reinserted but not attached to the "rescue" implants.

At 12 weeks postoperatively, the provisional restoration is removed and all implants are torqued to 35 Ncm. Radiographs are taken. If the implants tolerate the torque test, fabrication of the final restoration may commence (Figure 12.30).

USE OF CEMENT-RETAINED PROVISIONAL RESTORATIONS

The implant shoulders and internal configurations are cleared of blood and tissue. Solid abutments of the appropriate heights are placed with hand torque. Temporary cylinders are placed on the abutments. The acrylic shell is luted with acrylic to the temporary cylinders at the proper vertical dimension and bite, then removed from the mouth. It will be carved and polished extraorally. While this is occurring, either impression cylinders or healing covers are placed on the implants to avoid collapse of the soft tissues over the implants. The provisional restoration is fabricated, with care being taken to finish the acrylic to the shoulders of the implants. The implant covers are removed and the provisional restoration is seated and cemented. Care is taken to remove all excess cement (Figures 12.31a–b, 12.32a–d, and 12.33a–b).

If there is an angulation discrepancy, an implant level impression is taken, in order to select the proper components. A bite is captured and the impression is poured. Healing covers are placed on the implants. The casts are mounted. The appropriate abutments are selected and indexed with a jig, and the provisional restoration is fabricated. The patient returns to the dentist, who removes the healing covers and, with the aid of the jig, places the abutments with hand torque. If an angled abutment receives too much torque, the implant may rotate, which would alter the angulation of the abutment. Once the abutments are in place,

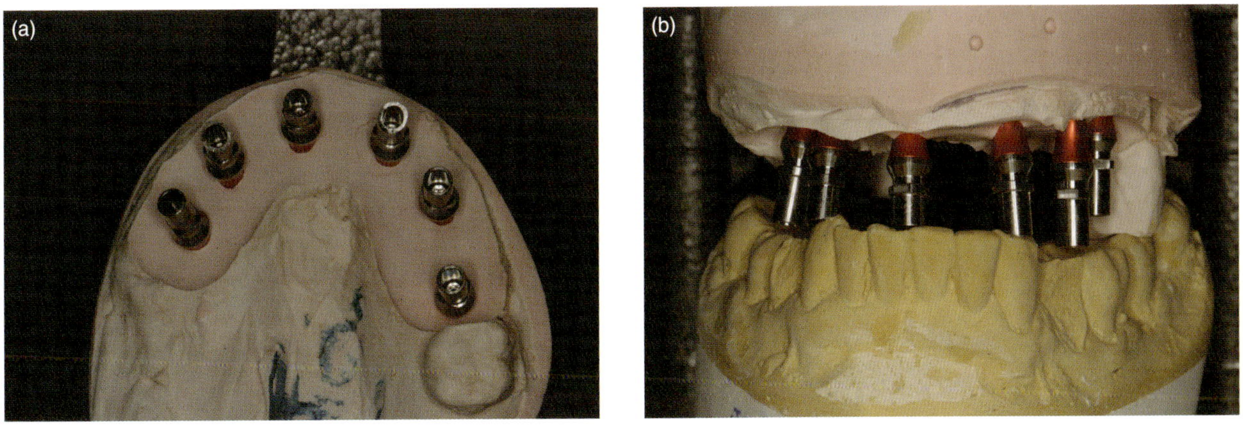

Figure 12.25 (a–b) Views of the master cast, articulated with occlusally reduced, screw-retained temporary cylinders.

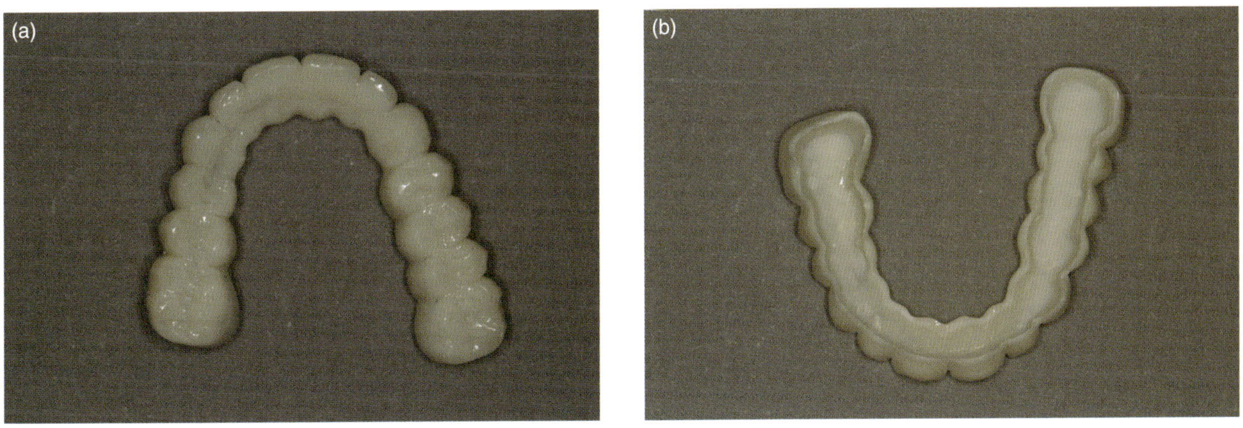

Figure 12.26 (a–b) A view of the hollow provisional shell.

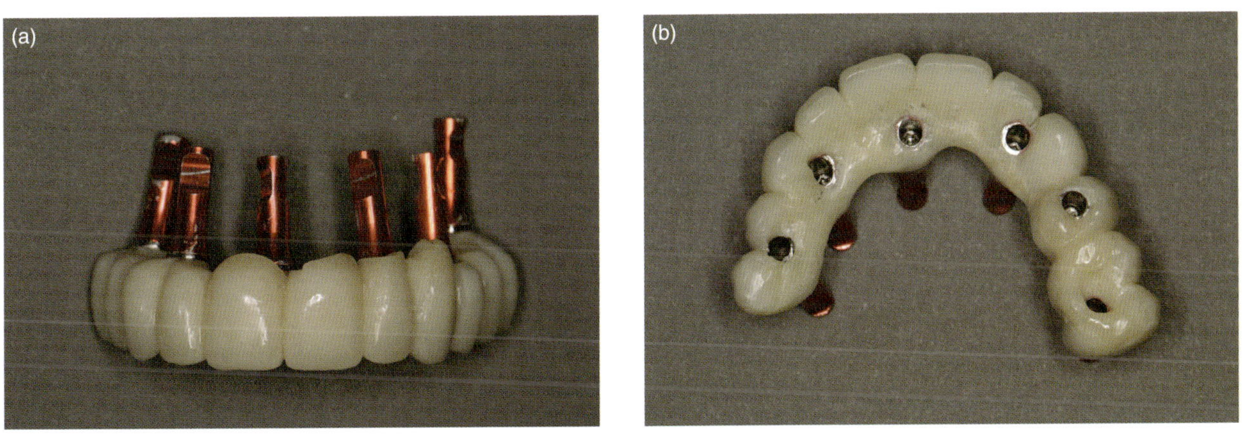

Figure 12.27 (a–b) Note the carved provisional with proper gingival contours.

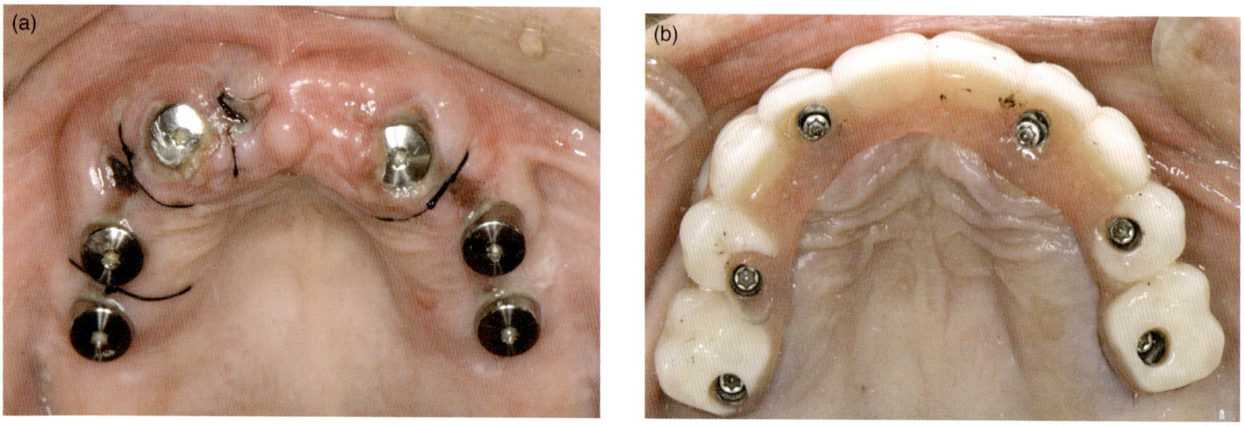

Figure 12.28 (a–b) Twenty-four hours after surgery, cover screws and sutures are in place and placement of the screw-retained provisional bridge is carried out.

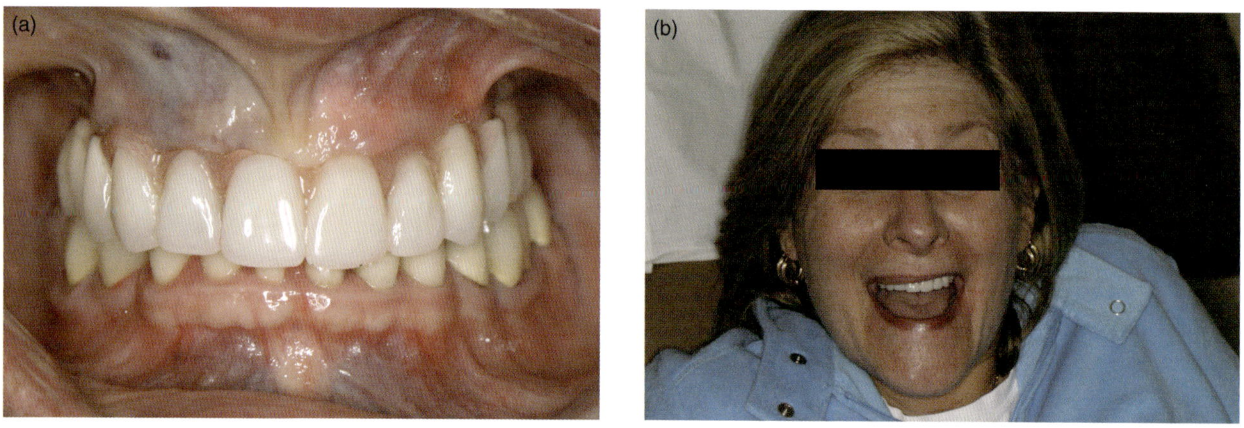

Figure 12.29 (a–b) A facial view after provisional bridge placement.

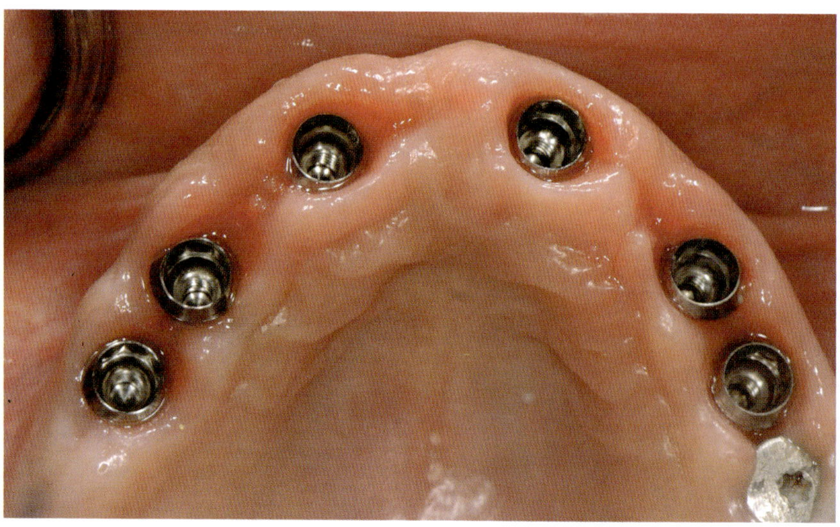

Figure 12.30 The healed tissue at 12 weeks.

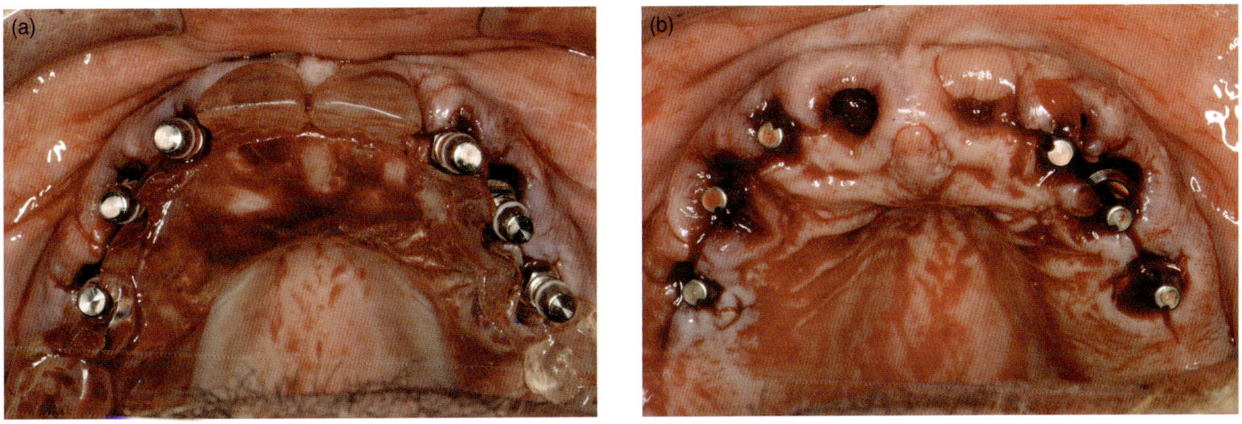

Figure 12.31 (a–b) Views of implant placement with the template; abutments are in place.

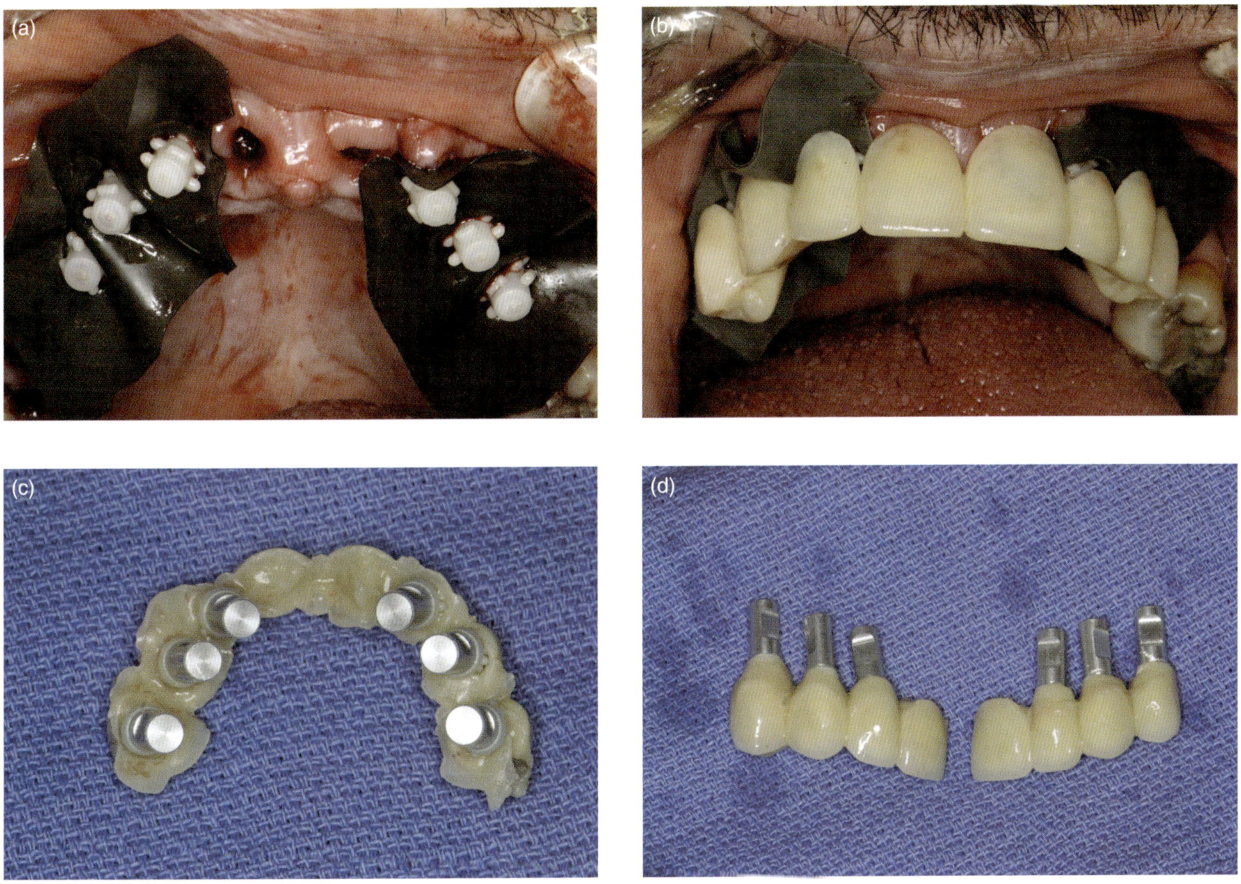

Figure 12.32 (a–d) Provisional bridge fabrication using the direct method on solid abutments: A rubber dam and temporary cylinders are placed; the shell is attached to the cylinders; removal of the shell demonstrates the divergence of the implants; the provisional bridge is fabricated in two segments which will be luted at the midline.

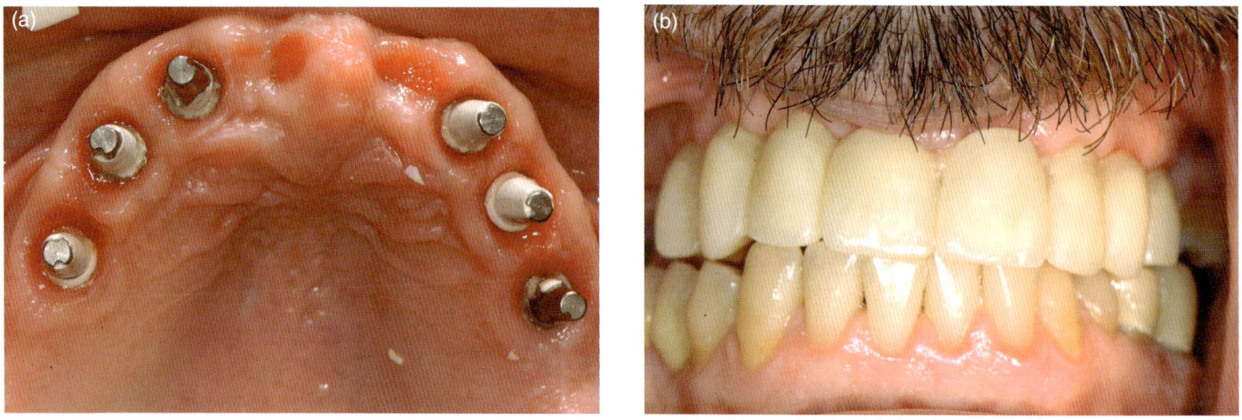

Figure 12.33 (a–b) Soft tissue healing at 12 weeks, and a facial view of the provisional bridge.

the provisional restoration is seated and cemented (Figures 12.34a–d, 12.35a–b, and 12.36a–b).

The patient follows the same dietary and postoperative instructions as previously outlined.

At 12 weeks postoperatively, radiographs are taken and the implants are torqued to 35 Ncm. If the patient is asymptomatic and all implants pass the torque test, final restoration of the implants may commence. In such cases, the soft tissues have healed around a properly contoured provisional restoration while the implants were integrating. Therefore, the final impression may now be taken.

Clinical Example One: Mandible

A 64-year-old male presents for evaluation of the mandible for immediate implant restoration. His chief complaint is pain in the mandible. The patient has had three full mouth rehabilitations in the past 40 years. Examination of the oral cavity reveals a full mouth of crowns and bridges. Unsplinted crowns are present on teeth numbers 18, 19, 20, 21, 28, 29, 30, and 31. A fixed bridge is present on teeth numbers 22–27.

The patient is medically compromised, having had a myocardial infarction in the past five years. He is being treated for atrial fibrillation. Among his many medications is Coumadin.

Periapical radiographs reveal extensive decay and bone loss throughout the mandible. Apical infections on teeth numbers 21 and 28 are evident. Teeth numbers 19, 26, and 30 demonstrate bone loss to their apices, compounded by failing endodontics. Caries is noted on teeth numbers 20, 22, and 27 (Figure 12.37).

The patient returned two weeks later with acute infections on teeth numbers 19, 21, 28, and 30. He was placed on a regimen of antibiotics. The teeth were extracted after Coumadin was stopped for three days (Figures 12.38a–b).

After a prosthetic workup, it was determined that the remaining mandibular teeth were hopeless except for numbers 18 and 31, which had a guarded prognosis. The treatment plan had to take into account the patient's extensive dental and medical history, including the risk involved in stopping blood thinners for each surgery. It was determined that immediate load implant therapy would be ideal for this patient. The treatment plan called for the placement of 6–8 implants, to be installed in the positions of teeth numbers 19, 21, 22, 23, 26, 27, 28, and 30.

Before surgery, a wax-up of final tooth positions would be established. From this wax-up a surgical template and provisional fixed restoration would be fabricated. Teeth numbers 18 and 31 would remain during implant placement, to stabilize the surgical template and maintain vertical dimension. The template would have the buccal halves of the teeth removed and a 2-mm vertical groove placed to guide the twist drill, in order to parallel the implants. After implant placement, solid abutments would be attached with hand torque. The cement-retained provisional restoration would be fabricated. The molars would then be extracted. Following 12 weeks of healing, the provisional restoration would be removed, and the final prosthesis would be constructed (Figures 12.39a–b).

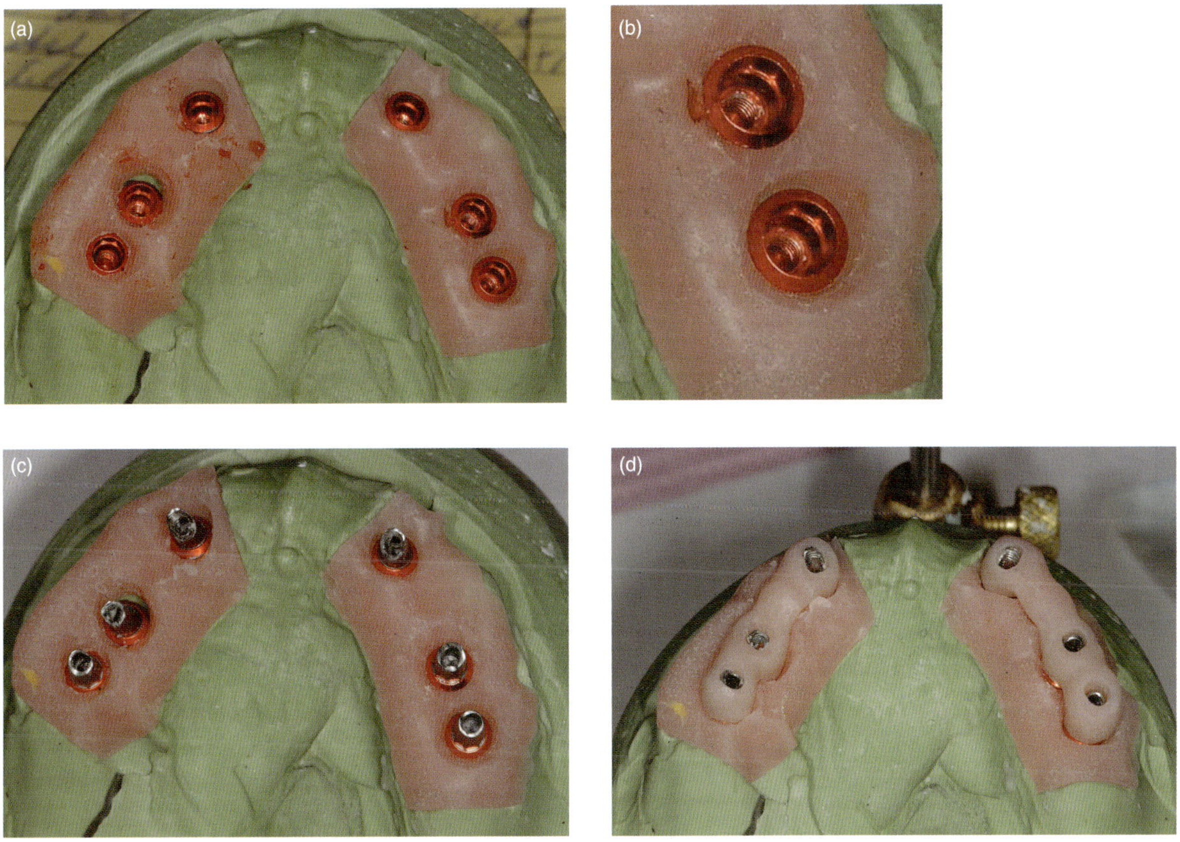

Figure 12.34 (a–d) The indirect technique for a cement-retained provisional bridge: A master cast of the indexed implants; a magnified view of the indexed implant; abutments are paralleled and a jig is fabricated.

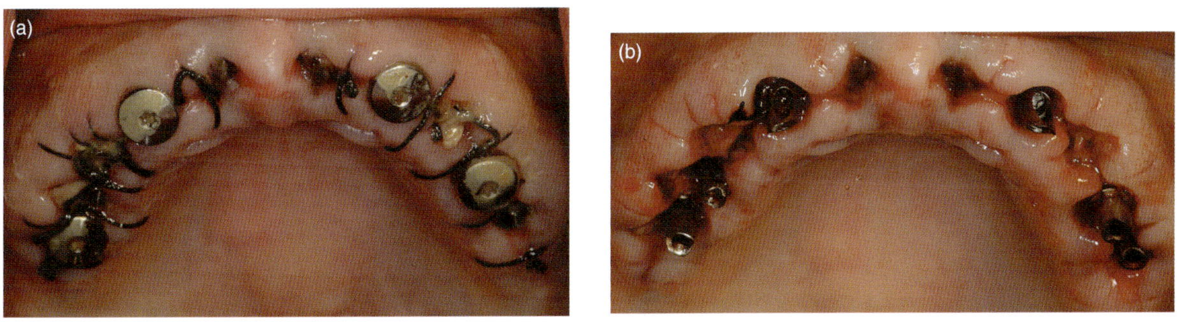

Figure 12.35 (a–b) A view 24 h after surgery with healing covers in place; abutments are placed with the aid of the jig.

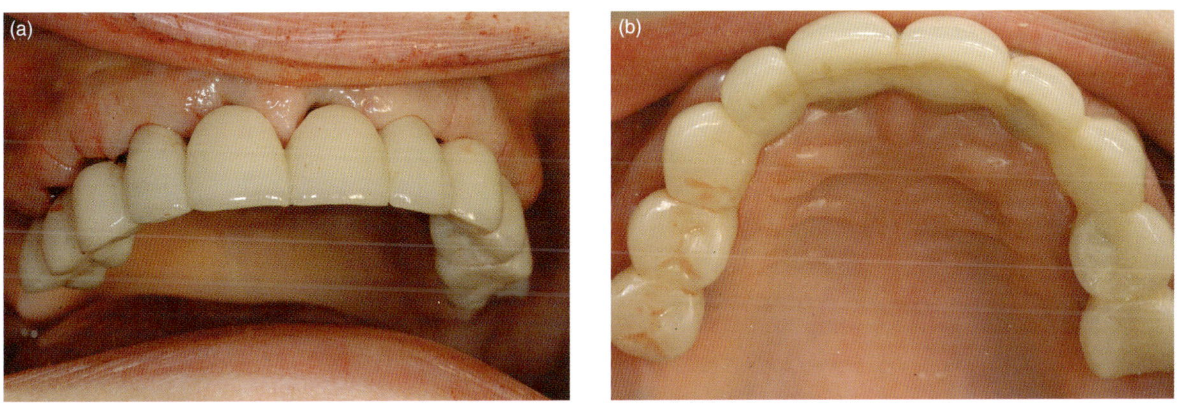

Figure 12.36 (a–b) The provisional bridge is placed over the abutments.

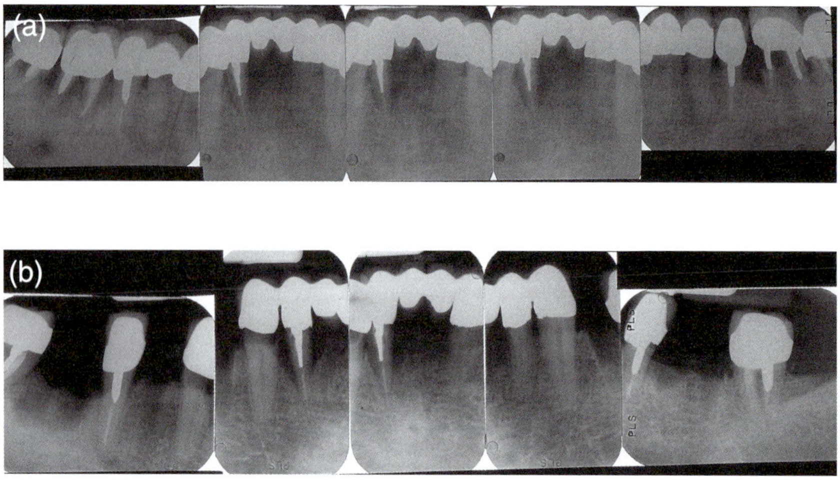

Figure 12.37 Radiographs of a 65-year-old patient at presentation, and 12 weeks later.

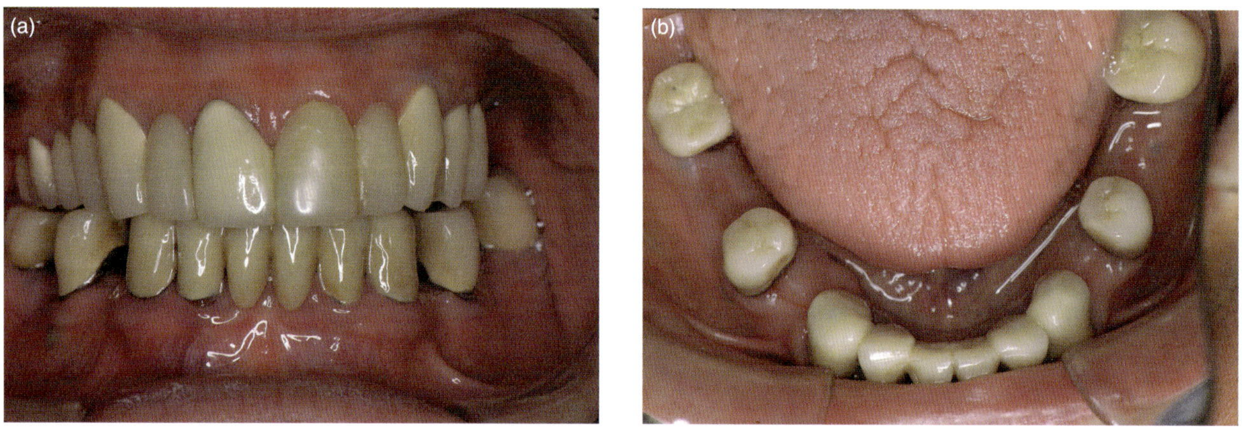

Figure 12.38 (a–b) The patient at 12 weeks after presentation.

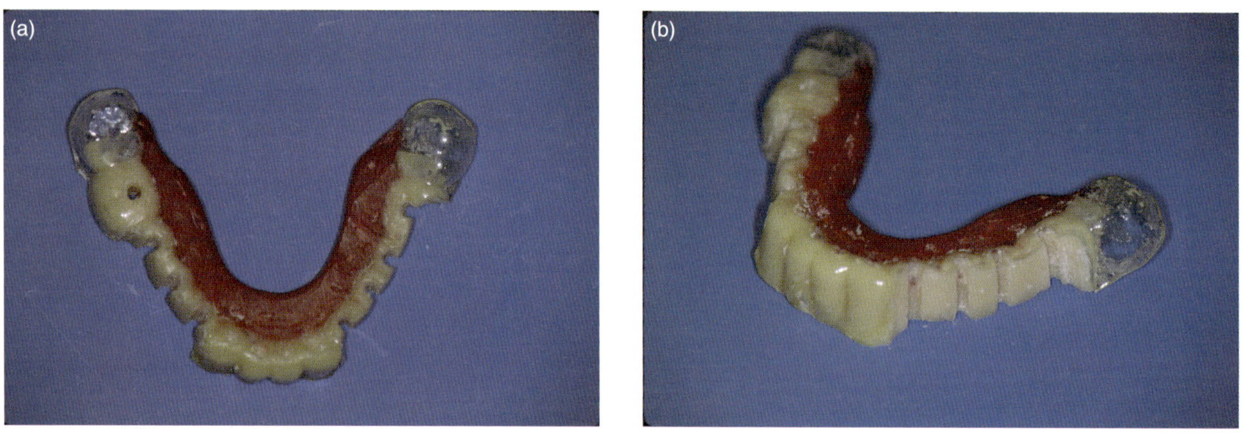

Figure 12.39 (a–b) A template of the waxed-up case is made to sit on the molars, with the buccal removed and a groove included for bur placement.

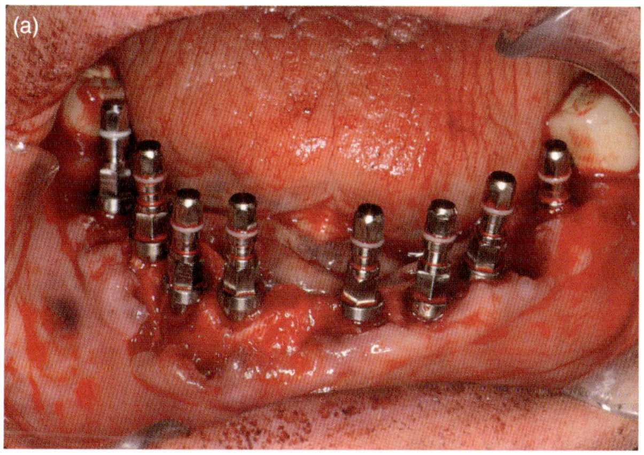

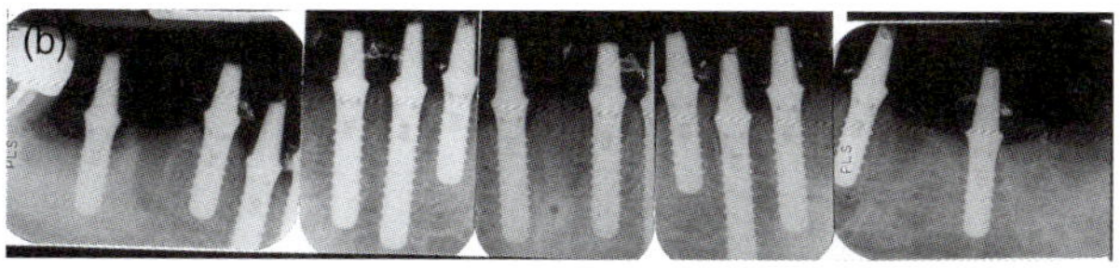

Figure 12.40 (a–b) Views of immediate implant placement in extraction sites, and radiographs taken immediately after placement.

On the day of surgery, the patient was premedicated with antibiotics. The patient was draped and the implant surgery commenced. The mucoperiosteal tissues of the mandible were infiltrated with local anesthesia. Teeth numbers 20, 22, 23, 26, 27, and 29 were extracted. The template was checked for stability in the mouth, new sharp burs were utilized during the procedure, in order to reduce chatter during site preparation. The anterior implant positions were prepared first, enabling easier parallel placement of the posterior implants on each side. Once the implants had been installed, any hard or soft tissues which impinged upon the placement of the temporary cylinders were removed. The temporary cylinders were attached and the flaps were loosely sutured (Figures 12.40a–b).

Fabrication of the provisional restoration commenced. The shell was placed over the temporary cylinders at the proper vertical dimension and was affixed to them with acrylic. The shell was removed, additional acrylic was added and the bridge properly contoured with appropriate emergence profiles and interproximal embrasures. It was returned to the mouth and the occlusion was verified. The provisional restoration was then polished. The molars were extracted and the bridge was cemented. Care was taken to remove all excess cement. The patient was prescribed an antibiotic and analgesic. Postoperative care included a soft diet for four weeks and oral hygiene beginning at one week postoperatively (Figures 12.41a–c).

The patient returned for suture removal at 7–14 days. The occlusion was checked over the next 2 weeks. The bridge was removed at 6 weeks to assess implant integration. There was no cement washout at any site and no implant movement or symptoms. At 12 weeks, the bridge was removed. The implants were checked for integration by torqueing the abutments clockwise and counterclockwise to 35 Ncm, and taking periapical radiographs (Figures 12.42a–b).

The patient now commenced with fabrication of the final prostheses. The prostheses were constructed in sections: two posterior segments and an anterior segment (Figures 12.43a–b, 12.44, 12.45a–b, and 12.46).

Clinical Example Two: Maxilla

A 57-year-old female presented for evaluation of her maxilla for implant reconstruction. She was unhappy with her esthetics and was aware of flaring of her incisors and gingival recession. The patient had been receiving routine dental care on a regular basis. Her past medical history was noncontributory and offered no obstacles to dental therapy (Figures 12.47a–d).

A full series of parallel periapical radiographs revealed a hopeless maxillary dentition (Figure 12.48). Teeth numbers 3, 4, 5, 6, 7, 8, 12, 14, and 15 had a poor prognosis. Teeth numbers 9, 10, 11, and 13 had a guarded prognosis. However, their longevity was questionable. It was determined that the patient required a full arch implant supported prosthesis to meet her functional and esthetic needs.

The patient was referred to the radiologist for a CAT scan. Evaluation of the CAT scan will permit selection of six implant sites. Two posterior and one anterior site must be found on each side of the arch. Assessment of the posterior maxilla revealed that an insufficient volume of bone was present at all molar positions. The four bicuspid sites were selected as potential implant sites, since at least 8 mm of apical bone height was available in these areas. The lateral incisor extraction sockets presented as ideal anterior locations, as sufficient bone volume was present for apical implant fixation (Figures 12.49a–b). Density measurements exceeded

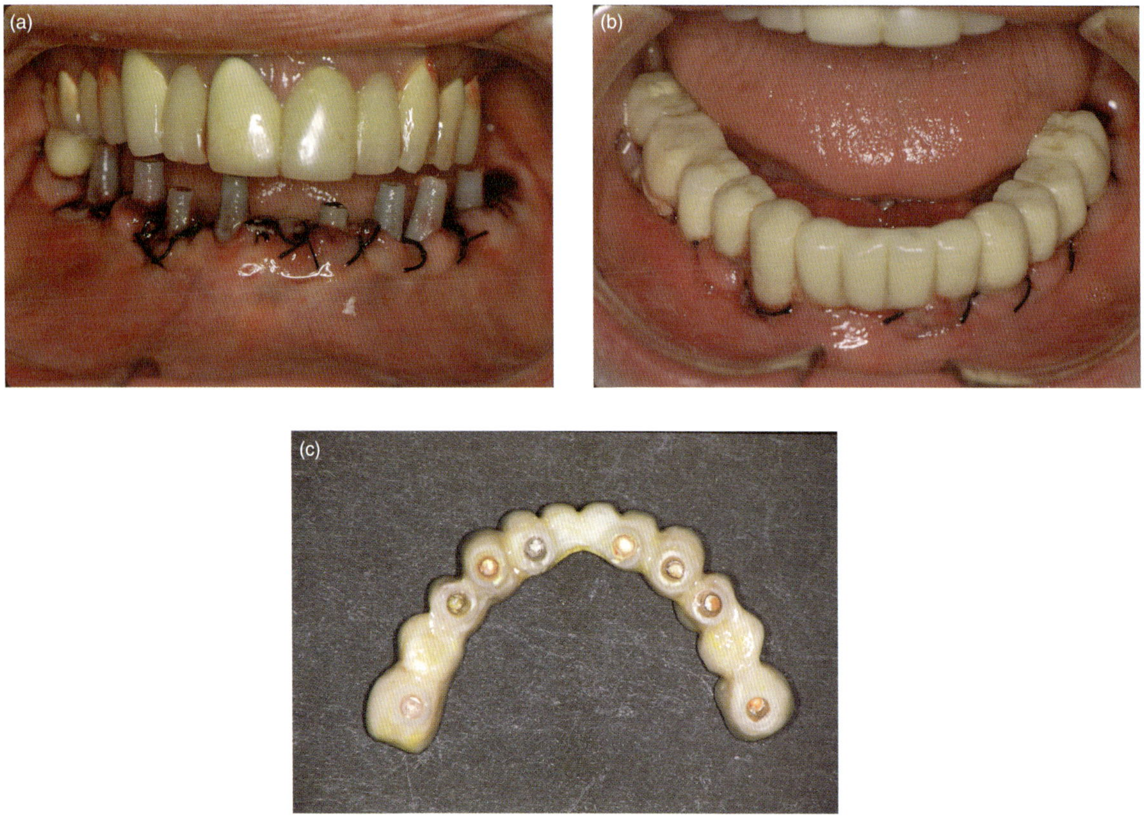

Figure 12.41 (a–c) Immediate fabrication of a cement-retained provisional over burn-out copings has been carried out; note the proper gingival contours.

minimum values at all sites, thereby permitting immediate implant loading (Figures 12.50a–c and 12.51). The three-dimensional views corroborated the treatment plan for a screw-retained provisional restoration, as the implants at positions 7 and 10 could be placed in palatal bone, with the screw-access holes emerging from the cingula. The bicuspid implants could be secured in the sockets with angulations which would emerge through the central fossae (Figures 12.52a–b).

The restorative dentist mounted the casts and waxed the teeth in the ideal esthetic and functional positions (Figures 12.53a–c and 12.56a–c). This wax-up was shown to the patient. Once it was acceptable, templates were fabricated (Figures 12.54a–b).

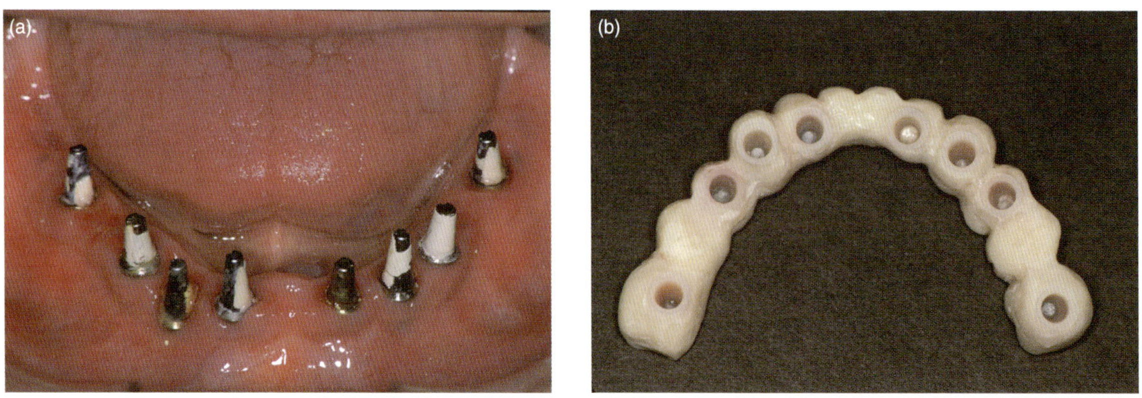

Figure 12.42 (a–b) Removal of the bridge at 12 weeks; there is no cement washout and the healed tissues are evident.

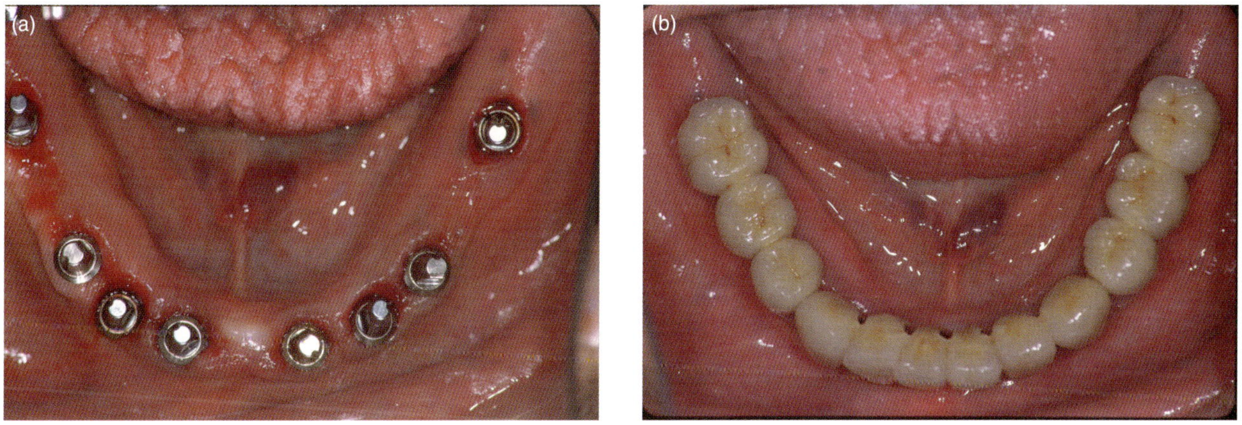

Figure 12.43 (a–b) Occlusal views of solid abutments and final case in three pieces: 19–21, 22–27, 28–30.

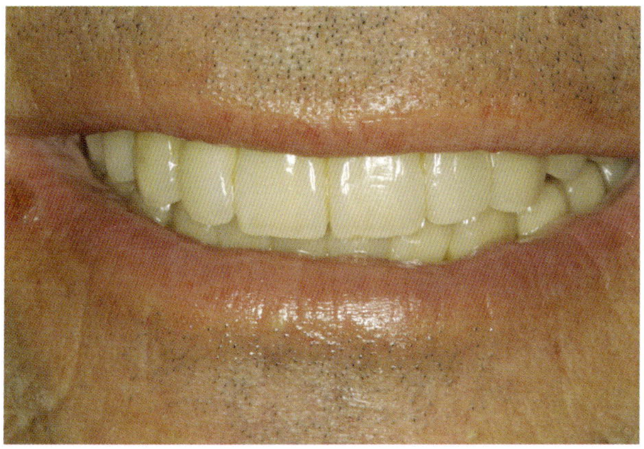

Figure 12.44 A facial view of the final case.

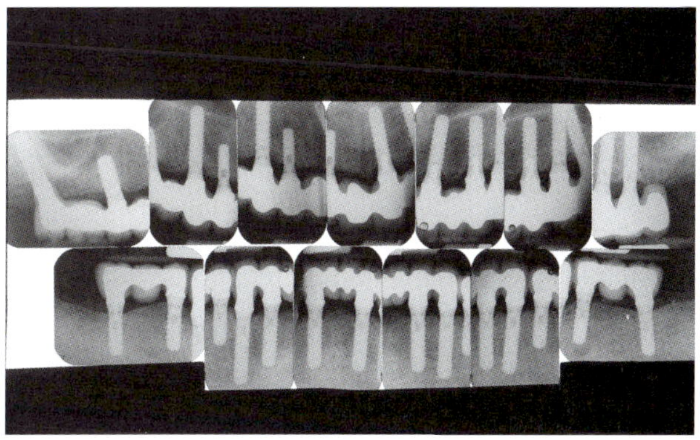

Figure 12.46 Radiographs taken at five years post therapy.

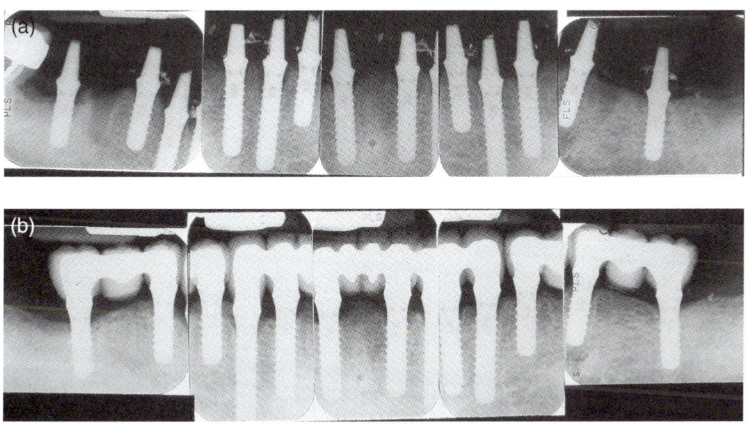

Figure 12.45 (a–b) A radiograph comparison of implants at placement and two years later.

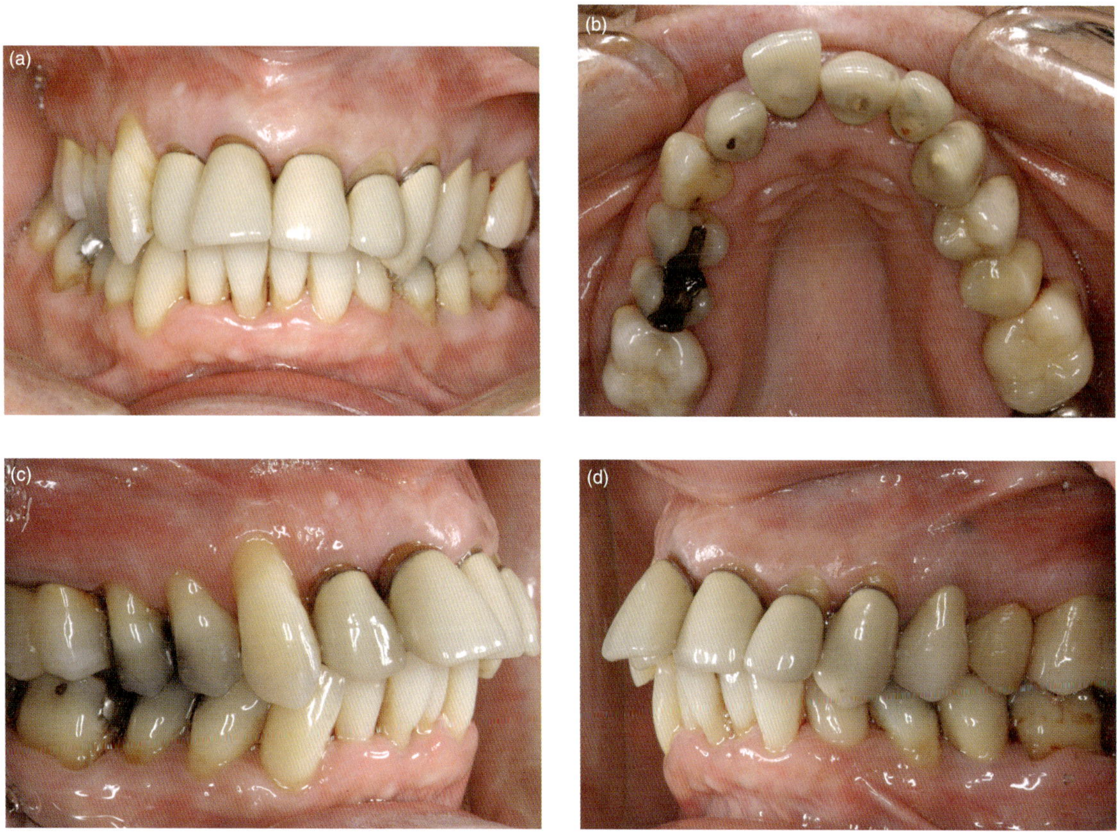

Figure 12.47 (a–d) Presentation views of a 57-year-old female.

Following template fabrication, the patient was ready for surgery. The preoperative protocols outlined above were followed. The teeth were extracted with as little trauma as possible, and implant placement commenced. The templates were utilized for proper implant positioning (Figures 12.55a–d). Once the implants were installed, the implant shoulders were checked to ensure that no hard or soft tissues prevented seating of the impression or temporary cylinders. A bone profiler

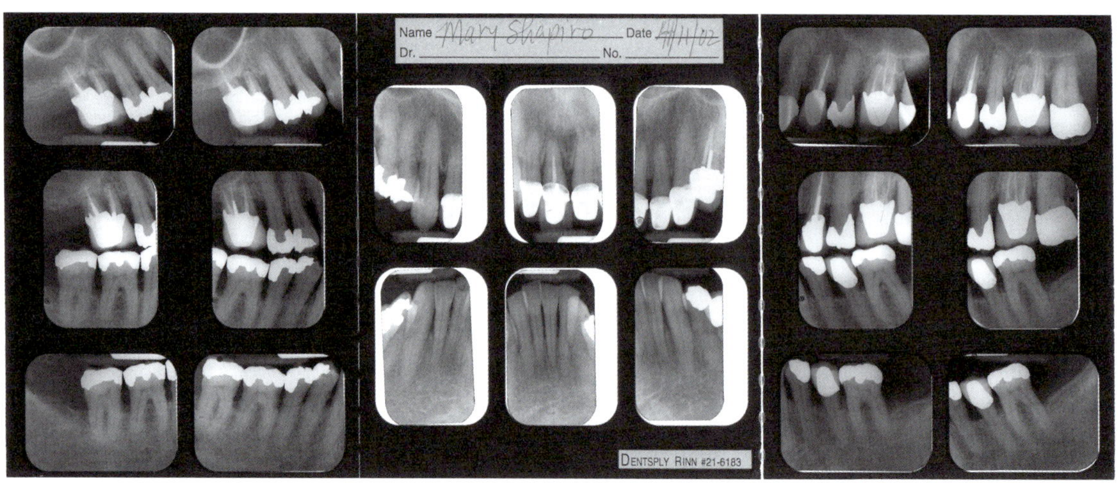

Figure 12.48 Full mouth periapical radiographs were taken at presentation.

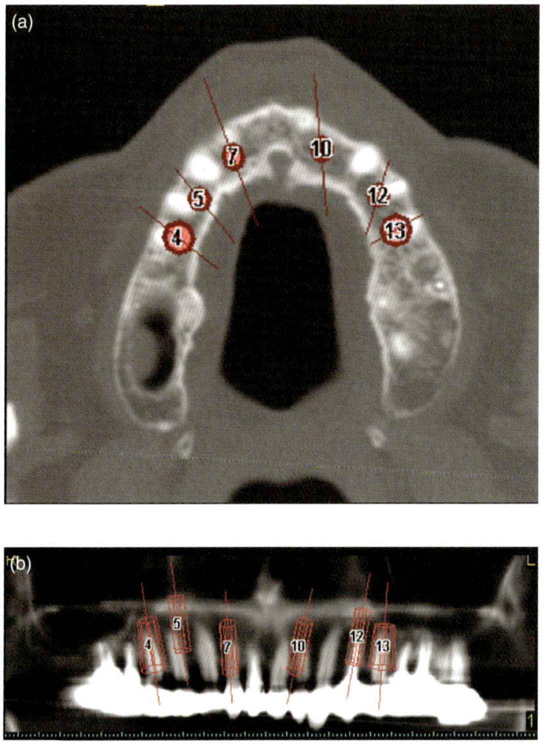

Figure 12.49 (a–b) Axial and panoramic views taken from the CT, with implant placement.

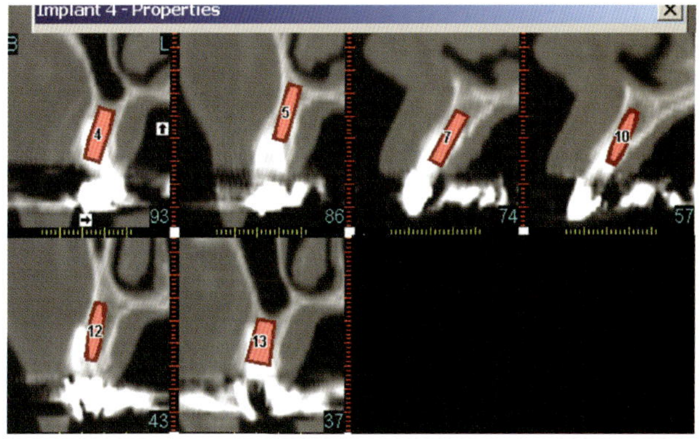

Figure 12.51 Oblique views of six selected sites: 4, 5, 7, 10, 12, 13.

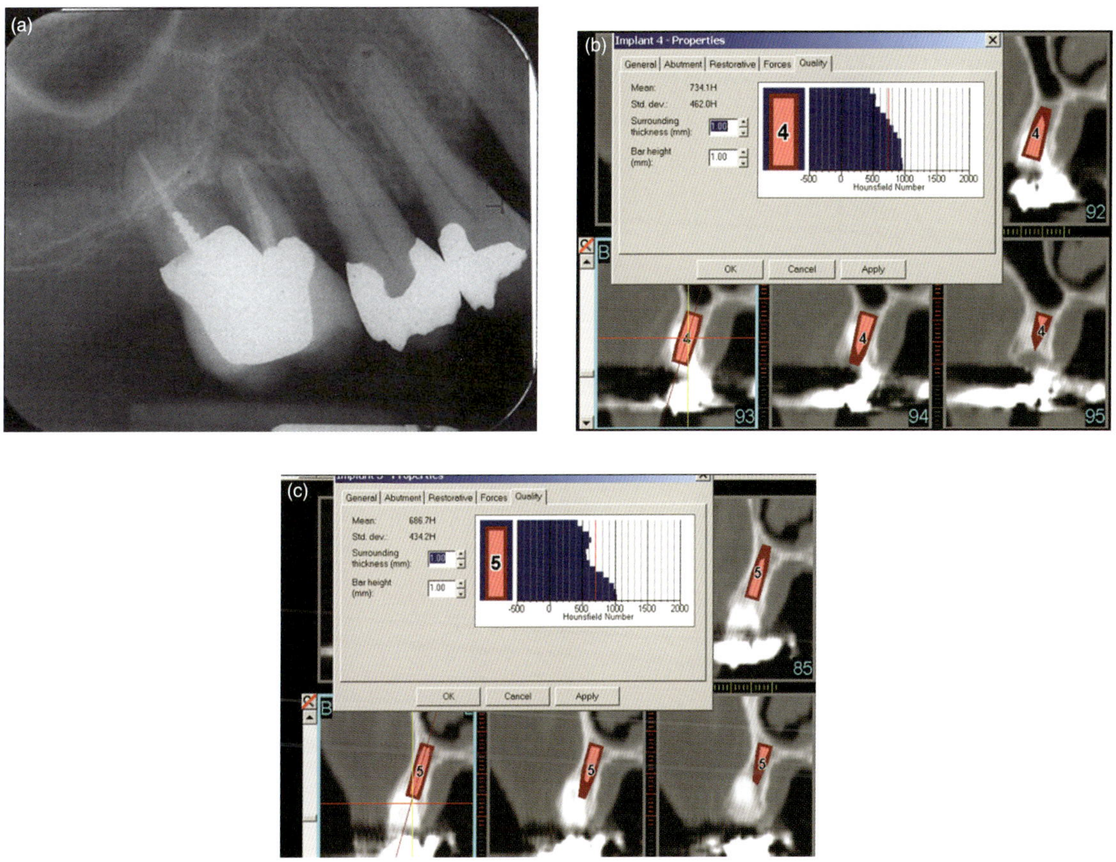

Figure 12.50 (a–c) Periapical views of the maxillary right bicuspids, and oblique CT views of 4 and 5, with density measurements.

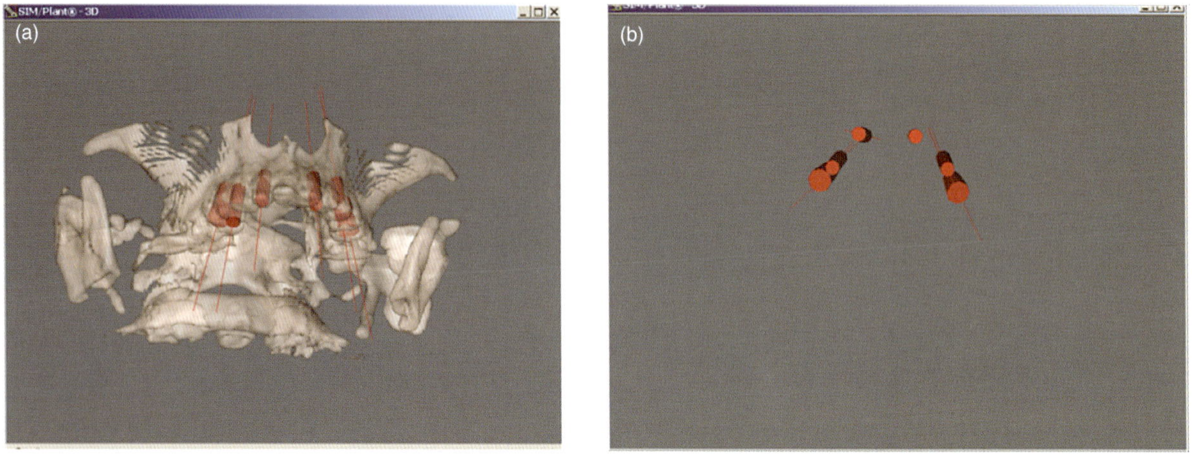

Figure 12.52 (a–b) Three-dimensional views of the maxilla and implants, with and without bone.

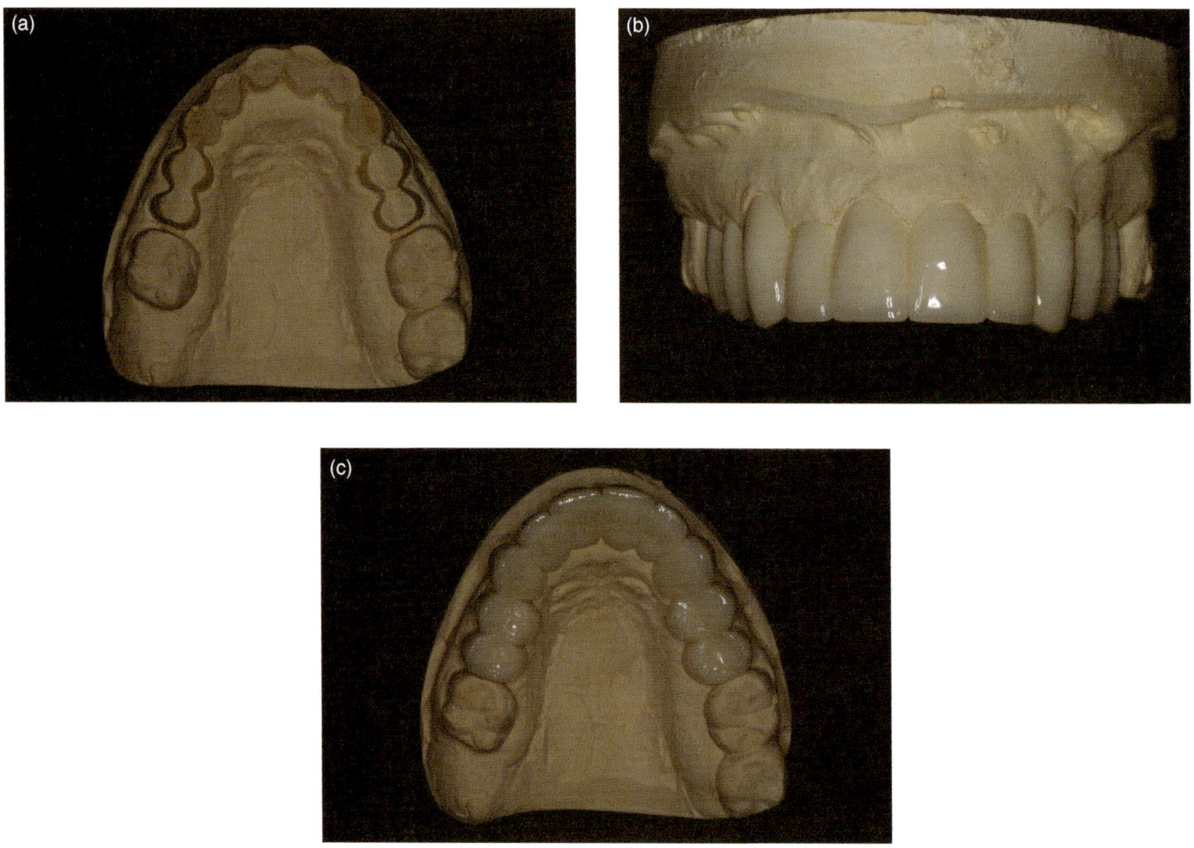

Figure 12.53 (a–c) A view of models showing cut-down of the teeth and a wax-up with the widened gingival third.

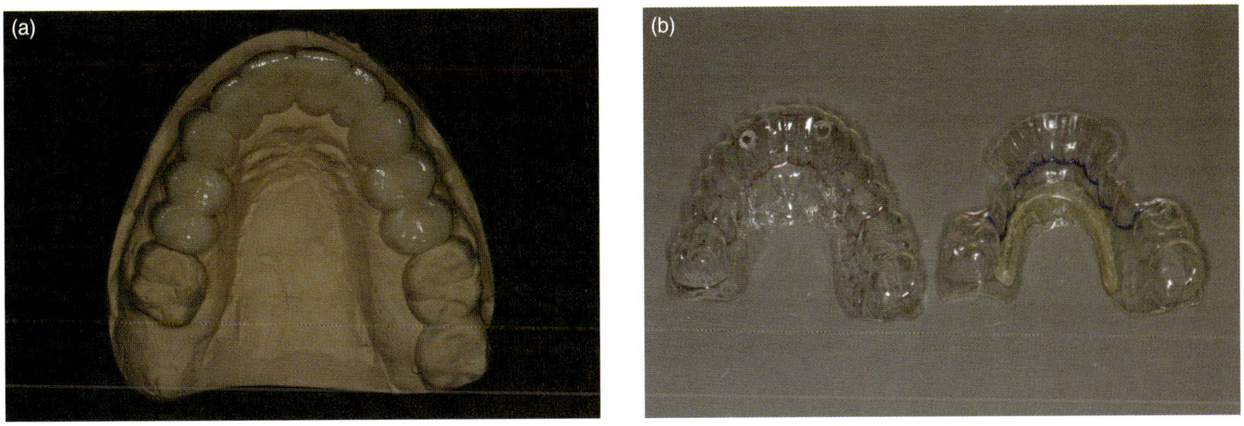

Figure 12.54 (a–b) Views of the waxed-up maxilla and the templates; clear stent and a buccally reduced templates.

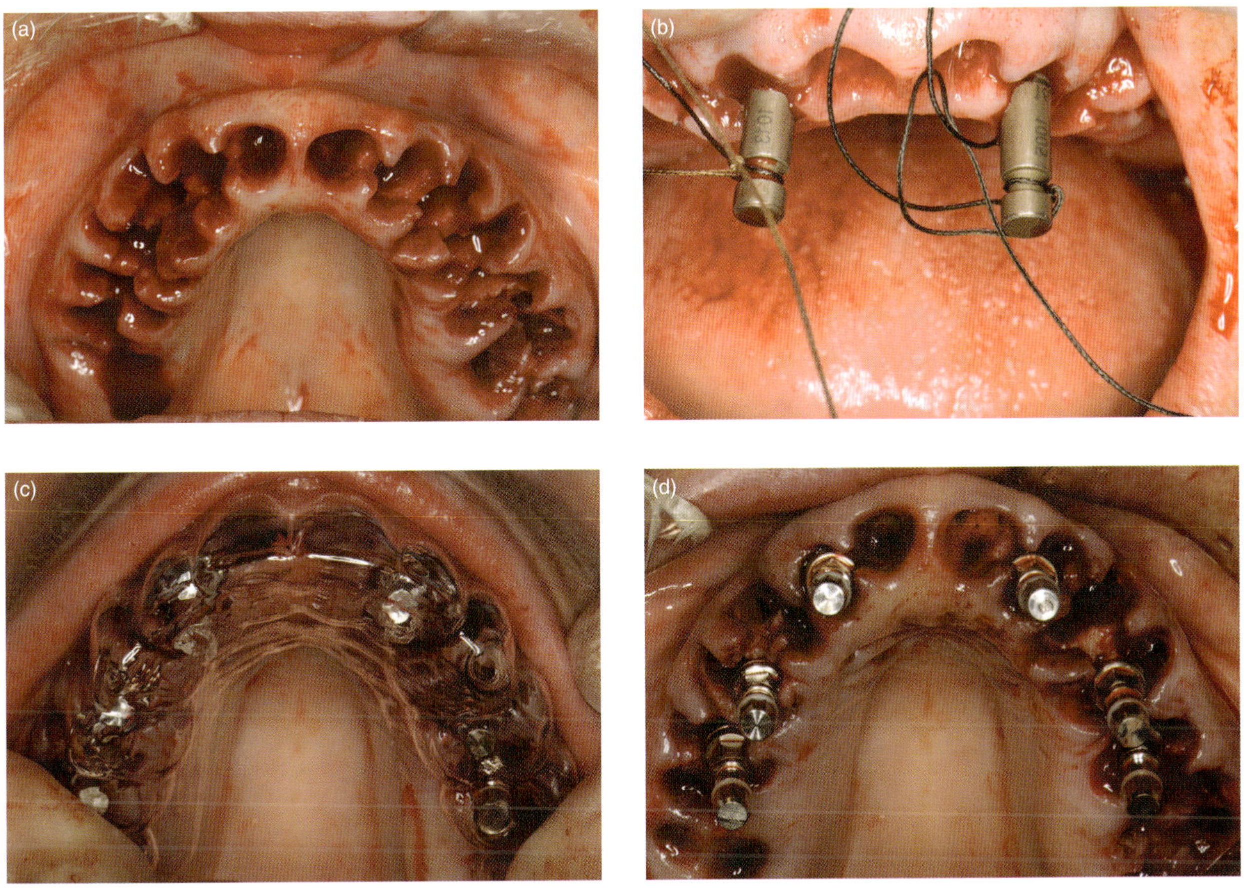

Figure 12.55 (a–d) Extraction of all maxillary teeth has been carried out; 3.5-mm indicators are placed at positions 7 and 10; a view of the template demonstrating proper implant positions; implants without the template.

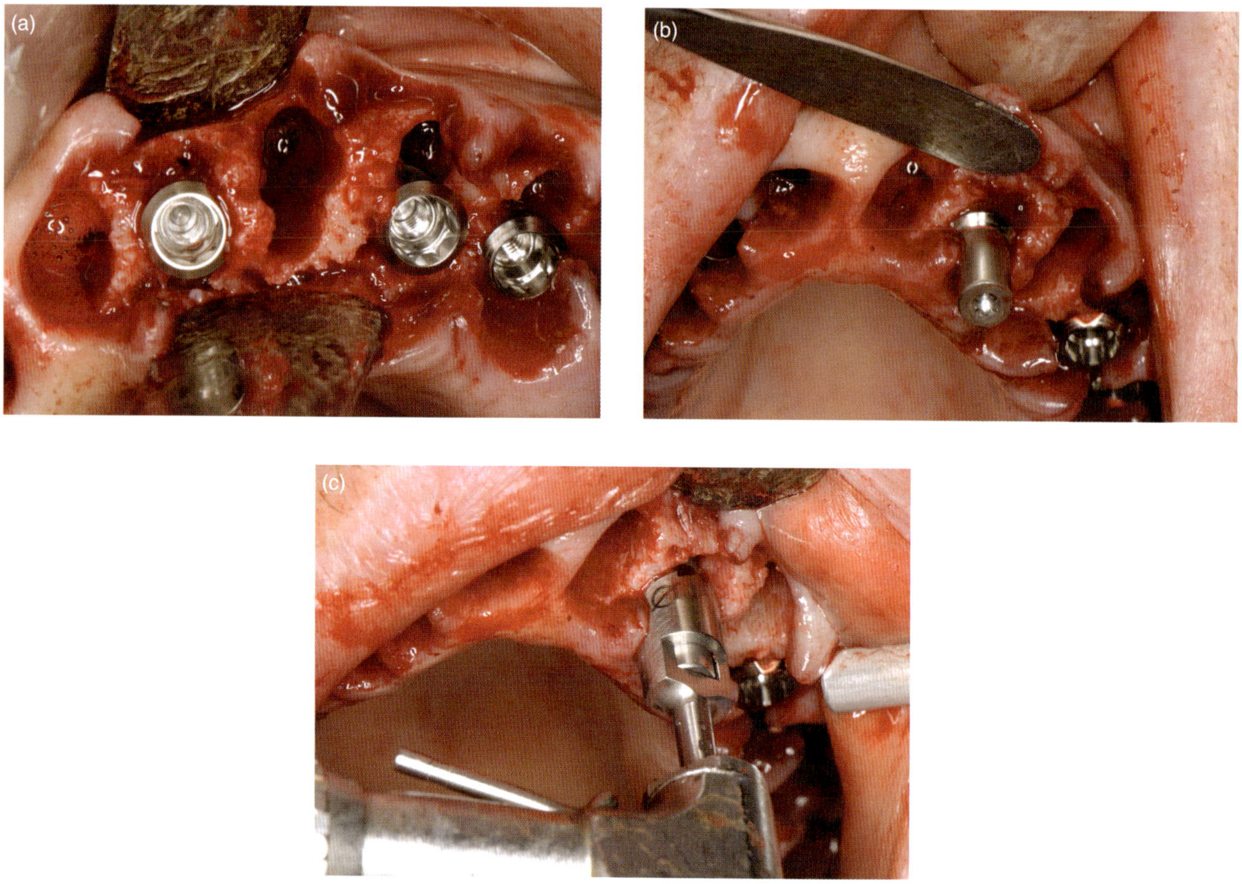

Figure 12.56 (a–c) Implants are in the sockets, with scalloped bone; a view of placement of the guide device; bone profiling is carried out to reduce impingement of the interproximal bone.

was used to remove any excess hard tissues (Figures 12.56a–c) which were present.

A bite registration was taken. Solid abutments were loosely screwed into the implants. A template which either sits on the remaining teeth, or has a positive seat on the palate, is used to help take a stable bite using a fast setting material (Figures 12.57a–d).

The impression cylinders were attached to the implants, with care being taken to ensure they were fully seated. The open tray was tried in and the impression was taken with a medium- to heavy-bodied impression material. After the impression was removed, it was checked to be sure that no impression cylinders moved in the impression (Figures 12.58a–c). Long healing covers, lubricated with petroleum jelly or Neosporin ointment, were screwed into the implants

The master cast was poured and mounted. Screw-retained temporary cylinders were attached to the master cast and the provisional restoration was fabricated (Figures 12.59a–c and 12.60a–d).

The provisional restoration was delivered to the patient in 24–48 h. The healing covers were removed and the provisional restoration was placed. The retaining screws were hand tightened (Figures 12.61a–c) and the occlusion was checked. Radiographs were taken to verify restoration seating (Figure 12.62). The patient was instructed in post-operative care, including a soft diet and use of a nightguard. Healing was followed for 12 weeks (Figures 12.63a–b).

When the bridge was removed 12 weeks post-operatively, completed soft and hard tissue healing was evident (Figures 12.64a–b). The implants were torqued to 35 Ncm in both clockwise and counter-clockwise rotations, to validate osseointegration. Radiographs were taken and the patient returned to the restorative dentist for fabrication of the final prosthesis.

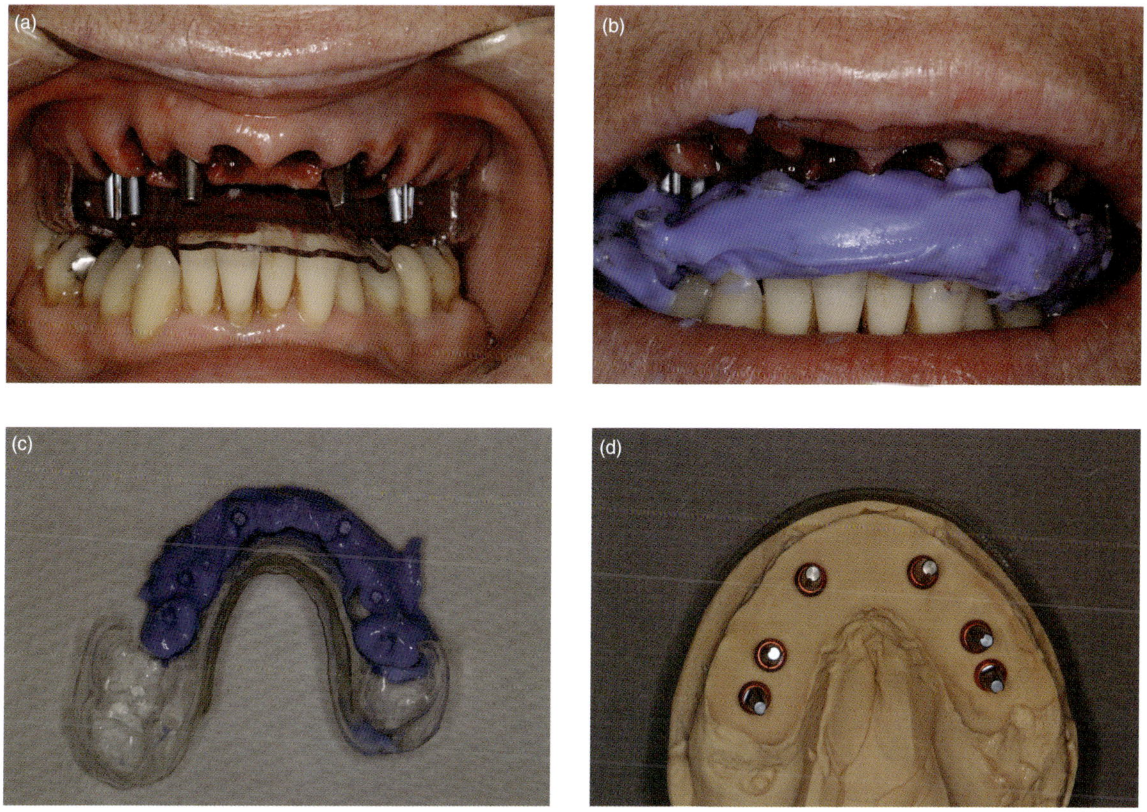

Figure 12.57 (a–d) Views of the bite registration; solid abutments in place to help stabilize the registration; the template with an occlusal stop; registration material injected; the registration removed; the cast with solid abutments ready to be mounted.

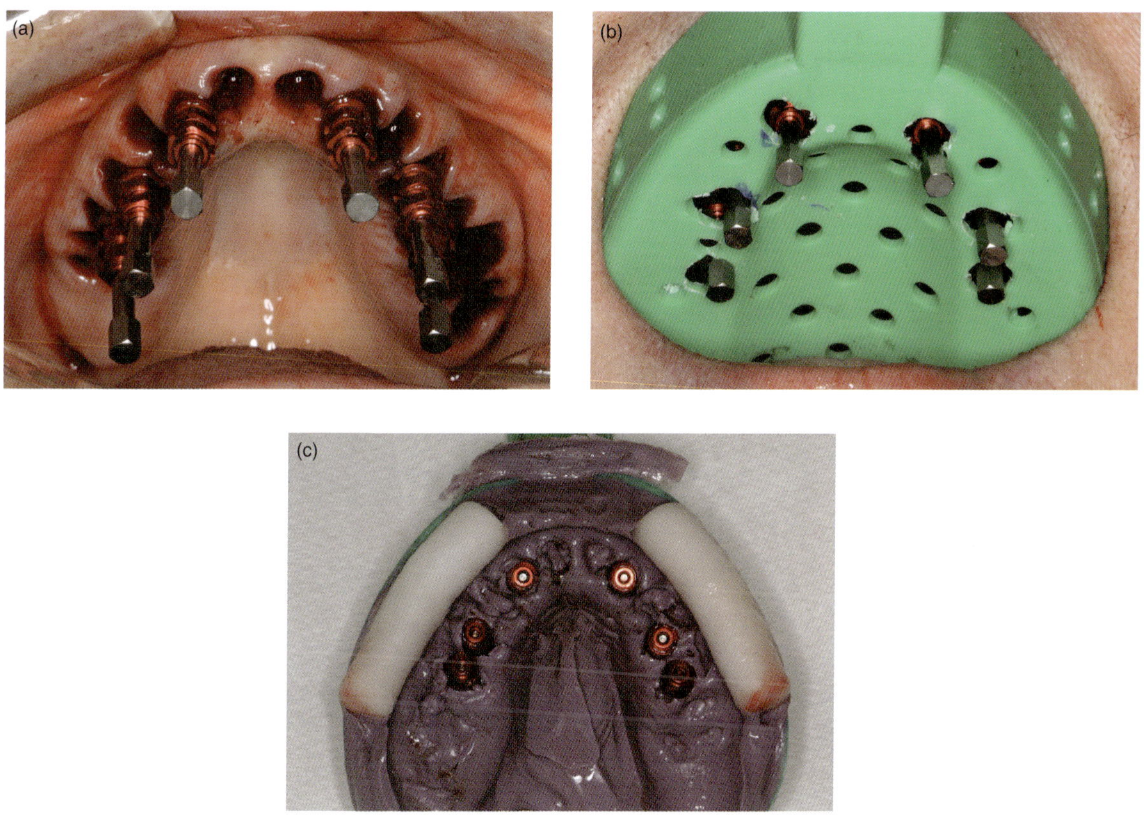

Figure 12.58 (a–c) Views of an open tray impression; cylinders in place, the tray fitted over the impression cylinders; the impression.

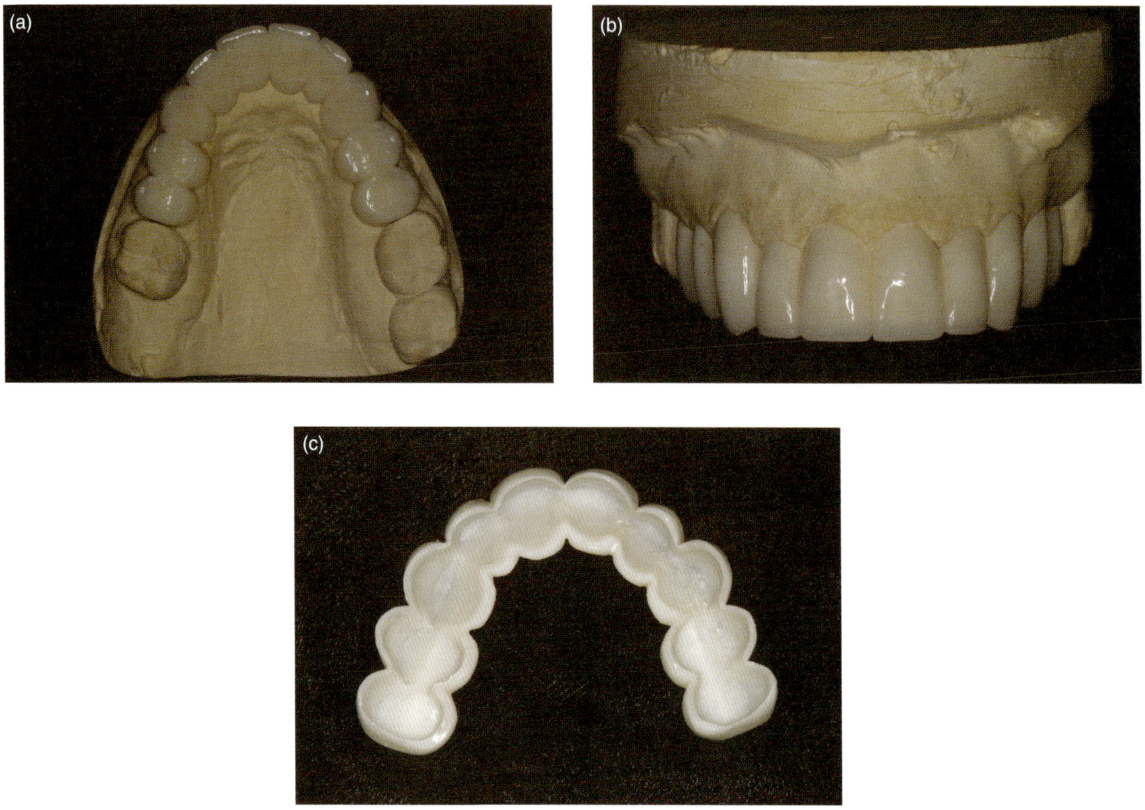

Figure 12.59 (a–c) A view of the provisional bridge with the gingival one-third widened.

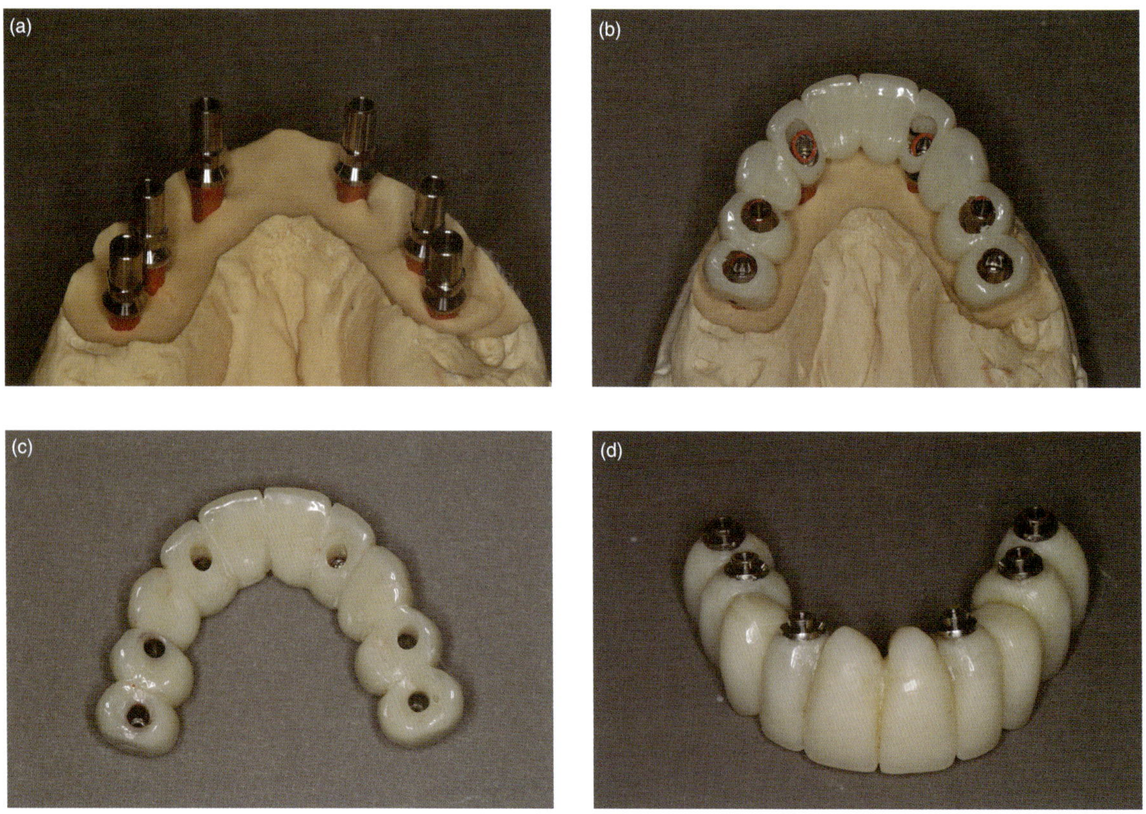

Figure 12.60 (a–d) Temporary cylinders are in place on the master cast; the provisional bridge is fitted over the cylinders; occlusal and tissue views of the fabricated provisional bridge.

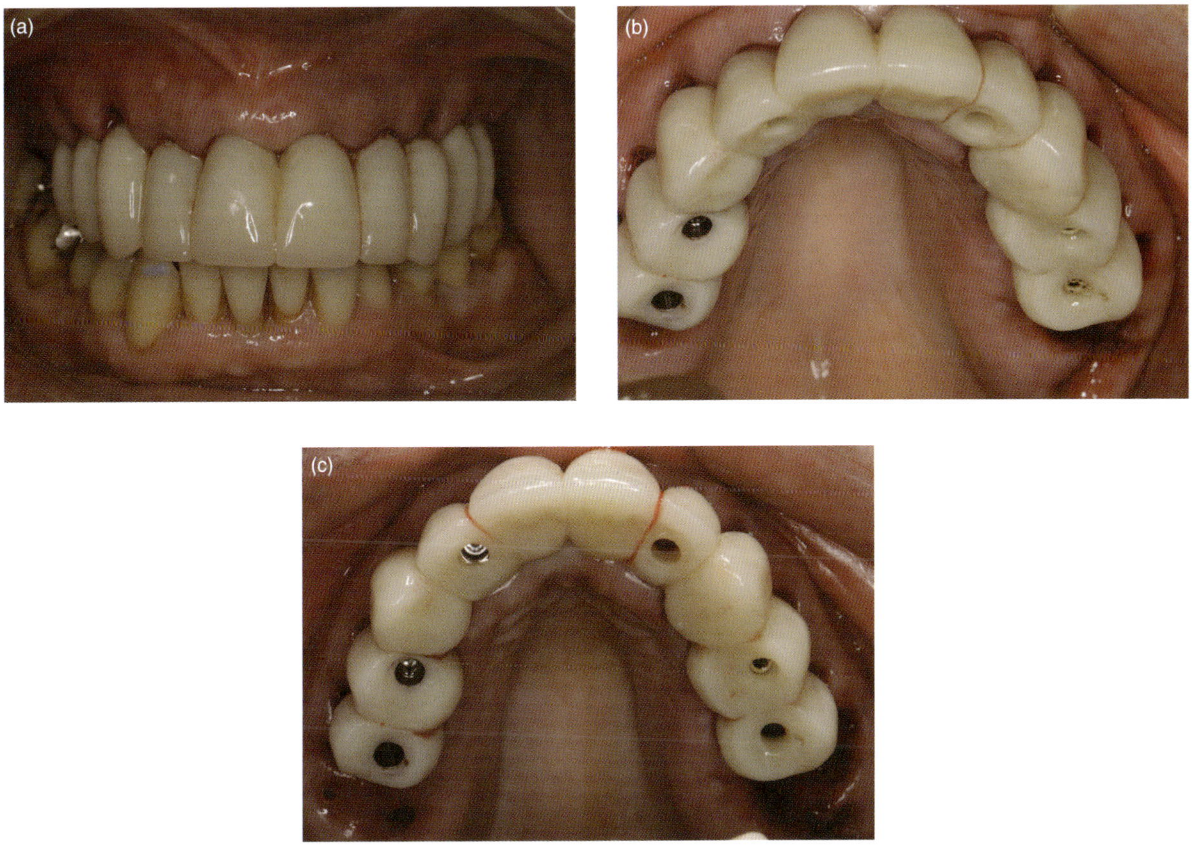

Figure 12.61 (a–c) The provisional bridge is placed 24-h postimplant insertion: buccal and occlusal views.

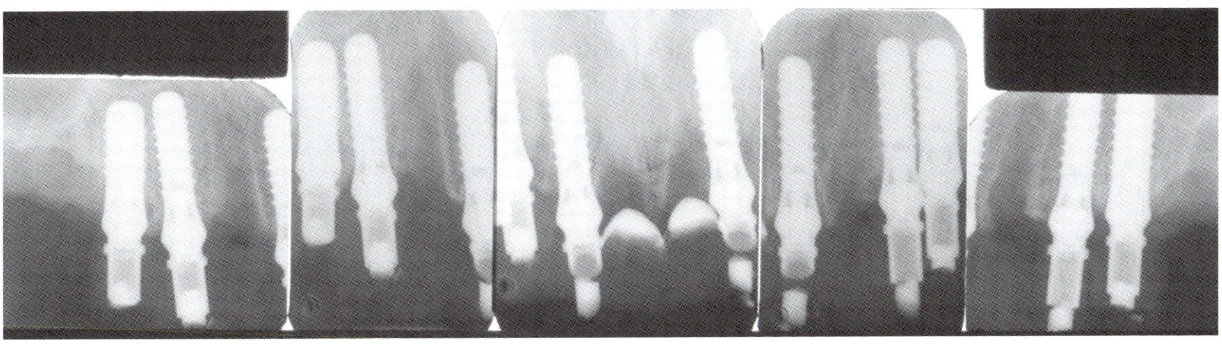

Figure 12.62 A radiograph is taken 24-h postsurgery to verify seating of the provisional bridge.

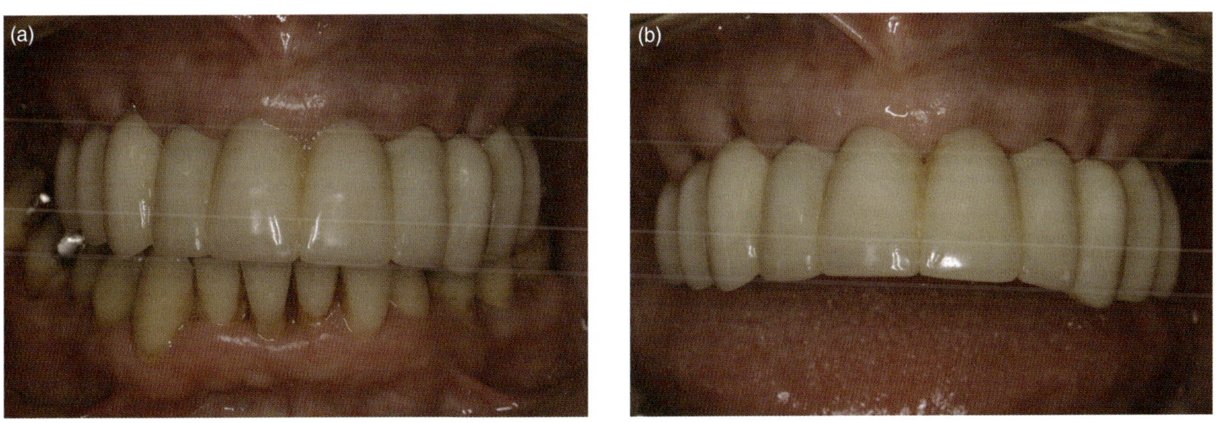

Figure 12.63 (a–b) A view of the four-week healing around the provisional bridge.

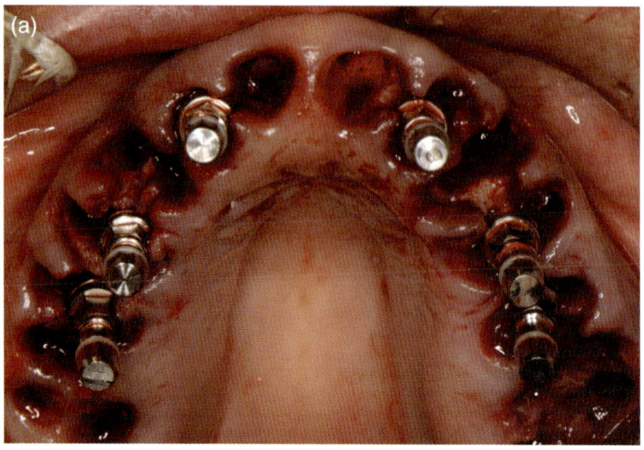

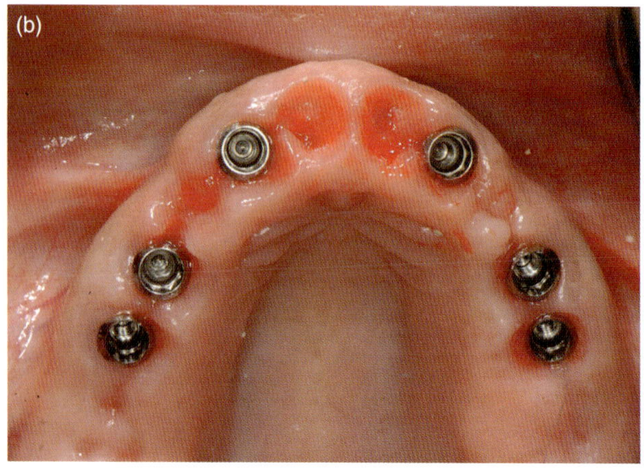

Figure 12.64 (a–b) Views of the implants at placement; the healed tissue at 12 weeks.

As a cement-retained final prosthesis was planned, solid abutments were selected and the prosthesis was fabricated (Figures 12.65a–d, 12.66a–d, and 12.67a–d).

Clinical Example Three: Full Mouth Restoration

A 65-year-old healthy female presented for implant evaluation. The patient had had many negative dental office experiences and was a dental phobic. She was therefore reluctant to treat her esthetic and functional problems. The patient had no medical condition which would limit her treatment.

Examination of the patient's oral cavity revealed hopeless maxillary and mandibular dentitions due to extensive bone loss. An arch size discrepancy, with significant maxillary resorption, was evident (Figures 12.68a–d). The patient was referred for maxillary and mandibular CAT scans. Before a prosthetic determination was made, the scans would confirm whether or not a sufficient volume of bone of adequate density was available for implant placement.

The mandibular CAT scan was evaluated for implant placement. Sufficient volume of bone was present between the mental foramina for implant placement. The mandibular canal was identified and outlined. From examination of the oblique CAT scan slices, it was established that 10 mm of bone was present superior to the inferior alveolar canal. Six sites were selected for implant installation; one implant placed above the canal, either at the first molar or second bicuspid position; one implant at the first bicuspid site and one implant in the lateral incisor region on each side. The cuspid site was not considered because of the volume of the socket (diameter and depth). In addition, the retained cuspid would be helpful with implant placement and bite registration (Figures 12.69a–b).

The maxilla displayed significant resorption in a palatal direction. However, 8 mm of bone could be found at six sites between teeth numbers 4 and 13. Bone density in these areas exceeded minimum values. The three-dimensional view demonstrated the inclination of the implants. This information was discussed with the prosthodontist (Figures 12.70a–b and 12.71a–b).

The patient had a significant gag reflex, making accurate record taking difficult. It was impossible to take preliminary impressions without IV sedation. After consultation with the prosthodontist, surgeon, and patient, it was decided that the most predictable and expedient therapy would be most prudent for the patient. This meant that each arch would be treated in an immediate load manner. The treatment plan involved placing the patient under IV sedation. At that time, all mandibular teeth would be extracted except the cuspids, which would aid in implant placement and taking of a bite registration. The implants would be installed, and a bite would be taken using the cuspids as vertical stops. The cuspids would then be extracted. An open tray impression of the implants would be taken, healing covers placed and a maxillary impression taken. The impressions and bite registration would be sent to the laboratory, where a screw-retained mandibular provisional

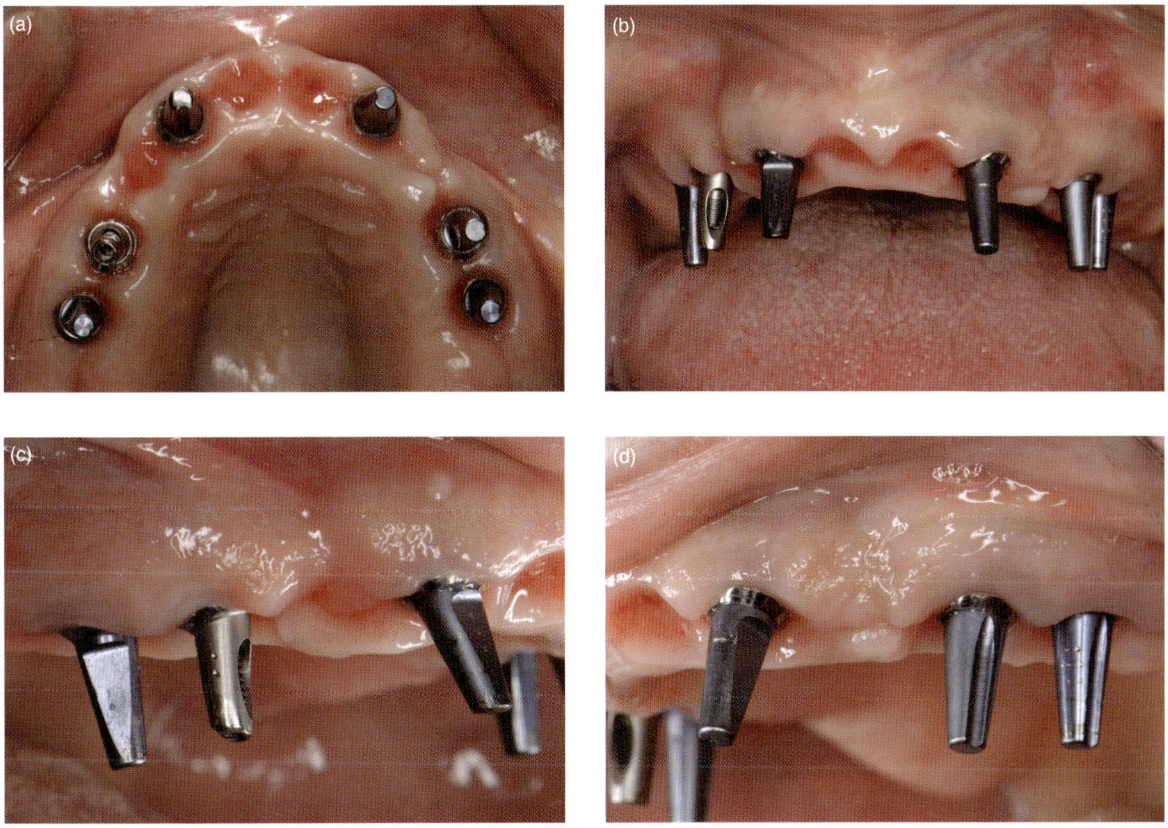

Figure 12.65 (a–d) Views of abutments placed on integrated implants at 12 weeks. The bridge to be fabricated in three sections.

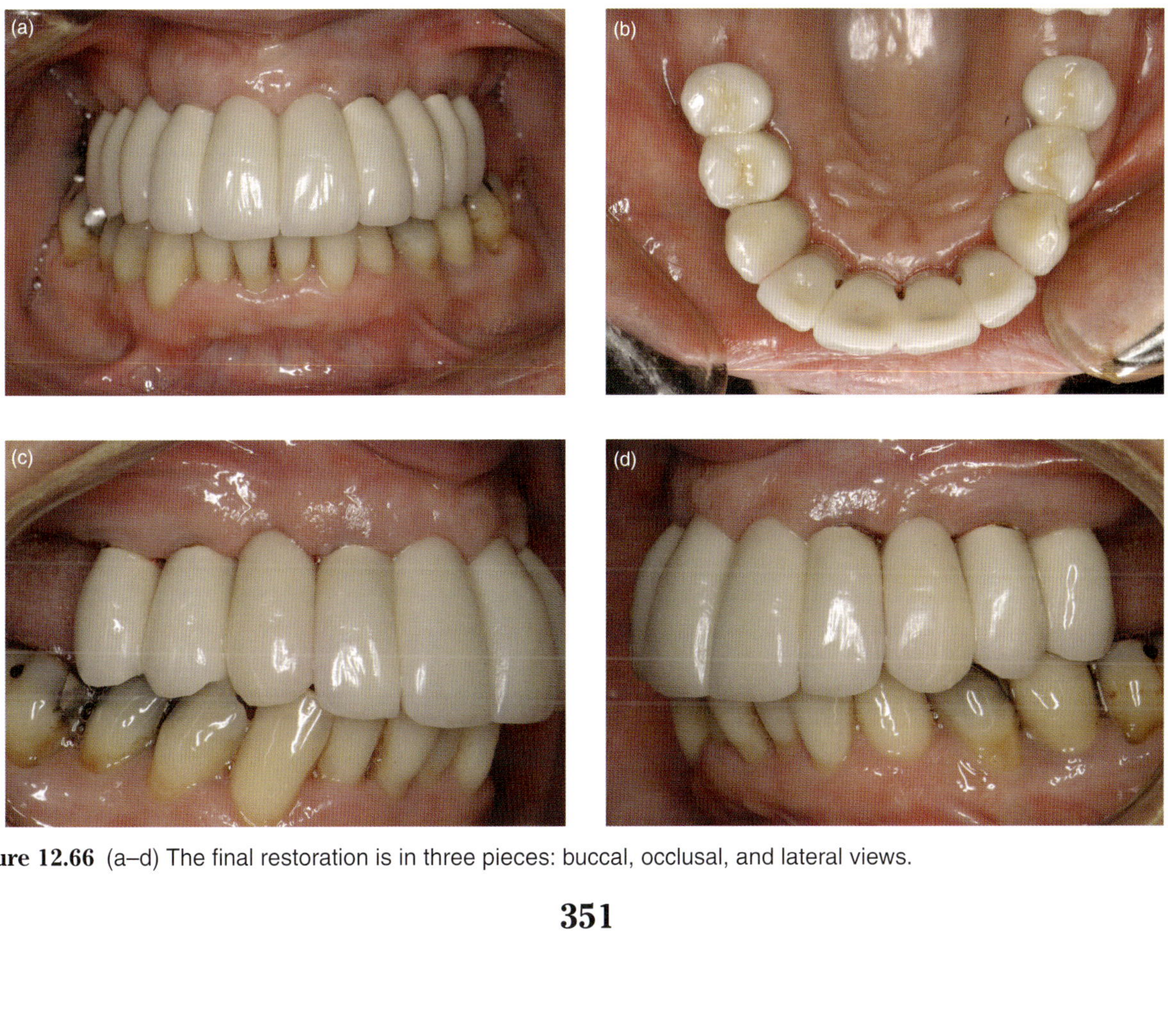

Figure 12.66 (a–d) The final restoration is in three pieces: buccal, occlusal, and lateral views.

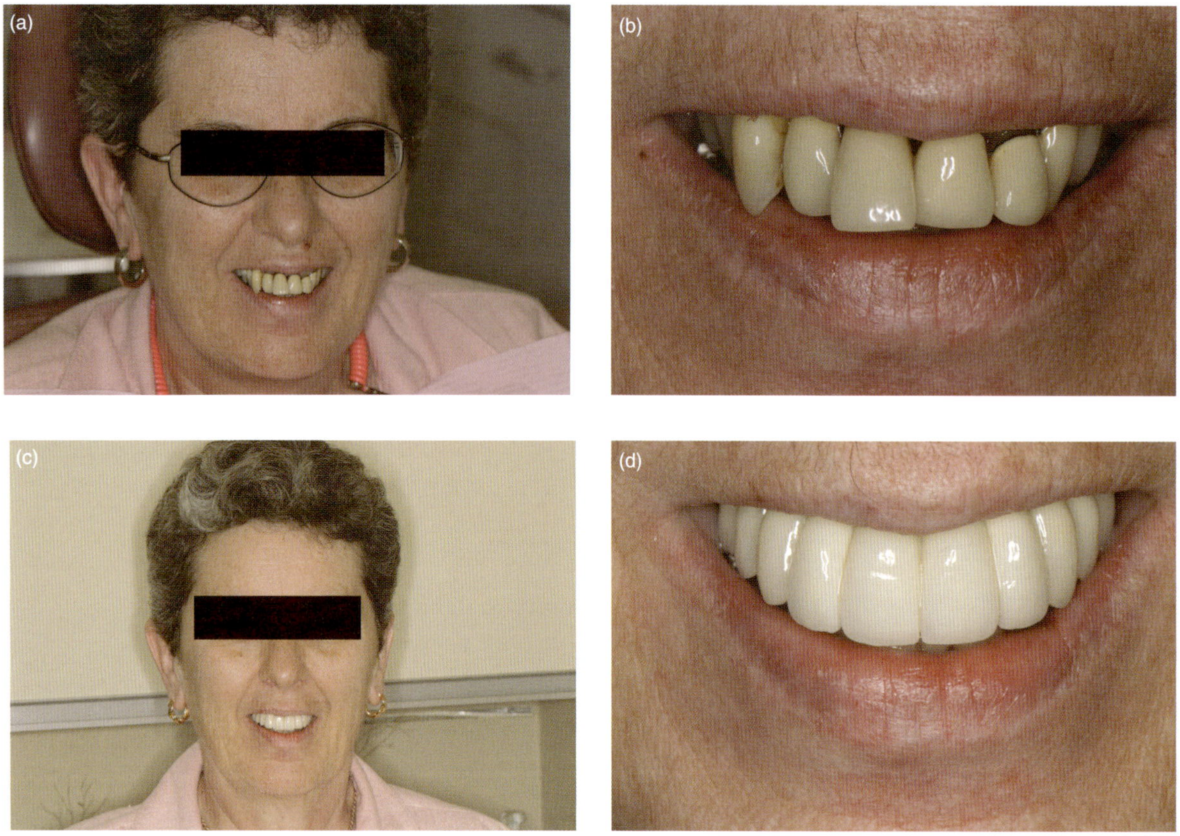

Figure 12.67 (a–d) Before and after: full face and closeup views.

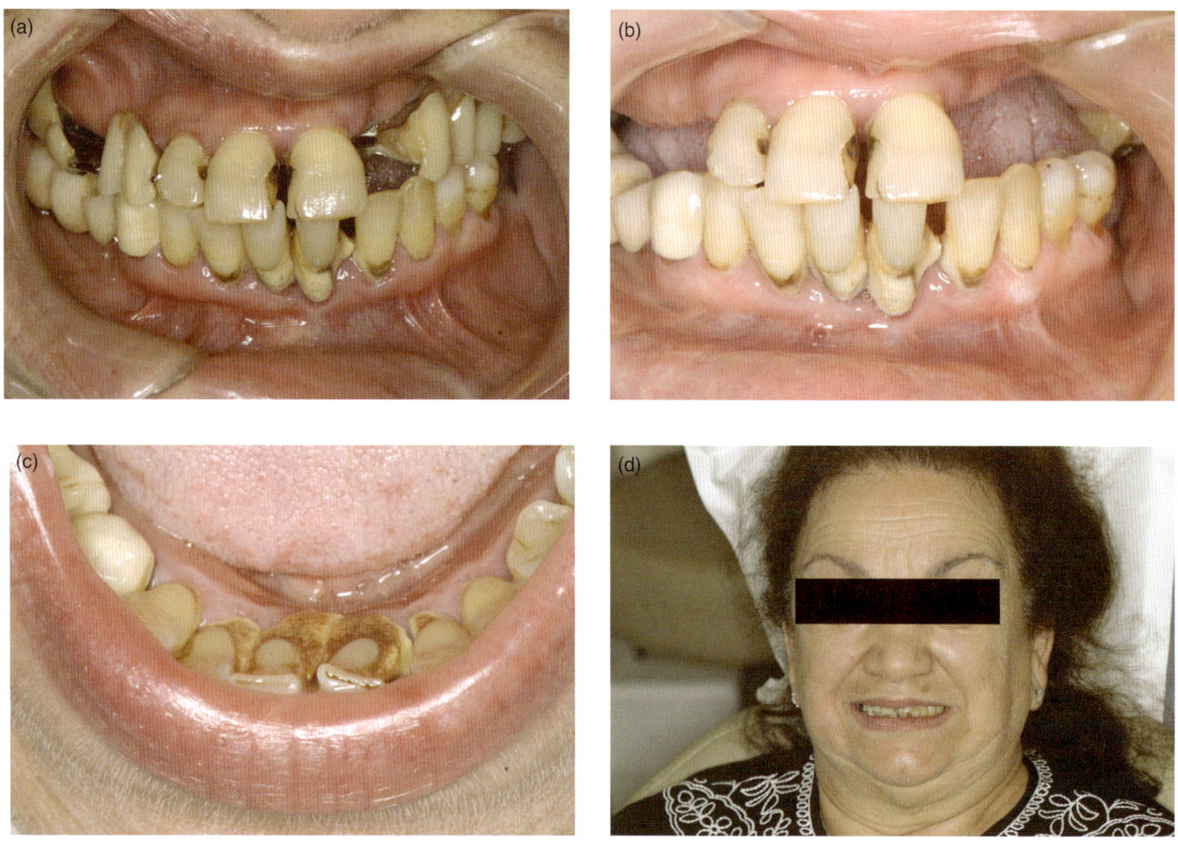

Figure 12.68 (a–d) A 65-year-old healthy female at presentation: full face, closeup, and occlusal views.

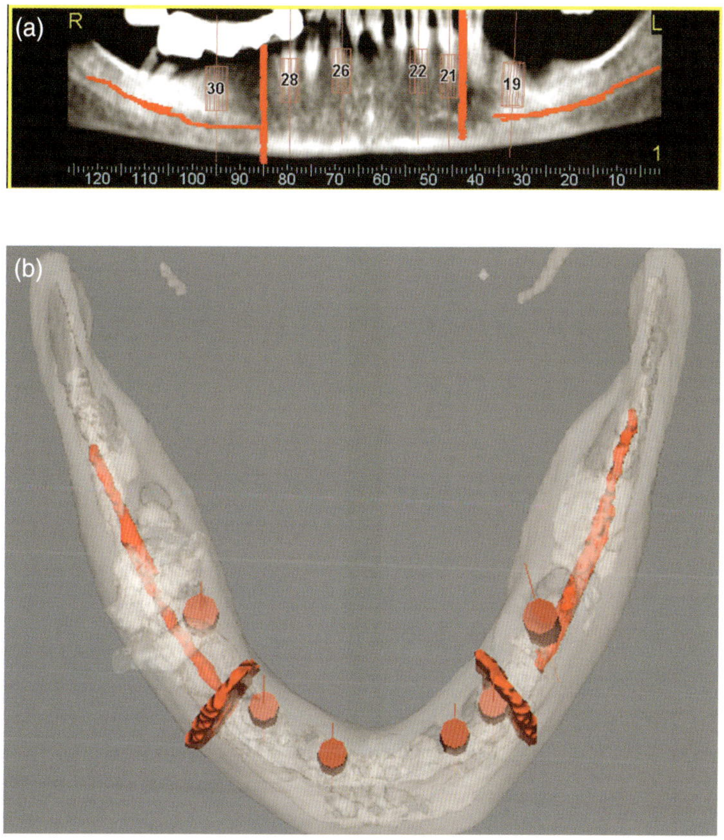

Figure 12.69 (a–b) A panorex view from a CT, with the canal outlined and implant positions determined; a three-dimensional occlusal view with the implants in place.

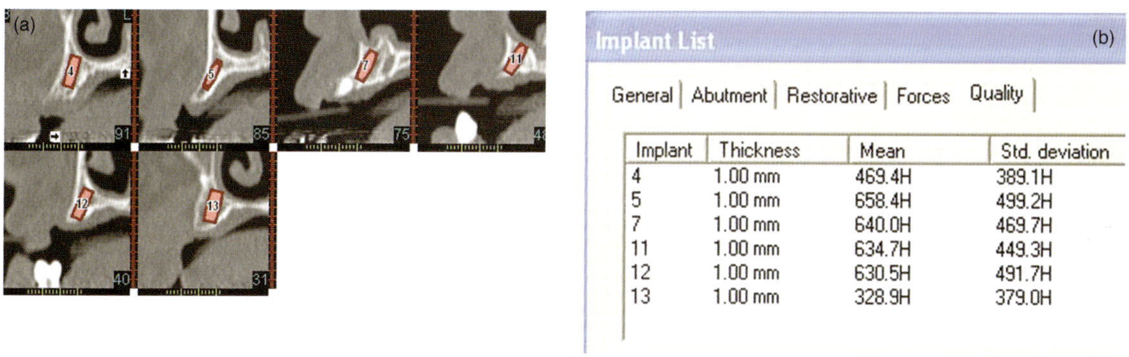

Implant	Thickness	Mean	Std. deviation
4	1.00 mm	469.4H	389.1H
5	1.00 mm	658.4H	499.2H
7	1.00 mm	640.0H	469.7H
11	1.00 mm	634.7H	449.3H
12	1.00 mm	630.5H	491.7H
13	1.00 mm	328.9H	379.0H

Figure 12.70 (a–b) A view of the implant positions in the maxilla, with density measurements and oblique sections.

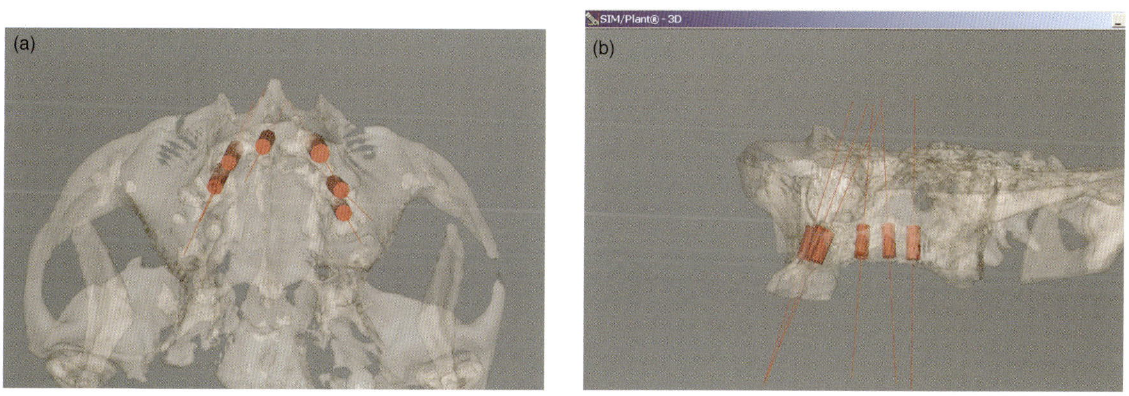

Figure 12.71 (a–b) Three-dimensional views of the maxilla demonstrate the divergence of the implants between the right and left sides.

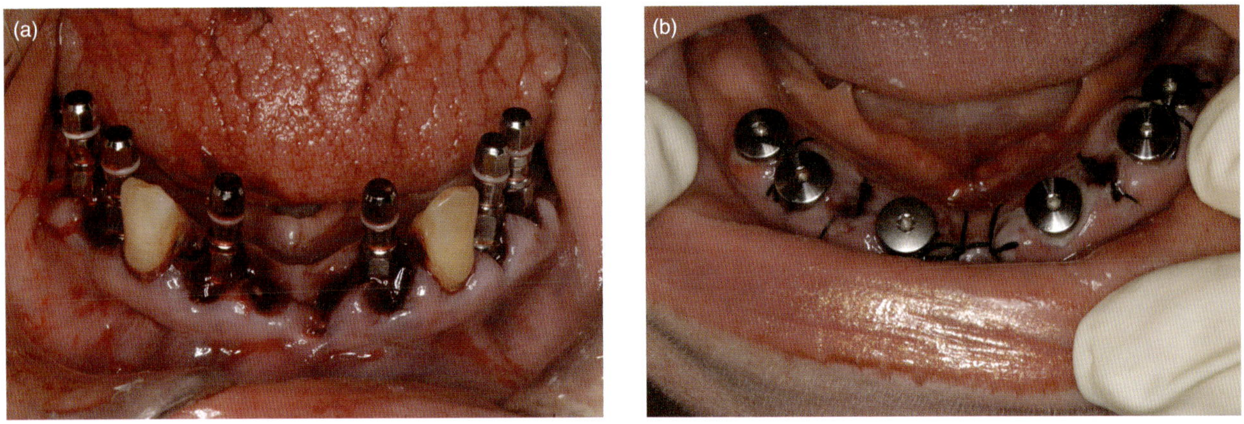

Figure 12.72 (a–b) Placement of mandibular implants has been carried out, with retention of teeth numbers 22 and 27 to aid in implant placement and bite registration; healing covers are placed after a bite registration and impression are taken.

restoration would be fabricated against a waxed-up maxilla, based upon the mounting. A template for the maxillary implants would then be fabricated for proper implant positioning for a screw-retained case, which would occur after the mandibular provisional restoration was in place.

Treatment proceeded as planned. The mandible was treated first. The retention of the cuspids during surgery aided in implant alignment and bite registration (Figures 12.72a–b). The provisional restoration was inserted 24 h postoperatively (Figures 12.73a–b and 12.74a–b). The impression of the upper arch taken during the mandibular surgery permitted fabrication of the appropriate template. Maxillary implants were installed with the aid of the stent, which was also used to take the bite registration (Figures 12.75a–d). The provisional restoration was inserted 24 h postimplant insertion (Figures 12.76a–d). Minimal occlusal adjustment was required. The patient healed without untoward sequelae (Figure 12.77).

At 12 weeks after maxillary surgery, the provisional restorations were removed (Figures 12.78a–b). The implants were torqued, tested to 35 Ncm in both clockwise and counterclockwise directions, and radiographs were taken. All 12 implants had integrated. The final prostheses were constructed as segmental units (Figures 12.79a–d, 12.80a–d, 12.81a–c, 12.82a–d, and 12.83).

COMPLICATIONS

Complications are minimized by following the described protocols. However, complications do still occur. Implant loss due to micromotion is the most

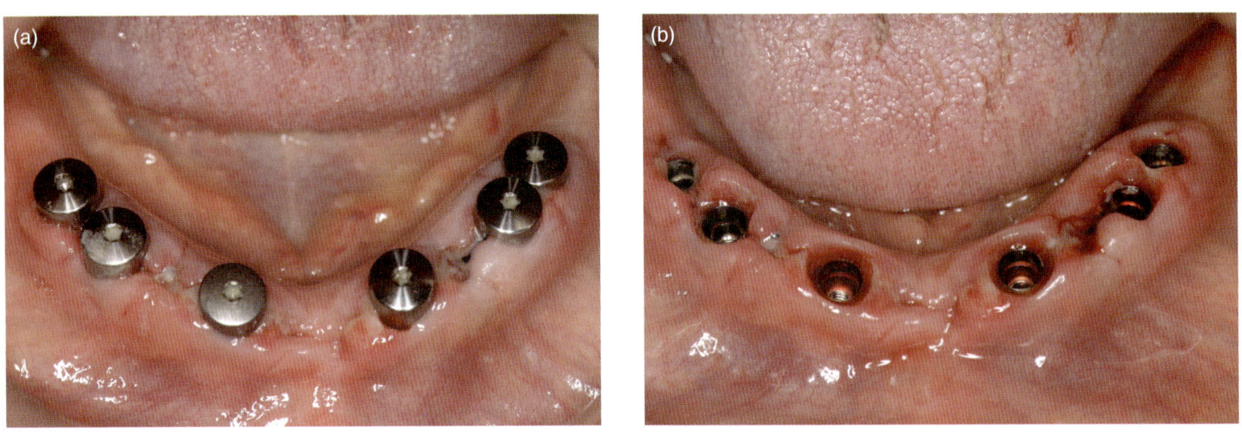

Figure 12.73 (a–b) Twenty-four hours postoperative, healing covers are removed to effect provisional bridge placement.

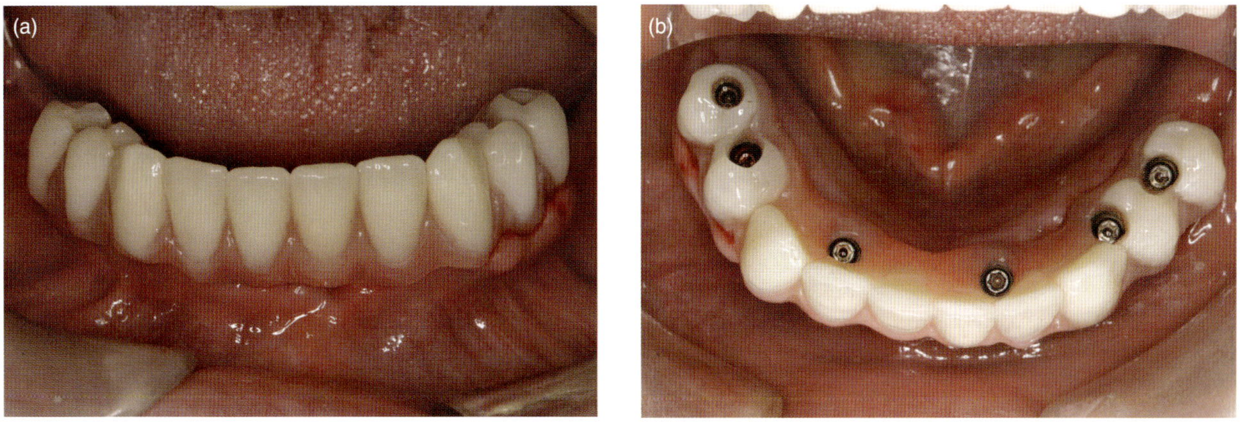

Figure 12.74 (a–b) The mandibular provisional bridge is placed.

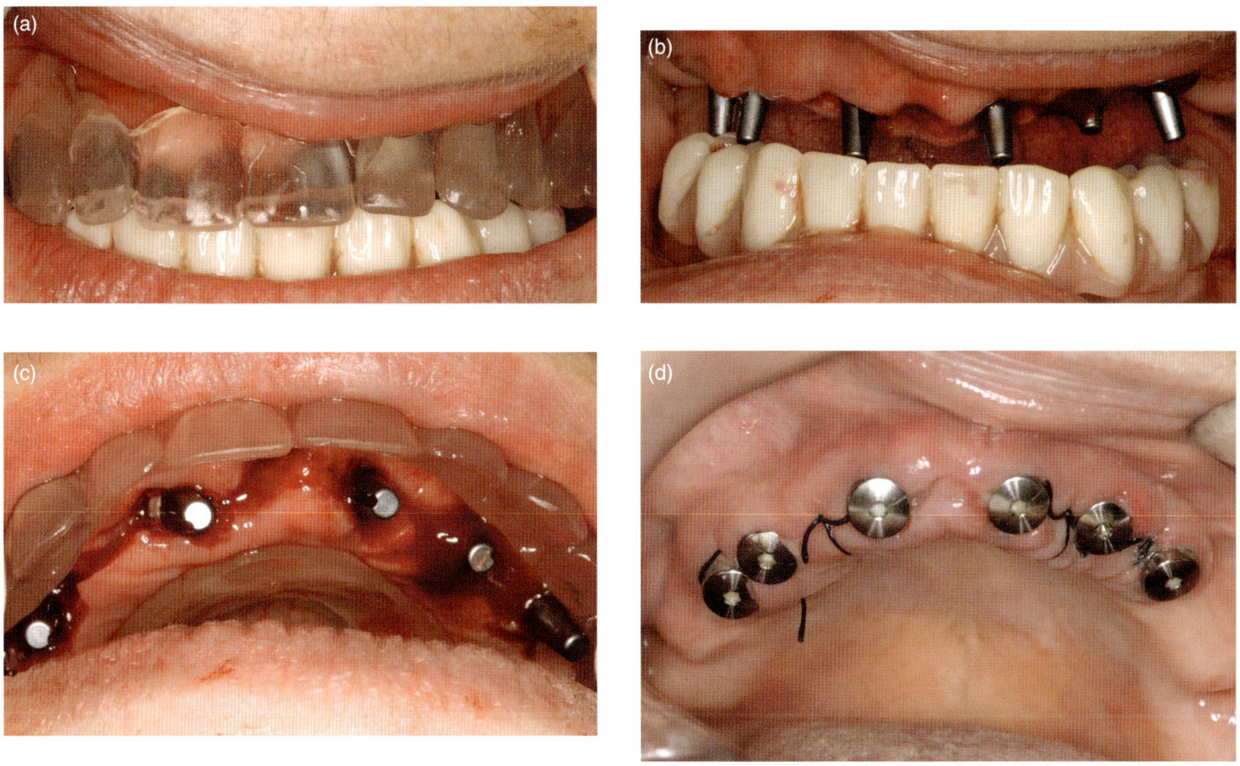

Figure 12.75 (a–d) Views of the maxillary template; solid abutments for bite registration; healing covers.

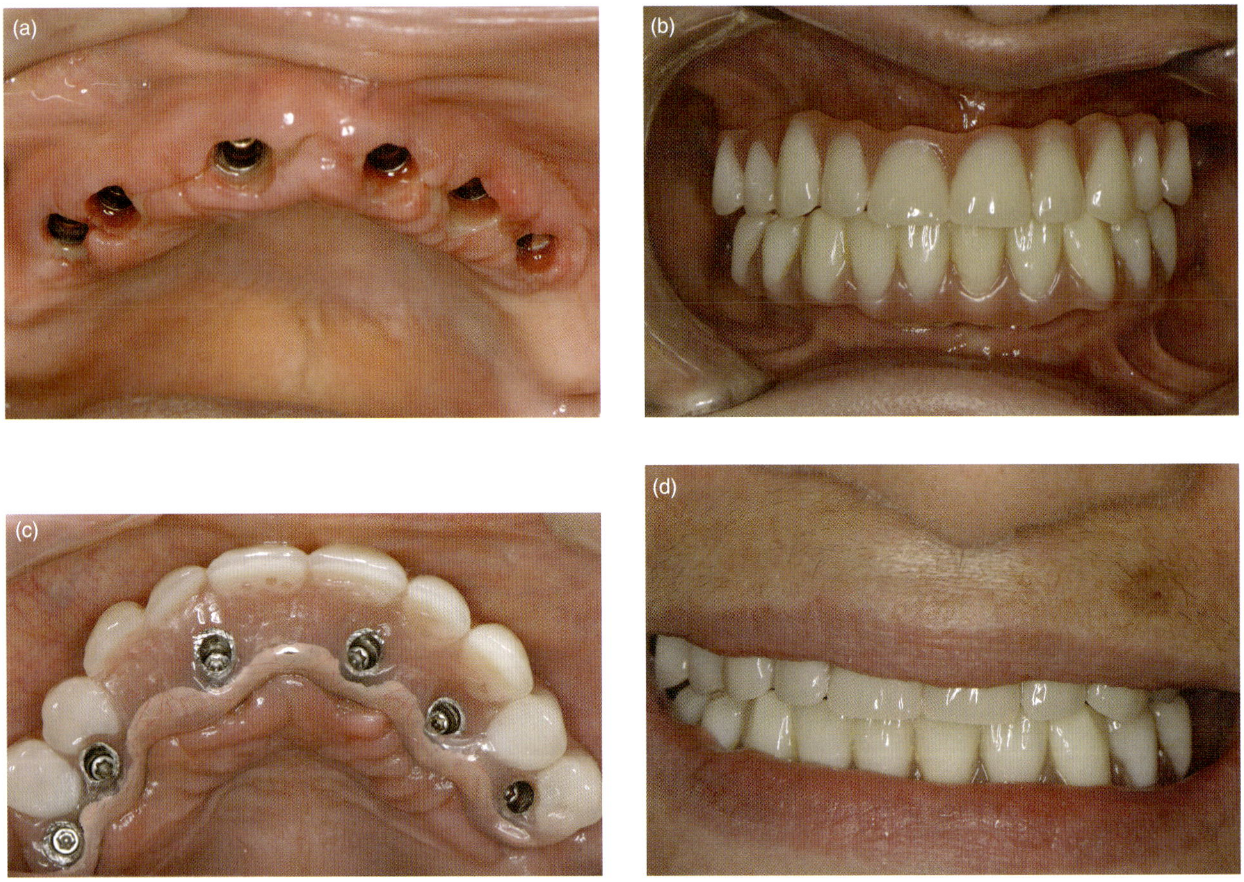

Figure 12.76 (a–d) Delivery of the maxillary provisional bridge at 24 h: healing cover removal; bridge delivery; the patient's smile.

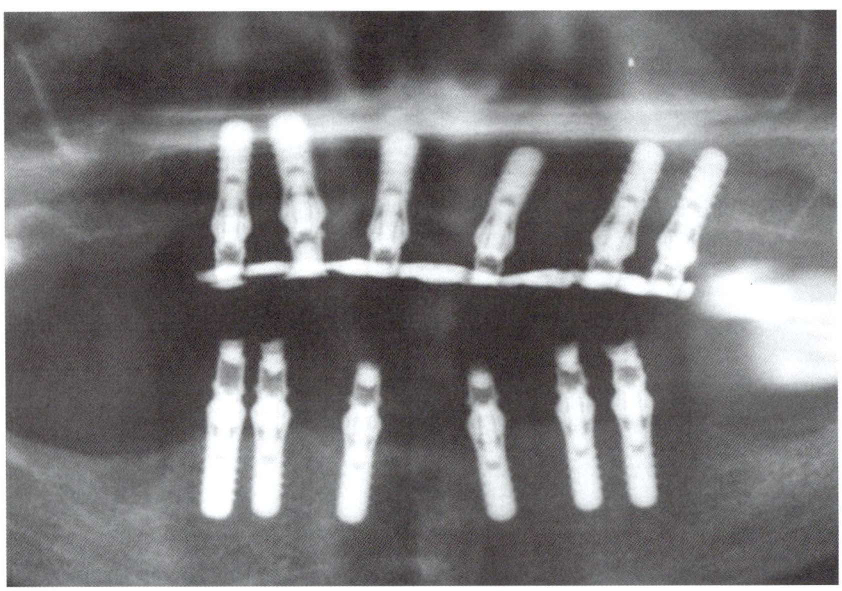

Figure 12.77 A panorex taken during implant healing.

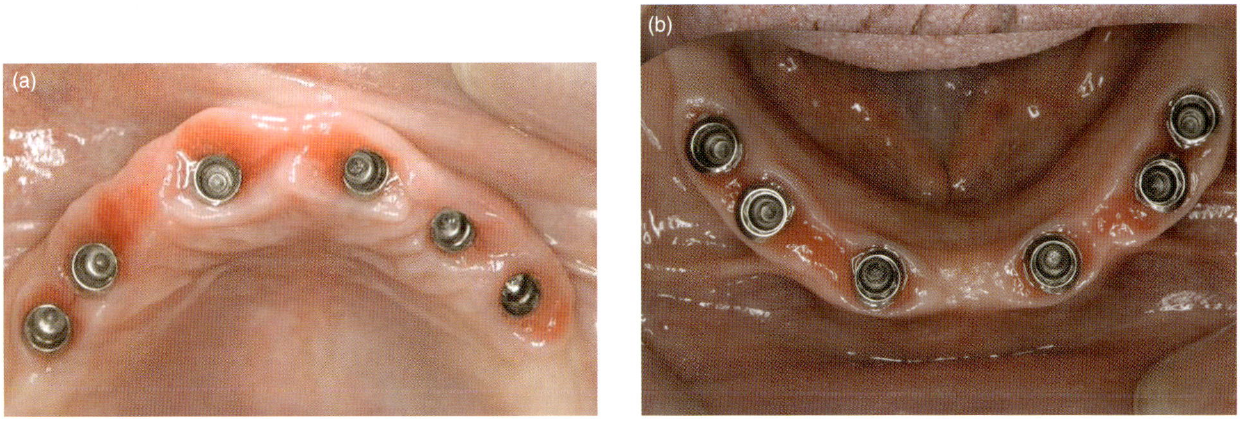

Figure 12.78 (a–b) The healed tissues at 12 weeks.

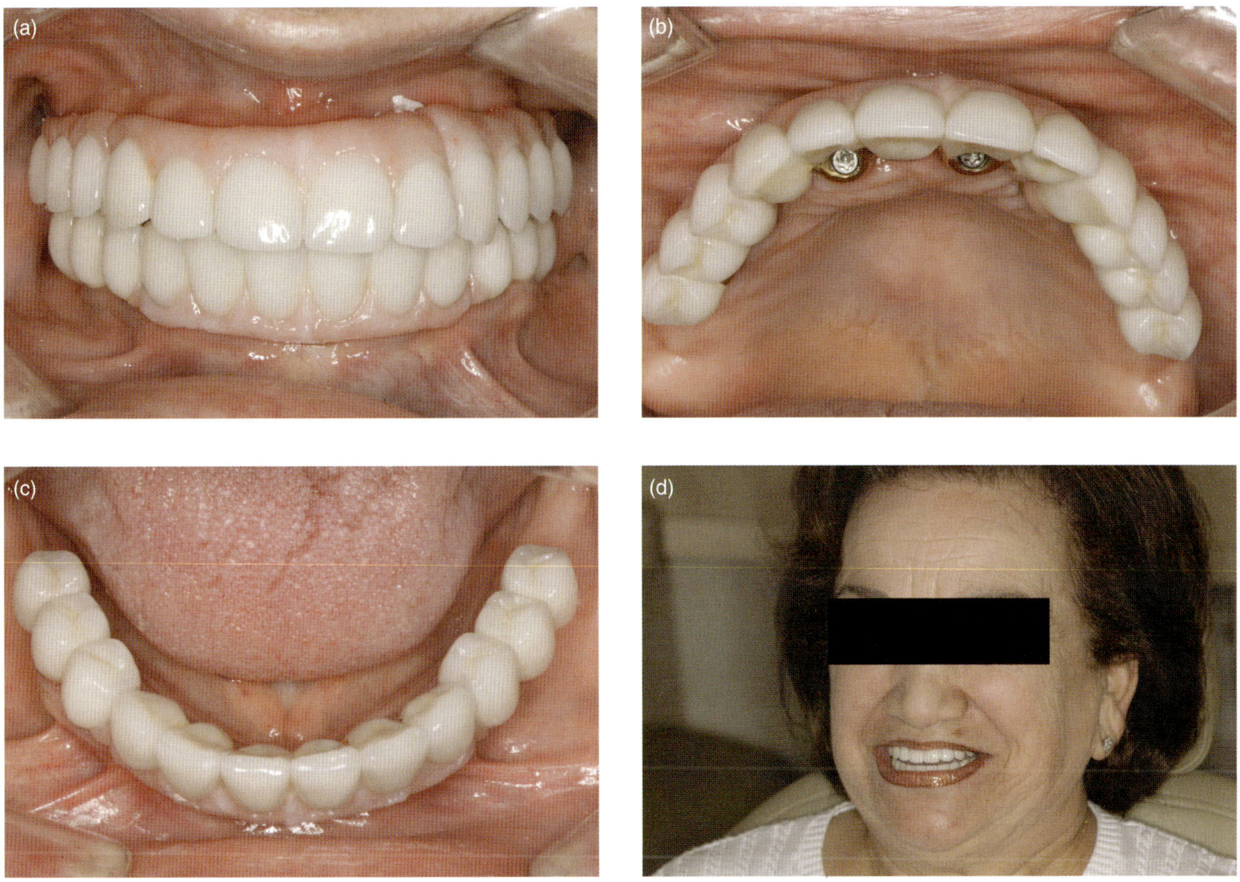

Figure 12.79 (a–d) The final restorations in each arch are in three pieces: anterior and two posterior sections.

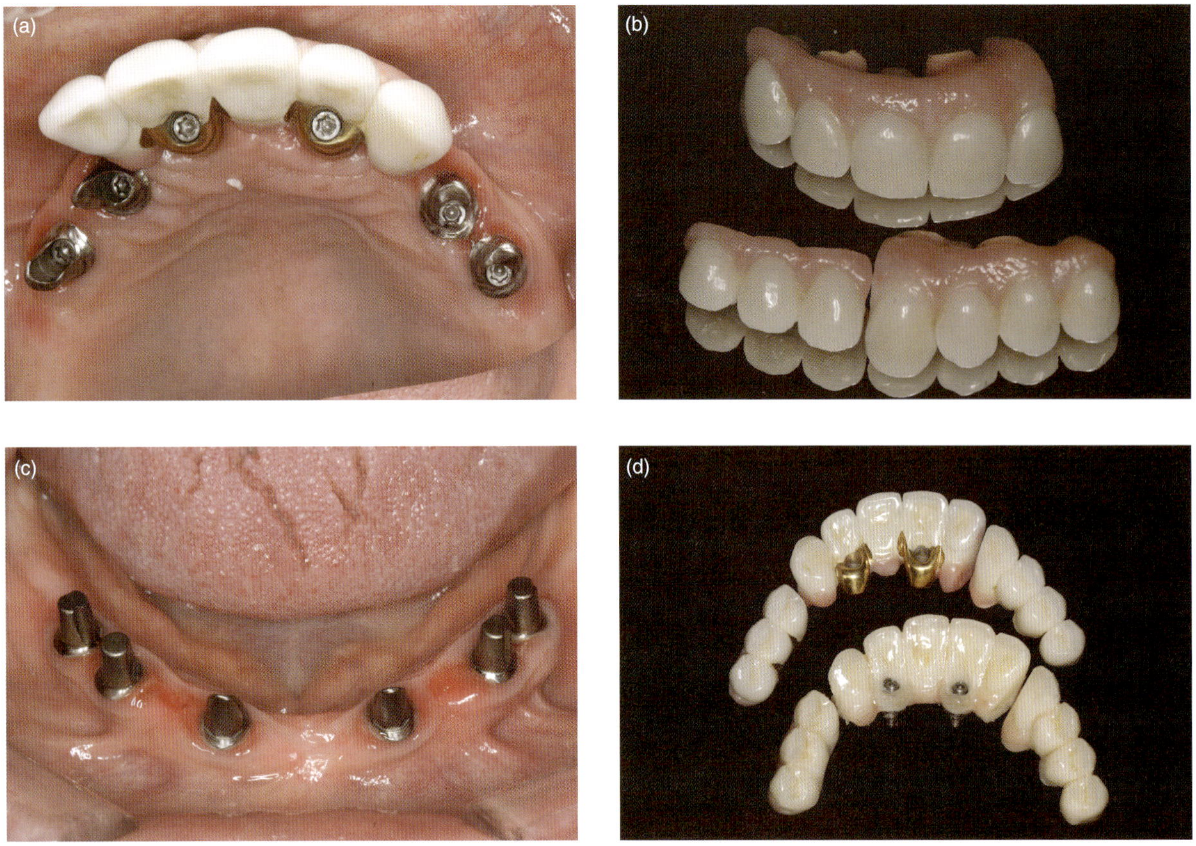

Figure 12.80 (a–d) The final cases are each in three pieces.

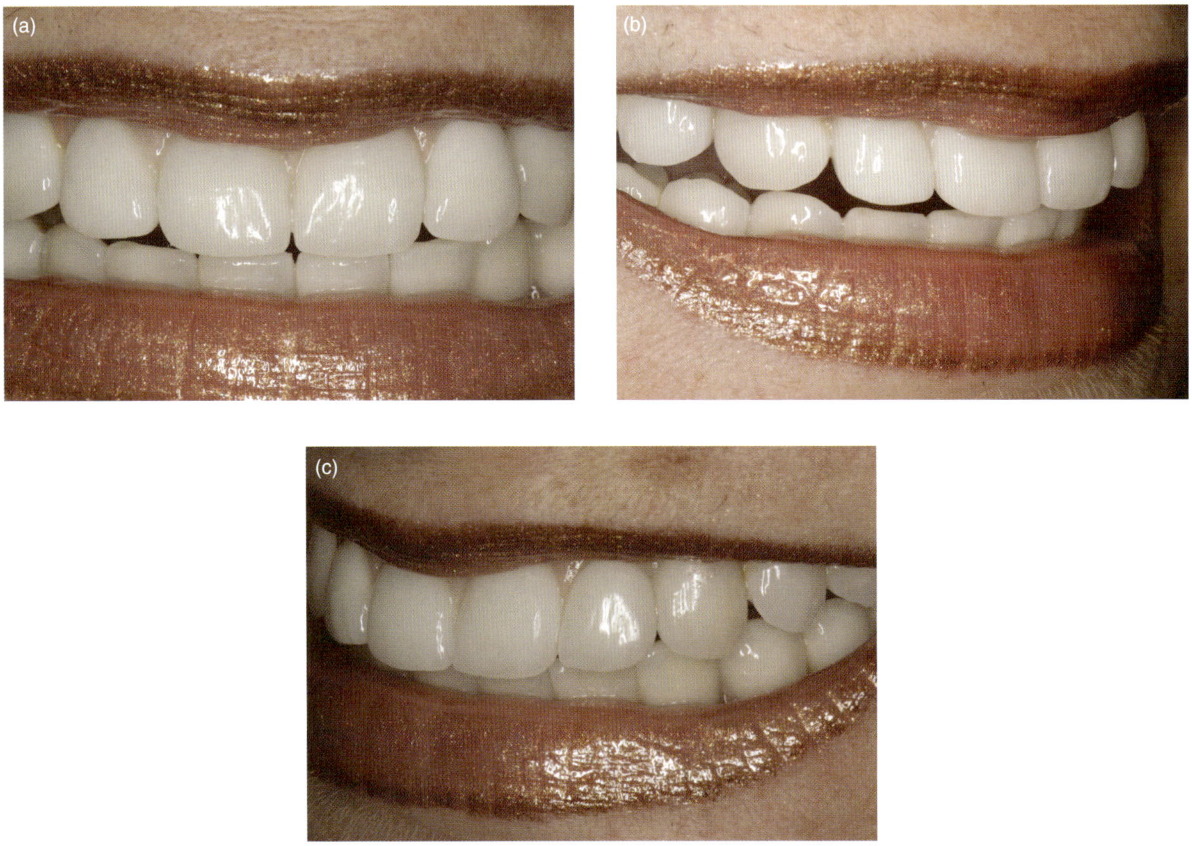

Figure 12.81 (a–c) The smile of the final case.

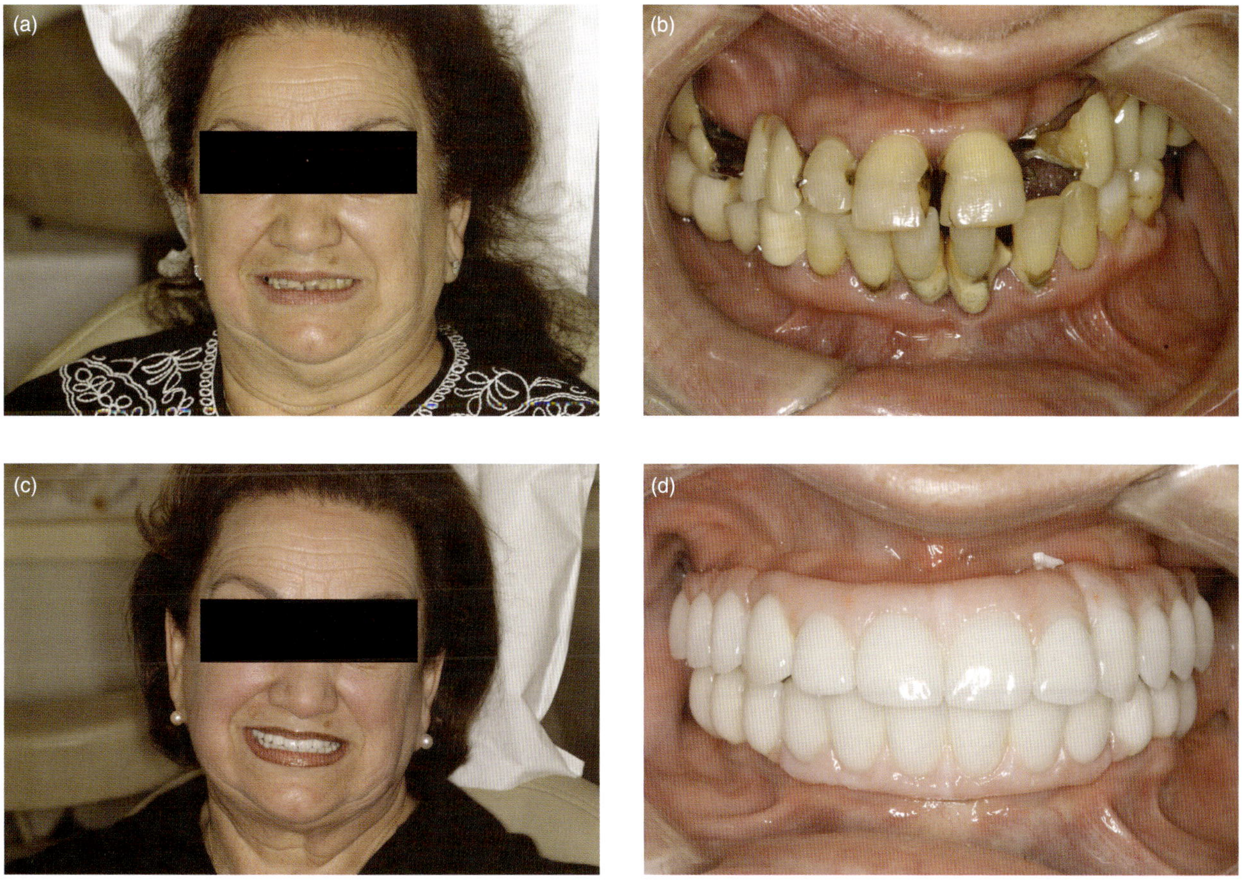

Figure 12.82 Before and after: full face and closeup views.

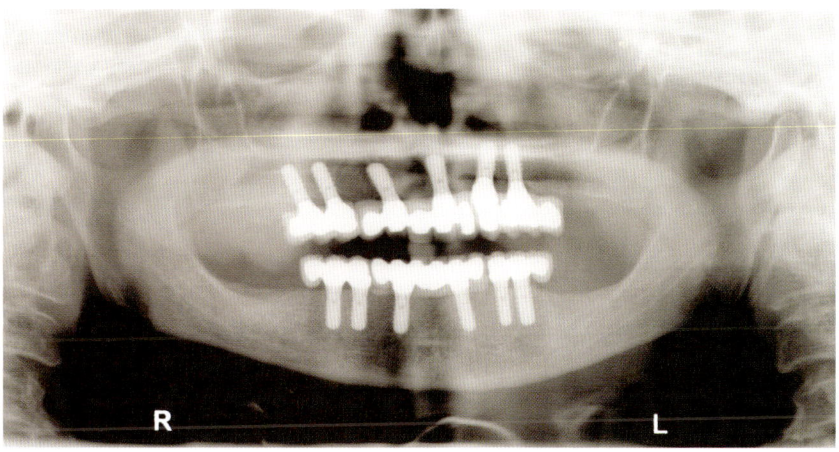

Figure 12.83 A panorex of the final case.

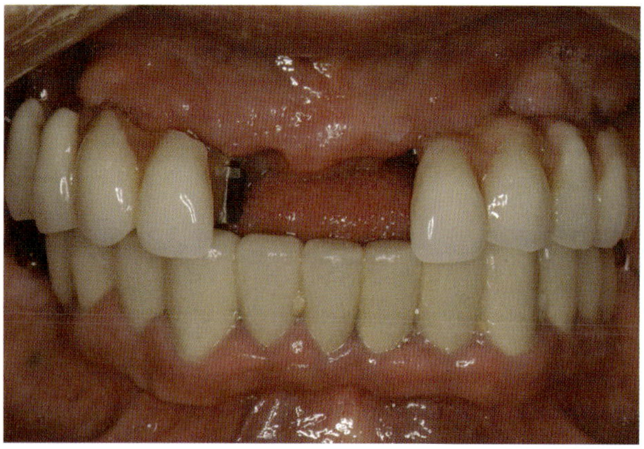

Figure 12.84 A fractured bridge due to lack of patient compliance in avoiding hard food before implant integration has occurred.

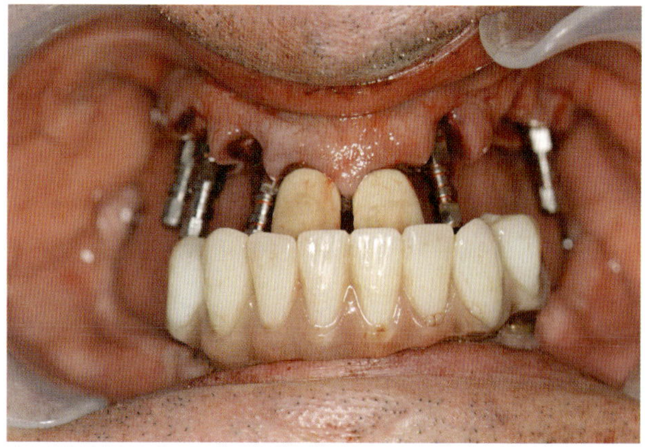

Figure 12.85 Implants have been placed in a patient with a Class 3 occlusion.

common untoward occurrence. Most often, such movement is due to lack of restoration passivity and/or patient compliance. If care is not taken to fabricate a passive provisional restoration, implants will become mobile. The restoration should remain in place for six weeks before it is removed and the implants are checked. The patient should be examined either weekly or biweekly during the first month to ensure that cement does not washout or screws do not loosen. Such occurrences are signs of an improperly fitting prosthesis, which could lead to micromotion and implant loss.

Before the implants are placed, patients are instructed regarding diet and care after immediate implant loading. They are told to follow a soft diet for four weeks and are cautioned that one bite into a hard substance could jeopardize the final result and cause implant loss (Figure 12.84.) If the patient evidences parafunctional habits, nightguards are fabricated.

Since the largest size implant is never used, if an implant is lost, it can be replaced with a wider or longer implant. The restoration may then be reinserted. Six weeks of healing is then necessary. This delay does not impact the timing of the final prosthesis insertion, as 12 weeks of integration is generally needed for soft tissue maturation with immediate implant placement and loading.

If multiple implants are lost it may not be possible to use the transitional fixed prosthesis. In such a situation, a denture must be fabricated. This sequella is usually due to improper treatment planning. For example, in the case of a Class 3 occlusion, immediately loading a full maxilla leaves only the anterior implants in function and unable to tolerate the occlusal load (Figures 12.85–12.90).

Conclusions

This technique has been successfully employed in over 200 arches. Cumulative implant success rates exceed 97% in the mandible and 92% in the maxilla. The outlined immediate load protocol permits patients who are losing their dentitions to be transitioned into implants and remain in fixed dentitions, while not having to undergo multiple surgeries and provisional restorations.

The major cause of implant failure is micromotion during healing. This micromotion is created by patients eating a hard diet during the first four to

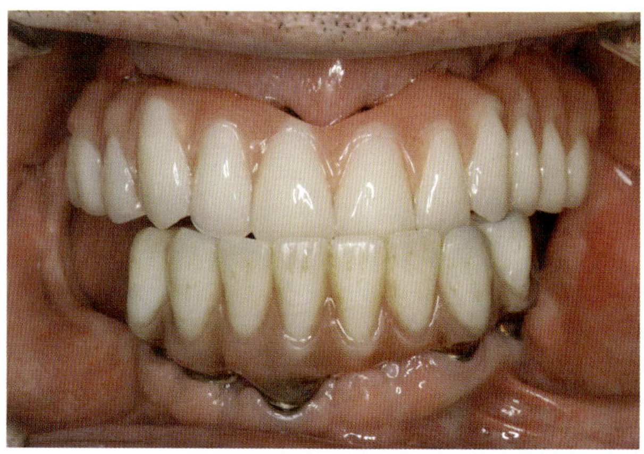

Figure 12.86 The immediate provisional bridge has been placed with only anterior contact.

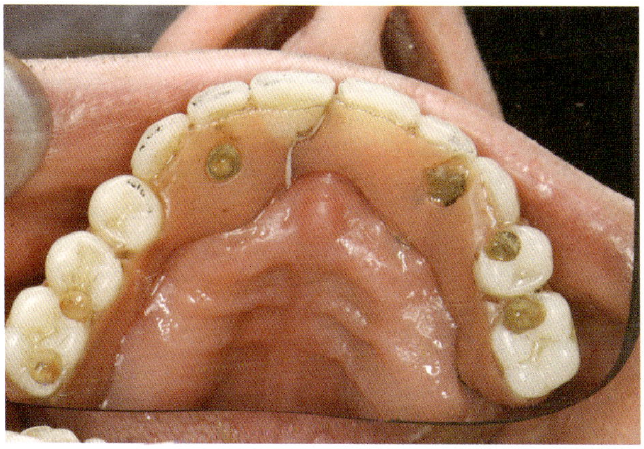

Figure 12.87 A view of the fractured bridge at four weeks.

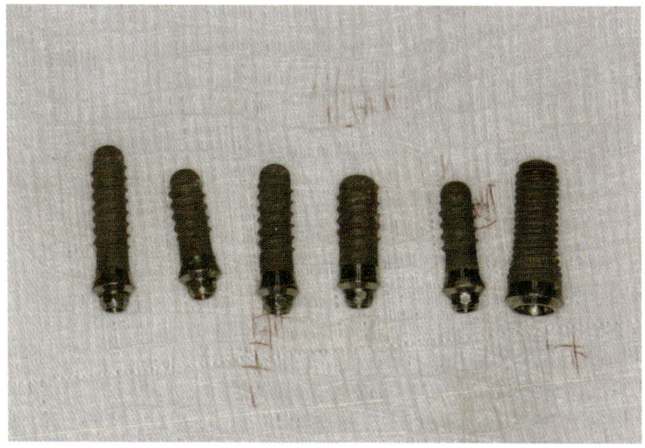

Figure 12.89 Loss of all implants at four weeks has occurred.

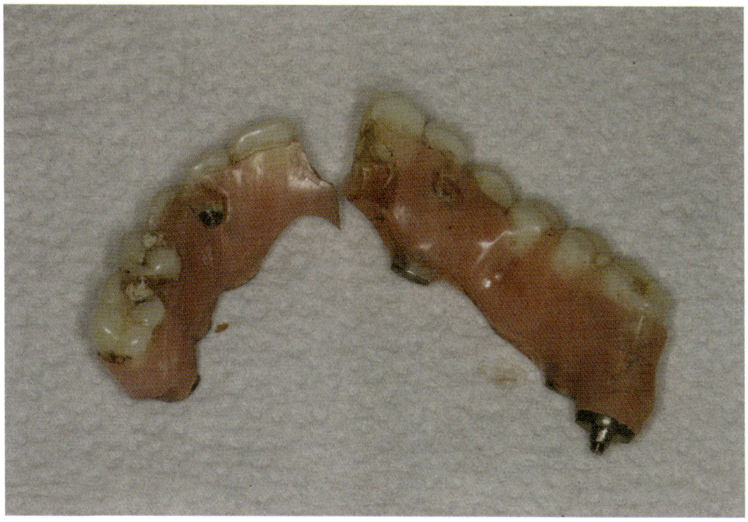

Figure 12.88 An occlusal view of the fractured bridge at four weeks.

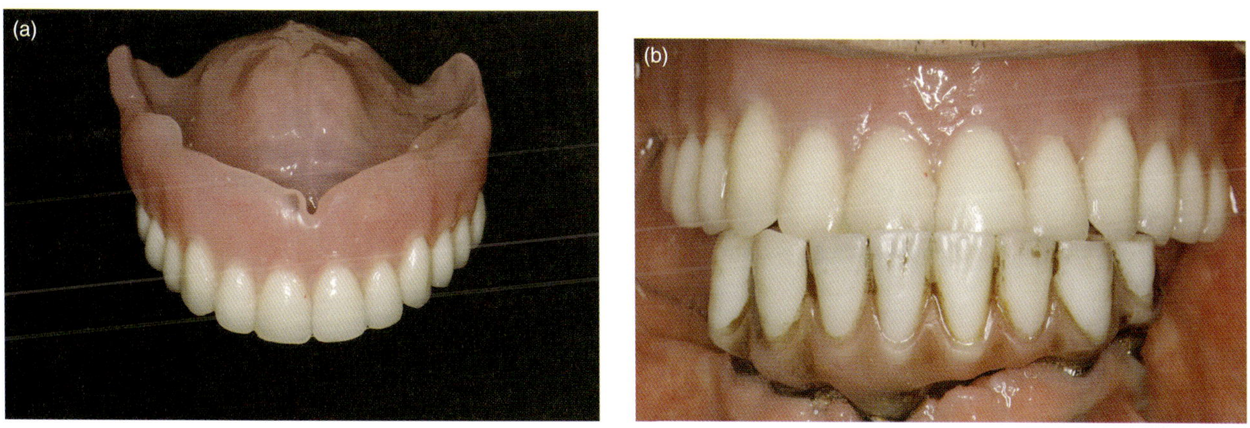

Figure 12.90 A rescue denture was fabricated for the patient to use, while new implants healed.

six weeks after implant placement, or is due to an improperly fitted provisional restoration. Full arch immediate implant loading, with cross-arch splinting, eliminates this concern.

Extensive presurgical planning is vital to ensure a successful treatment outcome. If an implant or even two implants fail to integrate, they may be replaced while the patient continues to wear the provisional restoration.

The utilization of two surgical templates offers the convenience of being able to prepare osteotomy sites while visualizing the bur with the buccal half of the template cut away. Templates with sleeves offer the benefit of a fixed position for the bur. This approach works well with a fully edentulous arch. However, in patients who are losing multiple teeth, sites may be lost after extraction due to fracture of buccal and/or interproximal bone. If this occurs, a fixed template with sleeves would be rendered useless.

Utilizing a prefabricated shell from an articulated waxed-up cast provides many treatment options. If implant position or angulation change from the initial plan, the shell may still be employed. Increases or decreases in pontic sizes are easy to accommodate. In a prefabricated provisional restoration, these adaptations are more difficult to achieve, if not impossible.

A predictable protocol has been developed to transform an arch of hopeless teeth into a fixed implant prosthesis utilizing immediately placed, immediately loaded implants (Tables 12.4 and 12.5).

Table 12.4 Criteria for screw versus cement-retained provisional restorations.

- Method of choice is always screw retained—less traumatic and more accurate
  - Inability to get implants and/or abutments parallel—must screw retain
  - Discrepancy in heights of implant shoulders—screw retain
  - Discrepancy in heights of buccal and lingual tissues—screw retain
  - Ability to atraumatically remove bridge during healing—screw retain
- Dentist comfortable with fabricating cementable prosthesis—cementable prosthesis

Table 12.5 Criteria for indirect versus direct prosthesis.

- Immediate delivery of prosthesis a must—direct
- Accuracy—indirect
- Atraumatic—indirect

References

1. Adell R, Lekholm U, Rockler B, and Branemark PI. 1981. A 15-year study of osseointegrated implants in the treatment of the edentulous jaw. *Int J Oral Surg* 10: 387–416.
2. Szmukler-Moncler S, Salama H, Reingewirtz Y, and Dubruille JH. 1998. Timing of loading and effect of micromotion on bone-dental implant interface: Review of experimental literature. *J Biomed Mater Res* 43: 192–203.
3. Schnitman PA, Wohrle PS, Rubenstein JE, DaSilva JD, and Wang NH. 1997. Ten-year results for Branemark implants immediately loaded with fixed prostheses at implant placement. *Int J Oral Maxillofac Implants* 12:495–503.
4. Beagle JR. 2006. The immediate placement of endosseous dental implants in fresh extraction sites. *Dent Clin North Am* 50:375–389.
5. Buser D, Nydegger T, Hirt HP, Cochran DL, and Nolte LP. 1998. Removal torque values of titanium implants in the maxilla of miniature pigs. *Int J Oral Maxillofac Implants* 13:611–619.
6. Buser D, Broggini N, Wieland M, et al. 2004. Enhanced bone apposition to a chemically modified SLA titanium surface. *J Dent Res* 83:529–533.
7. Park JY and Davies JE. 2000. Red blood cell and platelet interactions with titanium implant surfaces. *Clin Oral Implants Res* 11:530–539.
8. Masuda T, Yliheikkila PK, Felton DA, and Cooper LF. 1998. Generalizations regarding the process and phenomenon of osseointegration. Part 1: In vivo studies. *Int J Oral Maxillofac Implants* 13:17–29.
9. Geng JP, Tan KB, and Liu GR. 2001. Application of finite element analysis in implant dentistry: A review of the literature. *J Prosthet Dent* 85:585–598.
10. Holmgren EP, Seckinger RJ, Kilgren LM, and Mante F. 1998. Evaluating parameters of osseointegrated dental implants using finite element analysis—a two-dimensional comparative study examining the effects of implant diameter, implant shape, and load direction. *J Oral Implantol* 24:80–88.
11. Himmlova L, Dostalova T, Kacovsky A, and Konvickova S. 2004. Influence of length and diameter on stress distribution: A finite elemental analysis. *J Prosthet Dent* 91:20–25.

12. Fugazzotto PA, Beagle JR, Ganeles J, Jaffin R, Vlassis J, and Kumar A. 2004. Success and failure rates of 9 mm or shorter implants in the replacement of missing maxillary molars when restored with individual crowns: Preliminary results 0 to 84 months in function. A retrospective study. *J Periodontol* 75:327–332.
13. Hansson S. 2000. Implant–abutment interface: Biomechanical study of flat top versus conical. *Clin Implant Dent Rel Res* 2:33–41.
14. Norton MR. 1997. An in vitro evaluation of the strength of an internal conical interface compared to a butt joint interface in implant design. *Clin Oral Implants Res* 8:290–298.
15. Jaffin R and Berman C. 1991. The excessive loss of Branemark fixtures in type IV bone: A 5-year analysis. *J Periodontol* 62:2–4.
16. Trisi P, Rao W, and Rebaudi A. 1999. A histometric comparison of smooth and rough titanium implants in human low-density jawbone. *Int J Oral Maxillofac Implants* 14:689–698.
17. Godfredson K, Berglundh T, and Lindhe J. 2001. Bone reactions adjacent to titanium implants subjected to static load. A study in the dog (I). *Clin Oral Implants Res* 12:1–8.
18. Godfredsen K, Berglundh T, and Lindhe J. 2001. Bone reactions adjacent to titanium implants with different surface characteristics subjected to static load. A study in the dog (II). *Clin Oral Implants Res* 12:196–201.
19. Nedir R, Bischof M, Szmukler-Moncler S, Bernard JP, and Samson J. 2004. Predicting osseointegration by means of implant primary stability. *Clin Oral Implants Res* 15:520–528.
20. Jaffin RA, Kumar A, and Berman CL. 2004. Immediate loading of dental implants in the completely edentulous maxilla: A clinical report. *Int J Oral Maxillofac Implants* 19:721–730.
21. Ganeles J, Rosenberg MM, Holt RL, and Reichman LH. 2001. Immediate loading of implants with fixed restorations in the completely edentulous mandible: Report of 27 patients from a private practice. *Int J Oral Maxillofac Implants* 16:418–426.

Chapter 13

The Rehabilitation of the Edentulous Maxillary Jaw Utilizing Dental Implant Therapy

Anthony J. Dickinson, BDSc, MSD

Outline

Maxillary edentulism can be for most people a debilitating disorder. The loss of one's upper teeth not only compromises the ability of the person to function adequately and comfortably, but also has ongoing negative effects on facial appearance. Diet is invariably compromised, with effects on the general health. Self-esteem is diminished, and the quality of life is reduced.

Conventional removable full upper dentures have improved over time and may provide an adequate, but not entirely satisfactory, replacement for missing teeth and associated hard and soft tissues. With the introduction and scientific establishment of the biologic response of a functional anklyosis to titanium implants when placed into the human jawbones, many patients now have a treatment alternative to the conventional denture.

However, it is salient to bear in mind: "Patient's don't want implants . . . they want teeth" (attributed to Prof Graham White, Sheffield, UK). Dental implants only provide a fixation mechanism to allow a tooth or set of teeth to be anchored in the jaw. Whilst dental implants have offered an expanded range of treatment options to partially and fully edentulous patients, the technique and required procedures have increased the necessary diagnostic, planning, and technical skills of dental practitioners.

For patients who are managed with a comprehensive, careful, and if necessary, interdisciplinary approach to treatment, the outcomes can be extremely rewarding—some say "life changing" (Figures 13.1a–d). We must seek to avoid, for a range of reasons, some patients feeling that they were better served with their previous conventional removable appliance.

There are essentially two options when considering the use of dental implants for the rehabilitation of the edentulous maxillary jaw: The fixed implant-retained prostheses; alternatively, an implant retained/supported removable prostheses. These are further subclassified in Table 13.1.

Each category, with either subclassification, can be considered to have both advantages and disadvantages, which should be considered and evaluated for each patient (Table 13.2). Following the appropriate clinical, radiological, and diagnostic data being collected and analyzed, a decision as to the most beneficial therapeutic plan should be made in consultation with the patient.

Initial Diagnostic Criteria for Treatment Selection

In determining the appropriate management of a patient, several key diagnostic criteria must be identified and evaluated. There are factors that pertain to the patient—their presenting condition and health; as well as operator factors. Management of a patient involves the interaction of the subsets of diagnosis, treatment, and maintenance; the outcome of each being determined by the skill, experience, and critical analysis of the operator or team of operators when management is interdisciplinary. It is essential that management, not simply treatment, be undertaken to achieve the best outcome for the patient.

As such, there are key patient and operator factors that must be identified and evaluated in consideration of the rehabilitation of the edentulous (or soon to be edentulous) maxillary jaw. These can be considered as risk factors in case selection.

PATIENT RISK FACTORS: GENERAL

Presenting Condition

It is imperative to determine what the patients themselves believe to be the reasons they seek your advice. For patients who have previously been rendered edentulous in the maxilla and have had continued dissatisfaction through a series of conventional full upper dentures, it may be clear as to what they seek. Alternatively, a patient with periodontally compromised maxillary teeth may not have yet psychologically reached a position to accept loss of his or her natural teeth; but coincidentally desires a more pleasing appearance or improved function.

A patient's presentation, in words of their choosing, reveals much in so far as the operator's further direction for inquiry. Initially, the operator should ascertain the patient's concept of their problem and what understanding they have of their likely management requirements. Questions to garner information on the history of the patient's edentulism, the success of past and current prostheses, and any previous treatments performed in an attempt to address the presenting complaint, are important and often enlightening.

When a patient is unclear of what problems exist, cannot articulate what they want or are unaware of the implications of previously suggested plans of management, a measured, stepwise process is judicious in reaching and presenting a considered management plan.

Medical History

A thorough medical history is essential prior to any examination or invasive procedures being undertaken. It is outside the scope of this chapter to provide detailed analysis of the implications of various medical conditions and prescribed or nonprescribed medications that may affect the dental

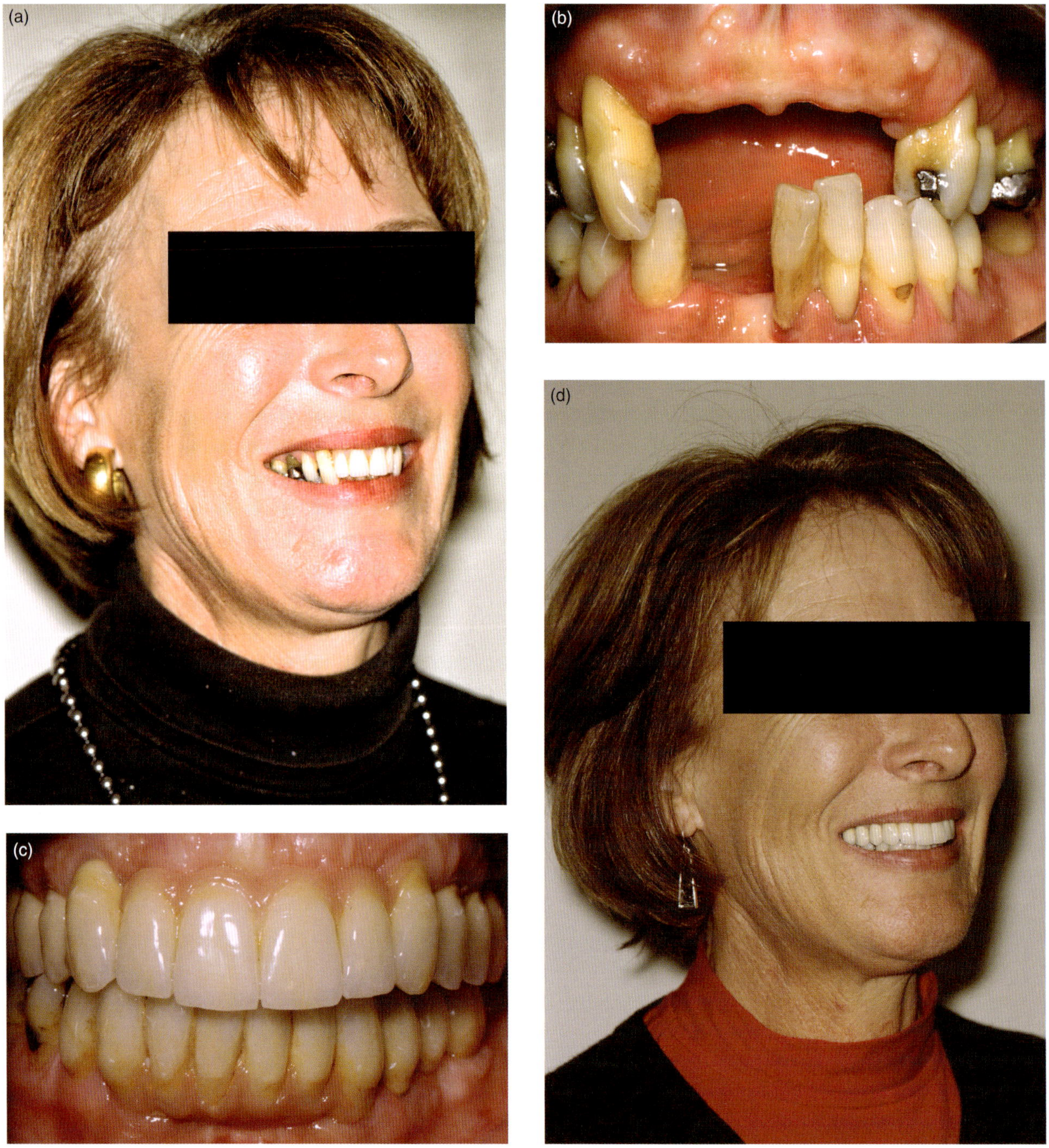

Figure 13.1 (a–c) Preoperative views of the appearance and failing dentition in a 55-year-old female. (d) Facial view following oral rehabilitation involving replacement of all remaining maxillary teeth with implant-retained fixed dental prostheses, and partial replacement of the diseased mandibular teeth.

Table 13.1 Options for rehabilitation of the edentulous maxilla.

Implant-retained fixed prosthesis
Type 1: Congruent implant-tooth prostheses
Type 2: Noncongruent implant-tooth prostheses
Implant retained/supported removable prosthesis
Single-implant retention
Splinted-implant retention via a bar

management of a patient. For the patient under evaluation for dental implant therapy, it is essential that the patient be healthy. Absolute contraindications include: acute myocardial infarction (within the prior six months), acute cerebral vascular accident, and immunosuppression. They are required to be free of any uncontrolled systemic disease or acute infections and not currently requiring cytotoxic medications. Other medications directed at the management of circulatory or endocrine disorders or disturbances should be carefully investigated.

Medications for the management of psychological and psychiatric conditions should signal a deeper consideration of the patient's medical condition. Mental illness, particularly when not well controlled, may impair the patient's ability to cope with what is invariably a demanding plan of management, or to harbor unrealistic expectations of the outcomes of the treatment.

Patient Age

Within our current understanding there is no contraindication to the use of dental implants for the restoration of a patient's maxillary dentition on the basis of advanced age alone. Many patients have more complex medical histories simply as a consequence of their advancing years. Patients who have been edentulous in the maxilla and worn conventional full dentures since their youth often present with advanced resorption of the maxillary alveolar bone, which in itself may significantly complicate their management.

Table 13.2 Fixed versus removable prostheses—advantages and disadvantages.

Maxillary fixed implant prostheses	Maxillary removable implant prostheses
Advantages • Patient's sense of "natural" teeth • Improved intraoral sense without palatal mucosal coverage • Improved function • No mucosal loading • Established high survival rates	**Advantages** • Can restore lost ridge form • Allows greater variance in tooth position • Allows for greater lip and facial support in the prosthesis • Generally, patient's home care less complex • Potentially easier maintenance • May benefit elderly patients who require living assistance • Often less implants required • Function improved • Potentially reduced mucosal loading
Disadvantages • May not adequately reconstitute the ideal of the maxillary alveolar arch form with the prosthesis • Patient's home care more complicated • More complex surgical and technical demands required • Esthetic outcome may not meet patient's expectation • Potentially more complicated maintenance and repair	**Disadvantages** • Must have sufficient inter-arch space to allow the incorporation of required retentive elements whilst providing for sufficient strength in the removable prosthesis • The patients replacement dentition remains removable • Anticipated higher maintenance requirements

The necessary posttreatment maintenance may influence the type of therapy in the management of an elderly patient. The design of an implant-retained prosthesis to facilitate ease of patient oral home care and simpler correction of any technical complications, assumes greater importance in older patients.

Reason for Tooth Loss—Susceptibility to Periodontal Disease

Patients may loose their natural dentitions over short or extended time intervals, segmentally or wholly; in a single event, as a consequence of oral disease or trauma. As discussed elsewhere, the physiologic bone resorption and remodeling that occurs following tooth loss can vary greatly in its effect on the shape of the edentulous maxilla.

Areas which have been edentulous for greater periods of time can be anticipated to have increased resorptive bone remodeling. Esthetic considerations in planning the maxillary implant rehabilitation will be influenced by advanced areas of bone resorption in the edentulous anterior maxilla, when compared to the posterior ridge.

Advanced periodontal destruction associated with the remaining teeth in the maxilla will result in a significant reduction of available bone in the jaw following tooth loss (Figures 13.2a–d). There is also evidence that patients who show a high susceptibility to periodontal disease, particularly when combined with chronic and heavy cigarette smoking, are at increased risk of biological complications, including early loss of the dental implant, when undertaking dental implant therapy.

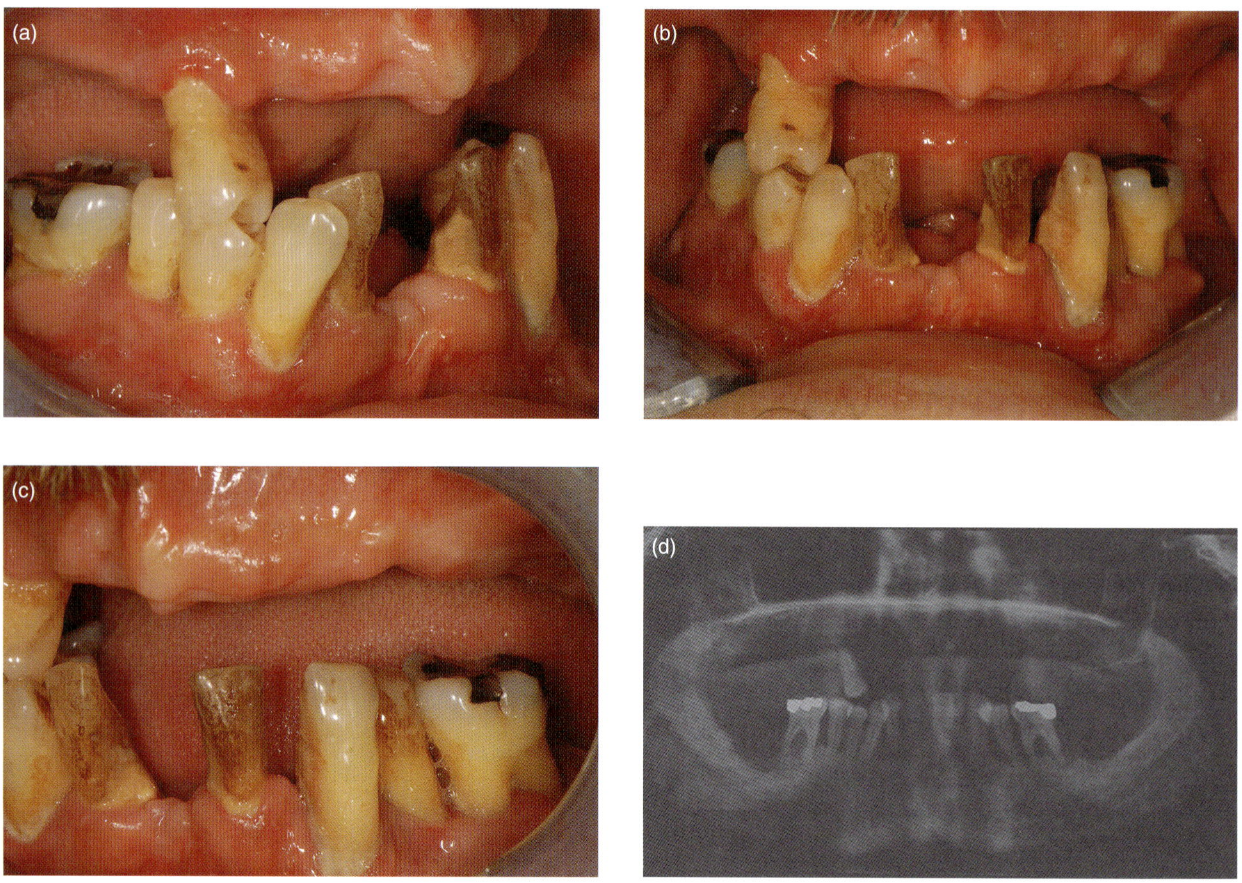

Figure 13.2 (a–c) Preoperative intraoral views of an edentulous maxillary jaw (except for a single premolar and multiple missing and compromised teeth in the lower jaw) in a 36-year-old male with a history of a chronic heavy cigarette smoking habit and who shows a high susceptibility to periodontal disease. (d) A Panorex film of the same patient.

Patient's Expectation of Treatment—Esthetics Versus Function

To achieve a successful outcome the expectation of the patient must be achieved. It is the role of the operator to inform and educate the patient during the diagnostic and planning phases as to realistic expectations of the outcomes of the procedures to be undertaken. We should rely on published evidence when comparing therapeutic options and informing patients as to the risks and possible complications associated with each and any of the therapies being considered.

A greater challenge exists in developing a realistic expectation of the esthetic outcomes of the treatment. Patient expectations are often fashioned by many factors outside the control or influence of the operator. Each patient's clinical presentation varies from that of another patient requiring consideration of implant therapy in the maxillary jaw. Patients also rarely understand the consequences of the physiological changes the maxillary jaw has undergone as a result of tooth loss, and the effects such changes have on the operator's ability to provide restitution of normal hard and soft tissue architectures. It is imperative that the operator understands the expectations the patient harbors.

Of equal importance is the operator's ability to understand the parameters of the therapy being considered as a consequence of the limitations of the biological aspects, prosthetic materials, and the operator's own skill and competence. In an interdisciplinary approach to a patient's management, each operator (including the technical staff involved) must understand and work within their skill level or competence.

The operator responsible for the prosthesis must accept the ultimate responsibility for the planning and outcome, as it is not implants but teeth the patient desires. This is the person who must invest time in understanding the patient's expectations and determining whether these expectations are realistic biologically and esthetically, and within the skill of the operators and the interdisciplinary team. This is also the person who will be required to undertake required maintenance and attend to technical complications.

PATIENT RISK FACTORS: SPECIFIC

Facial—Extraoral Analysis

Lip Lines

- Incisal display
- Upper lip/alveolar mucosal junction
- Activity of the upper and lower lips

The upper and lower lips frame the teeth when we speak and smile, and thus exert a powerful influence on our appearance. The teeth complete the effect as the lips spring to action through the activity of the facial musculature—particularly the *muscularis obicularis oris*, revealing a healthy, balanced, and attractive compliment of anterior teeth. An irregular, interrupted series of projections are uncomplimentary to the face and general appearance. The greater the amount of the teeth that are exposed by the lips, the more challenging tooth replacement becomes when considering an implant-retained prosthesis.

Careful assessment of the extent of dental display commences during the consultation discussion with the patient. The parameters of lip activity can be assessed from the "rest" position through to the display when the patient enunciates the letter "e." As teeth are lost and ridge resorption ensues, tooth replacement positions may have to be altered. Additionally, as a person ages, the activity of the circular oral musculature reduces and tends to result in a reduced display of the maxillary anterior teeth and an increased display of their antagonists.

Emphasis must be given to the position of the most inferior border of the alveolar mucosa overlying the anterior maxillary ridge. In patients where this border is beneath the upper lip when fully elevated, the options for implant-retained prostheses increase and the esthetic risk factors reduce. Conversely, the visual display of the mucosa from under the upper lip demands that the interface of the prosthesis and the soft tissue becomes part of the esthetic challenge.

When there is an existing prosthesis in place, an assessment needs to be made of its adequacy with respect to the patient's perception of their appearance, and the technical quality of the appliance. The contribution to the lip and midfacial support from the existing denture tooth position and the volume and extension of the flange can most accurately be assessed though a new trial setup, excluding the labial and buccal flanges (i.e., a diagnostic prosthesis). This data alone may determine whether the patient would be most appropriately treated with a fixed or removable prosthesis (Figures 13.3a–g).

Facial—Intraoral Analysis

- Ridge shape (vertical/horizontal/transverse dimensions)
- Ridge axis
- Inter-arch distance
- Adequacy of the existing denture
- Condition of the remaining dentition
- Existing levels of periodontal disease and destruction
- Mandibular dentition

The intraoral analysis includes a complete assessment of all soft and hard tissues of the oral cavity. Of particular significance is the dimension of the maxillary arch: This dimension can be preliminarily assessed from an inspection of the fitting surface of the existing denture with respect to the arch form of the attached teeth. The vertical dimension of the maxilla will relate to the display from under the upper lip. Any canting of the ridge should be noted. The available distance between the maxillary alveolar mucosa and the opposing dentition requires assessment and recording.

The definitive analysis can be more accurately completed following full data collection and the visualization of diagnostic casts when correctly mounted at the vertical dimension which is appropriate for the definitive restoration (Figures 13.4a–c).

Radiographic Analysis

A routine radiographic screening can be adequately undertaken with an accurate orthopantomographic film (OPG). Advances now permit high-quality digital formatting of these films to provide more highly defined and contrasted images of the jaws. Where the maxillary jaw under examination is fully edentulous, an OPG will provide the operator with information concerning the position and size of the maxillary sinus spaces, the nasal floor, and a reasonable estimate of the vertical height of the residual alveolar ridge. This data, in conjunction with accurately mounted diagnostic casts, can provide sufficient information for an initial assessment.

In the case of a partially dentate jaw (where the prognosis of the remaining dentition is guarded or poor) accurate periapical films, particularly in the areas of the remaining teeth, will provide greater information and reduce the likelihood of error due to image distortion or the "burnout" sometimes found associated with metallic restorative materials in retained teeth.

In many patients requiring rehabilitation of the maxillary dentition, a more detailed radiographic analysis is indicated. Sectional tomography utilizing cone-beam computer-enhanced tomography (CBCT) allows accurate and detailed radiological images of the facial skeleton. The CBCT provides undistorted, accurate cross-sectional, axial, coronal, sagittal, and panoramic views allowing three-dimensional interpretation and measurement of the jaw. By utilizing this information and in conjunction with clinical data, more careful planning of implant placements is achieved (Figures 13.5a–b).

OPERATOR RISK FACTORS: SPECIFIC

Diagnostic Classification for Treatment Selection

From the completed diagnostic assessment for dental implant therapy an operator should be able to determine the degree of difficulty associated with each aspect of the intended treatment. In the case of the restoration of the edentulous maxilla, the factors previously discussed will lead the operator to a subjective judgment as to whether the proposed plan is straightforward, advanced or complex (SAC). The Swiss Society of Oral Implantology adopted this classification system in 1999 and more recently the classification has been expanded and detailed by the International Team for Implantology (ITI).

Significant emphasis must be placed on the skill and experience of the members of the team in interdisciplinary management. The multiple factors to be considered in all planning decisions, and the esthetic importance of the outcome, will determine that the restoration of the edentulous maxilla must be either an advanced or complex undertaking.

Visualization of Treatment Outcome (Goals)

Ultimately, the operator must present the proposed plan of management to the patient as a formal case

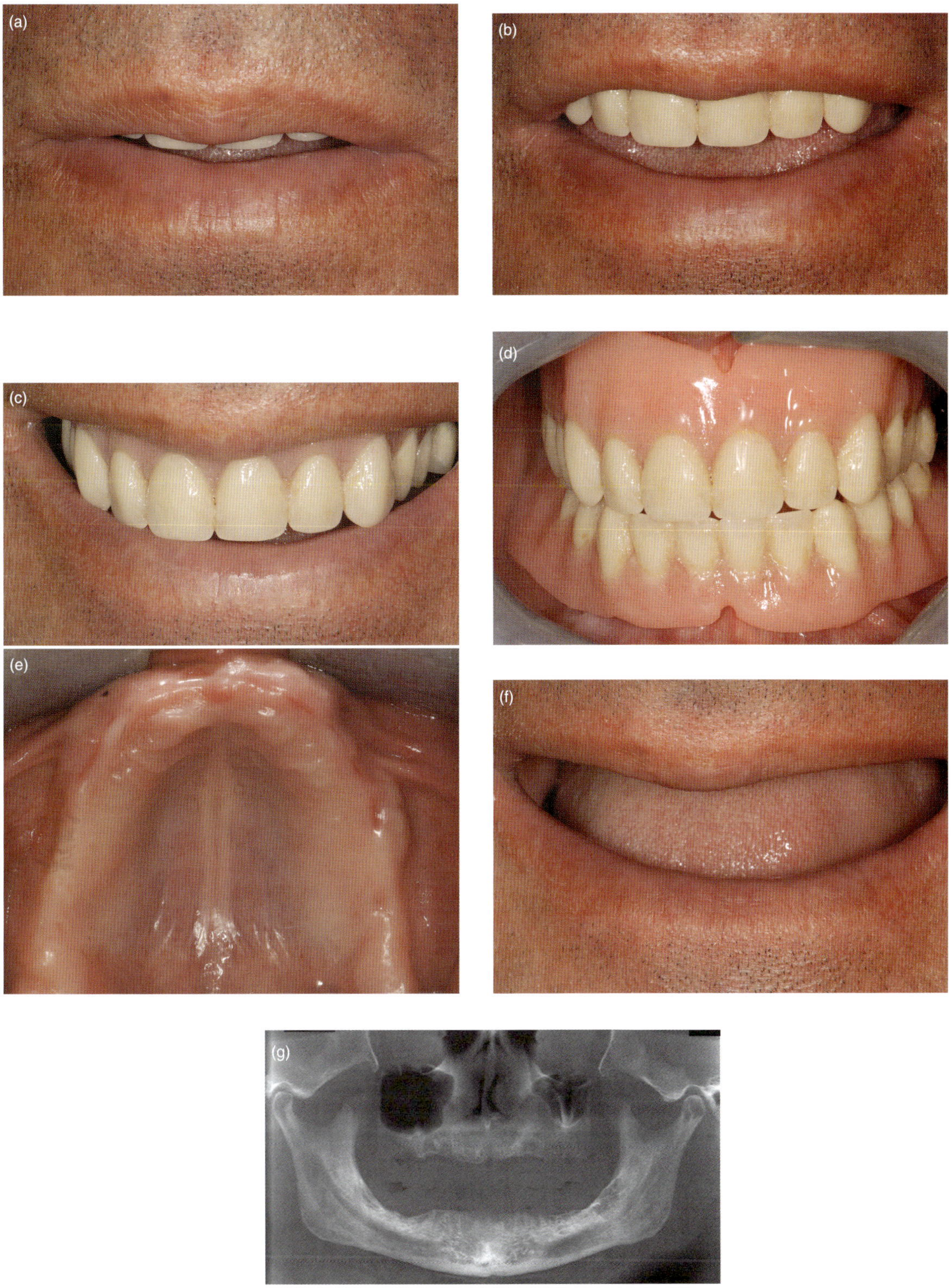

Figure 13.3 (a–c) A preoperative extraoral evaluation of the appearance of the existing fully removable prostheses for a 46-year-old male. The lips are relaxed in (a), during speech in (b), and smiling in (c). (d) An intraoral view of the existing fully removable prostheses. (e) An intraoral view of the maxillary edentulous ridge. (f) The lip position when smiling following removal of the prostheses. The lower border of the mucosa of the edentulous maxillary ridge is not seen from the upper elevation of the upper lip. This observation allows for consideration of either a Type 1 or Type 2 fixed dental prosthesis as the junction between the prosthesis and the alveolar mucosa will not be seen from beneath the lip. (g) Digital OPG of the edentulous arches.

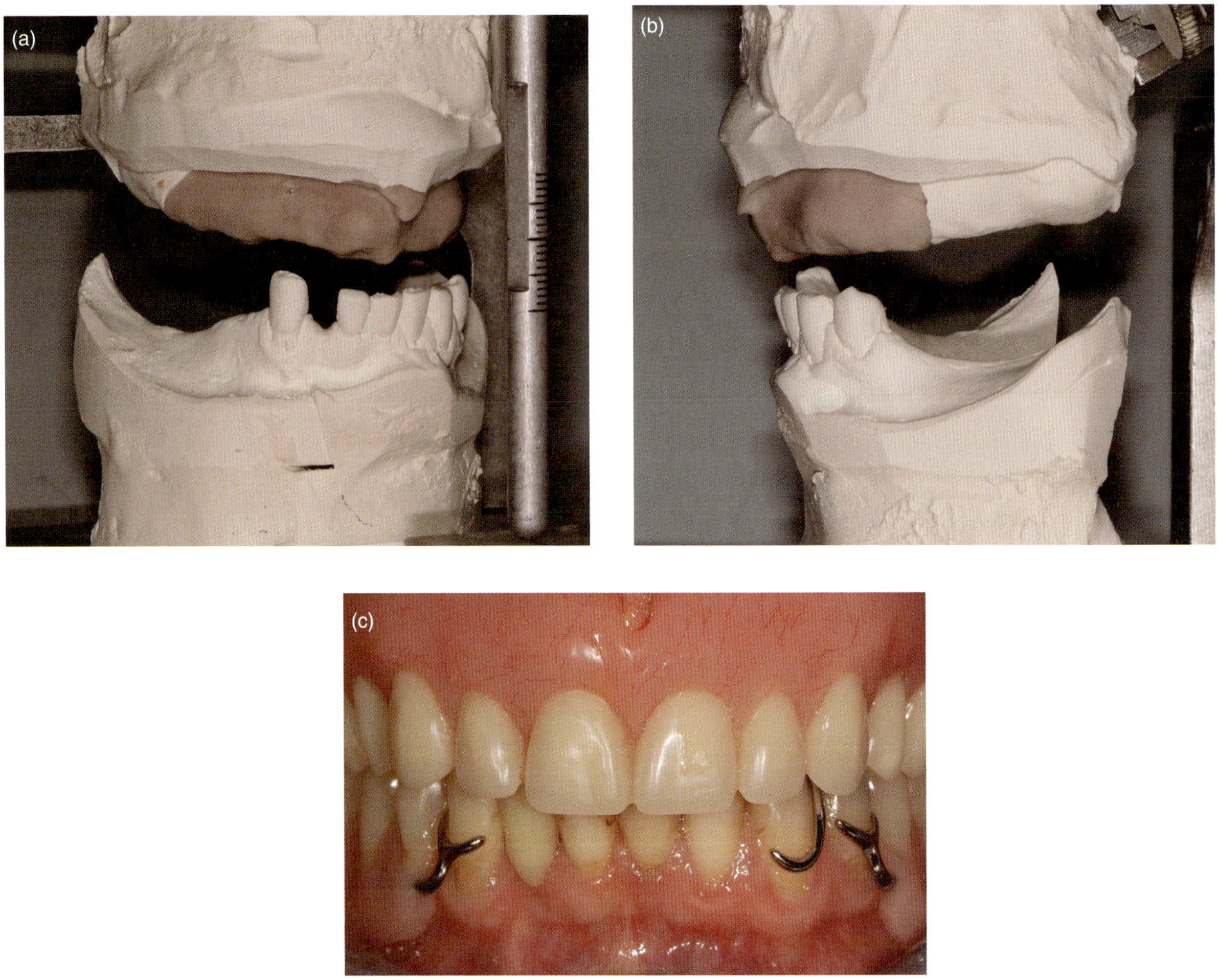

Figure 13.4 (a–b) Mounting of the casts has been accomplished using a facebow transfer and a semi-adjustable articulator. This will most accurately allow for final analysis of the inter-arch distance and permits a final diagnostic setup to be created. Consideration is then made of whether an implant overdenture can be considered in the possible treatment options. (c) A facial view of the intraoral appearance of the existing upper dental prosthesis in the intercuspal position, with the lower natural teeth and adjunctive partial removable partial dental prosthesis.

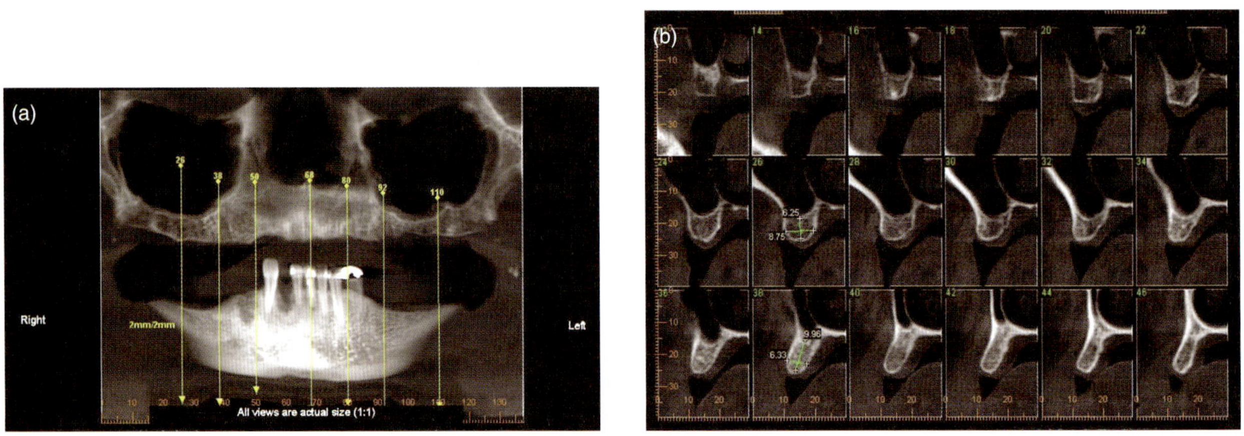

Figure 13.5 (a) Cone-beam computer-enhanced tomography (CBCT) panographic view with computer-generated sections at 1 mm intervals. (b) Details of the tomographic sectional views at 1 mm intervals from the right side of the edentulous maxilla. These views provide clear and detailed analysis of the architecture of the jaw-bone with recorded measurements at predetermined sections. As the images are at an "actual size," dimensions are able to be identified for any further section.

presentation that may include a selection of, or all the visual data that had been previously collected.

This diagnostic data can be used as a visual aid to assist the patient's comprehension of the proposed plan. It is vital to this discussion that the operator has established, based on the clinical, radiological and diagnostic information attained, a visualization of the outcomes of the proposed therapy. In advanced cases, the operator must ensure that the patient has a similar expectation of the treatment outcomes and understands the procedures that are involved.

In complex cases, the operator will be required to carefully explain the anticipated outcomes of the various stages that by necessity are components of complex therapy. Both the operator and patient need to appreciate the importance of assessing the outcome of each stage of therapy prior to finalizing the expectations of the final outcome. As an example, where the patient requires bony augmentation procedures as a component of the rehabilitation of the jaw prior to implant placement, an assessment of the outcome of this procedure alone forms an important determinate of the likely ultimate treatment outcomes.

ADDITIONAL OPERATOR RISK FACTORS

There are several additional factors that the operator must assess for each patient's therapy. They involve a determination of:

- The sequence of treatment:
  - Sequential extraction and implant placement
  - Sequential implant placement
- Level of clinical "tolerance" in selection and surgical placement sites
- Timing of placement (immediate/early/ delayed)
- Type of implants to be used
- Loading protocol (immediate/early/delayed)
- Type and design of definitive prosthesis
- Anticipated maintenance protocols

Each of these operator factors will be discussed with reference to the specific types of prostheses later in the chapter.

Restorative Options for Dental Implant Therapy in the Maxillary Jaw

IMPLANT-RETAINED FIXED PROSTHESIS

Classification

Type 1: Congruent implant-tooth prostheses
Type 2: Noncongruent implant-tooth prostheses

The rehabilitation of the edentulous maxilla utilizing dental implants can be undertaken using either a fixed or removable prosthesis. Implant-retained fixed dental prostheses (I-R FPDs) can be classified as screw-retained (retrievable) or cemented (may be retrievable).

I-R FPDs can also be classified with respect to the relationship of the prosthesis to the residual ridge and the position of the implants supporting and retaining the prosthesis. An I-R FPD may be designed to allow the prosthetic teeth to exit the alveolar mucosa in a similar relationship to that of a natural tooth and its supporting periodontium. An example is the result attained by a successful single implant-retained tooth replacement. As such, each dental implant must be placed in a precise position that provides *congruence* between the position of the restorative head of the implant and the prosthetic tooth, with no requirement for prosthetic soft tissue augmentation on the prosthesis. This is designated as—Type 1: *Congruent implant-tooth* (I-T) prosthesis (Figures 13.6a–c).

Alternatively, the residual ridge form is often reduced in its vertical, horizontal, and transverse dimensions as a consequence of the reason for the tooth loss combined with normal physiologic remodeling following tooth extraction. There no longer is, nor can be established, a direct exit of the prosthetic teeth, in their correct esthetic and functional positions, from the alveolar mucosa. There will be a need to incorporate prosthetic augmentation of the deficient mucosa. The implant position is then determined more by the bony anatomy and the biomechanical factors that influence stress distribution through the prosthesis when under load. Greater consideration will be given to the restorative heads being within the buccopalatal dimension of the design of the prosthesis, and less regard to the precise tooth position. Such a prosthesis is designated as—Type 2: *Noncongruent implant-tooth* (I-T) prosthesis (Figures 13.7a–c).

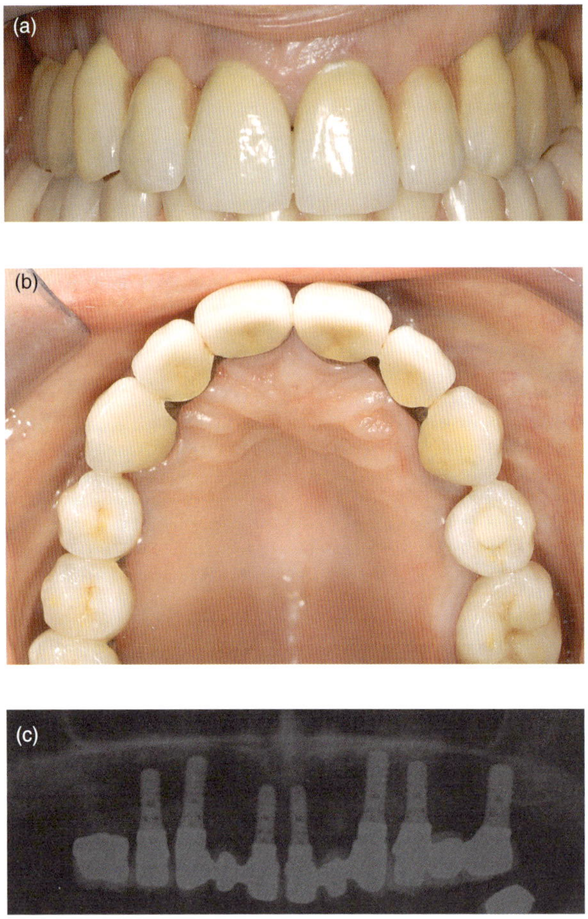

Figure 13.6 (a) A postoperative intraoral view of full maxillary implant segmental reconstruction for a 52-year-old female. (b) a mirror view of a maxillary arch segmental reconstruction, demonstrating a Type 1 congruent full-arch rehabilitation. (c) OPG postoperative radiograph demonstrating the number and position of the dental implants placed to provide simple and segmented prostheses.

The outcome of the treatment with either a Type 1 congruent I-T prosthesis or Type 2 noncongruent I-T prosthesis will be influenced by several factors. The former is indicated when the prosthetic teeth can be placed in direct contact with the alveolar mucosa. In such a case, the dimensional change of the edentulous maxilla must be minimal. The Type 2 noncongruent I-T prosthesis is indicated where the prosthetic tooth position is required to be horizontally and/or vertically distant from the residual edentulous maxilla. When the therapy is carefully planned and precisely undertaken, either approach may provide very acceptable and pleasing outcomes for patients.

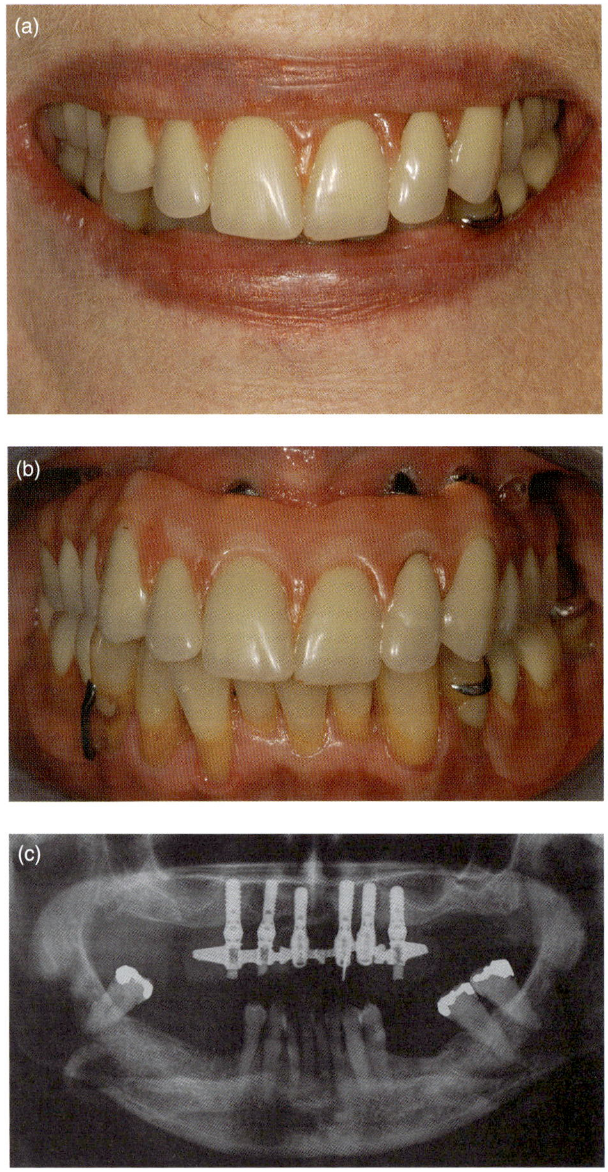

Figure 13.7 (a) Smile appearance at a six-year postoperative review of a Type 2 noncongruent I-T prosthesis in a 65-year-old female. (b) Intraoral appearance at a six-year postoperative review of a Type 2 noncongruent I-T prosthesis. (c) The OPG view at the six-year review.

Implant-Retained Fixed Prosthesis—Materials

Both Type 1 and Type 2 I-T prostheses can be fabricated using various materials and techniques. For Type 1, the most esthetic result is generally obtained using ceramo-metal technology. However, when the design of the prosthesis is a one-piece full arch restoration, there may be an inverse relationship between the size of the prosthesis and the quality of the fit to the implants or their abutments, when fabricated using standard techniques.

This problem can be ameliorated in various ways, including a segmental design, providing for smaller segments that are individually constructed and function as individual restorations within the full-arch rehabilitation. Additionally, larger segments can be constructed in parts and either soldered—pre- or postceramic application, or joined via an interlinked attachment and luted together at the time of insertion of the prosthesis. Alternatively, prefabricated collars that form the direct screw-retained interface between the implants and the prosthesis can be luted into the completed ceramo-metal reconstruction at the time of insertion.

Metal-reinforced/acrylic hybrid prostheses may be used in Type 1 reconstructions, but have a greater indication in Type 2 prosthesis designs. The hybrid prosthesis was the original recommended design for fixed implant restorations in both upper and lower arch reconstructions. Technical improvements over time have allowed for improved esthetics and treatment outcomes and a reduction in technical complications as a consequence of clinical function.

The reduced ability to create esthetic excellence in the individual tooth forms and the necessity for greater material bulk as a consequence of the inferior physical properties of the acrylic, often restricts the use of the hybrid prosthesis in Type 1 designs. With the further refinement of CAD-CAM technologies, machined multi-unit metal frameworks to be screw-retained directly to the implants has improved the available treatment options (Figures 13.8a–b).

Computer-aided framework design and fabrication provides the potential to overcome many of the inaccuracies that are inherent in traditional lost wax/casting techniques. More recently, all-ceramic (Zirconia) frameworks have been constructed using computer-aided technologies. Further analysis of longer-term results of these prostheses in function will be required prior to their becoming a predictable treatment alternative.

TYPE 1: CONGRUENT I-T PROSTHESIS

Type 1 prostheses may be successfully utilized in patients who are fully edentulous at the time of presentation, or in those who present with a failing partial dentition. The optimal esthetic outcome is more likely when the prosthesis is constructed using metal-ceramic technology. The process allows for a single full-arch construction, but is more preferable as several individual segments. The prosthesis may be screw-retained, cemented or combined when a segmental restoration is utilized (Figures 13.9a–e).

The advantages and disadvantages of these various options are summarized in Table 13.3.

Such cases are invariably complex (under the SAC classification) and usually require an experienced interdisciplinary team. When considering a congruent I-T prosthesis, there are several key issues that require particular analysis. These are summarized in Table 13.4 and then subsequently discussed in further detail.

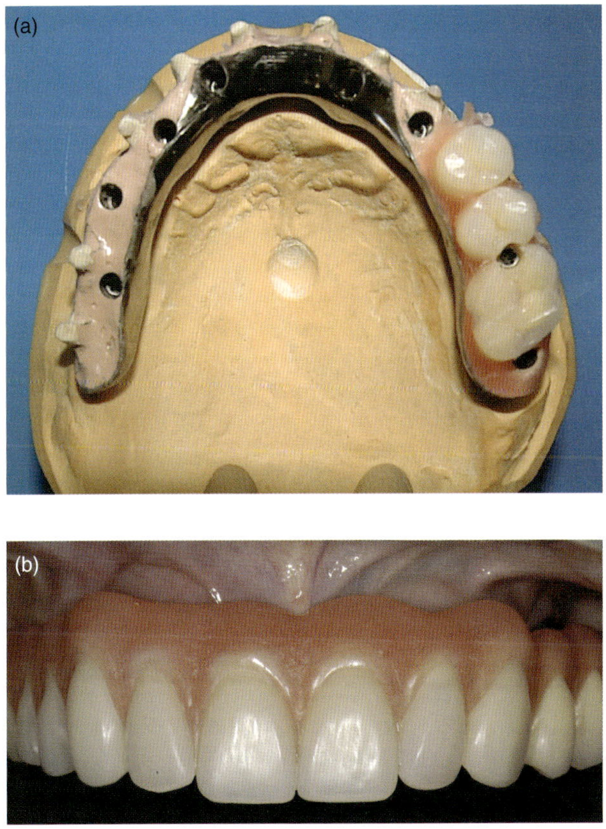

Figure 13.8 (a) An occlusal view of the master cast and CAD-CAM (Procera) full maxillary framework (Courtesy of Dr G. Burt). (b) An intraoral view of the completed Type 2 noncongruent prosthesis directly screw-retained (Courtesy of Dr G. Burt).

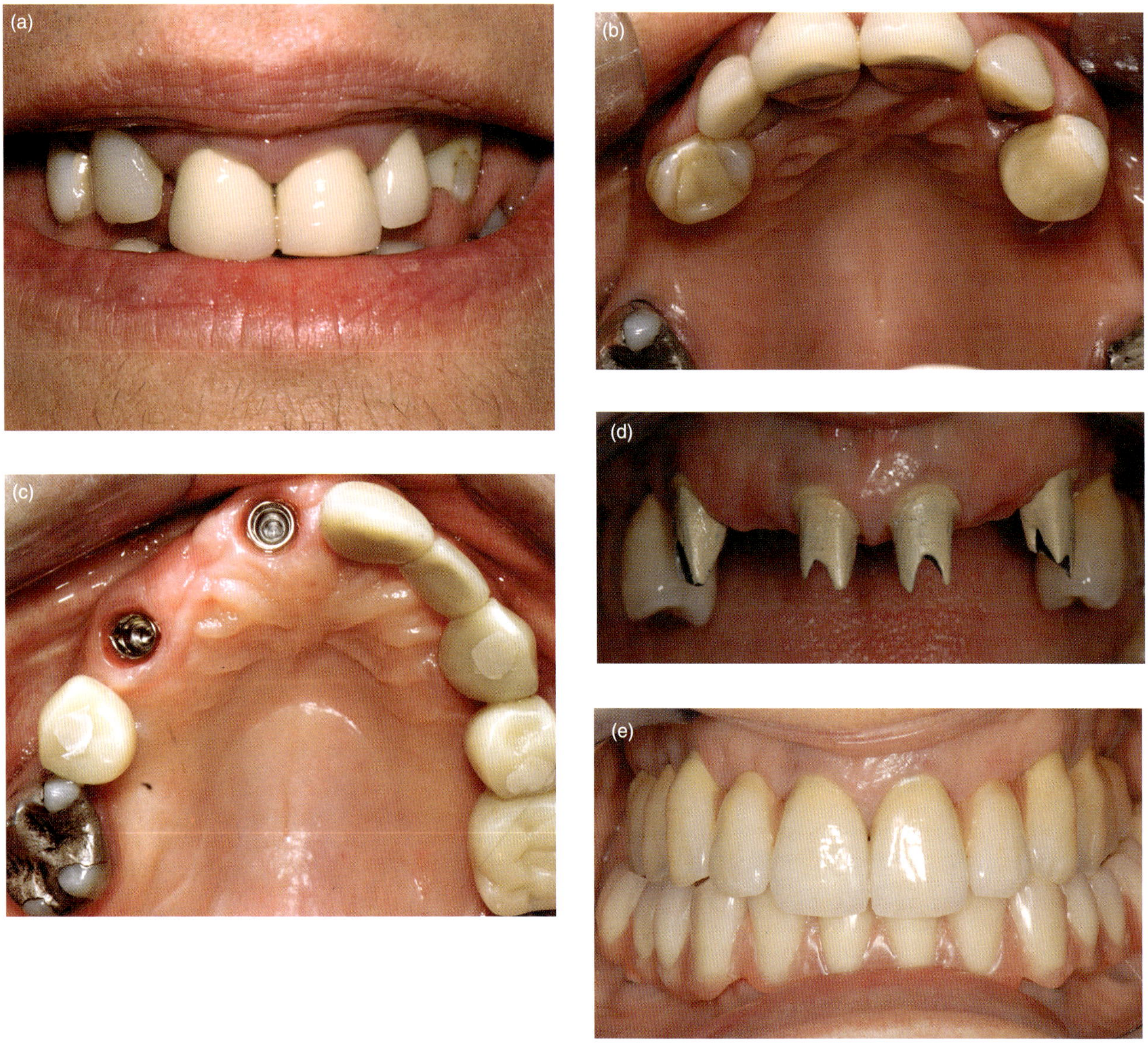

Figure 13.9 (a) The smile of patient preoperatively. Note the slight vertical maxillary excess with an increased display of the soft tissues, and the irregular number and position of the remaining maxillary dentition. (b) An occlusal view preoperatively. (c) The occlusal view at the provisional stage of therapy, demonstrating a segmental approach to the planned Type 1 congruent definitive prostheses. (d) A facial view of the definitive custom-fabricated ceramo-metal meso-structures, provide the support for the definitive three units FPD being cemented. (e) A facial view of the definitive segmental, porcelain-fused-to-metal FPDs.

Clinical and Radiographic Diagnostic Criteria Are More Demanding

As a consequence of the critical nature of implant position, both clinical and radiographic diagnostic analyses are more demanding. A complete and accurate definitive tooth setup must be established and verified intraorally. The try-in confirms the relationships of the necks of the teeth to the alveolar mucosa in the areas where the implants are to be placed, as well as in the sites where pontics are planned. The trial appliance is constructed without a labial or buccal flange so as to ascertain any negative effect the proposed prosthesis will exert on upper lip support. The patient's existing conventional full denture provides enhancement to the support of the upper lip; the loss of such support, if required, may not be acceptable to the patient.

Table 13.3 Segmental compared to full-arch congruent I-T prostheses.

Segmental restorations (ceramo-metal reconstruction)	Full-arch prostheses (ceramo-metal reconstruction)
Advantages • Greater flexibility for prosthetic design • Reduces noncompatible axial alignments of implants • Offers several options for the design of the prosthesis • Improved access for patient's home care • Reduced technical inaccuracy due to the shorter span lengths • Allows a staged approach to management where indicated • Mixed fixation to the implants (screw-retained and cemented) possible • Technical complications can be managed more easily; limited to the affected segment • A biological failure (loss of implant) will require reconstruction of the affected segment only	**Advantages** • Shared cross-arch loading of all implants in function • Rigid design • Loss of implant may only require modification of the existing prosthesis • Immediate restoration and loading possible
Disadvantages • Often implants must be placed adjacent to each other • Immediate restoration and loading may require a full-arch provisional restoration attached to selected implants • Possible localized increased implant loading	**Disadvantages** • Nonaxial alignment of implants increases complexity of design of the definitive restoration • Technical complication in any area will require removal of the entire prosthesis • Addition or repair of ceramic material may affect other parts of the prosthesis • Increased technical complexity in fabrication • Reduced accuracy of fit—may predispose to ceramic fracture • May complicate or compromise patient's home care • Does not allow a staged approach to patient management • Increased clinical maintenance protocol should periodic removal of the prosthesis be indicated

In the partially dentate individual, ideal prosthetic design may dictate tooth positions that vary from those that the remaining natural teeth occupy at the time of the patient's presentation. Initial treatment may necessitate one or more extractions prior to verifying the desired ultimate prosthetic tooth position. Additionally, where an occlusal plane cant exists, or posterior teeth are required to be replaced to provide for a change in the vertical dimension of occlusion, a staged approach is recommended. A Type 2 or delayed approach with respect to the timing of implant placement will be advantageous in such a case (Figures 13.10a–b).

Detailed radiographic information will be required to more thoroughly investigate each of the proposed implant sites prior to determining the most desirable sites, and designating the types of implants which are most appropriate. CBCT or similar computer-assisted images will be required. When available, computer-assisted planning software and navigational surgical units may also assist in ensuring desired implant positioning.

Table 13.4 Summary of key issues in Type 1 congruent implant-retained fixed prostheses.

- Clinical and radiographic diagnostic criteria more demanding
- Precise surgical placement of the implant required
- Accurate surgical positioning guide required
- Need for intermediate prosthetic mucosal replacement (ceramic/acrylic)
- Careful design of the prosthesis—segmental restorations
- Esthetic considerations of implant supported teeth and pontics
- The soft tissue prosthetic interface
- Materials selection—costs and expected esthetic outcome

Implant Position Determination and Surgical Placement Are Critical to the Final Esthetic Outcome

The critical issue in the esthetic success of a Type 1 congruent I-T prosthesis is precise surgical placement of each of the dental implants. At the time of surgery, the surgeon must know and be able to visualize the positions of the teeth as they will be on the definitive prosthesis.

The three-dimensional concept of implant placement described by Buser (*ITI Treatment Guide*, Vol. 1, 2006, Quintessence Publications) in relation to the placement of dental implants in a single-tooth site must be adhered to. Where implants are to be placed adjacent to one another, adequate distance must be allowed between the restorative heads of the implants to provide for a stable inter-implant mucosa to be established and maintained. This distance should usually not be less than 3 mm, but may vary depending upon the type of implants placed. There is limited tolerance, particularly in the mesiodistal positioning of the implant, as minor deviations from the ideal axial position may significantly compromise tooth position or tooth contour in the final prosthesis. This is particularly important for implant placement in the anterior maxilla.

The operator responsible for the surgical placement of the implants must be a skilled surgeon with advanced experience in implant surgery and soft and hard tissue management.

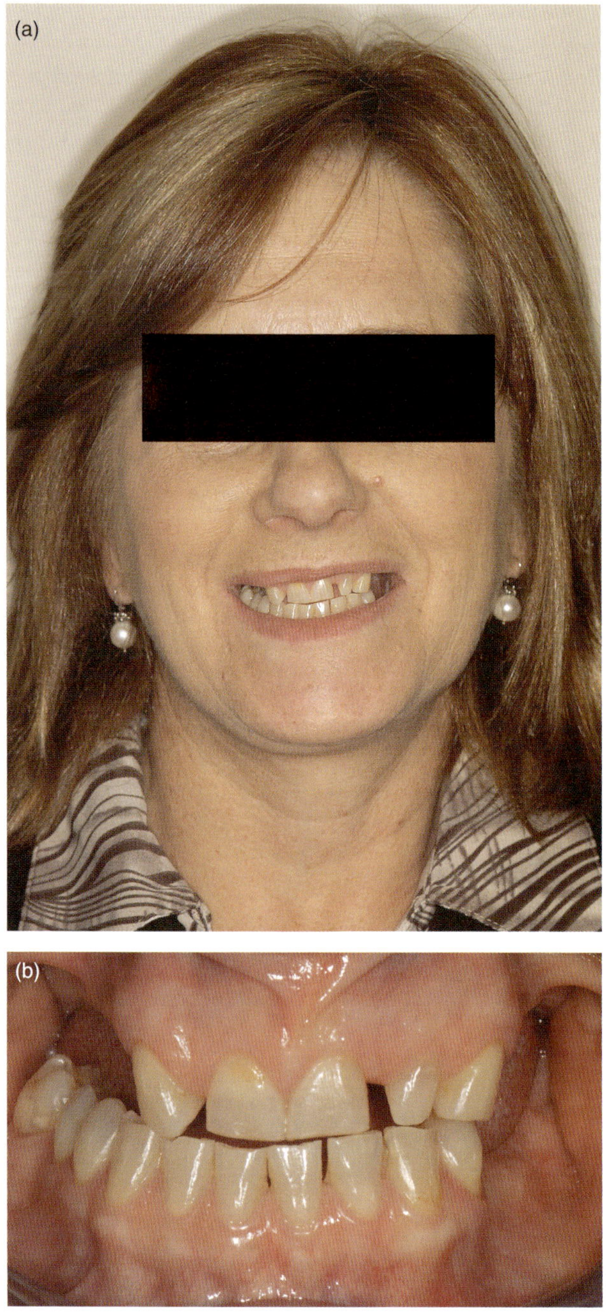

Figure 13.10 (a) A full facial view of a 56-year-old female patient preoperatively. Note the cant of the maxillary teeth and deviated midline. (b) An anterior intraoral view.

The Use of a Surgical Guide (Stent)

A carefully constructed and accurate surgical guide must be used at the time of surgery. The guide should provide the precise axial tooth position and mucosal margin of the anticipated exit profile of the prosthetic tooth. The guide should be designed in consultation with the operator who is to undertake the surgical component of the patient's management. As a minimum, the guide should:

- identify the exact positions and shapes of the teeth to be constructed in the definitive congruent I-T prosthesis
- demonstrate the relationship of the necks of the teeth to the overlying mucosa
- identify the palatal or occlusal access holes that should align to the restorative heads of the implants, or angle correction abutments (should these be anticipated) following placement
- use tooth shapes that are anatomically aligned to natural teeth rather than diminutive commercial denture teeth, particularly in the posterior sextants of the maxilla
- allow for mucosal flap elevation and retraction when in place
- be stable when placed; provision for rigid fixation in the fully edentulous maxilla is often required
- allow full access and visualization of surgical instrumentation
- provide directional holes that indicate ideal placement positions, and secondary positions should these be required (Figures 13.11a–c)

ADDITIONAL CONSIDERATIONS

Implant Design—Bone Level or Trans-Mucosal

Commercially available dental implants with documented evidence of survival may be of either a bone level or trans-mucosal design. From the restorative perspective, the design and diameter of the restorative interface (head) of the implant is of greatest importance in the prosthetic design. Biomechanically, long-term stability of the joint between the implant and its abutment requires a tapered internal connection. It appears that improved biological stability with resultant reduced bone loss may also result from an internal fixation design with an abutment–implant interface that demonstrates a slightly reduced abutment diameter when compared to the head of the implant.

For Type 1 congruent I-T prostheses, it is desirable to have a similar head diameter to the restorative tooth size at the various fixation points between the prosthesis and the implants. This aids in the creation of biologically acceptable and esthetically pleasing emergence through the mucosa of the various prosthetic teeth from their congruent implants. Thus the type of dental implants to be utilized in the various designed sites should be decided with both restorative and surgical input. The restorative operator must consider the implications of implant selection for each site, being ultimately responsible for the design, construction, and placement of the definitive prosthesis. The surgeon will own the responsibility to choose the most appropriate intraosseous body for the designated bony site that provides the preferred restorative head. The selection of a bone level design compared to a transmucosal design will depend upon several factors, and should take into consideration the desire to provide for simplicity in prosthetic design.

Timing of Placement

In the fully edentulous maxilla between six and eight dental implants can often be placed coincidently. The former teeth sites are usually well healed, or have been allowed to heal for sufficient time following extraction to allow adequate soft and hard tissue healing.

In the partially dentate maxilla a dental implant may be placed into the tooth socket immediately following tooth removal. The implant should not be placed at the time of tooth removal if the residual ridge morphology precludes attainment of primary stability of an appropriately sized implant in the desired restorative position.

In patients who have high esthetic expectations procedures that reduce risk are preferred. Therefore, immediate placement in sockets of misaligned or malpositioned teeth is contraindicated when the desired outcome is a congruent I-T prosthesis.

Staged Treatment

The partially dentate maxilla may be managed through a staged approach to the complete replacement of the missing and existing natural teeth when using a Type 1 congruent I-T prosthesis. Following the necessary diagnostic and planning phases and appropriate periodontal therapy for the remaining teeth, staged surgical placement of implants can be undertaken. A segmental restorative plan allows for various stages of the maxillary rehabilitation

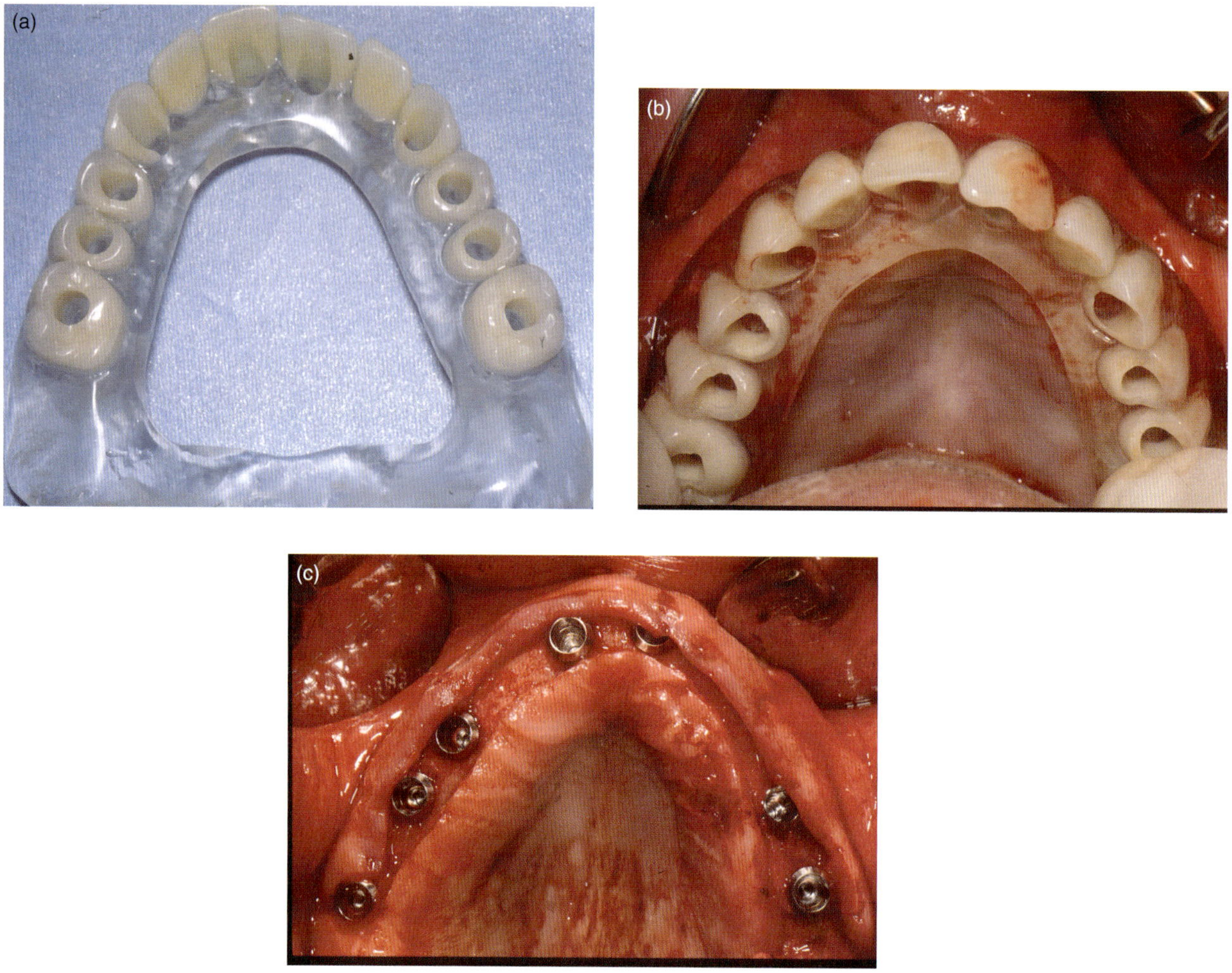

Figure 13.11 (a) Prepared surgical guide (stent) for placement of multiple implants in the maxilla to provide for a Type 1 congruent FPD. (b) Surgical guide in situ prior to flap elevation. (c) Occlusal view of flap elevation and implant placement having used the prepared surgical guide.

to proceed while being cognizant of, but without compromise to, the final planned outcome.

The advantages of such an approach are related to the ability for some patients to better manage the physiological and psychological challenges of losing all of their upper teeth; providing an often simpler healing phase with a transitional prosthesis, and the ability to provide for a more rapid improvement of appearance, function, and patient comfort. Fixed provisional segmental prostheses are sometimes used, thus allowing modifications in the definitive prosthetic design should appearance, function, maintenance or phonetics dictates.

A staged approach does increase the time over which treatment takes place, and by definition involves an increased number of surgical stages. Such an approach is contraindicated if the teeth designated for later extraction are unable to be stabilized with periodontal therapy, or where the tooth or teeth positions would compromise the desired implant placement or final prosthesis design.

Loading Protocols and the Transition Phase

There are a number of examples of immediate loading (in a full-arch form) of the edentulous maxilla in the literature, which report the procedure, techniques, and early outcomes. Fewer studies document longer-term survival and complication. However, objective analyses of esthetic outcomes when prostheses are placed at the time of surgical implant placement are lacking.

Alternatively, early loading, being defined as a restoration in contact with the opposing dentition and placed at least 48 h after implant placement but not later than three months postimplant placement, can be supported (when using implants with a roughened titanium intraosseous surface) in the edentulous maxilla (Proceedings of the Third ITI Consensus Conference, *JOMI*, Vol. 19 (Supplement):75–114; 2004). From an esthetic point of view, there appears to be a low risk of a negative outcome when single tooth implant-retained provisional crowns are placed six weeks following implant placement. The early placement of well-fitting short-span provisional restorations in segments around the arch is to be recommended as a precursor to the definitive ceramo-metal restoration in a Type 1 congruent I-T prosthesis.

Considerations of Implant and Pontic Positioning for Optimal Esthetics

When planning the restoration in the anterior region of the maxilla, several factors must be balanced in determining the most desirable implant positions to achieve the optimal esthetic outcome. These factors include:

- the areas that provide sufficient volume of alveolar bone
- the desired tooth positions in the definitive prosthesis
- the volume and architecture of the alveolar mucosa
- the relationship of the upper lip position to the planned restoration on smiling and the crest of the alveolar mucosa
- the importance of visual bilateral symmetry around the maxillary dental midline

Clinical observation has demonstrated that it is often difficult to recreate the scalloped soft tissue architecture that accompanies a healthy natural dentition when using multiple dental implants. Adjacent implant restorations are at present unpredictable with respect to the postrestoration interproximal soft tissue contours. The tissue-type and relationship of the periodontal supporting tissues and a natural tooth are quite different from those between the mucosa and an implant-retained restoration. Thus, in the edentulous anterior maxilla, the esthetic outcome can often be optimized by placement of fewer implants, spaced adequately to provide pontic sites.

The use of a ceramo-metal pontic or pontics in the restoration allows greater variation in the ability to recreate the desired tooth–soft tissue relationship. In areas where the alveolar mucosa is of sufficient volume, an ovate design of the apical area allows the pontic to be seated into the mucosa and provide the appearance of a scalloped architecture. The interproximal tissue does not extend as far coronally as that between two natural teeth, but does change the flattened alveolar mucosa covering on the ridge to a scalloped form. Figures 13.12a–b demonstrate this effect in the anterior maxilla of a partially dentate patient.

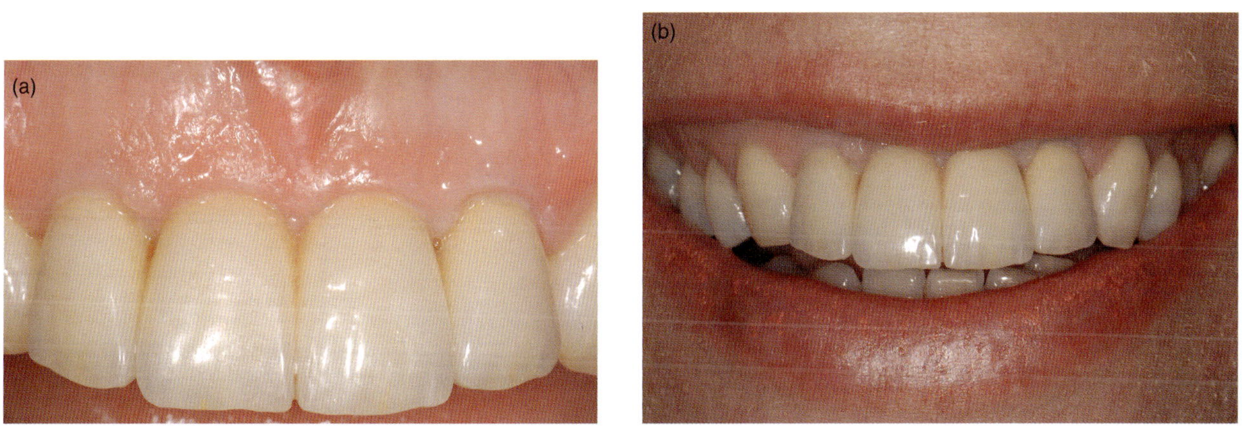

Figure 13.12 (a) A facial view of a four-unit Type 1 congruent FPD supported by two dental implants (in the maxillary lateral incisor sites) in a partial edentulous patient demonstrating adequate, but not ideal, interproximal soft tissue architecture around the pontics of the FPD. (b) A smile view of same patient.

Alternatively, where two or more pontics exist between implant abutment crowns, the limited addition of soft-tissue colored ceramic can provide an esthetically pleasing illusion of a natural soft tissue architectural form around the prosthetic teeth. This colored ceramic can either be limited to the interproximal gingival embrasure alone; with the neck of the pontic seated on the alveolar mucosa, or extended in the form of a narrow, thin flange apical to the neck of the pontic to allow a balanced tooth form to be created. In both situations, the restoration can be constructed to achieve a bilaterally symmetrical appearance of the prosthetic soft tissue.

The utilization of soft-tissue colored ceramic also obviates the need for additional surgical attempts to augment deficient alveolar mucosa. Whilst augmentation may provide for an improved result, the precise outcome of surgical intervention aimed at vertical enhancement of the ridge form is at best unpredictable.

The critical issue when considering the addition of soft-tissue colored ceramic is the relationship of the upper lip at the point of its highest elevation, and the inferior crest of the alveolar mucosa. To esthetically "hide" the soft-tissue colored ceramic–mucosal junction, it must be placed just superiorly to the upper elevation of the upper lip upon smiling. This junction must not be exposed when the patient smiles. Such extension also allows the necks of the pontic teeth to be correctly positioned independent of an existing nonideal ridge contour (Figures 13.13a–c).

The extension should not be confused in design with a conventional denture flange; it should be short, thin, and taper out onto the tissue in to a thin sharp edge. The extension should be constructed using a matching tissue colored ceramic

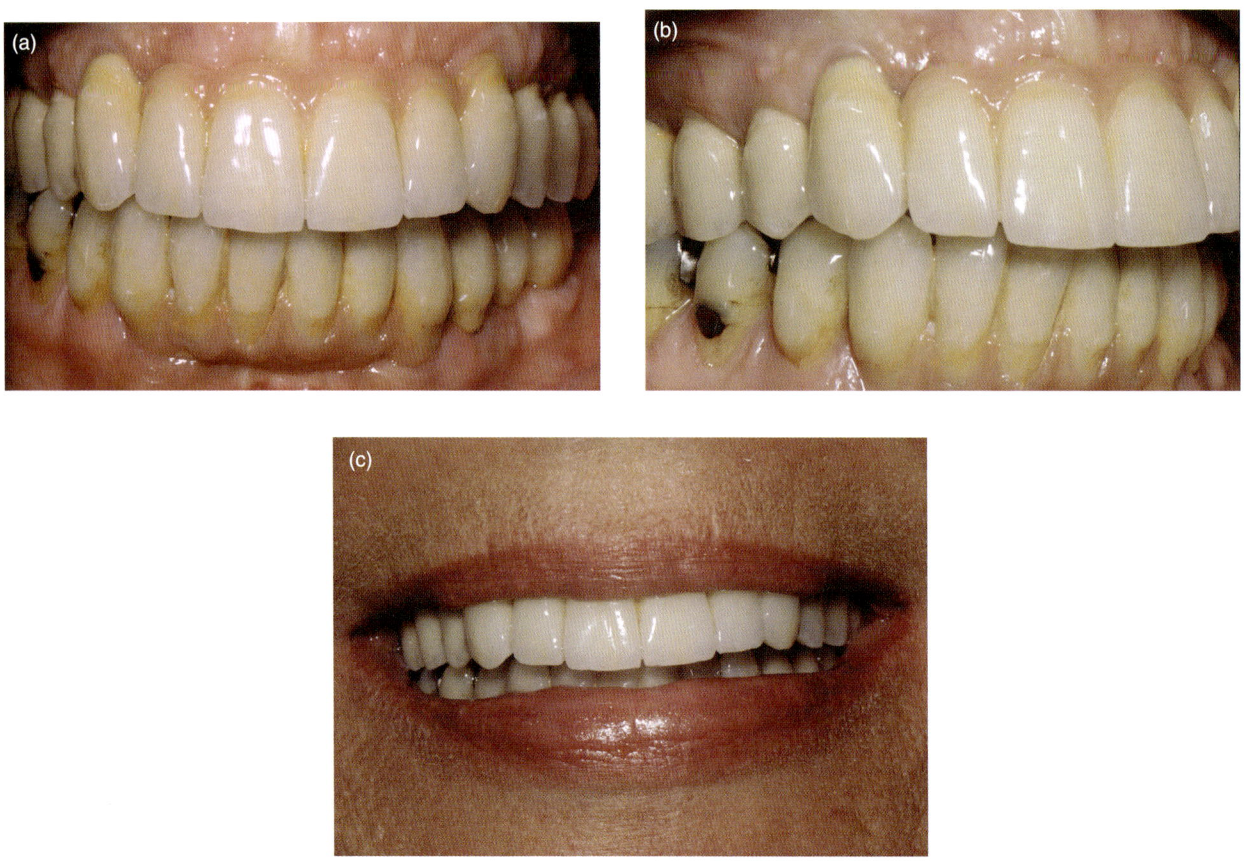

Figure 13.13 (a–b) A facial and right-facial intraoral views of the completed FPD utilizing a ceramic "flange" in the pontic regions of the lateral incisor replacement teeth. The ceramic "flange" provides for an artificial architecture that mimics natural contours and esthetics. (c) A smile view of the same patient demonstrating the "masking" of the ceramic "flange" under the upper lip at its highest elevation.

and thinned to an almost transparent appearance to allow the natural mucosal color to "blend" with the margin.

Design Options for Type 1 Congruent I-T Prostheses Using Segmental Restorations

Option 1: The placement of eight implants allows for the construction of four individual three-unit FPDs; with two three-unit FPDs replacing the anterior six teeth (Figure 13.14).

Option 2: The placement of eight implants allows for the construction of four individual three-unit FPD; with two three-unit FPDs replacing the anterior six teeth and utilizing single-unit distal-extension cantilever pontics (premolar size) bilaterally in the posterior FPDs (Figure 13.15).

Option 3: The placement of eight implants allows for the construction of one anterior four-unit FPD to replace the incisor teeth*; single implant-retained restorations to replace the cuspid teeth, and two three-unit FPDs replacing the posterior teeth (Figure 13.16).

Option 4: The placement of six implants allows for the construction of one anterior four-unit FPD to replace the incisor teeth* and two three-unit FPDs replacing the posterior teeth (Figure 13.17).

Option 5: The placement of six implants allows for the construction of one anterior six-unit FPD to replace the incisor and cuspid teeth*

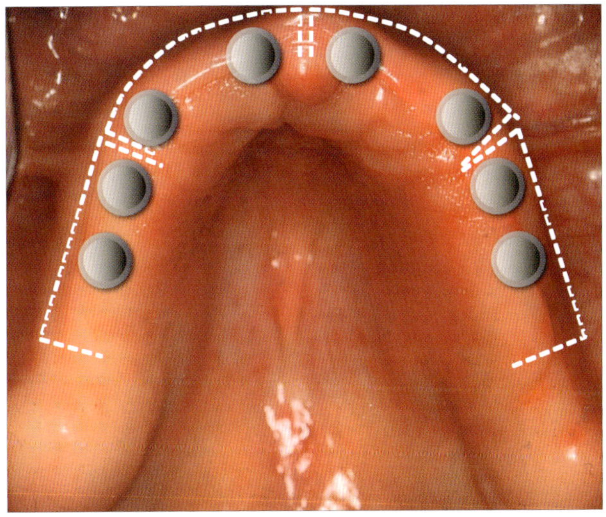

Figure 13.15 The placement of eight implants allows for the construction of four individual three-unit FPDs; with two three-unit FPDs replacing the anterior six teeth and utilizing single-unit distal-extension cantilever pontics (premolar size) bilaterally in the posterior FPDs.

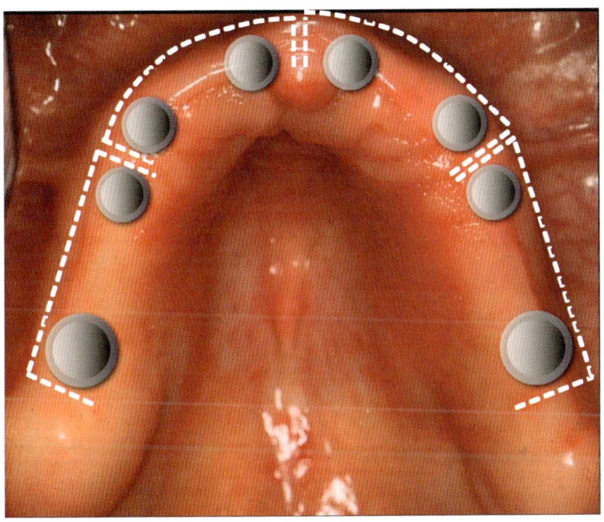

Figure 13.14 The placement of eight implants allows for the construction of four individual three-unit FPDs; with two three-unit FPDs replacing the anterior six teeth.

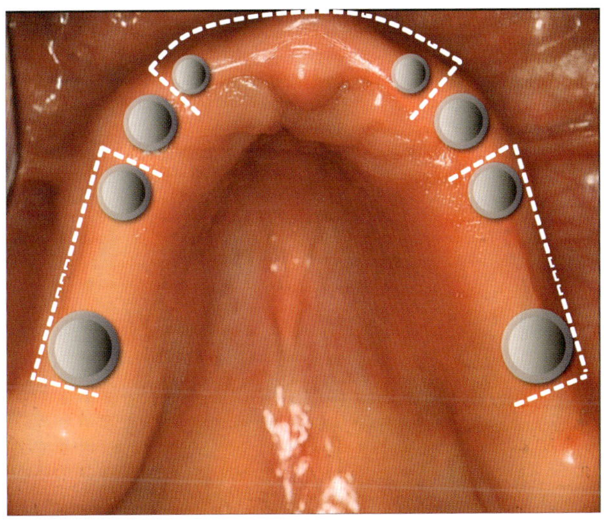

Figure 13.16 The placement of eight implants allows for the construction of one anterior four-unit FPD to replace the incisor teeth*; single implant-retained restorations to replace the cuspid teeth, and two three-unit FPDs replacing the posterior teeth.

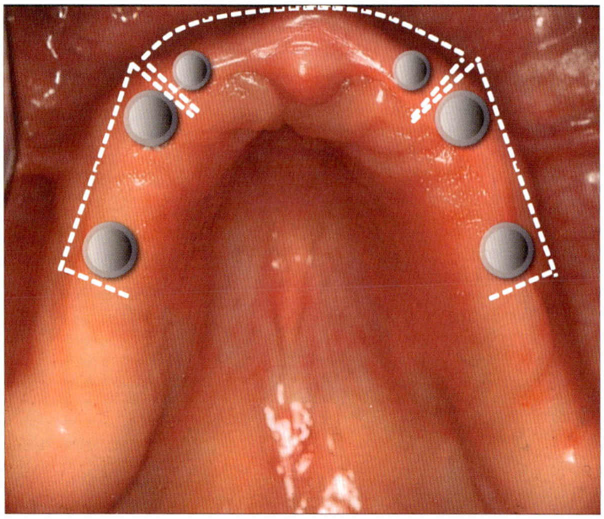

Figure 13.17 The placement of six implants allows for the construction of one anterior four-unit FPD to replace the incisor teeth* and two three-unit FPDs replacing the posterior teeth.

and two three-unit FPDs replacing the posterior teeth, without the use of a cantilever distal extension (Figure 13.18).

Option 6: The placement of six implants allows for the construction of one anterior six-unit FPD to replace the incisor and cuspid teeth* and two three-unit FPDs replacing the posterior teeth, utilizing single-unit distal-extension cantilever pontics (premolar size) bilaterally (Figure 13.19).

(*There may be an esthetic requirement to include some interproximal soft-tissue colored ceramic in the gingival embrasures between the pontics to provide optimal result.)

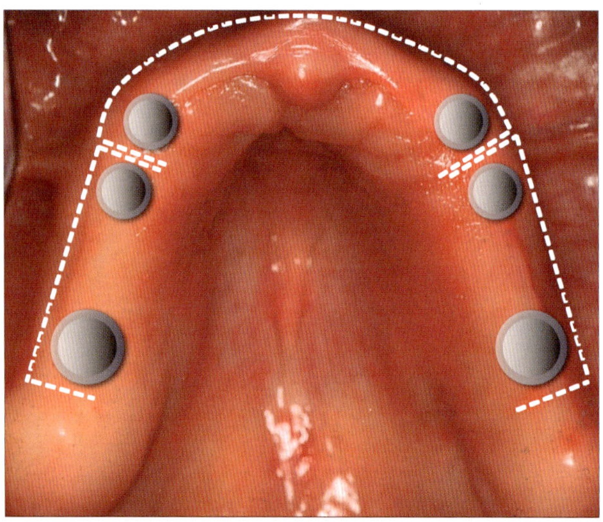

Figure 13.18 The placement of six implants allows for the construction of one anterior six-unit FPD to replace the incisor and cuspid teeth* and two three-unit FPDs replacing the posterior teeth without the use of a cantilever distal extension.

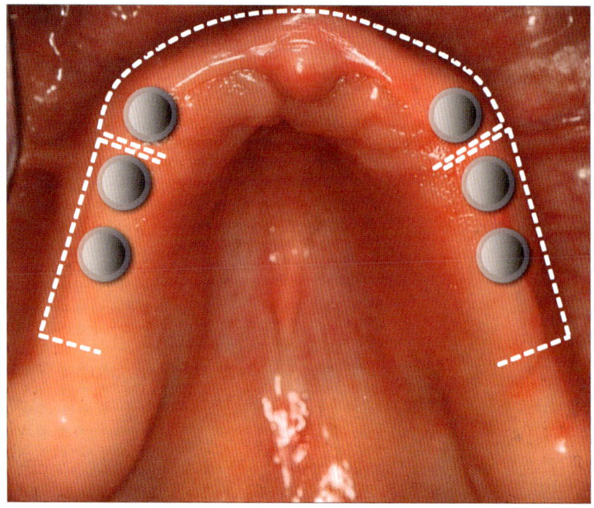

Figure 13.19 The placement of six implants allows for the construction of one anterior six-unit FPD to replace the incisor and cuspid teeth* and two three-unit FPDs replacing the posterior teeth, utilizing single-unit distal-extension cantilever pontics (premolar size) bilaterally.

An example of a clinical case representing the rehabilitation of the edentulous maxilla utilizing dental implants and segmental FPDs is demonstrated in Figures 13.20a–d (and previously seen in Figure 13.13). This example provides for implant placement in positions similar to those in Option 6. Such a therapeutic approach was indicated in this patient as there was an anterior open bite and thus little load applied to the anterior segmental prosthesis. Additionally, complex ridge reconstitution required for implant placement in the incisor region is avoided.

TYPE 2: NONCONGRUENT I-T PROSTHESIS

The Type 2 noncongruent I-T prosthesis is indicated where the prosthetic tooth position is required to be horizontally and/or vertically distant from the residual edentulous maxilla. A diagnostic setup establishes the distance between the necks of the teeth in their desired positions and the alveolar

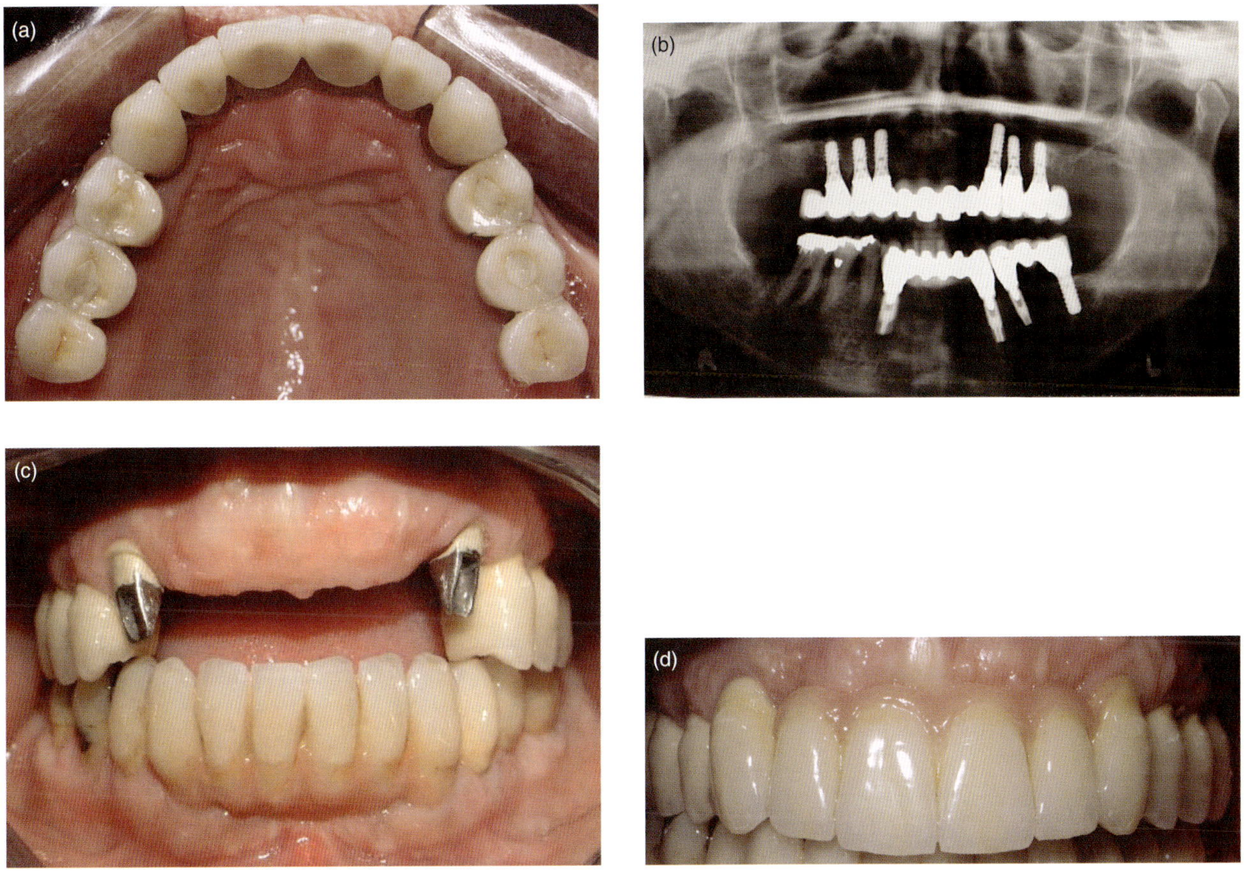

Figure 13.20 (a) An occlusal view of FPDs utilizing the therapeutic Option 6: A six-unit anterior FPD with two separate posterior segments comprising three-unit FPDs (each inclusive of a single distal cantilever extension) being directly screw-retained. (b) A postoperative OPG radiograph. (c) An anterior view demonstrating the ceramo-metal meso-structures in place, prior to the cementation of the anterior six-unit FPD. (d) Facial view of the completed reconstruction.

ridge. As a consequence of the necks of the teeth being distanced from the ridge form, the prosthetic teeth cannot exit directly from the mucosa. In such a case, there is always additional soft-tissue colored prosthetic material required between the mucosa and the prosthetic teeth.

The general principles for patient analysis outlined above for the determination of the Type 1 congruent I-T prosthesis are equally relevant when the definitive prosthesis does not allow the implants to be congruent with specific prosthetic tooth positions on the prosthesis. The Type 2 noncongruent I-T prosthesis has the advantage of being able to be constructed in either ceramo-metal or metal-reinforced acrylic (i.e., a hybrid prosthesis). With the ongoing development of CAD-CAM technology, milled metal and all-ceramic frameworks are being utilized as further extensions of fabrication techniques. Regardless of the technique employed, it remains essential that the junction between the soft-tissue colored prosthetic material and the alveolar mucosa be superior to the highest elevation of the upper lip upon smiling (Figures 13.21a–d).

Key issues

Clinical and Radiographic Diagnostic Criteria Are Less Demanding

Implant positioning is not as critical as for the Type 1 prosthesis. A complete and accurate definitive tooth setup must still be established and verified intraorally. The try-in confirms the distances between the necks of the teeth and the alveolar mucosa in the areas where the implants are to be placed. Where there are areas of advanced resorption,

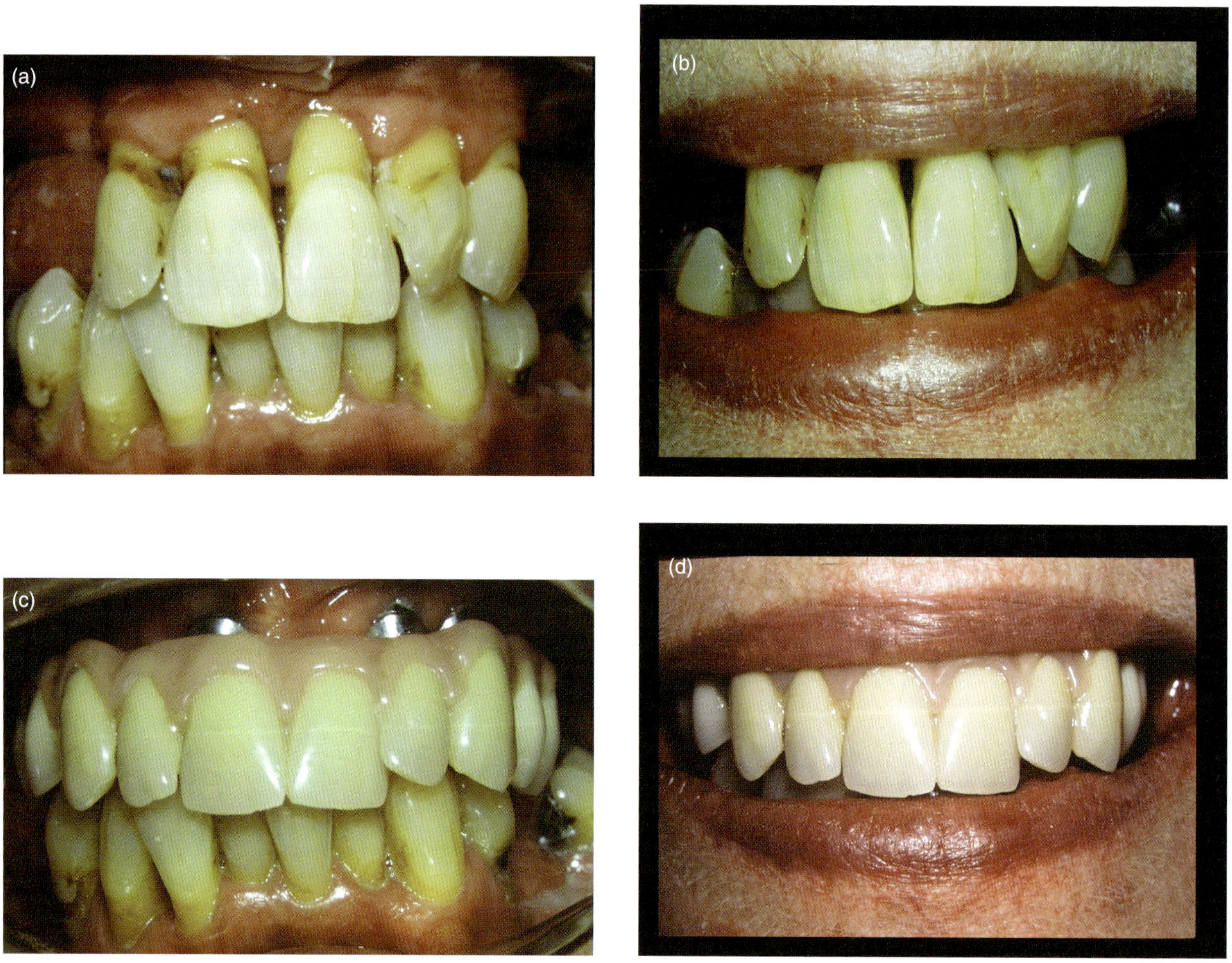

Figure 13.21 (a) A facial view of the preoperative state of a 65-year-old female patient with terminal remaining five anterior maxillary teeth. (b) Lip positions during smiling indicating that the remaining ridge mucosa lies superior to the upper lip position. (c) A view of the completed Type 2 noncongruent FPD. (d) The patient's smile, confirming the nonappearance of the junction of the prosthesis and the alveolar mucosa.

particularly in the anterior ridge, pontics should be planned. The trial appliance will have a slight labial or buccal flange. It should not extend into the vestibule. Upper lip support will be provided predominately by the teeth.

An appropriate radiographic analysis is required to confirm the proposed implant sites prior to final determination of the most suitable positions, and designation of the types of implants most appropriate. CBCT or similar computer-assisted images may be required where the residual ridge width is in question. When available, computer-assisted planning software and navigational surgical units may also assist.

Determination of Implant Position

A Type 2 noncongruent I-T prosthesis requires a distribution of dental implants around the maxillary ridge that will allow for the predetermined prosthesis design to be attached and distribute functional loading. At the time of surgery, the surgeon is still required to visualize the positions of the teeth as they will be on the definitive prosthesis. Positions should be chosen that allow the implants to be placed in adequate bony sites, be spaced from one another for improved patient home care, and provide screw access holes through the occlusal and palatal aspects of the prosthesis. In most cases, the relationship of the head diameter of the implants to the tooth types (and thus sizes) on the prosthesis is of less importance.

The operator responsible for the surgical placement of the implants must be a skilled surgeon with adequate understanding of implant surgery and soft and hard tissue management.

The Use of a Surgical Guide (Stent)

A carefully constructed and accurate surgical guide must again be fabricated and used at the time of surgery. The guide should provide a replica of the final prosthesis to demonstrate tooth position in relation to the bony ridge form. Its aim will be to allow the various implants to be placed in such a manner as to provide the simplest connection within the prosthetic design.

ADDITIONAL CONSIDERATIONS

Implant Design and Number

As the esthetics of the definitive Type 2 noncongruent I-T prosthesis depends less upon the interface of the mucosa and the prosthetic connection to the implant, the type of implant to be utilized is not as critical. The points relating to the design of the restorative connection, as outlined above, remain valid. Where the implant-prosthetic connection is concealed under the upper lip, as is the indication for the Type 2 prosthetic design, implant selection can be made to optimize the biological response and facilitate maintenance. As such, a transmucosal implant design is usually preferred. Where the prosthesis is constructed as a reinforced metal-acrylic hybrid, the need to have acrylic extending submucosally will be reduced. Further, when the restorative interface is at, above or minimally below the mucosal margin, more accurate clinical determination of the fit of the prosthesis is possible.

Between four and eight implants are required to adequately support a Type 2 maxillary prosthesis. The determination of the number of implants to be placed is based upon several factors, including the ability to distribute the implants around the arch, the opposing dentition, the prosthetic design (with four implants a segmental restoration is not possible) and the desire to provide adequate space between each implant.

Staged Treatment and the Transition Phase

For the fully edentulous patient, the simultaneous placement of the required number of implants is common. In the partially dentate maxilla, for reasons similar to those discussed for the patient planned for a Type 1 prosthesis, a staged approach to the complete replacement of remaining natural teeth using a Type 2 noncongruent I-T prosthesis may be considered.

This approach is particularly beneficial when both the extractions of the remaining teeth and the implant placements can be staged. The simplest approach is to extract nonstrategic teeth, with the retained teeth prepared to allow for a tooth-supported fixed partial denture. Alternatively, a removable partial appliance being supported by the unprepared retained teeth is another option. Several dental implants are then placed in the appropriate sites, whether they be existing edentulous sites, extraction sockets, or partially healed sockets in a Type 2 or delayed approach.

Following the required healing time, impressions are made and the provisional implant-supported prosthesis is fabricated, allowing for attachment to the implants yet to be placed. This appliance also acts as a definitive surgical guide and is best utilized when the final implants are to be placed in more critical sites. The remaining teeth are subsequently removed, additional implants are placed (either immediate placement or delayed as a Type 2 procedure) and the provisional prosthesis is linked to these implants and screw-retained in situ. The definitive prosthesis can then be fabricated at the appropriate time. The clinician may also evaluate the functional and esthetic parameters as afforded by the provisional appliance. Such a staged approach has several advantages, which are listed in Table 13.5.

Figures 13.22a–f demonstrate a case managed with a Type 2 noncongruent I-T prosthesis, in this case fabricated in metal-ceramics. The patient, a 64-year-old male, demonstrates a moderately high risk of technical complications from parafunctional activity. He has a shortened mandibular arch, with the majority of his posterior teeth absent. He declined treatment in his lower jaw. Therapy was therefore limited to replacement of his maxillary teeth.

Staged extraction of the remaining maxillary teeth was undertaken, using three strategic teeth

Table 13.5 Advantages of a maxillary rehabilitation utilizing a staged implant placement protocol.

- The surgical phase is simplified for the patient, as two less extensive procedures are required
- The physiological and psychological challenges of losing the natural upper teeth are better managed
- There is often a simpler healing phase with a transitional prostheses
- An immediate restoration is provided at the time of the second surgical placement of implants
- There is reliance on a combination of previously integrated implants as well as the just placed implants, when loading is introduced through immediate prosthesis placement
- A more accurate and simpler construction of the immediately placed prosthesis is possible
- Functional and esthetic assessment of the prosthetic design prior to construction of the definitive prosthesis can be carried out
- Although the provisional is usually a full-arch construction, it still allows for a definitive segmental restorative design

as temporary abutments for a transitional FPD during the two stages of implant placements. Once the initial implants placed had successfully integrated, a provisional implant-supported FPD was constructed and placed followed by the placement of the final implants. Later the definitive metal-ceramic prosthesis was constructed; being screw-retained to custom-fabricated gold cylinders via transversal (or lateral) screws. Individual pressed ceramic crowns were constructed and individually luted on the rigid "tooth-form" projections on the framework.

The eight-year following and radiographs are demonstrated in Figures 13.23a–d. During this time, one of the pressed ceramic crowns has required replacement as a result of cracking. The design facilitates this type of repair as the individual crown can be replaced without the removal of the prosthesis, using conventional "tooth-based" crown and bridge procedures.

Loading Protocols

Following an extensive review of the literature, and as a result of the third ITI Consensus Conference, there are considered sufficient studies on early loading to allow clinical recommendations to be published. Four or more implants supporting a fixed restoration on a framework that rigidly connects the implants should be employed. The implants should be characterized by a roughened titanium intraosseous surface, and be allowed to heal for at least six weeks. The implant sites should be characterized by types 1, 2, or 3 bone quality.

Implant-Retained Fixed Prosthesis—Summary

A comparison of the advantages and disadvantages between Type 1 and Type 2 FPDs are presented in summary form in Table 13.6. These factors need to be considered on a case-by-case basis to allow analysis of the best option for any particular patient presentation.

Maintenance Considerations

All fixed prostheses will require maintenance as a consequence of technical complications. These complications may be implant-related, connection-related or suprastructure-related. The associated soft tissues and supporting alveolar bone are also at risk of biologic complications, including mucositis, peri-implantitis, and general soft tissues complications. Possible complications of both a biologic and technical nature are summarized in Table 13.7.

When completing Type 1 or Type 2 fixed prostheses, the operator must be aware of the risks of such complications. Provision for the management of complications must be considered in the planning phase. Screw retention of the prosthesis will allow retrieval to more easily address peri-implant and soft tissue complications. Segmented restorations may have some or all individual segments cement-retained, as a segment will likely to have less complicated access for a site-specific biologic problem.

All patients must be offered a specific program of maintenance following successful implant

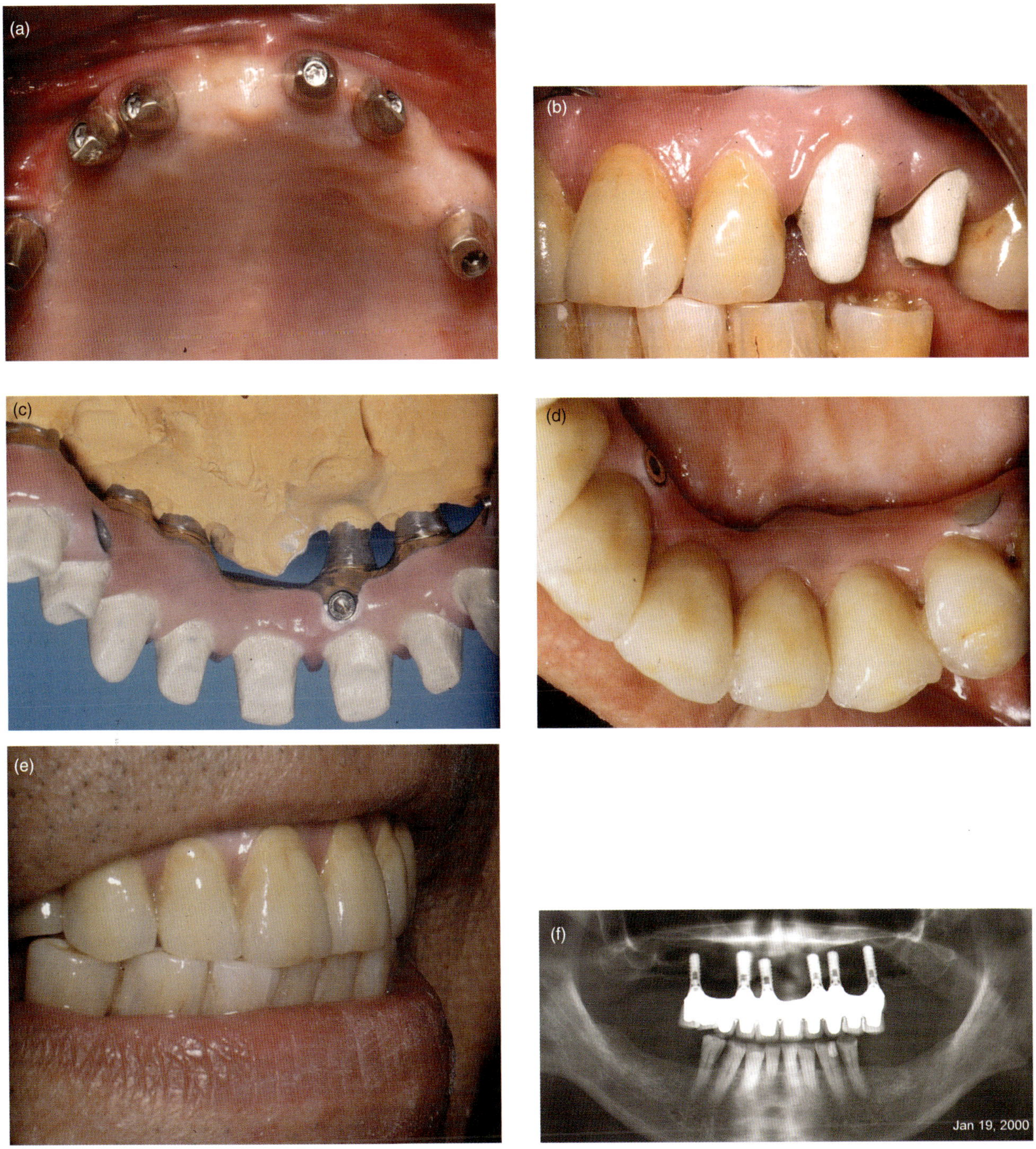

Figure 13.22 (a) An occlusal view of custom-fabricated gold meso-structures, screw-retained to the implant–abutment assemblies of the integrated trans-mucosal implants prior to the placement of the definitive suprastructure. (b) An intraoral view of the left facial aspect of the Type 2 noncongruent metal-ceramic FPD in place, demonstrating the opaqued metal "preparations" onto which the pressed all-ceramic crowns are luted. (c) A view of the metal-ceramic framework on the master cast. (d) A palatal view of the prosthesis, which demonstrates the design position of transverse screws. (e) Postoperative view of patient with lips in an exaggerated smile position. (f) A postoperative OPG.

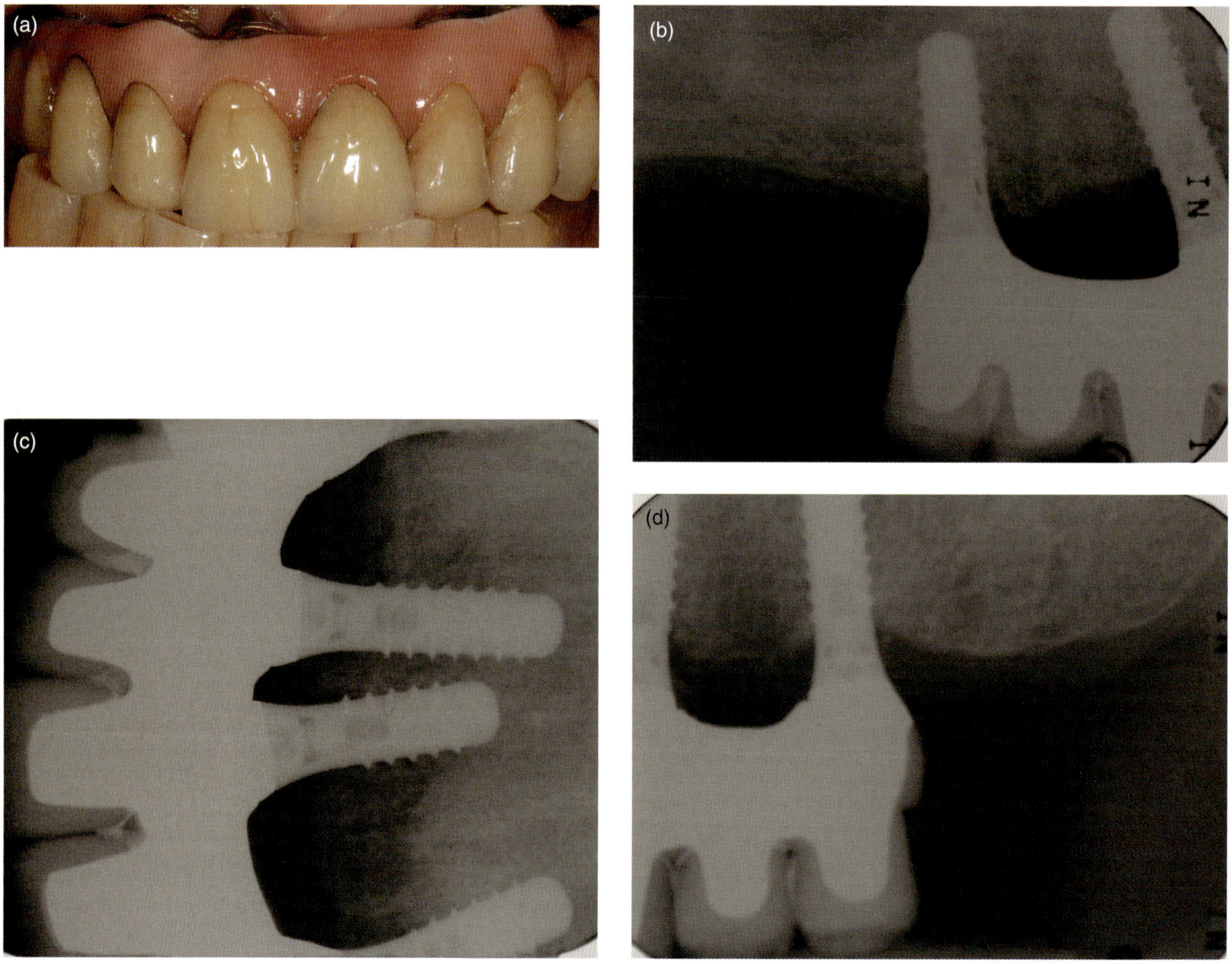

Figure 13.23 (a) A facial view of the Type 2 noncongruent FPD, at the eight-year review. (b–d) Eight-year radiographs demonstrate adequate maintenance of bone levels.

therapy. The combined incidence of biologic and technical complications has been assessed as approximately 50% of cases after five years of function.

Bruxism is a recognized risk factor in the increased incidence of technical complications. Patients who demonstrate evidence of such parafunctional activity should be warned of the likely incidence of various technical complications. The actual risk is associated with several factors, including the material used in the prosthesis construction, the design of the prosthesis and the opposing dentition. Design features, beyond conventional screw-retained (i.e., transocclusal and transverse) frameworks can be incorporated into the design to provide for less involved correction of a likely incident. Such a design feature was illustrated in the patient case previously presented in Figures 13.22a–f.

There is also a recognized high incidence of technical complications associated with metal-reinforced acrylic Type 2 FPDs. These complications can involve the regular fracturing of the teeth (both adhesive and cohesive), fracturing of the pink acrylic supporting material, and prosthesis fracture. The resin-based teeth will eventually wear and require replacement—the rate being individually determined by the parafunctional activity and force of the each patient.

It is wise to identify the likelihood of such complications at the time that the presentation of

Table 13.6 A comparison of the Type 1 and Type 2 fixed prostheses.

Type 1 congruent I-T prosthesis	Type 2 noncongruent I-T prosthesis
Advantages • Can provide excellent esthetic outcome • The use of segmental restorations are indicated; simplifies construction • Tooth–mucosal interface created to imitate natural anatomy • Pontics can be placed with very good adaptation to mucosa • Often multiple design options that can accommodate for variation in the suitability of implant bony sites	**Advantages** • Greater scope in choosing implant sites • Greater tolerance in surgical implant placement • Able to distance implants to improve patient access for home care • Compensation of missing alveolar ridge form possible with prosthetic material • Generally screw-retention provides for simpler maintenance • Various material options available • Often cheaper option compared to a Type 1 ceramo-meal prosthesis
Disadvantages • Requires very precise implant positioning • Requires highly skilled operators and team • Technically demanding • Patient's home care can be complicated • Minor deviation in implant placement positions or alignment may have significant negative effects on esthetic outcome	**Disadvantages** • Shape of prosthesis is influenced by the position of the implants • Potential for phonetic complications • Often constructed in one piece • Often high costs • May require scheduled removal at maintenance appointments to allow for thorough evaluation and cleaning

the treatment options is being made to the patient. A decision to proceed with such therapy should be made in the knowledge it is likely that there will be a higher incidence of technical complications and maintenance requirements.

Table 13.7 Possible maintenance complications.

Biologic complications

- Mucositis: Localized lesion without bone loss around an osseointegrated implant
- Peri-implantitis: Localized lesion including bone loss around an osseointegrated implant
- Soft tissue complications: Fistula, excessive swelling, hyperplasia, etc.

Technical complications

- Implant-related: Fracture
- Connection-related: Screw loosening, fracture
- Suprastructure-related: Framework, veneer, loss of retention (in cemented restorations), tooth displacement, excessive wear

IMPLANT RETAINED/SUPPORTED REMOVABLE PROSTHESIS

Patients who are prepared to continue with a removable maxillary prosthesis but seek an improvement in the function and comfort of the appliance are a group who can be considered for removable implant-retained and/or supported prosthetic rehabilitations of their maxillary jaws.

Conversely, some patients are not suitable for either Type 1 or Type 2 fixed design options, and see the implant-enhanced removable option as an improvement when compared to a conventional denture. There are many advantages to providing such therapy, as have been summarized earlier. The challenge is to determine the most appropriate prosthetic design for each patient. It must be a design which will address the presenting concerns of the patient and provide the enhancements that are expected.

The Role of Implants in a Removable Prosthesis

Dental implant therapy employed in either jaw to provide a removable prosthesis is aimed at improving retention, stability and/or support. While these elements are rarely mutually exclusive, identifying the patient's dissatisfaction with any functional aspect of their existing conventional full denture will provide an indicator as to the most appropriate design to eliminate the problem in the new removable prosthesis. A basic comparison is summarized in Table 13.8.

Dental implants can be used either individually with retentive abutments or splinted via a bar form. Individual use utilizing two implants is common in the lower jaw. Individual abutments are placed that provide for a retentive patrix that engages a corresponding matrix placed in the removable prosthesis. These are either a near-spherical shape (e.g., retentive anchors) or a wide disc that provides a dual internal and external retentive configuration (Locator®) (Figures 13.24a–b). Other retentive designs exist, such as magnets.

Table 13.8 Implant supported/retained maxillary removable prosthesis.

Single retentive elements
For retention primarily, but does improve stability of the prosthesis
Limited use in maxilla: 2 implants are rare/4 implants are possible, but there are limitations
Can utilize various retentive designs
Indicated where primary problem with existing denture is retention
Alveolar mucosa continues to provide primary support for functional loading
Maintenance requirements
Splinted bar-retained
Four implants are required
Adequate inter-arch distance is for required prosthetic elements
Placement is effective for retention and provides a reduced mucosal loading
Bar design—determines the distribution of the functional load between the bar and the alveolar mucosa
Maxillary prosthesis design—assessment of resilience of alveolar mucosa determines requirement for palatal coverage
Maintenance requirements

Each of these elements provides, as its primary function, enhanced retention. There is also a coincident improvement in the stability of the prosthesis. However, there is little effect on support, as the attachment (patrix–matrix) design provides for resilience between the parts, thus allowing the prosthesis to continue to require support from the underlying maxillary mucosa. Only after the quality of the mucosal-denture base fit deteriorates does the support for the functional occlusal loading transfer to a greater extent to the implants; something that should be corrected with a readaptation of the denture base.

When implants are splinted together using a cast, soldered or welded bar, retentive matrices are also incorporated into the prosthesis. The circumferential shape of the bar will be determined by the extent of functional loading that the prosthesis must transmit to the implants through the bar. The mucosal area under the extension of the bar will not be loaded, thus the bar will provide retention (through the retentive clips that engage the bar), improved stability and support. The bars share the load in conjunction with the mucosa in areas where the denture base is in contact with mucosa beyond the bar extension.

Diagnostic Criteria: Clinical and Radiographic

The key issues in determining the clinical indications for implant therapy using a removable prosthesis are:

- the need to provide additional support to the facial middle one-third beyond that provided by the residual maxillary ridge, and
- sufficient area of available space between the maxillary alveolar mucosa and the proposed internal surface of the denture base for the required implant connections and associated hardware to fabricate the bar and the prosthesis.

Where the teeth are required to be placed beyond the vertical, horizontal, and transverse dimensions

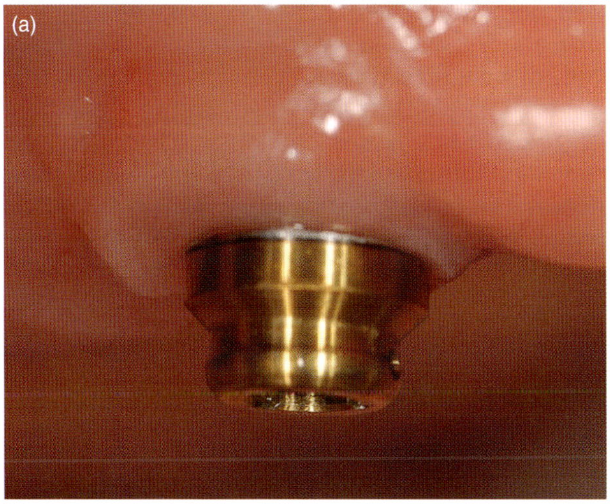

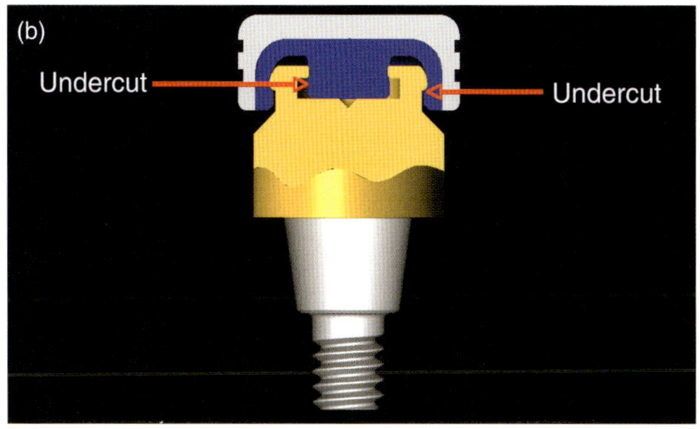

Figure 13.24 (a) A clinical view of a Locator® attachment in place in an edentulous maxillary jaw. (b) A diagrammatic representation of the Locator® attachment with the plastic matrix engaging the metal patrix. Divergence of greater than 10° (20° between implants) can be accommodated with a modification of the design of the matrix, that then only engages the external retentive feature.

of the residual ridge form, there is an immediate need to provide additional prosthetic augmentation of the arch. Such augmentation is simply provided through the use of a removable prosthesis.

Infrequently the presenting complaint of the patient is exclusively related to retention in their conventional full maxillary denture. Usually the resorptive changes that have occurred in the edentulous maxilla lead to reduced stability in function, or the alveolar mucosa is unable to absorb the functional loading transmitted through the conventional appliance.

Recommended management involves the placement of four dental implants in the edentulous maxilla to provide for a removable prosthesis. The implants may be restored with individual retentive elements. More commonly, the implants are splinted with a bar. There is a need for not less than 15 mm between the alveolar ridge and the denture base to allow for the incorporation of a bar structure and the attendant retentive elements. This requirement will be less when a nonsplinted (individual elements) implant-retained appliance can be utilized.

The preferred sites for implant placements are in the anterior and premolar areas of the maxilla. The available bone in these area is usually adequate, except when either the maxillary sinus has enlarged vertically and anteriorly, or when there has been significant bone loss in the anterior maxilla (as in the abnormally advanced bone resorption seen in the "combination syndrome" patient).

SINGLE RETENTIVE ELEMENTS

As the use of this procedure is limited to patients whose problem relates primarily to a lack of retention (the maxillary mucosa and underlying alveolar bone is of sufficient volume and resiliency to maintain stability and support), this therapy has limited use in maxilla. In such cases, the use of four dental implants with individual retentive elements is most effective. On rare occasions two may be used.

In one such instance, a 54-year-old male patient, being a person who derived his income predominately from being engaged as a public speaker, felt concerned that he could loose his conventional full upper denture whilst presenting. The ridge form was adequate and the patient had no other complaints. He had worn a full denture for many years, and the present prosthesis was satisfactory in normal function. The patient's residual maxillary ridge did not permit a Type 1 or Type 2 fixed option, due to an inadequacy of the residual bone volume. He declined bone grafting to permit the placement of multiple implants.

Following appropriate clinical and radiographic analysis, it was determined that the placement of two implants in the cuspid regions, with the view to placing individual retentive elements, would provide a solution to his concern regarding confidence in the retention of the conventional full denture. Whilst this is an unusual presentation, and a treatment that is not recommended as a routine modality, it demonstrates the principle of the use of individual implants to enhance the retention of a conventionally designed full upper denture (Figures 13.25a–d).

When four dental implants can be placed in the maxilla, the management decision exists as to whether to prescribe a Type 2 fixed I-T prosthesis or an implant-retained overdenture. In addition to the two key issues previously listed, there are several additional factors to evaluate: The occlusal forces the appliance will need to withstand, the opposing dentition, and the desires of the patient

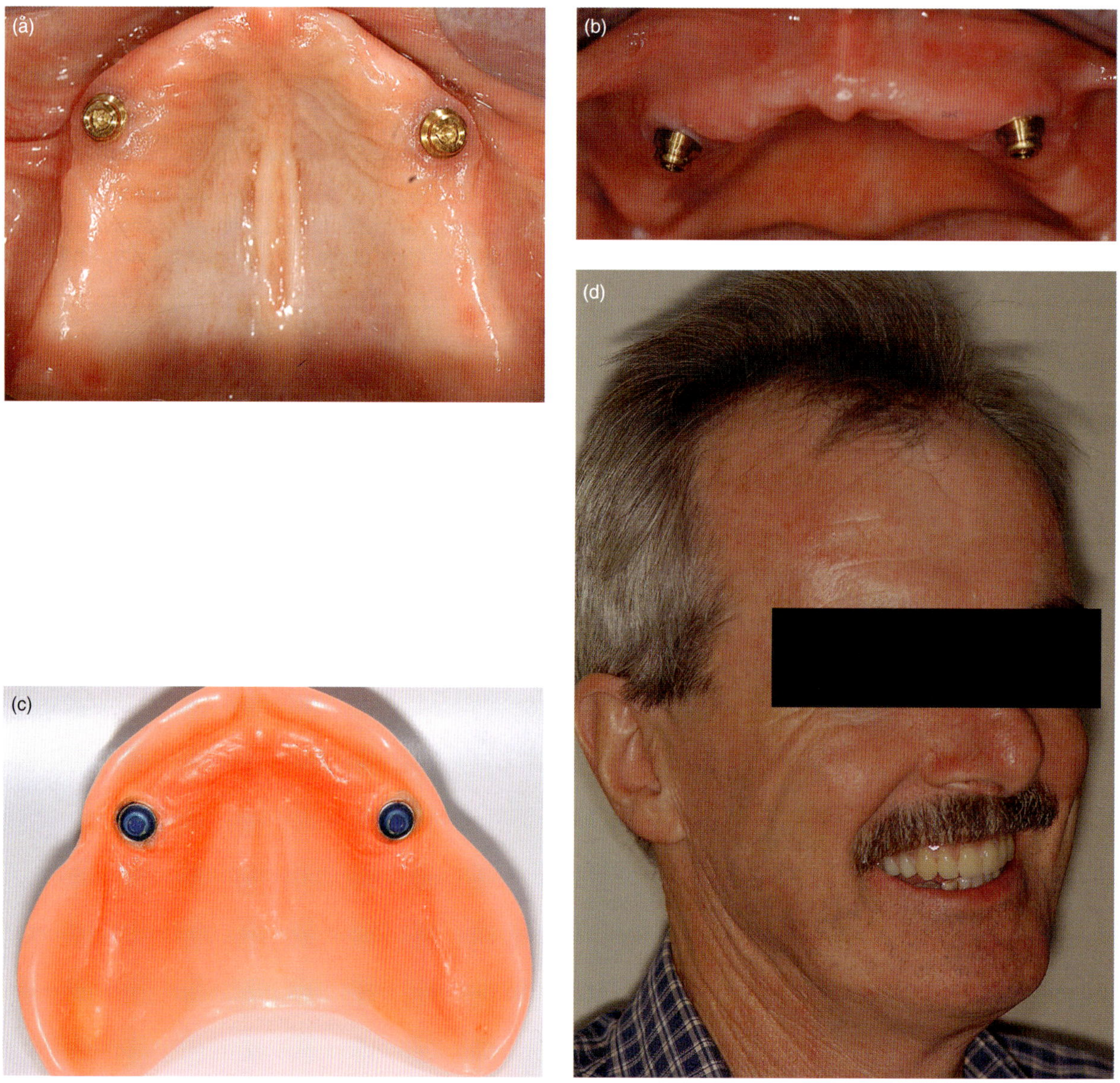

Figure 13.25 (a) An occlusal view of the edentulous maxillary arch with two implants and Locator® attachments placed. (b) A facial view of the edentulous maxilla, demonstrating the divergence of the axial alignment of the implants and abutments. As this is not greater than 20°, standard matrices can be utilized. (c) The fitting surface of the conventionally designed denture, incorporates the light retentive plastic matrices in the metal housings processed into the denture base. (d) The full facial view of the patient postoperatively.

with respect to surgical intervention and their understanding of the likely outcome.

The placement of four dental implants in the maxilla, with individual retentive elements attached, can provide optimal retention and a marked increase in the stability of a removable prosthesis. The implant placements do need to be sufficiently distributed around the arch form to allow optimal cross-arch and anteroposterior distribution of the occlusal loading.

An example of such therapy is illustrated in the case of a 65-year-old male in Figures 13.26a–c. The patient was concerned with the continuing fractures of his conventional full upper prosthesis. The lower jaw was compromised, with an inadequate lower removable partial denture replacing the missing posterior teeth and retained by the remaining six lower anterior natural teeth. The lower jaw was managed with the extraction of the remaining, lower teeth and the placement of six dental implants. This approach allowed for the construction and placement of two three-unit posterior FPDs and a six-unit anterior FPD.

The retentive elements chosen for the four implants placed in the maxilla were the Locator® system, as it provided the necessary compensation for the divergent axes of the implants. The maxillary jaw often demonstrates a pattern of resorption of the alveolar processes after tooth loss that dictates divergent axes when dental implants are placed around the arch. As a consequence, when individual retentive elements are to be used, the

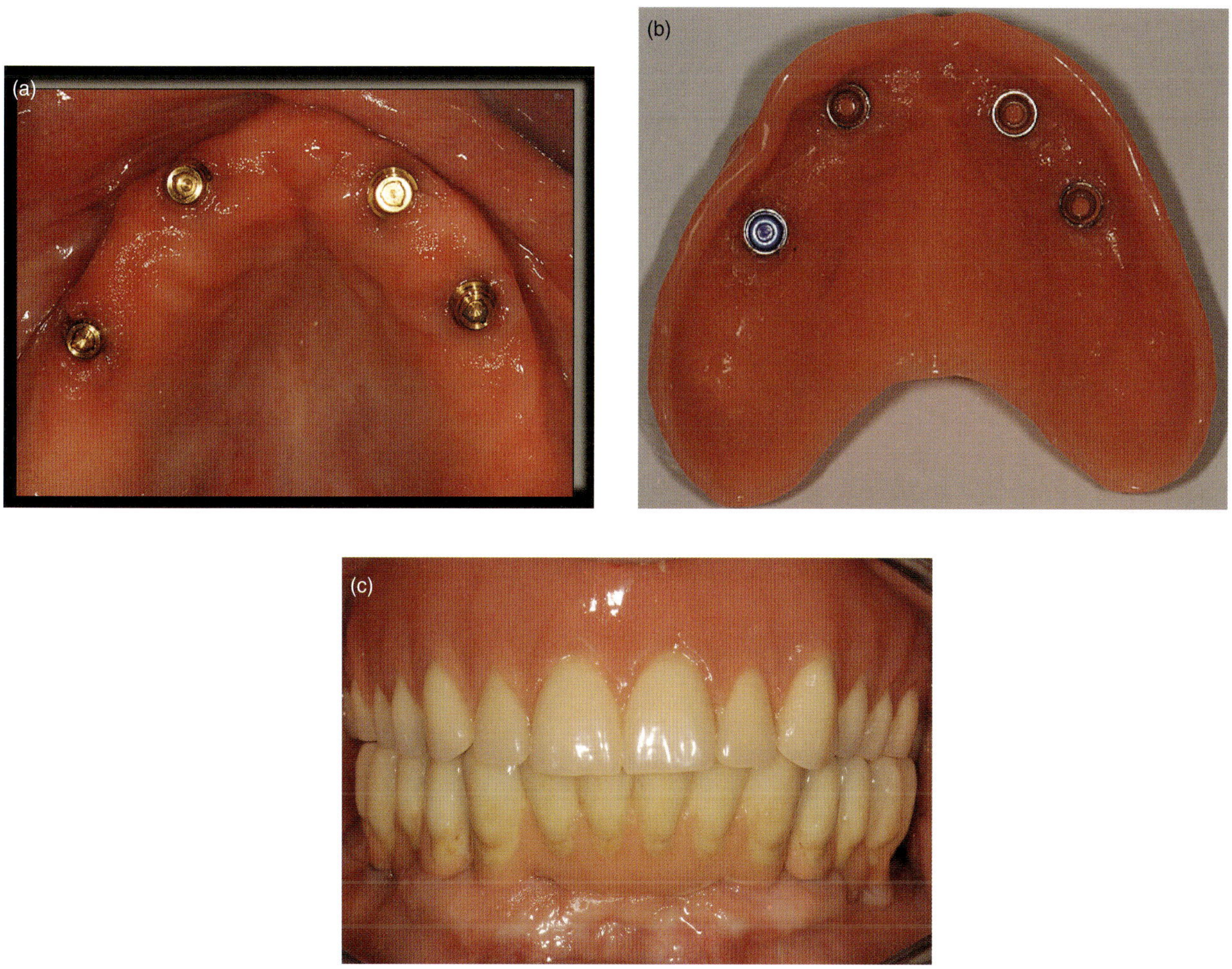

Figure 13.26 (a) An occlusal view of the edentulous jaw with the four implants and Locator® attachments in place. (b) The fitting surface of the conventionally designed denture incorporates the retentive plastic matrices in the metal housings processed into the denture base. (c) A facial view of the completed rehabilitation.

system chosen must allow for such divergence whilst maintaining its effectiveness as a retentive element. The Locator® system provides for a resilient plastic matrix that allows up to 40° of divergence between the axes of the implants. The housing inside the removable prosthesis allows for easy removal and replacement of the matrices, as required over time.

SPLINTED BAR-RETAINED PROSTHESIS

Where improved stability and support against functional loading of the mucosa is required in addition to increased retention, a splinted bar-retained prosthesis is indicated. In the maxillary arch, a minimum of four implants is required to effectively undertake this procedure.

The implants should be placed around the arch form to allow for adequate anteroposterior distribution of the load. Implant placement positions should be selected to allow for sufficient bar length between the abutments, to provide for retentive clips of adequate length. To maximize this distance between the anterior and posterior implants, and to avoid the anatomical restrictions that maxillary sinus extensions may introduce, the implants in the posterior maxilla may be distally inclined; engaging adequate bone anterior to the sinus, yet providing an exit through the mucosa at a point further distal.

The design of the removable prosthesis will depend upon the extension and circumferential shape of the bar, and to what extent the bar, and as a consequence the implants, will be loaded

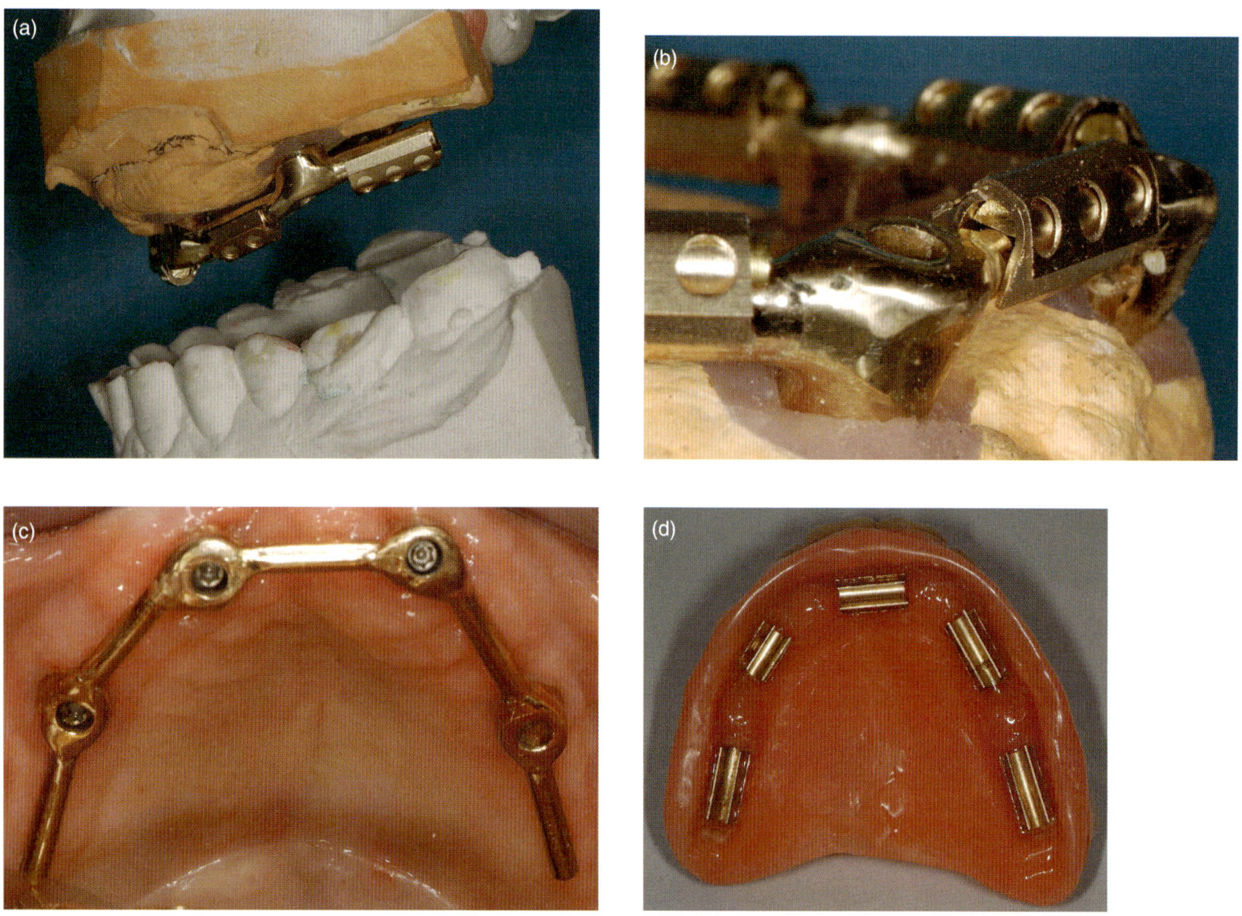

Figure 13.27 (a) A view of the mounted master cast with bar and clips attached. (b) A more detailed view of the clasp–bar assembly, with the set spacer between to provide for vertical and some rotational resiliency. (c) A palatal view demonstrating the bar design having been placed. Note the distal extension that will provide increased retention and remove the denture base from the poor-quality mucosal ridge in this area. (d) The fitting surface of the conventionally designed denture incorporates the retentive assemblies.

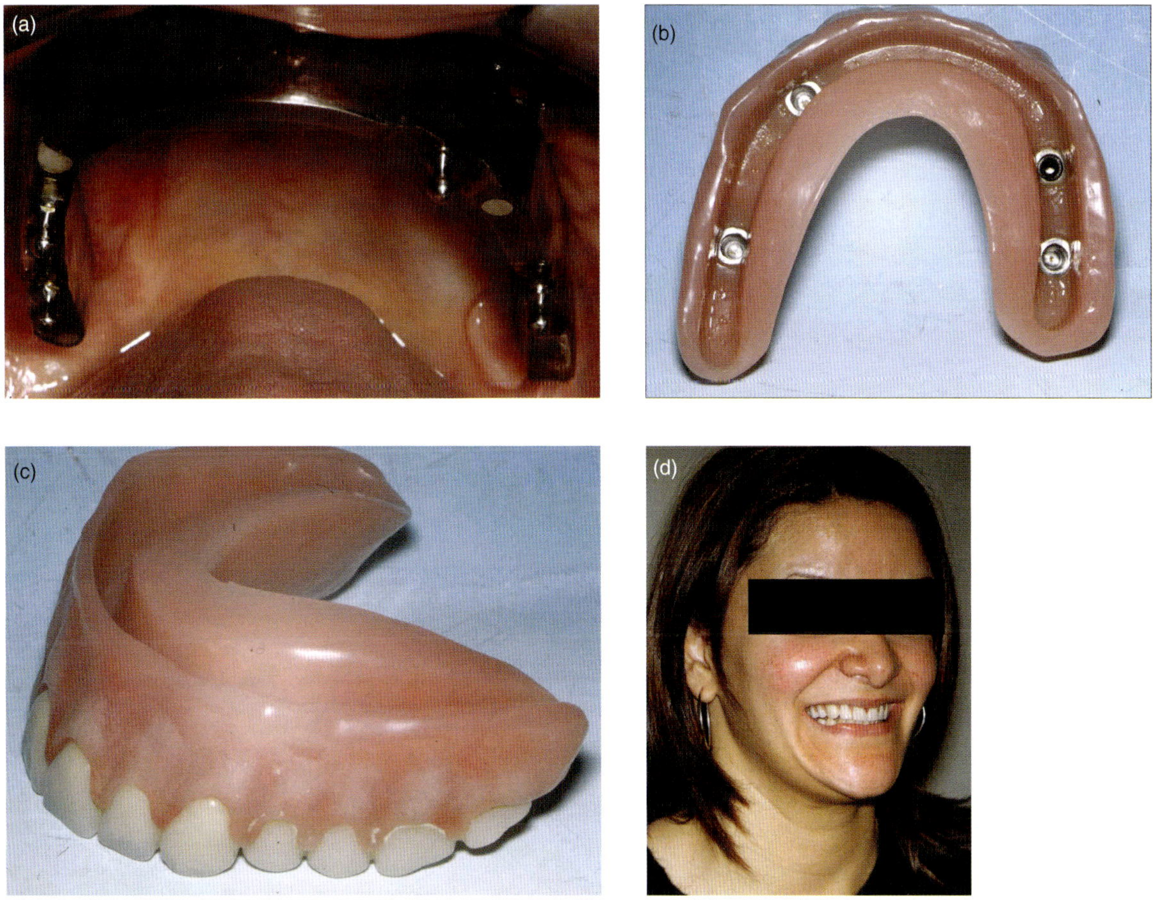

Figure 13.28 (a) A palatal view of the bar having a wide rectangular cross-section. In doing so, the entire maxillary ridge form isconstituted. Four additional retentive ball-shaped anchors provide a mechanism of increasing the retention of the prosthesis. (b) The fitting surface of the prosthesis, at the time of review required only one rubber "o" ring to optimize the retention. (c) The definitive prosthesis. (d) A full facial view of the 30-year-old female patient four years posttreatment.

as compared to the load shared by the alveolar mucosa. The shape of the bar can vary from round to ovoid to a rectangular cross-section. In the case illustrated in Figure 13.27, the patient has a Class III skeletal relationship. As such the removable prosthesis will be predominately loaded in a vertical direction. Round and ovoid bars provide for resilience in the potential movements of the denture. The retentive clips are spaced from the bar to permit vertical movement under functional loading (Figure 13.27b). The extension of the bar with the use of cantilevered distal extensions may further enhance its effectiveness (Figures 13.28c–d).

Where the form of the residual maxillary arch is more significantly compromised, the bar should be designed to accept a greater role in the stability of the prosthesis and support for the functional loading. A bar with a rectangular cross-section facilitates this function. Ultimately, in the severely resorbed maxilla, the bar may need to effectively replace the vertical extension of the ridge, thus providing a complete rim into which the removable prosthesis is anchored (Figures 13.28a–d).

Conclusions

Dental implant therapy can offer patients an improved quality of life. Of critical importance in considering such therapy is the ability of the dental professional to conduct a comprehensive evaluation, with appropriate consideration of the patient's presenting problems. The edentulous maxilla presents biologic, technical, and esthetic challenges. Each of these challenges needs to be identified and addressed. Not only what the proposed therapeutic management involves, but also what the implications are for the patient's subsequent and future management, must be considered.

To ensure a successful outcome, whether providing a fixed or removable implant-supported maxillary prosthesis, all interdisciplinary components of the patient's therapeutic management must be undertaken within the competency of each operator, and the patient's consent to such therapy must be accompanied by realistic expectations of the outcomes of the therapy.

Index

“Our definition of success is limited by our perception of possibilities.”

– Gerald M. Kramer

“There are some things you do and some things you do not do.”

– Confucius